Stem Cells and Cancer Stem Cells

Stem Cells and Cancer Stem Cells
Volume 2

For other titles published in this series, go to
www.springer.com/series/10231

Stem Cells and Cancer Stem Cells
Volume 2

Stem Cells and Cancer Stem Cells

Therapeutic Applications in Disease and Injury

Edited by

M.A. Hayat
Distinguished Professor
Department of Biological Sciences,
Kean University, Union, NJ, USA

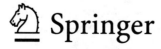

Editor
M.A. Hayat
Department of Biological Sciences
Kean University
Union, NJ, USA
ehayat@kean.edu

ISBN 978-94-007-2015-2   e-ISBN 978-94-007-2016-9
DOI 10.1007/978-94-007-2016-9
Springer Dordrecht Heidelberg London New York

Library of Congress Control Number: 2011933477

© Springer Science+Business Media B.V. 2012
No part of this work may be reproduced, stored in a retrieval system, or transmitted in any form or by any means, electronic, mechanical, photocopying, microfilming, recording or otherwise, without written permission from the Publisher, with the exception of any material supplied specifically for the purpose of being entered and executed on a computer system, for exclusive use by the purchaser of the work.

Printed on acid-free paper

Springer is part of Springer Science+Business Media (www.springer.com)

"Although touched by technology, surgical pathology always has been, and remains, an art. Surgical pathologists, like all artists, depict in their artwork (surgical pathology reports) their interactions with nature: emotions, observations, and knowledge are all integrated. The resulting artwork is a poor record of complex phenomena."

Richard J. Reed MD

Preface and Introduction

It is recognized that scientific journals and books not only provide current information but also facilitate exchange of information, resulting in rapid progress in the medical field. In this endeavor, the main role of scientific books is to present current information in more detail after careful additional evaluation of the investigational results, especially those of new or relatively new therapeutic methods and their potential toxic side-effects.

Although subjects of diagnosis, cancer recurrence, resistance to chemotherapy, assessment of treatment effectiveness, including cell therapy and side-effects of a treatment are scattered in a vast number of journals and books, there is need of combining these subjects in single volumes. An attempt will be made to accomplish this goal in the projected seven-volume series of Handbooks.

In the era of cost-effectiveness, my opinion may be minority perspective, but it needs to be recognized that the potential for false-positive or false-negative interpretation on the basis of a single laboratory test in clinical pathology does exist. Interobserver or intraobserver variability in the interpretation of results in pathology is not uncommon. Interpretative differences often are related to the relative importance of the criteria being used.

Generally, no test always performs perfectly. Although there is no perfect remedy to this problem, standardized classifications with written definitions and guidelines will help. Standardization of methods to achieve objectivity is imperative in this effort. The validity of a test should be based on the careful, objective interpretation of the tomographic images, photomicrographs, and other tests. The interpretation of the results should be explicit rather than implicit. To achieve accurate diagnosis and correct prognosis, the use of molecular criteria and targeted medicine is important. Equally important are the translation of molecular genetics into clinical practice and evidence-based therapy. Translation of medicine from the laboratory to clinical application needs to be carefully expedited. Indeed, molecular medicine has arrived.

Although current cancer treatment methods have had an important impact on cancer-related morbidity and mortality, the cure rates are modest. On the other hand, cell-based therapy has the potential to treat human conditions not treatable with available pharmaceutical agents, radiation, surgery, chemotherapy or hormonal therapy. Stem cells present important opportunity to elucidate manifold aspects of molecular biology and potential therapeutic strategies, especially in the areas of cancer and tissue/organ injuries. In other words, stem cell field has tremendous potential in deciphering the molecular pathways involved in human diseases. Some stem cell therapies already are being clinically used routinely; for example in leukemic therapy. Human stem cells also have the potential for application in regenerative medicine, tissue engineering, and in vitro applications in drug discovery and toxicity testing. Stem cells represent populations of primal cells found in all multicellular organisms, which have the capacity to form a variety of different cell types.

A brief statement on the difference between tissue specific stem cells and embryonic stem cells is in order. Tissue specific stem cells (adult or somatic stem cell) can be isolated from a range of organs and tissues from fetal or adult organisms. These cells have a limited life span, senescence during in vitro propagation, and are multipotent; thus, can be differentiated into a limited number of specialized cells. Embryonic stem cells, on the other hand, are isolated from the inner cell mass of a fertilized egg that has been cultured in vitro to match the blastocyst stage (5–7 days post-fertilization). These cells possess infinite capacity to proliferate in vitro provided maintained in an appropriate condition. The advantage of these cells is that they are pluripotent and can give rise to any fetal or adult cell type.

This is volume 2 of the seven-volume series, *Stem Cells and Cancer Stem Cells: Therapeutic Applications in Disease and Injury*. A stem cell is defined as a cell that can self-renew and differentiate into one or more specialized cell types. A stem cell may be pluripotent, which is able to give rise to the endodermal, ectodermal, and mesodermal lineages; an example is embryonic stem cells. A stem cell may be multipotent, which is able to give rise to all cells in a particular lineage; examples are hematopoietic stem cells and neural stem cells. A stem cell may be unipotent, which is able to give rise to only one cell type; an example is keratinocytes. These types of stem cells are discussed in this volume.

A cancer stem cell is a cell type within a tumor that possesses the capacity of self-renewal and can give rise to the heterogeneous lineages of cancer cells that comprise the tumor. In other words, a cancer stem cell is a tumor initiating cell. A unique feature of a cancer stem cell is that although conventional chemotherapy will kill most cells in a tumor; cancer stem cells remain intact, resulting in the development of resistance of therapy.

As stated above, given that human embryonic stem cells possess the potential to produce unlimited quantities of any human cell type; considerable focus has been placed on their therapeutic potential. Because of the pluripotency of embryonic stem cells, they have been used in various applications such as tissue engineering, regenerative medicine, pharmacological and toxicological studies, and fundamental studies of cell differentiation. The formation of embryoid bodies, which are three-dimensional aggregates of embryonic stem cells, is the initial step in the differentiation of these cells. Embryonic stem cells can differentiate into derivatives of three germ layers: the endoderm, mesoderm, and ectoderm. Therefore, embryoid body culture has been widely used as a trigger for the in vitro differentiation of embryonic stem cells.

Support and development of the stem cell field, especially the application of human embryonic stem cells, mesenchymal stem cells, hematopoietic stem cells, gliosarcoma stem cells, intestinal stem cells, thyroid stem cells, and cancer stem cells, in cancer and other diseases and tissue/organ repair (regeneration), are described. The damage or injury of living tissues is a major challenge during adult life in humans. Enhancing the regenerative potential of cells devoted to tissue repair (the stem cells) either endogenous or supplied from outside, is one of the most important challenges and developments in the medical field. This aspect of therapy is discussed in detail in this volume.

Ischemia is one of the diseases discussed in this volume. Ischemic heart diseases represent one of the major causes of morbidity and death worldwide. Cell based therapies are useful for cardiac regeneration following ischemic heart disease. The finding that heart contains a reservoir of resident stem and progenitor cells, has opened new perspectives in the biology of cardiac regeneration, suggesting the exploration of experimental procedures aimed at in vitro expansion of cardiac stem cells for in vivo transplantation. Hematopoietic stem cells, mesenchymal stem cells, or neural stem cells have been successfully used for the treatment of experimental stroke. Human marrow stem cells show promise as a potential therapy for restoration of function after ischemic stroke. Some of these procedures are detailed in this volume.

Another example of the therapy for a disease discussed in this volume is repairing retina using transplantation. Other examples of therapies using stem cells detailed in this volume include bone defects and acute myocarditis. Methods for the isolation of bone marrow stromal cells from bone marrow, induced pluripotent stem cells, human embryonic stem cells, and cancer stem cells are presented. The rational for transplantation of normal stem cells is included.

Hematopoietic stem cell transplantation is increasingly being performed in patients with malignancies, non-malignant hematological disorders, and autoimmune diseases. Renal injury is a common complication after such treatment, and is associated with high morbidity and mortality. Renal insufficiency and proteinuria are the symptoms of this injury. Both acute kidney injury and chronic kidney disease can occur after hematopoietic stem cell transplantation. Such renal injury is thought to be caused by antibody-mediated endothelial cell injury in chronic graft-versus-host disease. Chronic graft-versus-host disease, a frequent complication of bone marrow transplantation, occurs among 30–50% of bone marrow recipients. This disease is characterized by skin, gut, and liver involvement. Treatment of this disease using allogenic mesenchymal stem cells is described in this volume.

A new promising medical scenario has been discovered by using nanotechnology that provides unique opportunities of building and/or modifying biomaterials and scaffolds with specific, functional molecules and/or drugs carried by nanoscale fibers or particles. This technology facilitates delivery, for example of drugs at the desired sites in precise amounts.

By bringing together a large number of experts (oncologists, neurosurgeons, physicians, research scientists, and pathologists) in various aspects of this medical field, it is my hope that substantial progress will be made against terrible human disease and injury. It is difficult for a single author to discuss effectively the complexity of diagnosis, therapy, including tissue regeneration. Another advantage of involving more than one author is to present different points of view on a specific controversial aspect of cancer cure and tissue regeneration. I hope these goals will be fulfilled in this and other volumes of the series. This volume was written by 116 contributors representing 15 countries. I am grateful to them for their promptness in accepting my suggestions. Their practical experience highlights their writings, which should build and further the endeavors of the readers in this important area of disease. I respect and appreciate the hard work and exceptional insight into the nature of cancer and tissue injury provided by these contributors. The contents of the volume are divided into four subheadings: Stem Cells, Cancer Stem Cells, Diseases, and Tissue Repair (Regeneration) for the convenience of the reader.

It is my hope that subsequent volumes of the series will join the first two volumes in more complete understanding of this medical field. There exists a tremendous, urgent demand by the public and the scientific community to address to cancer diagnosis, treatment, cure, and hopefully prevention and therapy for tissue injuries. In the light of existing cancer calamity and disabilities, government funding must give priority to eradicating deadly malignancies over military superiority.

I am thankful to Dr. Dawood Farahi and Dr. Kristie Reilly for recognizing the importance of medical research and publishing through an institution of higher education.

Union, New Jersey M.A. Hayat
April 2011

Contents

Part I Stem Cells 1

1. **Isolation of Bone Marrow Stromal Cells from Bone Marrow by Using a Filtering Device (Method)** 3
   Tomoki Aoyama and Junya Toguchida

2. **Hematopoietic Stem Cell Frequency Estimate: Statistical Approach to Model Limiting Dilution Competitive Repopulation Assays** 13
   Thierry Bonnefoix and Mary Callanan

3. **Characteristics of Cord Blood Stem Cells: Role of Substance P (SP) and Calcitonin Gene-Related Peptide (CGRP)** 27
   Massoumeh Ebtekar, Somayeh Shahrokhi, and Kamran Alimoghaddam

4. **A New Concept of Stem Cell Disorders, and the Rationale for Transplantation of Normal Stem Cells** 37
   Susumu Ikehara

5. **Differentiation of Human Embryonic Stem Cells into Functional Hepatocyte-Like Cells (Method)** 43
   Takamichi Ishii

6. **Stem Cell Mobilization: An Overview** 51
   Alessandro Isidori and Giuseppe Visani

7. **Status and Impact of Research on Human Pluripotent Stem Cells: Cell Lines and Their Use in Published Research** 61
   Peter Löser, Anke Guhr, Sabine Kobold, Anna M. Wobus, and Andreas Kurtz

8. **Gliosarcoma Stem Cells: Glial and Mesenchymal Differentiation** .. 75
   Ana C. deCarvalho and Tom Mikkelsen

9. **Generation of Induced Pluripotent Stem Cells from Mesenchymal Stromal Cells Derived from Human Third Molars (Method)** 83
   Yasuaki Oda, Hiroe Ohnishi, Shunsuke Yuba, and Hajime Ohgushi

10	**Self-renewal and Differentiation of Intestinal Stem Cells: Role of Hedgehog Pathway**	95
	Nikè V.J.A. Büller, Sanne L. Rosekrans, and Gijs R. van den Brink	
11	**Hematopoietic Stem Cell Repopulation After Transplantation: Role of Vinculin**	103
	Tsukasa Ohmori and Yoichi Sakata	
12	**Static and Suspension Culture of Human Embryonic Stem Cells**	111
	Guoliang Meng and Derrick Rancourt	
13	**Generation of Marmoset Induced Pluripotent Stem Cells Using Six Transcription Factors (Method)**	119
	Ikuo Tomioka and Erika Sasaki	
14	**MYC as a Multifaceted Regulator of Pluripotency and Reprogramming**	127
	Keriayn N. Smith and Stephen Dalton	

Part II Cancer Stem Cells ... 135

15	**Human Thyroid Cancer Stem Cells**	137
	Veronica Catalano, Antonina Benfante, Giorgio Stassi, and Matilde Todaro	
16	**Tumor Stem Cells: CD133 Gene Regulation and Tumor Stemness**	145
	Kouichi Tabu, Tetsuya Taga, and Shinya Tanaka	
17	**Cripto-1: A Common Embryonic Stem Cell and Cancer Cell Marker**	155
	Maria Cristina Rangel, Nadia P. Castro, Hideaki Karasawa, Tadahiro Nagaoka, David S. Salomon, and Caterina Bianco	

Part III Diseases ... 167

18	**Treatment of Heart Disease: Use of Transdifferentiation Methodology for Reprogramming Adult Stem Cells**	169
	Milán Bustamante, Macarena Perán, Juan Antonio Marchal, Fernando Rodríguez-Serrano, Pablo Álvarez, and Antonia Aránega	
19	**Rat Mesenchymal Cell CD44 Surface Markers: Role in Cardiomyogenic Differentiation**	185
	Tze-Wen Chung and Ming-Chia Yang	
20	**Stroke Therapy Using Menstrual Blood Stem-Like Cells: Method**	191
	Maria Carolina Oliveira Rodrigues, Svitlana Garbuzova-Davis, Paul R. Sanberg, Júlio C. Voltarelli, Julie G. Allickson, Nicole Kuzmin-Nichols, and Cesario V. Borlongan	
21	**Spontaneous Cerebral Stroke in Rats: Differentiation of New Neurons from Neural Stem Cells**	199
	Tatsuki Itoh, Kumiko Takemori, Motohiro Imano, Shozo Nishida, Masahiro Tsubaki, Shigeo Hashimoto, Hiroyuki Ito, Akihiko Ito, and Takao Satou	

22	Neurogenesis in the Cerebral Cortex After Stroke	211
	Yukiko Kasahara, Takayuki Nakagomi, Tomohiro Matsuyama, and Akihiko Taguchi	
23	Ex Vivo Expanded Hematopoietic Stem Cells for Ischemia	219
	Jingwei Lu, Reeva Aggarwal, Vincent J. Pompili, and Hiranmoy Das	
24	Breast Cancer Risk: Role of Somatic Breast Stem Cells	231
	John A. Eden	
25	Cellular Replacement Therapy in Neurodegenerative Diseases Using Induced Pluripotent Stem Cells	241
	Takayuki Kondo, Ryosuke Takahashi, and Haruhisa Inoue	
26	Treatment of Graft-Versus-Host Disease Using Allogeneic Mesenchymal Stem Cells	249
	Sun U. Song	
27	Adult Neurogenesis in Etiology and Pathogenesis of Alzheimer's Disease	259
	Philippe Taupin	

Part IV Tissue Repair (Regeneration) ... 267

28	Generating Human Cardiac Muscle Cells from Adipose-Derived Stem Cells	269
	Rodney Dilley, Yu Suk Choi, and Gregory Dusting	
29	Mesenchymal Stem Cells and Mesenchymal-Derived Endothelial Cells: Repair of Bone Defects	277
	Jian Zhou and Jian Dong	
30	Omentum in the Repair of Injured Tissue: Evidence for Omental Stem Cells	283
	Ignacio García-Gómez	
31	Human Embryonic Stem Cells Transplanted into Mouse Retina Induces Neural Differentiation	291
	Akira Hara, Hitomi Aoki, Manabu Takamatsu, Yuichiro Hatano, Hiroyuki Tomita, Toshiya Kuno, Masayuki Niwa, and Takahiro Kunisada	
32	Stem Cells to Repair Retina: From Basic to Applied Biology	299
	Muriel Perron, Morgane Locker, and Odile Bronchain	
33	Heterogeneous Responses of Human Bone Marrow Stromal Cells (Multipotent Mesenchymal Stromal Cells) to Osteogenic Induction	307
	Hideaki Kagami, Hideki Agata, Yoshinori Sumita, and Arinobu Tojo	
34	Adipose-Derived Stem Cells and Platelet-Rich Plasma: Implications for Regenerative Medicine	315
	Natsuko Kakudo, Satoshi Kushida, and Kenji Kusumoto	
35	Skeletal Muscle-Derived Stem Cells: Role in Cellular Cardiomyoplasty	323
	Tetsuro Tamaki	

36 **Cardiac Regenerative Medicine Without Stem Cell Transplantation** 331
Carlo Ventura and Vincenzo Lionetti

37 **Allogeneic Transplantation of Fetal Membrane-Derived Mesenchymal Stem Cells: Therapy for Acute Myocarditis** 341
Shin Ishikane, Hiroshi Hosoda, Kenichi Yamahara, Makoto Kodama, and Tomoaki Ikeda

38 **Patients with Cancer or Hematopoietic Stem Cell Transplant: Infection with 2009 H1N1 Influenza** 351
Gil Redelman-Sidi

Index 361

Contents of Volume 1

1. Pluripotent Human Stem Cells: An Overview
2. Complexity of Tumor Angiogenesis and Stem Cells
3. Stem Cells Like Astrocytes: Various Roles
4. Neural Crest Cell-Derived Tumors: An Overview
5. Therapeutic Neural Stem Cells for Brain Tumor Therapy
6. Brain Tumors: Role of Neural Cancer Stem Cells
7. Targeting Cancer Stem Cells with Phytochemicals: Inhibition of the Rat C6 Glioma Side Population by Curcumin
8. Glioma Patients: Role of CD133 Stem Cell Antigen
9. Cancer Stem Cells in Brain Gliomas
10. Primary Glioma Spheroids: Advantage of Serum-Free Medium
11. Tumorigenesis of Glioma-Initiating Cells: Role of Sox11
12. Glioma-Initiating Cells: Interferon Treatment
13. Is CD133 the Appropriate Stem Cell Marker for Glioma?
14. Cancer Stem Cells in Glioblastoma
15. Glioblastoma-Derived Cancer Stem Cells: Treatment with Oncolytic Viruses
16. Cancer Stem Cells in Medulloblastoma
17. Transplantation of Embryonic Stem Cells Results in Reduced Brain Lesions
18. Allogenic Hematopoietic Stem Cell Transplantation Followed by Graft-Versus-Host Disease: Role of Adenosine A_{2A} Receptor
19. Umblical Cord Blood and Alpha-3 Fucosyl Transferase-Treated Haematopoietic Stem Cells for Transplantation
20. Bone Marrow-Derived Stem Cell Therapy for Myocardial Infarction
21. The Use of Mesenchymal Stem Cells in Orthopedics

Contributors

Hideki Agata Tissue Engineering Research Group, Division of Molecular Therapy, The Advanced Clinical Research Center, The Institute of Medical Science, The University of Tokyo, Tokyo 108-8639, Japan

Reeva Aggarwal Cardiovascular Stem Cell Research Laboratories, Davis Heart and Lung Research Institute, Columbus, OH 43210, USA

Kamran Alimoghaddam Hematology, Oncology and Stem Cell Transplantation Research Center, Tehran University of Medical Sciences, Tehran, Iran

Julie G. Allickson Cryo-Cell International, Inc., Tampa, FL, USA

Pablo Álvarez Biopathology and Medicine Regenerative Institute (IBIMER), FIBAO, University of Granada, 18012, Granada, Spain

Hitomi Aoki Department of Tissue and Organ Development, Gifu University Graduate School of Medicine, 1-1 Yanagido, Gifu 501-1194, Japan

Tomoki Aoyama Human Health Sciences, Graduate School of Medicine, Kyoto University, Sakyo-ku, Kyoto 606-8507, Japan, blue@hs.med.kyoto-u.ac.jp

Antonia Aránega Biopathology and Medicine Regenerative Institute (IBIMER), Granada, Spain, aranega@ugr.es

Antonina Benfante Laboratory of Cellular and Molecular Pathophysiology, Department of Surgical and Oncological Sciences, University of Palermo, 90127 Palermo, Italy

Caterina Bianco Mammary Biology and Tumorigenesis Laboratory, Center for Cancer Research, National Cancer Institute, National Institutes of Health, Bethesda, MD, USA, biancoc@mail.nih.gov

Thierry Bonnefoix INSERM, U823, Université Joseph Fourier-Grenoble I, UMR-S823, Institut Albert Bonniot, Grenoble, France, and Pole de Recherche, CHU de Grenoble, France, Grenoble, F-38706, France, Thierry.bonnefoix@ujf-grenoble.fr

Cesario V. Borlongan Department of Neurosurgery and Brain Repair, College of Medicine, Center of Excellence for Aging and Brain Repair, University of South Florida, Tampa, FL, USA, cborlong@health.usf.edu

Odile Bronchain Laboratory of Neurobiology and Development, UPR CNRS 3294, Université Paris-Sud, Orsay, Paris, France

Nikè V.J.A. Büller Department of Gastroenterology & Hepathology, Tytgat Institute for Liver and Intestinal Research, Academic Medical Center, Amsterdam, The Netherlands

Milán Bustamante Biopathology and Medicine Regenerative Institute (IBIMER), Granada, Spain

Mary Callanan INSERM, U823, Université Joseph Fourier-Grenoble I, UMR-S823, Institut Albert Bonniot, Grenoble, France, and Onco-Hematology Genetics Unit, Plateforme Hospitalière de Génétique Moléculaire des Tumeurs, Department of Hematology, Onco-Genetics and Immunology, Pôle de Biologie, CHU de Grenoble, France, Grenoble, F-38706, France, mary.callanan@ujf-grenoble.fr

Nadia P. Castro Mammary Biology and Tumorigenesis Laboratory, Center for Cancer Research, National Cancer Institute, National Institutes of Health, Bethesda, MD, USA

Veronica Catalano Laboratory of Cellular and Molecular Pathophysiology, Department of Surgical and Oncological Sciences, University of Palermo, 90127 Palermo, Italy

Yu Suk Choi O'Brien Institute, Fitzroy, VIC 065, Australia

Tze-Wen Chung Department of Chemical and Material Engineering, National Yunlin University of Science & Technology, Dou-Liu, Yunlin 640, Taiwan, ROC, twchung@yuntech.edu.tw

Stephen Dalton Department of Biochemistry and Molecular Biology, Paul D. Coverdell Center for Biomedical and Health Sciences, University of Georgia, Athens, GA 30602, USA, sdalton@uga.edu

Hiranmoy Das Cardiovascular Stem Cell Research Laboratories, Davis Heart and Lung Research Institute, Columbus, OH 43210, USA, Hiranmoy.das@osumc.edu

Ana C. deCarvalho Hermelin Brain Tumor Center, Neurosurgery Research, E&R 3052, Henry Ford Hospital, Detroit, MI 48202, USA, ana@neuro.hfh.edu

Rodney Dilley O'Brien Institute, Fitzroy, VIC 065, Australia, rdilley@unimelb.edu.au

Jian Dong Department of Orthopaedic Surgery, Zhongshan Hospital, Fudan University, Shanghai 200032, China, Dong.jian@zs-hospital.sh.cn

Gregory Dusting O'Brien Institute, Fitzroy, VIC 065, Australia

Massoumeh Ebtekar Department of Immunology, Faculty of Medical Sciences, Tarbiat Modares University, Tehran, Iran, ebtekarm@modares.ac.ir

John A. Eden School of Women and Children's Health, Royal Hospital for Women, Randwick, NSW 2031, Australia, j.eden@unsw.edu.au

Svitlana Garbuzova-Davis Department of Neurosurgery and Brain Repair, College of Medicine, Center of Excellence for Aging and Brain Repair, University of South Florida, Tampa, FL, USA

Ignacio García-Gómez Laboratory of Cell Therapy, Autonoma University-La Paz University Hospital (idiPAZ), P.C. 28046 Madrid, Spain, biogarc@yahoo.es

Anke Guhr Roberts Koch Institute, DGZ-Ring1, D-13086 Berlin, Germany

Akira Hara Department of Tumor Pathology, Gifu University Graduate School of Medicine, 1-1 Yanagido, Gifu 501-1194, Japan, ahara@gifu-u.ac.jp

Shigeo Hashimoto Division of Pathology, PL Hospital, Osaka, Japan

Yuichiro Hatano Department of Tumor Pathology, Gifu University Graduate School of Medicine, 1-1 Yanagido, Gifu 501-1194, Japan

Hiroshi Hosoda Department of Biochemistry, National Cardiovascular Center Research Institute, Suita, Osaka 565-8565, Japan

Tomoaki Ikeda Department of Regenerative Medicine and Tissue Engineering, National Cardiovascular Center Research Institute, Suita, Osaka 565-8565, Japan, tikeda@hsp.ncvc.go.jp

Susumu Ikehara First Department of Pathology, Kansai Medical University, Moriguchi City, Osaka 570-8506, Japan, ikehara@takii.kmu.ac.jp

Motohiro Imano Department of Surgery, Kinki University School of Medicine, Osaka, Japan

Haruhisa Inoue Center for iPS Cell Research and Application, Kyoto University, Kyoto, Japan, haruhisa@cira.kyoto-u.ac.jp

Takamichi Ishii Department of Surgery, Graduate School of Medicine Kyoto University, 54 Kawahara-cho Shogoin Sakyo-ku, Kyoto, 606-8507, Japan, taishii@kuhp.kyoto-u.ac.jp

Shin Ishikane Department of Regenerative Medicine and Tissue Engineering, National Cardiovascular Center Research Institute, Suita, Osaka 565-8565, Japan

Alessandro Isidori Hematology and Stem Cell Transplant Center, San Salvatore Hospital, Pesaro, Italy, aisidori@gmail.com

Akihiko Ito Department of Pathology, Kinki University School of Medicine, Osaka, Japan

Hiroyuki Ito Department of Biomedical Engineering, Faculty of Biology-Oriented Science and Technology, Kinki University, Wakayama, Japan

Tatsuki Itoh Department of Pathology, Kinki University School of Medicine, Osaka, Japan, tatsuki@med.kindai.ac.jp

Hideaki Kagami Tissue Engineering Research Group, Division of Molecular Therapy, The Advanced Clinical Research Center, The Institute of Medical Science, The University of Tokyo, Tokyo 108-8639, Japan, kagami@ims.u-tokyo.ac.jp

Natsuko Kakudo Department of Plastic and Reconstructive Surgery, Kansai Medical University, Moriguchi 570-8506, Japan, kakudon@takii.kmu.ac.jp

Hideaki Karasawa Mammary Biology and Tumorigenesis Laboratory, Center for Cancer Research, National Cancer Institute, National Institutes of Health, Bethesda, MD, USA

Yukiko Kasahara Department of Cerebrovascular Disease, National Cardiovascular Center, Suita, Osaka 565-8565, Japan

Sabine Kobold Roberts Koch Institute, DGZ-Ring1, D-13086 Berlin, Germany

Makoto Kodama Department of Pathology, National Cardiovascular Center, Osaka, Japan

Takayuki Kondo Center for iPS Cell Research and Application, Kyoto University, Kyoto, Japan

Takahiro Kunisada Department of Tissue and Organ Development, Gifu University Graduate School of Medicine, 1-1 Yanagido, Gifu 501-1194, Japan

Toshiya Kuno Department of Tumor Pathology, Gifu University Graduate School of Medicine, 1-1 Yanagido, Gifu 501-1194, Japan

Andreas Kurtz Berlin Brandeburg Center for Regenerative Therapies, Berlin, Germany; Seoul National University, Seoul, Korea

Satoshi Kushida Department of Plastic and Reconstructive Surgery, Kansai Medical University, Moriguchi 570-8506, Japan

Kenji Kusumoto Department of Plastic and Reconstructive Surgery, Kansai Medical University, Moriguchi 570-8506, Japan

Nicole Kuzmin-Nichols Saneron CCEL Therapeutics, Inc., Tampa, Florida

Vincenzo Lionetti Unit of Molecular and Translational Medicine, Laboratory of Molecular Biology and Stem Cell Engineering, Cardiovascular Department, National Institute of Biostructures and Biosystems, University of Bologna, 40138 Bologna, Italy

Morgane Locker Laboratory of Neurobiology and Development, UPR CNRS 3294, Université Paris-Sud, Orsay, Paris, France

Peter Löser Roberts Koch Institute, DGZ-Ring1, D-13086, Berlin, Germany, loeserP@rki.de

Jingwei Lu Cardiovascular Stem Cell Research Laboratories, Davis Heart and Lung Research Institute, Columbus, OH 4321, USA

Juan Antonio Marchal Department of Human Anatomy and Embryology, Faculty of Medicine, University of Granada, Granada, Spain

Tomohiro Matsuyama Institute for Advanced Medical Sciences, Hyogo College of Medicine, Hyogo, Japan

Guoliang Meng Department of Biochemistry and Molecular Biology, Faculty of Medicine, University of Calgary, Calgary, AB, Canada, T2N 4N1

Tom Mikkelsen Hermelin Brain Tumor Center, Neurosurgery Research, E&R 3052, Henry Ford Hospital, Detroit, MI 48202, USA

Tadahiro Nagaoka Mammary Biology and Tumorigenesis Laboratory, Center for Cancer Research, National Cancer Institute, National Institutes of Health, Bethesda, MD, USA

Takayuki Nakagomi Institute for Advanced Medical Sciences, Hyogo College of Medicine, Hyogo, Japan

Shozo Nishida Kinki University School of Pharmaceutical Sciences, Osaka, Japan

Masayuki Niwa Medical Science Division, United Graduate School of Drug Discovery and Medical Information Sciences, Gifu University, 1-1 Yanagido, Gifu 501-1194, Japan

Yasuaki Oda Tissue Engineering Research Group, Health Research Institute, National Institute of Advanced Industrial Science and Technology (AIST), Amagasaki City, Hyogo 661-0974, Japan, y-oda@aist.go.jp

Hajime Ohgushi Tissue Engineering Research Group, Health Research Institute, National Institute of Advanced Industrial Science and Technology (AIST), Amagasaki City, Hyogo 661-0974, Japan, hajime-ohgushi@aist.go.jp

Tsukasa Ohmori Research Division of Cell and Molecular Medicine, Center for Molecular Medicine, Jichi Medical University, Shimotsuke, Tochigi 329-0498, Japan, tohmori@jichi.ac.jp

Hiroe Ohnishi Tissue Engineering Research Group, Health Research Institute, National Institute of Advanced Industrial Science and Technology (AIST), Amagasaki City, Hyogo 661-0974, Japan

Macarena Perán Biopathology and Medicine Regenerative Institute FIBAO (IBIMER), Granada, Spain

Muriel Perron Laboratory of Neurobiology and Development, UPR CNRS 3294, Université Paris-Sud, Orsay, France, Muriel.perron@u-psud.fr

Vincent J. Pompili Cardiovascular Stem Cell Research Laboratories, Davis Heart and Lung Research Institute, Columbus, OH 43210, USA

Derrick Rancourt Department of Biochemistry and Molecular Biology, Faculty of Medicine, University of Calgary, Calgary, AB, Canada T2N 4N1, rancourt@ucalgary.ca

Maria Cristina Rangel Mammary Biology and Tumorigenesis Laboratory, Center for Cancer Research, National Cancer Institute, National Institutes of Health, Bethesda, MD, USA

Gil Redelman-Sidi Memorial Sloan-Kettering Cancer Center, New York, NY 10065, USA, redelmansidi@hotmail.com

Maria Carolina Oliveira Rodrigues Department of Neurosurgery and Brain Repair, College of Medicine, Center of Excellence for Aging and Brain Repair, University of South Florida, Tampa, FL, USA

Fernando Rodríguez-Serrano Department of Human Anatomy and Embryology, Faculty of Medicine, University of Granada, Granada, Spain

Sanne L. Rosekrans Department of Gastroenterology & Hepathology, Tytgat Institute for Liver and Intestinal Research, Academic Medical Center, Amsterdam, The Netherlands

Yoichi Sakata Research Division of Cell and Molecular Medicine, Center for Molecular Medicine, Jichi Medical University, Shimotsuke, Tochigi 329-0498, Japan

David S. Salomon Mammary Biology and Tumorigenesis Laboratory, Center for Cancer Research, National Cancer Institute, National Institutes of Health, Bethesda, MD, USA

Paul R. Sanberg Department of Neurosurgery and Brain Repair, College of Medicine, Center of Excellence for Aging and Brain Repair, University of South Florida, Tampa, FL, USA

Erika Sasaki Central Institute for Experimental Animals, Kawasaki, Kanagawa 216-0001, Japan; School of Medicine, Keio University, Tokyo, Japan; PRESTO Japan Science and Technology Agency, Tokyo, Japan, esasaki@ciea.or.jpm

Takao Satou Department of Pathology, Kinki University School of Medicine, Osaka, Japan

Somayeh Shahrokhi Department of Laboratory Sciences, School of Medicine, Lorstan University of Medical Sciences, Khorram Abad, Iran

Keriayn N. Smith Department of Biochemistry and Molecular Biology, Paul D. Coverdell Center for Biomedical and Health Sciences, University of Georgia, Athens, GA 30602, USA

Sun U. Song Clinical Research Center, Inha University School of Medicine, Incheon, Korea 400-711, sunuksong@inha.ac.kr

Giorgio Stassi Laboratory of Cellular and Molecular Pathophysiology, Department of Surgical and Oncological Sciences, University of Palermo, 90127 Palermo, Italy, gstassi@gmail.com

Yoshinori Sumita Department of Regenerative Oral Surgery, Unit of Translational Medicine, Graduate School of Biomedical Sciences, Nagasaki University, Nagasaki 852-8523, Japan

Kouichi Tabu Department of Stem Cell Regulation, Medical Research Institute, Tokyo Medical and Dental University, 1-5-45, Yushima, Bunkyo-ku, Tokyo 113-8510, Japan, k-tabu.scr@mri.tmd.ac.jp

Tetsuya Taga Department of Stem Cell Regulation, Medical Research Institute, Tokyo Medical and Dental University, 1-5-45, Yushima, Bunkyo-ku, Tokyo 113-8510, Japan, taga.scr@mri.tmd.ac.jp

Akihiko Taguchi Department of Cerebrovascular Disease, National Cardiovascular Center, Suita, Osaka 565-8565, Japan, taguchi@ri.ncvc.go.jp

Ryosuke Takahashi Department of Neurology, Graduate School of Medicine, Kyoto University, Kyoto, Japan

Manabu Takamatsu Department of Tumor Pathology, Gifu University Graduate School of Medicine, 1-1 Yanagido, Gifu 501-1194, Japan

Kumiko Takemori Department of Food and Nutrition, Faculty of Agriculture, Kinki University, Higashiōsaka, Osaka, Japan

Tetsuro Tamaki Muscle Physiology and Cell Biology Unit, Division of Basic Clinical Science, Department of Regenerative Medicine, School of Medicine, Tokai University, Isehara, Kanagawa 259-1143, Japan, tamaki@is.icc.u-tokai.ac.jp

Shinya Tanaka Laboratory of Cancer Research, Department of Pathology, Hokkaido University Graduate School of Medicine, N15, W7, Kita-ku, Sapporo 060-8638, Japan, tanaka@med.hokudai.ac.jp

Philippe Taupin School of Biotechnology, Dublin City University, Dublin 9, Ireland, philippe.taupin@dcu.ie

Masahiro Tsubaki Kinki University School of Pharmaceutical Sciences, Osaka, Japan

Matilde Todaro Laboratory of Cellular and Molecular Pathophysiology, Department of Surgical and Oncological Sciences, University of Palermo, 90127 Palermo, Italy

Junya Toguchida Institute for Frontier Medical Sciences, Kyoto University, Sakyo-ku, Kyoto 606-8507, Japan

Ikuo Tomioka Central Institute for Experimental Animals, Kawasaki, Kanagawa 216-0001, Japan; School of Medicine, Keio University, Tokyo, Japan, tomioka@ciea.or.jp

Arinobu Tojo Division of Molecular Therapy, The Advanced Clinical Research Center, The Institute of Medical Science, The University of Tokyo, Tokyo 108-8639, Japan

Hiroyuki Tomita Department of Tumor Pathology, Gifu University Graduate School of Medicine, 1-1 Yanagido, Gifu 501-1194, Japan

Gijs R. van den Brink Department of Gastroenterology & Hepathology, Tytgat Institute for Liver and Intestinal Research, Academic Medical Center, Amsterdam, The Netherlands, g.r.vandenbrink@amc.nl

Carlo Ventura Laboratory of Molecular Biology and Stem Cell Engineering, Cardiovascular Department, National Institute of Biostructures and Biosystems, S.Orsola-Malpighi Hospital (Pavilion 21), University of Bologna, 40138 Bologna, Italy, Carlo.ventura@unibo.it

Giuseppe Visani Hematology and Stem Cell Transplant Center, San Salvatore Hospital, Pesaro, Italy

Júlio C. Voltarelli Ribeirão Preto School of Medicine, University of São Paulo, Ribeirão Preto, São Paulo, Brazil

Anna M. Wobus Leibniz Institute of Plant Genetics and Crop Plant Research, Gatersleben, Germany

Kenichi Yamahara Department of Regenerative Medicine and Tissue Engineering, National Cardiovascular Center Research Institute, Suita, Osaka 565-8565, Japan

Ming-Chia Yang Department of Surgery, National Taiwan University Hospital, National Taiwan University College of Medicine, Taipei, Taiwan, ROC

Shunsuke Yuba Tissue Engineering Research Group, Health Research Institute, National Institute of Advanced Industrial Science and Technology (AIST), Amagasaki City, Hyogo 661-0974, Japan

Jian Zhou Department of Orthopaedic Surgery, Zhongshan Hospital, Fudan University, Shanghai 200032, China

Part I
Stem Cells

Chapter 1

Isolation of Bone Marrow Stromal Cells from Bone Marrow by Using a Filtering Device (Method)

Tomoki Aoyama and Junya Toguchida

Abstract Bone marrow stromal cells (BMSCs) include cells with multi-directional differentiation potential, such as the mesenchymal stem cells (MSCs). For clinical use, it is important to develop safe and efficient methods of isolating BMSCs from the bone marrow. A new concept is to use a filtering device that selectively traps BMSCs from bone marrow aspirates based on its affinity to the filter material. The cells are then recovered by a retrograde flow in a closed system. This method is more efficient, faster, and easier to use than the density gradient method. Because this method is performed in a closed system without centrifugation, no biologically clean area is required, giving this method a great advantage in clinical applications.

Keywords Bone marrow stromal cells · Mesenchymal stem cells · Multipotent adult progenitor cells · Mononuclear cells · Red blood cells · Ethylenediaminetetraacetic acid

Introduction

Bone marrow stromal cells (BMSCs) contain cells with multi-directional differentiation potential, which are designated as mesenchymal stem cells (MSC) (Caplan, 1991), multipotent adult progenitor cells (MAPC) (Jiang et al., 2002), marrow-isolated adult multilineage inducible (MIAMI) cells (D'Ippolito et al., 2004),

T. Aoyama (✉)
Human Health Sciences, Graduate School of Medicine, Kyoto University, Sakyo-ku, Kyoto 606-8507, Japan
e-mail: blue@hs.med.kyoto-u.ac.jp

or multilineage-differentiating stress-enduring (Muse) cells (Kuroda et al., 2010). It is not yet clear whether these cells are distinct, overlapping, or even identical. In spite of such ambiguity, BMSC-derived multipotent cells have been used in various fields of regenerative medicine, because they can be isolated and propagated without difficulty. However, there are some points of concern, especially when these cells are used for clinical applications. Several methods of isolating BMSCs from bone marrow have been reported, most of which consist of 2 steps. The first step is to separate mononuclear cells (MNCs) from red blood cells (RBCs), which otherwise prevent the initial growth of MNCs upon ex vivo culturing (Horn et al., 2008). In the second step, BMSCs are separated from the hematopoietic MNCs based on their property to adhere to plastic dishes. The most popular method for the first step is density-gradient centrifugation by using sucrose gradients (Bøyum, 1964; Peterson and Evans, 1967). The aqueous solution containing sucrose, commercially available as Ficoll-Parque™ ($\rho = 1.077$ g/mL), is sterile, has low endotoxin content, and is guaranteed to maintain high viability of the separated cells (>90%). The density gradient methods, however, require skill and time. Alternatively, RBCs can be burst by treatment with ammonium chloride, potassium bicarbonate, or ethylenediaminetetraacetic acid (EDTA) (Horn et al., 2008). The number of MNCs obtained by this method has been shown to be higher than those obtained by the density gradient centrifugation methods (Horn et al., 2008). Both methods need chemicals to separate BMSCs. Finally, centrifugation with low gravity can also separate MNCs from RBCs (Caterson et al., 2002). While this method does not use chemical solutions, it does employ centrifugation.

We have developed a new method to isolate MNCs that uses neither chemical solutions nor centrifugation (Ito et al., 2010). A cell separation-by-filtering method has been used in various fields. For example, nonwoven fabrics are used to trap leukocytes (Takenaka, 1996). Because pure mechanical trapping based on cell size will damage cell membranes, we were interested in developing a filter that will trap BMSCs by their affinity to the material. BMSCs attach to plastic materials (Pittenger et al., 1999) and have an affinity for hydrophilic materials (Kim et al., 2007). In this chapter, we describe the methods to isolate BMSCs from bone marrow by using filtering devices.

Harvesting Bone Marrow

Bone marrow can be harvested from the pelvic bones of human, dog, goat, and pig. It is important to note that the volume of bone marrow aspirated from 1 portal should remain within the set limit to avoid contamination of the peripheral blood (in case of humans, it is 15–20 mL). To obtain more samples, either additional portals or portals on contralateral sites should be used. When using smaller mammals such as rabbit, rat, and mouse, the bone marrow is harvested from long bones. In this chapter, the method of obtaining bone marrow from the human iliac crest is described.

Materials

Reagents:

Heparin (10,000 U/mL)
Lidocaine (for local anesthesia)

Supplies:

Bone marrow harvesting needle (Medical Device Technologies Inc., USA)
Sterile plastic disposable syringe: 20 mL (for local anesthesia) and 30 mL
Sterile needle: 23G (for local anesthesia)
Disinfectant
Sterile drape

Equipment:

Operating table

Space:

Operating room

Methods

Have the patient or volunteer lie face down on the operating table.
Disinfect the area surrounding the posterior iliac crest with disinfectants.
Drape the area surrounding the posterior iliac crest.
Apply a local anesthesia to the posterior iliac crest.
Prepare a 30-mL syringe with 1 mL heparin.
Insert the bone marrow harvesting needle into the iliac crest, and attach the heparinized syringe.
Aspirate 10–20 mL of bone marrow by rapid pulling. Note that slow pulling can contaminate the sample with peripheral blood.
To prevent clotting, agitate the syringe immediately.

Filtering Device 1 (BASIC-SET)

Bone Marrow MSC Separation Device/BASIC-set contains minimum supplies. The sample is processed in open air. Therefore, an operating room or biohazard cabinet is needed for processing. Processing is quite easy for the BASIC-set. Thus, the BASIC-set enables on-demand processing at the operating table.

Materials

Reagents:

Sterilized physiological saline (100 mL) for priming and washing
Sterilized physiological saline (50 mL) for cell harvesting

Supplies:

Bone marrow MSC separation device BASIC-set (KANEKA CO., Osaka, Japan)
Sterilized filter (pore size, 70 μm)
4 sterile plastic disposable syringes (Luer-Slip or Luer-Lok type; 50 mL)
Priming syringe (Luer-Slip or Luer-Lok type; 50 mL)

Bone marrow fluid syringe (Luer-Slip or Luer-Lok type; 50 mL)

Washing solution syringe (Luer-Slip or Luer-Lok type; 50 mL)

Cell harvest solution syringe (ONLY Luer-Slip; 50 mL)

Waste solution container (150 mL)

Cotton alcohol pads

Equipment:

Syringe pump

Space:

Operating room or biohazard cabinet

Methods

Preparing the syringes (see Note 8.1)

Priming solution: Load the priming syringe with 50 mL of physiological saline solution.

Bone marrow fluid: Filter the bone marrow fluid through the sterilized filter, and load the bone marrow fluid syringe with that fluid; *see* Note 8.2.

Washing solution: Load the washing solution syringe with 30 mL of physiological saline solution.

Cell harvest solution: Load the accompanying Luer-Lok syringe with 50 mL of physiological saline solution; *see* Note 8.3.

Set-up (Fig. 1.1a)

Detach the cap on the column inlet, and connect the accompanying Luer-Lok joint to the nozzle on the column inlet.

Detach the cap on the column outlet, connect the accompanying 3-way cock to the nozzle on the column outlet, and detach the cap at the male-taper end of the 3-way cock.

Remove the cap located on the downstream port of 3-way cock.

Priming (Fig. 1.1b)

Connect the priming syringe to the Luer-Lok joint, and open the flow channel of the 3-way cock (Fig. 1.1b).

Tilt the assembled syringe and column, and gently push the syringe to deliver the solution, while removing air from within the column (Fig. 1.1b); *see* Note 9.4.

After removing all the air, position the assembled syringe and column horizontally, and deliver the remaining priming solution. Collect the fluid passed through the column into the waste solution container.

Close the flow channel for the 3-way cock, while tilting the assembled syringe and column.

With the Luer-Lok joint filled with physiological saline, remove only the syringe.

Processing the bone marrow fluid (Fig. 1.1c)

Orient the column vertically (point the column outlet down). Connect the bone marrow fluid syringe to the Luer-Lok joint, and allow it to stand for 3 min; *see* Notes 8.5 and 8.6.

Open the flow channel on the 3-way cock, and process the bone marrow fluid through the column at a rate of 6 mL/min, equivalent to 2 drops/s; *see* Note 8.7.

Collect the solution passed through the column into the waste solution container. After processing the bone marrow fluid, close the flow channel of the 3-way cock.

With the Luer-Lok joint filled with bone marrow fluid, remove only the syringe.

Washing (Fig. 1.1d)

Connect the washing solution syringe to the Luer-Lok joint, and open the flow channel of the 3-way cock.

Deliver the washing solution at a rate of 6 mL/min, equivalent to 2 drops/s, to wash out the unwanted cells within the column (Fig. 1.1d). Collect the fluid passed through the column into the waste solution container.

Close the flow channel on the 3-way cock (by rotating it 90° clockwise) after all the washing solution has been delivered.

Remove only the syringe.

Turn the column upside down, remove the air filter on the accompanying cell harvest bag, and connect it to the Luer-Lok joint.

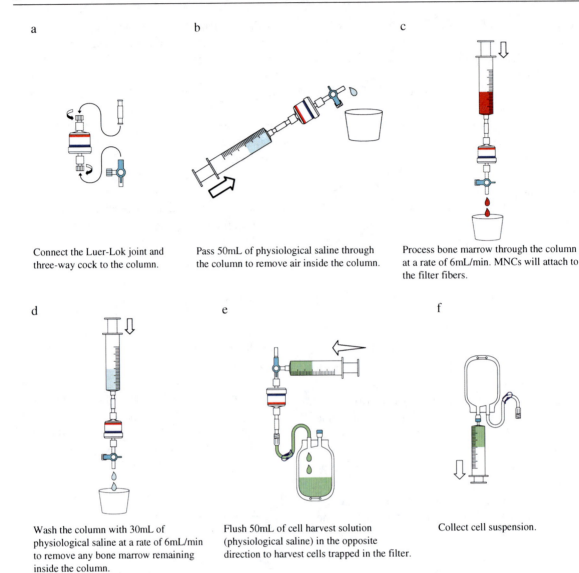

Fig. 1.1 Processing protocol for the filtering device (BASIC-Set)

Injecting the cell-harvest solution (Fig. 1.1e)

- Remove the cap located at the side-connection point for the syringe on the 3-way cock.
- Connect the Luer-Lok syringe pre-filled with cell harvest solution.
- Confirm that the clamp on the tube connecting the cell harvest bag is open.
- Operate the 3-way cock.
- Flush the cell harvest solution manually (inject 50 mL of cell harvest solution in about 3 s), and harvest the cells trapped within the column into the cell harvest bag (Fig. 1.1e); see Note 8.8.
- Close the flow channel on the 3-way cock.
- Close the clamp on the tube connecting the cell harvest bag circuit.
- Remove the cell harvest bag from the Luer-Lok joint.

Collecting the cell harvest solution (Fig. 1.1f)

Sterilize the cell harvest port with a sterile alcohol pad, and insert the cell harvest syringe into the port; see Note 8.9.
Collect the cell suspension (Fig. 1.1f).
Remove the syringe after collecting the suspension.

Notes

Remove any air from within the syringes before loading them with liquid (introducing air into the column may disrupt the flow of bone marrow).
A volume of up to 30 mL of bone marrow fluid can be used.
Take up the cell harvest solution in the accompanying syringe or in a syringe of an equivalent volume (50 mL). Using a syringe of a different volume may damage the circuit and may expose the operator to bone marrow fluid.
During priming, remove as much air as possible from inside the column. Priming from the bottom up will make this easier.
To orient the column vertically, hold the syringe and the column with a stand, a clamp, a syringe pump, or by hand.
Arrange the apparatus so that the column is orientated below the syringe. Allow it to stand still for 3 min to separate the oil (which may obstruct the column) within the bone marrow fluid. After 3 min, begin processing the bone marrow fluid.
When processing bone marrow fluid using a syringe pump, do not continue the process if the column gets obstructed. Continued use may result in damage to the connections and may cause the fluid to leak from the connections, potentially exposing the operator to direct contact with the bone marrow fluid. For this reason, never force delivery when you encounter unusual resistance.
If you encounter difficulty when pressing the syringe piston to deliver the cell harvest solution, the column may be obstructed. Try proceeding at a slower rate (e.g., injecting 50 mL of cell harvest solution in 10 s). Avoid excessive force. Stop delivery if you continue to encounter unusual resistance. Applying excessive force during this procedure may result in damage to the circuit and column and may expose the operator to direct contact with bone marrow fluid.

Connect a Luer-Slip-type syringe directly to the cell harvest port (without a needle).

Filtering Device 2 (ADVANCED-SET)

Bone Marrow MSC Separation Device/ADVANCED-set consists of a closed-line system. Theoretically, processing is possible in any space, but a clean area such as an operating room is recommended.

Materials

Reagents:

Sterilized physiological saline (100 mL) for priming and washing
Sterilized physiological saline (50 mL) for cell harvesting

Supplies:

Bone marrow MSC separation device ADVANCED-set (KANEKA CO., Osaka, Japan). The set consists of a Circuit set A (bone marrow bag, cell harvest bag, circuit, etc.) and Circuit set B (waste solution bag, circuit, etc.).
4 sterile plastic disposable syringes (Luer-Slip or Luer-Lok type; 50 mL)
Priming syringe (Luer-Slip or Luer-Lok type; 50 mL)
Bone marrow fluid syringe (Luer-Slip or Luer-Lok type; 50 mL)
Washing solution syringe (Luer-Slip or Luer-Lok type; 50 mL)
Cell harvest solution syringe (ONLY Luer-Slip; 50 mL)
Disinfectants (alcohol)
Cotton alcohol pads

Equipment:

Infusion stand
Infusion pump

Space:

Clean area is recommended.

Methods

Preparing the syringes (*see* Note 9.1)

Bone marrow fluid: Load the bone marrow fluid syringe with bone marrow fluid; *see* Note 9.2.

Cell harvest solution: Load the accompanying Luer-Lok syringe with 50 mL of physiological saline solution; *see* Note 9.3.

Set-up (Fig. 1.2a and b)

Close the clamp and roller clamp.

Close all 3-way cocks (i.e., A (downwards), B (downwards), C (cell harvest bag), D (injection port for cell harvest solution)), and E (air filter)). Orient 3-way cocks as shown in Fig. 1.2a.

Remove the column caps, the circuit cap at the connection to the column, and the air filter.

Connect the column to the circuit so that it is oriented. (Connect the column to match the red and

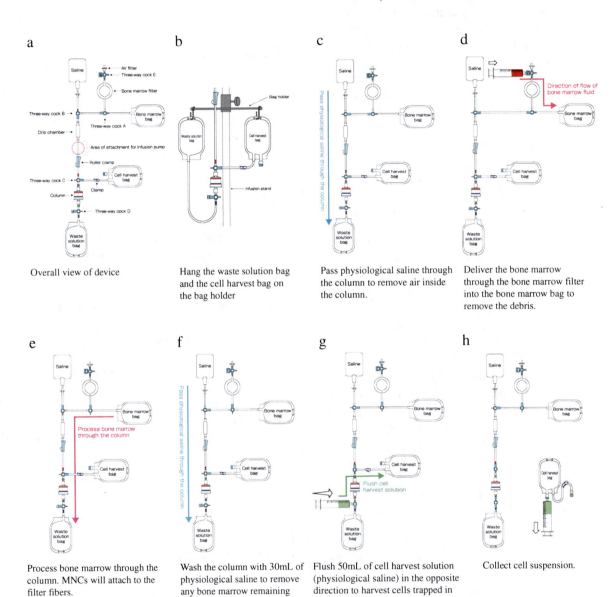

Fig. 1.2 Processing protocol for the filtering device (ADVANCED-Set)

blue markers on the column label to the red and blue tapes on the circuit, respectively).

Confirm once again that the column is connected properly to the circuit.

Hang the bone marrow and physiological saline bags on an infusion stand, and insert the spike into the physiological saline container.

Hang the waste solution and cell harvest bags on the bag holder, as shown in Fig. 1.2b; *see* Note 9.4, 9.5.

Close the port on the 3-way cock B on the side of the bone marrow bag (with the 3-way cock B oriented, as shown in Fig. 1.2b). Squeeze the drip chamber to empty it, and then, load it to about 70% with physiological saline; *see* Note 9.6.

Priming (Fig. 1.2c)

Open the roller clamp.

Once the waste solution bag is filled with physiological saline up to the blue priming solution line, close the roller clamp and the downstream port of the 3-way cock B.

Open the roller clamp, and squeeze the drip chamber to push air out of the column and into the waste solution bag.

Confirm that the air has been squeezed into the waste solution bag, and release the drip chamber. The physiological saline inside the waste solution bag will run into the column (Fig. 1.2c).

Close the roller clamp.

Injecting the bone marrow fluid (Fig. 1.2d)

Confirm that the downstream port of the 3-way cock A is closed. Confirm that the air-filter side port of the 3-way cock E is closed (confirm that the 3-way cocks A and E are oriented as shown in Fig. 1.2d).

After wiping the injection port for the bone marrow fluid of the 3-way cock E with a sterile alcohol pad, connect the bone marrow fluid syringe, inject all the bone marrow fluid (Fig. 1.2d), and then remove the syringe; *see* Note 9.7.

Connect the air injection syringe to the air filter, and close the bone marrow fluid injection side port of the 3-way cock E.

Inject air to flow through the air filter. Deliver all the bone marrow fluid remaining inside the bone marrow filter into the bag.

Remove the air injection syringe.

Processing the bone marrow fluid (Fig. 1.2e)

Attach the pump onto the infusion stand. Set the tube above the roller clamp to the infusion pump.

Close the bone marrow filter side port of the 3-way cock A (the 3-way cock A is oriented as shown in Fig. 1.2e).

Set the conditions for the infusion pump (flow rate: 6 mL/min). Close the physiological saline side port of the 3-way cock B (the 3-way cock B is oriented as shown in Fig. 1.2e), and open the roller clamp.

Turn on the infusion pump to initiate delivery of the bone marrow fluid; *see* Notes 9.8, 9.9.

Immediately after all the bone marrow fluid flows completely into the 3-way cock B, stop the infusion pump and close the bone marrow bag side port of the 3-way cock B (turned 90° clockwise); *see* Note 9.10.

Washing (Fig. 1.2f)

Turn on the infusion pump, and pass 30 mL of physiological saline at a flow rate equivalent to that used for processing the bone marrow fluid. After completing the delivery of the predetermined amount of physiological saline, stop the pump, and close the roller clamp.

Close the upstream side port of the 3-way cock C (turned 90° anti-clockwise).

Injecting the cell harvest solution (Fig. 1.2g)

Close the downstream port of 3-way cock D (the 3-way cock D is oriented as shown in Fig. 1.2g).

Remove the cap located on the injection port for cell harvest solution. Set the Luer-Lok syringe, previously filled with cell harvest solution, to the injection port for the cell harvest solution, and open the clamp (Fig. 1.2g).

Quickly inject the cell harvest solution manually (injecting 50 mL of cell harvest solution in about 3 s), to collect the cells trapped inside the column into the cell harvest bag; *see* Note 9.11.

Close the clamp.

Collecting the cell harvest solution (Fig. 1.2h)

Remove the cell harvest bag.

Sterilize the cell harvest port with a sterile alcohol pad, and insert the cell harvest solution syringe into the port; *see* Note 9.12.

Collect the cell suspension.
Remove the syringe after collecting.

Notes

Remove any air from within the syringes before loading them with liquid (introducing air into the column may disrupt the flow of bone marrow).

A volume of up to 30 mL of bone marrow fluid can be used.

Take up the cell harvest solution in either the accompanying syringe or a syringe of an equivalent volume (50 mL). Using a syringe of a different volume may damage the circuit and expose the operator to bone marrow fluid.

Adjust the position of the bag holder to orient the column vertically.

Set the cell harvest bag on the bag holder so that the cell harvest port points down.

Be careful to load the drip chamber with sufficient physiological saline, so that it does not run out while processing the bone marrow fluid.

A Luer-Slip-type of syringe should be connected directly to the injection port for bone marrow fluid (without a needle).

Running the infusion pump continuously in the presence of an obstruction present may result in damage to the circuit, potentially leading to the operator being directly exposed to bone marrow fluid. We recommend using an infusion pump with an alarm function to indicate obstructions/resistance.

If fluid delivery is halted because the empty alarm on the infusion pump is triggered before the bone marrow fluid reaches the drip chamber, disable the alarm and allow the bone marrow fluid to reach the drip chamber.

Stop the infusion pump after the fluid delivery is complete. Otherwise, damage to the circuit due to rising circuit pressure may expose the operator to bone marrow fluid.

If you encounter unusual resistance when pressing the piston of the syringe forward while delivering the cell harvest solution, the column may be obstructed. Try proceeding at a slower rate (e.g., injecting 50 mL of cell harvest solution in 10 seconds). Avoid excessive force. Stop delivery if you continue to encounter unusual resistance. Applying excessive force during this procedure may result in damage to the circuit and to the column, exposing the operator to direct contact with bone marrow fluid.

Connect a Luer-Slip-type syringe directly to the cell harvest port (without a needle).

Assessment

We compared the efficiency of using a filtering device to that of using the density gradient method, analyzing the time required for processing, the colony-forming unit (CFU) assay (Friedenstein et al., 1974), and fluorescence-activated cell sorting (FACS) analysis. The CFU assay and FACS analysis were performed, as previously reported (Pochampally, 2008; Gronthos, 2008).

Ten milliliters of bone marrow was aspirated from a 43-year-old female donor. Three milliliter of bone marrow was processed using either the filtering device (BASIC-set) or the density gradient method (Table 1.1.1). The processing time required 8 min for the filtering device, and 55 min for the density gradient method. The number of MNCs obtained by the filtering device (20.6×10^6) was higher than that obtained by the density gradient method (4.23×10^6). The number of contaminated RBCs was also higher in the filtering device (58.9×10^6) than in the density gradient method (2.25×10^6), suggesting that the selectivity of the density gradient method is superior to that of the filtering device. The results of the CFU assay showed that the efficiency of the filtering device was comparable to that of the density gradient method (Table 1.1.2). MNCs (2.5×10^5) isolated by each method were seeded on 25-cm^2 culture dishes and cultured for 2 weeks, and then, the number of colonies with a diameter of more than 4 mm was counted as CFU. The CFU was higher in MNCs isolated by the filtering device than those by the density gradient method (Table 1.1.2). Collection efficacy was calculated from the CFU assay (number of CFU × collection number of MNCs/number of cells number for the CFU assay/total number of MNCs). The collection efficacy was much higher in the filtering device than in the density gradient method.

Ten milliliters of bone marrow was aspirated from a 31-year-old male donor for FACS analysis. MNCs were isolated from 3 mL of bone marrow by either the filtering device (BASIC-set) or the density gradient method. MNCs (1×10^6) were incubated with each

Table 1.1 Assesment of filtering device. Cell processing efficacy was compared with density gradient method

1. Processing time and isolated cell numbers

	Processing time (min)	Total number of MNCs ($\times 10^6$)	Total number of RBC (10^6)
Bone marrow		62.7	7110
Filtering device	8	20.6	58.9
Density gradient	55	4.23	2.25

2. Colony forming units

	Number of CFUs	Total number of CFUs
Filtering device	20.0±3.6	26.3
Density gradient	13.7±1.5	3.7

3. Fluorescence activated cell sorting: Single staining

	CD10	CD90	CD106	CD166	CD271	STRO-1	CD34
Filtering device	30.9	1.33	1.87	2.41	1.09	10.2	0.64
Density gradient	22.9	0.27	1.48	0.6	2.02	7.5	1.75

4. Fluorescence activated cell sorting: Double staining

	CD10/CD271	CD90/CD166	CD90/CD271	CD106/STRO-1
Filtering device	0.21	0.17	0.13	1.19
Density gradient	0.13	0.05	0.09	0.34

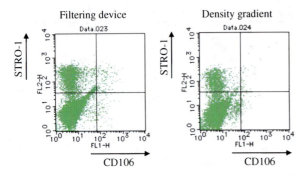

Fig. 1.3 Assessment of filtering devices by FACS analysis. 1×10^6 MNCs were stained for both CD106 and STRO-1

antibody against MSC-related cell surface markers (CD10, CD90, CD106, CD166, CD271, or STRO-1) or a hematopoietic cell surface marker (CD34), and processed for FACS analysis. With the exception of CD271, the number of cells positive for MSC-related cell surface markers was higher in the MSCs isolated by the filtering device than in those isolated by the density gradient method (Table 1.1.3). The number of CD34-positive cells was lower in MNCs isolated by the filtering device than in those isolated by the density gradient method. MNCs were double-stained with pairs of 2 MSC-related cell surface markers (Table 1.1.4), and the fraction of double-positive cells, particularly that of CD106/STRO-1 double-positive, was higher in MSCs isolated by the filtering device (Table 1.1.4, Fig. 1.3). It is reported that CD106/STRO-1 double-positive fractions contain cells with multi-differentiation property (Gronthos and Zannettino, 2008). These results suggest that the filtering device method is more efficient than the density gradient method for isolating MNCs that contain multi-potent cells.

Acknowledgements The authors thank Ms. M. Ueda and Mr. S. Yoshida for reviewing.

References

Bøyum A (1964) Separation of white blood cells. Nature 204:793–794
Caplan AI (1991) Mesenchymal stem cells. J Orthop Res 9: 641–650
Caterson EJ, Nesti LJ, Danielson KG, Tuan RS (2002) Human marrow-derived mesenchymal progenitor cells: Isolation, culture expansion, and analysis of differentiation. Mol Biotechnol 20:245–256
D'Ippolito G, Diabira S, Howard GA, Menei P, Roos BA, Schiller PC (2004) Marrow-isolated adult multilineage inducible (MIAMI) cells, a unique population of postnatal young and old human cells with extensive expansion and differentiation potential. J Cell Sci 117(Pt 14):2971–2981
Friedenstein AJ, Deriglasova UF, Kulagina NN, Panasuk AF, Rudakowa SF, Luri EA, Ruadkow IA (1974) Precursors for fibroblasts in different populations of hematopoietic cells as detected by the in vitro colony assay method. Exp Hematol 2:83–92
Gronthos S, Zannettino AC (2008) A method to isolate and purify human bone marrow stromal stem cells. Methods Mol Biol 449:45–57
Horn P, Bork S, Diehlmann A, Walenda T, Eckstein V, Ho AD, Wagner W (2008) Isolation of human mesenchymal stromal cells is more efficient by red blood cell lysis. Cytotherapy 10:676–685
Ito K, Aoyama T, Fukiage K, Otsuka S, Furu M, Jin Y, Nasu A, Ueda M, Kasai Y, Ashihara E, Kimura S, Maekawa T, Kobayashi A, Yoshida S, Niwa H, Otsuka T, Nakamura T, Toguchida J (2010) A novel method to isolate mesenchymal stem cells from bone marrow in a closed system using a device made by nonwoven fabric. Tissue Eng C Methods 16:81–91
Jiang Y, Jahagirdar BN, Reinhardt RL, Schwartz RE, Keene CD, Ortiz-Gonzalez XR, Reyes M, Lenvik T, Lund T, Blackstad M, Du J, Aldrich S, Lisberg A, Low WC, Largaespada DA, Verfaillie CM (2002) Pluripotency of mesenchymal stem cells derived from adult marrow. Nature 418:41–49
Kim MS, Shin YN, Cho MH, Kim SH, Kim SK, Cho YH, Khang G, Lee IW, Lee HB (2007) Adhesion behavior of human bone marrow stromal cells on differentially wettable polymer surfaces. Tissue Eng 13:2095–2103
Kuroda Y, Kitada M, Wakao S, Nishikawa K, Tanimura Y, Makinoshima H, Goda M, Akashi H, Inutsuka A, Niwa A, Shigemoto T, Nabeshima Y, Nakahata T, Nabeshima Y, Fujiyoshi Y, Dezawa M (2010) Unique multipotent cells in adult human mesenchymal cell populations. Proc Natl Acad Sci USA 107:8639–8643
Peterson EA, Evans WH (1967) Separation of bone marrow cells by sedimentation at unit gravity. Nature 214:824–825
Pittenger MF, Mackay AM, Beck SC, Jaiswal RK, Douglas R, Mosca JD, Moorman MA, Simonetti DW, Craig S, Marshak DR (1999) Multilineage potential of adult human mesenchymal stem cells. Science 284:143–147
Pochampally R (2008) Colony forming unit assays for MSCs. Methods Mol Biol 449:83–91
Takenaka Y (1996) Lymphocytapheresis. Artif Organs 20: 914–916

Chapter 2

Hematopoietic Stem Cell Frequency Estimate: Statistical Approach to Model Limiting Dilution Competitive Repopulation Assays

Thierry Bonnefoix and Mary Callanan

Abstract The competitive repopulation assay in recipients has emerged as the gold standard test that enables characterization of hematopoietic stem cells (HSCs) by their capacity for reconstitution of the lymphohematopoietic system. When combined with a limiting dilution design, this assay, termed limiting-dilution competitive repopulation assay (LDCRA) allows measurement of HSC numbers in vivo. Thus far, the statistical single-hit Poisson model (SHPM) has played a prominent role in analyzing LDCRAs to estimate HSC frequencies. This chapter presents a review of a new statistical method for analyzing LDCRAs, called multi-cell Poisson modeling, with aim to more accurately estimate the frequency of HSCs. Multi-cell Poisson models (MCPM) stand for a general family of Poisson models that extend the SHPM hypothesis, including the traditional SHPM as a special case of the model series. Through examples of re-analyses of LDCRAs from previously published papers, it is shown the ability of MCPM to model LDCRAs in comparison to the traditional SHPM. The results emphasize that MCPM can provide more reliable HSC frequency estimates than obtained from the exclusive use of the SHPM. It is concluded that the use of proper Poisson models alternative to the traditional SHPM appears as critical to ensure accurate HSC frequency estimates, and MCPM should be routinely used to model LDCRAs. More generally, MCPM provide substantial refinement in the art of modeling limiting dilution assays.

Keywords Hematopoietic stem cells · Limiting-dilution competitive repopulation assay · Multi-cell Poisson model · Single-hit Poisson model · Akaike's information criterion · Competitive repopulating units

Introduction

The hematopoietic stem cell compartment has recently been shown to be composed of multiple hematopoietic stem cell (HSC) subpopulations that are characterized by highly diverse cycling activity, self-renewal, differentiation behavior and repopulating activity as reflected in their repopulation kinetics in recipients (Purton and Scadden, 2007; Wilson et al., 2008; Roeder et al., 2008; Weissman and Shizuru, 2008; Morita et al., 2010). Moreover, it has become apparent that both extrinsic (prostaglandins, growth factors, cytokines) and intrinsic (transcription factors) mechanisms tightly govern HSC decisions of self-renewal and differentiation (North et al., 2007; Zon, 2008; Himburg et al., 2010). It must be emphasized that much of our knowledge regarding the hematopoietic stem cell box comes from experimental transplantation assays performed into lethally irradiated mice as recipients. To measure HSC functional potential, the gold standard method is the competitive repopulation assay (Purton and Scadden, 2007), which measures the repopulating activity of the unknown source of HSCs against a set known number of HSCs, allowing quantitation of HSCs as competitive repopulating units (CRUs). The frequency of HSCs (also

T. Bonnefoix (✉)
INSERM, U823, Université Joseph Fourier-Grenoble I, UMR-S823, Institut Albert Bonniot, Grenoble, France, and Pole de Recherche, CHU de Grenoble, France, Grenoble, F-38706, France
e-mail: Thierry.bonnefoix@ujf-grenoble.fr

termed as CRU frequency) is usually more accurately determined by using the limiting dilution competitive repopulation assay (LDCRA) (Szilvassy et al., 1990), which is a variation of the competitive repopulation assay. Especially, limiting dilution HSC transplantation enables a more sensitive functional study of small numbers of HSCs after transplantation into marrow-ablated recipient mice. In this limiting dilution assay, a series of dilutions of the unknown source of HSCs (donor test cells) are competed against a set number of competitor bone marrow cells. The number of mice negative for hematopoietic reconstitution in each cell dose is then measured, and HSC frequencies are routinely estimated within the traditional, well-known single-hit Poisson distribution (called the single-hit Poisson model; Taswell, 1981). To aid in data analysis of limiting dilution assays, the single-hit Poisson model (SHPM) has been implemented in two easily available software packages, L-Calc (StemCell Technologies) and ELDA software (Hu and Smyth, 2009); ELDA is available free online on http://bioinf.wehi.edu.au/software/elda/index.html. These programs calculate the frequency of HSCs within the donor test cell population, provide the 95% confidence intervals for these calculations, and can also be used to perform statistical comparison between two or more test samples.

Our goal is to present a new statistical modeling approach applied to LDCRAs, based on a family of Poisson models, called multi-cell Poisson models (MCPM) which stand for an extension of the SHPM hypothesis. The text is designed primarily for biologists involved in the analysis of limiting dilution transplantation data. This is the reason why the presentation is written in a nontechnical style and does not require familiarity with advanced statistics, and we hope that it will appeal to readers that prefer a simplest introduction to the art of multi-cell Poisson modeling than our earlier paper provides (Bonnefoix and Callanan, 2010). For instance, this text do not present the equations of the Poisson models and the maximum likelihood equations used to fit the models to limiting dilution data. As shown below, the concept of MCPM is easily understandable and the multi-cell Poisson modeling method does not require extensive computation. Unfortunately, no available software or program can perform this task at the present time (2011). However, crude limiting dilution data can be sent to the authors of this text for detailed analysis under the modeling methods presented here.

Modeling Limiting Dilution Competitive Repopulation Assays with Multi-cell Poisson Models: Concept and Principles

The objective of statistical analysis of LDCRAs is to extract all the information from the limiting dilution data to deduce an accuracy measure of the frequencies of HSCs able to repopulate the recipients. Hence, a crucial step in statistical analysis of LDCRAs is to use the best method to approximate some accuracy measures of HSC frequencies. In this regard, it is an outstanding consideration that the relative accuracy of the HSC frequency estimates does depend on the underlying statistical model. In the traditional approach, HSC frequency measure is estimated by the SHPM which posits that one transplanted HSC is sufficient to generate a progeny of detectable differentiated cells above a threshold value in recipients. However, there is no clear support for this statement, and it is receivable that more than one donor HSC may be necessary to provide detectable hematopoietic reconstitution in recipients above the threshold level for detection, usually 0.1–1% of donor-derived cells as routinely assessed by standard flow cytometric analysis (Purton and Scadden, 2007). Therefore, by ignoring this potential weakness of the SHPM, blindly applying the traditional SHPM-based statistical approach implemented in L-Calc and ELDA softwares can lead to biased (inaccurate) HSC frequency estimates. To address this issue, we have demonstrated that it is possible to more accurately quantitate HSCs, providing that the traditional SHPM is mathematically remodeled to turn to a new class of Poisson models termed multi-Cell Poisson models (MCPM) which take into account the possibility that one, but also more than one, stem cell(s) can be necessary to generate detectable hematopoietic reconstitution in recipients above the threshold level for detection achieved by standard methods (Bonnefoix and Callanan, 2010; Box 2.1; Fig. 2.1). In this context of multi-cell Poisson modeling, HSC frequency estimates are obtained by a mathematical procedure called "model averaging" performed across the set of all statistically plausible MCPM (Burnham and Anderson, 2002; Box 2.2; Fig. 2.2). It must be noted that the main feature of MCPM is that the resulting HSC frequency estimates, termed model-averaged HSC frequency estimates, are higher than those provided by the SHPM. This is the direct consequence of the ability of MCPM to take into account recipients falsely classified as negative for hematopoietic reconstitution, due to insufficient sensitivity of detection methods used to investigate hematopoietic reconstitution. Of note, a crucial step of the multi-cell Poisson modeling process is to check the statistical validity of the model-averaged HSC frequency estimate, ensuring that the MCPM holds for the LDCRA under examination (Box 2.3). Full methods that relate to model averaging based on the concept of model selection uncertainty and to the multi-cell Poisson modeling procedure are given in the books by Burnham and Anderson (2002), Anderson (2008) and in the paper by Bonnefoix and Callanan (2010).

Box 2.1 The Multi-cell Poisson Model Hypothesis

In limiting dilution competitive repopulation assays, recipients can be divided into three groups: (1) recipients that have received no HSC; (2) recipients that have received HSCs, but not in sufficient number to ensure detectable progeny of multilineage differentiated cells at time endpoint of analysis, due to insufficient sensitivity of detection methods (usually, flow cytometry) and (3) recipients that have received HSCs in sufficient number to ensure detectable progeny of multilineage differentiated cells at time endpoint of analysis.

The single-hit Poisson model (SHPM) posits that one transplanted HSC is sufficient to generate a progeny of differentiated cells above the threshold level of detection. The SHPM ignores the possibility that one, or even more than one, transplanted HSC(s) may not generate sufficient amount of differentiated cells to ensure their detection by conventional methods. The direct consequence is that a number of recipients may be falsely classified as negative for hematopoietic reconstitution at the time endpoint of analysis. In other words, the number of engrafted recipients is underestimated; it follows that the frequency of HSCs is underestimated.

The multi-cell Poisson model hypothesis posits that more than one transplanted HSC may be necessary to generate a progeny of differentiated cells above the threshold level of detection. Therefore, multi-cell Poisson models (MCPM) take into account the possibility that a number of recipients may have been falsely classified as negative at the time endpoint of analysis, because they may have received a number of HSCs less than the required number of HSCs necessary to generate sufficient amount of differentiated cells to ensure their detection by conventional methods. The direct consequence is that the frequency of HSCs estimated by MCPM is greater than estimated by the use of the SHPM, and the accuracy of the HSC frequency estimate is improved over that imposed by the exclusive use of the SHPM. In the case where one transplanted HSC is sufficient to generate a progeny of differentiated cells above the threshold level of detection, the MCPM series mathematically reduces to the SHPM.

The aim of this chapter is to provide several new examples that will help illustrate the use of MCPM in comparison to the traditional SHPM to more accurately approximate the unknown, true HSC frequencies. The modeled limiting dilution data are drawn from real competitive repopulating experiments of recently published papers studying the hematopoietic stem cell compartment in various situations, like the effect of gene deletion on HSC frequencies, in particular genes coding for transcription factors that can selectively regulate the expansion potential of HSCs. In numerous cases, model-averaged HSC frequencies resulting from the multi-cell Poisson modeling procedure are substantially different from those originally reported according to the traditional SHPM, leading to revise the biological conclusions made by the authors.

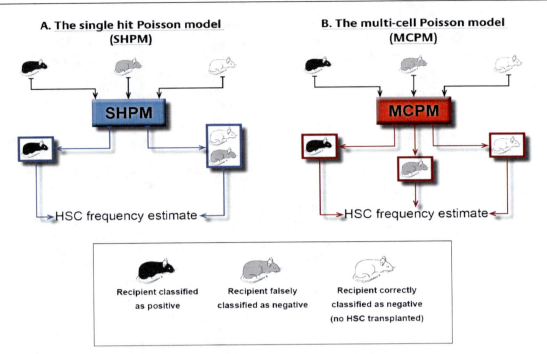

Fig. 2.1 Comparison of single-hit and multi-cell Poisson model hypotheses. The SHPM hypothesis ignores the possibility of recipients falsely classified as negative for hematopoietic reconstitution and hence computation of the HSC frequency estimate is based on two categories (*blue boxes*) of recipients: the positive recipients and the apparently negative recipients; by contrast, the MCPM hypothesis unmasks the recipients falsely classified as negative; it follows that HSC frequency estimate is based on three categories (*red boxes*) of recipients: the positive recipients, the recipients falsely classified as negative and the recipients truly classified as negative (no HSC transplanted)

Box 2.2 The Multi-Cell Poisson Modeling Method: Computation of Model-Averaged HSC Frequency Estimate

Let C be the minimal number of HSCs that must be transplanted to generate a detectable response (hematopoietic reconstitution) in recipients, C = 1,2, ... ,N. Each model from the MCPM family is featured by a given value of C; as example, the model with C = 2 means that at least 2 HSCs are required to detect hematopoietic reconstitution in recipients; of note, the first model of the MCPM series is the SHPM featured by C = 1. Given the limiting dilution transplantation data at hand, the first step of the multi-cell Poisson modeling process is to define a set of models from the MCPM series which are statistically plausible; the plausible models are also called the competing models. The confidence set of plausible models is based on likelihood and Akaike's information criterion (AIC) values obtained for each model of the MCPM series. However, the competing models are not equally plausible, i.e. some models are statistically more plausible than others, a situation giving rise to the concept of model selection uncertainty (Burnham and Anderson, 2002). Once the confidence set of plausible models has been selected, a quantity, called the Akaike weight, is calculated for every model of the set. Because it directly relates to the statistical plausibility of the model, the Akaike weight is also called the model probability. Next, the HSC frequency estimate is calculated for every plausible model, and this estimate is directly influenced by the Akaike weight for the model. Finally, based on every HSC frequency estimate, a model-averaged HSC frequency estimate, termed F_{MCPM}, is computed. An example of model selection, model selection uncertainty and model Akaike weights is given

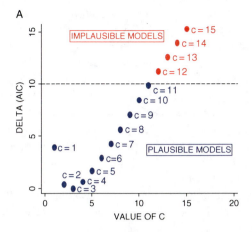

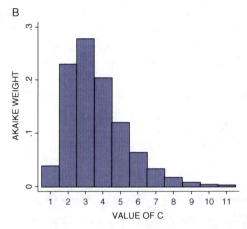

Fig. 2.2 Model-averaged HSC frequency estimate: selection of a set of plausible models among the MCPM family and calculation of Akaike weight relative to every plausible model of the set. This illustrating example is based on the LDCRA performed with 34⁻ KSL cells (recipients analyzed at 4 weeks post transplant) and presented in Table 2.5. (**A**) selection of a set of plausible models among candidate models: Delta (AIC) is the difference between the AIC value of the best model (i.e. the model with minimum AIC) and the AIC value of the candidate model; by convention, the AIC value of the best model is referred to as AIC = 0. Every model is identified by the corresponding value of C. As a rough guideline (Burnham and Anderson, 2002; Bonnefoix and Callanan, 2010), a confidence set of plausible MCPM (colored in *blue*) is defined as the models within 0–10 units of the best model in the data at hand; here this confidence set includes 11 models (C = 1 to C = 11), and therefore all 11 models are used to compute the model-averaged HSC frequency estimate. Models with delta (AIC) superior to 10 are considered as implausible (colored in *red*); (**B**) Akaike weight relative to every plausible model: the estimated best model is featured by C = 3 (weight = 0.279) whereas the less plausible model is featured by C = 11 (weight = 0.002). Of note, the traditional SHPM (featured by C = 1) has low plausibility with weight = 0.039. Given that Akaike weights are probabilities, Akaike weights across all competing models sum to 1

in Figure 2. In the special case where the SHPM is found to be the sole plausible model, the rendered HSC frequency estimate is termed F_{SHPM}.

Box 2.3 Checking the Statistical Validity of the Model-Averaged HSC Frequency Estimate (F_{MCPM})

Once MCPM have been fitted to the LDCRA under examination, it is essential to check that F_{MCPM}, the model-averaged HSC frequency estimate, is statistically significant, that is, significantly different from zero. To make this inference about F_{MCPM}, it is necessary to compute $USE(F_{MCPM})$, the unconditional standard-error for F_{MCPM}, where USE results from the joint use of the usual (called conditional) SE of every competing model (Burnham and Anderson, 2002); USE captures the variation in the HSC frequency estimate across competing models. Next, the ratio $F_{MCPM}/USE(F_{MCPM})$ is calculated. Assuming the standard normal distribution of the ratio $F_{MCPM}/USE(F_{MCPM})$, a value of the ratio $Z = F_{MCPM}/USE(F_{MCPM})$ equal to, or greater than, 1.96 usually means that the estimated F_{MCPM} is significantly different from 0, and it can be said that the estimated F_{MCPM} is statistically valid at the 5% level of significance. When the ratio $F_{MCPM}/USE(F_{MCPM})$ is inferior to 1.96 (*P*-value inferior to 0.05), the usual meaning is that the estimated F_{MCPM} is not significantly different from 0, and it is concluded that the multi-cell Poisson modeling procedure has failed to produce an applicable HSC frequency estimate, that is, the MPCM assumption is not viable. However, this guideline should not be interpreted rigidly. For example, there is no practical difference between a *P*-value of 0.044 and 0.056, even though only the former indicates that the estimated F_{MCPM} is significant at the 5% level. Of note, the appropriate *P*-value refers to a two-sided hypothesis test and is calculated as:

$$P\text{-value} = 2 \times (1 - \text{normal distribution}\ (Z))$$

where the expression "normal distribution (Z)" refers to the numerical output of the standard normal distribution given the value Z. As example, normal distribution (1.96) = 0.975 and therefore the related P-value = 0.05.

When the MCPM hypothesis is rejected, MCPM reduce to the SHPM that is considered as the unique plausible model; in this situation, HSC frequency estimate, termed F_{SHPM}, is based on the SHPM hypothesis.

Examples Illustrating Multi-cell Poisson Modeling of Limiting Dilution Competitive Repopulation Assays

Effect of Trp53/p16^{Ink4a}/p19^{Arf} Gene Deletion on the Frequency of Murine Hematopoietic Stem Cells

The molecular mechanisms that limit the proliferation capacity of multipotent progenitors and other more mature progenitors are not fully understood (Zon, 2008). In their paper, Akala et al. (2008) wished to know whether three pathways commonly repressed in cancer, namely $p16^{Ink4a}$, $p19^{Arf}$ and $Trp53$ have the ability to regulate self-renewal in blood cells. To do this, limiting dilution transplantation assay was done to determine the frequencies of bone marrow cells (BMC) responsible for long-term haematopoietic reconstitution in wild-type mice in comparison to mutant mice genetically deficient for $p19^{Arf}$, $p16^{Ink4a}$ $p19^{Arf}$, $Trp53$ and $p16^{Ink4a}$ $p19^{Arf}$ $Trp53$. Based on the SHPM hypothesis, HSC frequency estimate in $p19^{Arf-/-}$, $Trp53^{-/-}$ and $p16^{Ink4a-/-}$ $p19^{Arf-/-}$ BMC responsible for long-term reconstitution (measured 20 weeks after transplantation) was not significantly different from that of wild-type mice. However, HSC frequency estimate in triple mutant $p16^{Ink4a-/-}$ $p19^{Arf-/-}$ $Trp53^{-/-}$ BMC was 11.8-fold higher than that of wild-type BMC, and the authors concluded that triple deletion of $p16^{Ink4a}$, $p19^{Arf}$ and $Trp53$ caused a striking increase in the frequency of long-term blood repopulating cells. Reanalyzing the limiting dilution data along to multi-cell Poisson modeling shows that HSC frequency estimates have been underestimated by a factor of 2.48 for wild-type, 2.13 for $p19^{Arf-/-}$ and 2.89 for $p16^{Ink4a-/-}$ $p19^{Arf-/-}$ BMC (Table 2.1). For $Trp53^{-/-}$ and $p16^{Ink4a-/-}$ $p19^{Arf-/-}$ $Trp53^{-/-}$ BMC, HSC frequency estimates remain unchanged because the SHPM is the sole plausible Poisson model. Model-averaged HSC frequency estimates in $p19^{Arf-/-}$ and $p16^{Ink4a-/-}$ $p19^{Arf-/-}$ BMC are not far from the frequency observed in wild-type bone marrow, supporting the previous conclusion based on the SHPM that deletion of these genes does not affect the frequency of repopulating stem cells. By contrast, the model-averaged HSC frequency estimate in triple mutant $p16^{Ink4a-/-}$ $p19^{Arf-/-}$ $Trp53^{-/-}$ BMC is only 4.9-fold higher than that of wild-type BMC (instead of 11.8-fold higher based on the SHPM assumption), weakening the main conclusion of Akala et al. (2008) that triple deletion of $p16^{Ink4a}$, $p19^{Arf}$ and $Trp53$ causes an arresting increase in the frequency of long-term blood repopulating cells by removing constraints limiting self-renewal of stem cell subsets.

Effect of the Vent-Like Homeobox Gene VENTX on the Frequency of Human Hematopoietic Stem Cells

It has been reported that homeobox HOX genes play a significant role in the development of normal hematopoietic progenitor cells by amplifying the human hematopoietic stem cell pool (Buske et al., 2002). In their recent paper, Rawat et al. (2010) investigated a role for the vent-like homeobox gene $VENTX$ in normal and malignant myelopoiesis. Functional analyses confirmed that aberrant expression of $VENTX$ in normal CD34$^+$ human progenitor cells perturbs normal hematopoietic development, promoting generation of myeloid cells and impairing generation of lymphoid cells in vitro and in vivo. However, based on LDCRAs and single-hit Poisson modeling, HSC frequency estimates were 1/41,500 in control, GFP-transduced CD34$^+$ BMC and 1/74,000 in $VENTX$-transduced CD34$^+$ BMC, and the difference was reported as not significant by the authors. In line with this statement, we did not found any significant difference as assessed

Table 2.1 Comparison of HSC frequencies estimated by SHPM and MCPM fitting to limiting dilution competitive repopulation assays (LDCRAs) aimed to examine the impact of deleting $p19^{Arf}$, $Trp53$, $p16^{Ink4a}$ $p19^{Arf}$ and $p16^{Ink4a}$ $p19^{Arf}$ $Trp53$ on long-term engraftment of murine HSCs

LDCRA[a]	F_{SHPM}[b]	Number of plausible models (values of C[c])	$Z = F_{MCPM} / USE(F_{MCPM})$[d]	P-value (Z)	MCPM hypothesis	F_{MCPM}	F_{MCPM} / F_{SHPM}
Wild type BMC $n = 42$[e]	1/92,049	8 (C = 1 to C = 8)	2.02	0.0433	Accepted	1/37,188	2.48
$p19^{Arf-/-}$ BMC $n = 51$	1/55,072	5 (C = 1 to C = 5)	2.13	0.0331	Accepted	1/25,967	2.13
$Trp53^{-/-}$ BMC $n = 16$	1/50,317	1[f]	NA	NA	Rejected	NA	NA
$p16^{Ink4a-/-}$ $p19^{Arf-/-}$ BMC $n = 38$	1/53,002	9 (C = 1 to C = 9)	2.09	0.0366	Accepted	1/18,328	2.89
$p16^{Ink4a-/-}$ $p19^{Arf-/-}$ $Trp53^{-/-}$ BMC $n = 29$	1/7,657	11 (C = 1 to C = 11)	1.66	0.097	Rejected	NA	NA

[a] All statistical reanalyzes of LDCRAs were based on the crude limiting dilution data presented in Supplementary Table 2 of Akala et al. (2008); the genotype of mice is stated in the column; BMC: bone marrow cells; LDCRAs were performed with whole BMC; mice that had more than 1% donor-derived (CD45.2 phenotype) cells in both lymphoid and myeloid subpopulations as measured 20 weeks after transplantation by flow cytometry were considered to be repopulated by donor cells.
[b] HSC frequency estimate based on the traditional SHPM assumption and reported by the authors.
[c] C, is the minimum number of HSCs necessary to promote detectable hematopoietic reconstitution in recipients; the plausible models are selected based on model likelihood values and related model Akaike's information criterion (AIC) values.
[d] F_{MCPM} is the model-averaged HSC frequency estimate based on the MCPM assumption; USE is the unconditional standard-error for F_{MCPM}.
[e] n, is the total number of recipients in the LDCRA.
[f] The traditional SHPM (featured by C = 1) is the most plausible model, i.e. no other candidate Poisson model from the MCPM series can plausibly compete with the SHPM, as outlined by unacceptably large likelihood and AIC values of every candidate model with C superior to 1. See Boxes 2.1, 2.2, and 2.3 and Bonnefoix and Callanan (2010) for further details regarding the methodology, especially the selection of plausible (competing) models and the computation of USE(F_{MCPM}). NA: not applicable due to rejection of the MCPM assumption.

by a standard likelihood ratio test based on the SHPM hypothesis (P-value = 0.22). The authors concluded that *VENTX*-enforced expression did not show any significant impact on the stem cell pool as assayed in vivo, and therefore *VENTX* appeared to be more involved in myeloid differentiation pathways than in stem cell development. In addition, knockdown of *VENTX* in human acute myeloid leukemia cell lines, which displayed aberrantly high expression of *VENTX*, strongly inhibited their proliferative potential, supporting the possibility that aberrant expression of *VENTX* might contribute to human myeloid leukemogenesis. In Table 2.2, it can be seen that MCPM fitting is acceptable for the LDCRA performed with GFP-transduced CD34+ BMC, resulting in increasing the difference in HSC frequency estimates between GFP-transduced CD34+ BMC (which is now 1/33,000 according to MCPM fitting) and *VENTX*-transduced CD34+ BMC (which remains to be 1/74,000 because the SHPM is found to be the unique plausible model). The ratio of HSC frequency estimates between GFP-transduced CD34+ BMC and *VENTX*-transduced CD34+ BMC increase from 1.78 (based on SHPM fitting) to 2.24 (based on MCPM fitting), denoting a 26% increase in the HSC frequency estimate difference between the 2 LDCRAs. These findings reinforce the conclusion of the authors that *VENTX* is not a positive regulator of the primitive growth activity of human hematopoietic progenitor cells. This is in clear contrast to stem-cell–associated *HOX* genes such as *HOXB4*, which has been shown to expand the human hematopoietic stem-cell pool (Buske et al., 2002).

Table 2.2 Comparison of HSC frequencies estimated by SHPM and MCPM fitting to LDCRAs aimed to examine the impact of the enforced expression of the homeobox gene *VENTX* on short-term engraftment of human HSCs

LDCRA[a]	F_{SHPM}[b]	Number of plausible models (Values of C[c])	$Z = F_{MCPM} / USE(F_{MCPM})$[d]	P-value (Z)	MCPM hypothesis	F_{MCPM}	F_{MCPM} / F_{SHPM}
VENTX-transduced CD34⁺ BMC n = 27[e]	1/74,042	1[f]	NA	NA	Rejected	NA	NA
GFP-transduced CD34⁺ BMC n = 24	1/41,571	2 (C = 1 and C = 2)	2.13	0.0331	Accepted	1/32,927	1.275

[a] All statistical reanalyzes of LDCRAs were based on the crude limiting dilution data presented in Supplementary Table S4 of Rawat et al. (2010); mice that had more than 0.025% donor-derived (human) cells in both lymphoid (CD19) and myeloid (CD15) subpopulations as measured 6 weeks after transplantation by flow cytometry were considered to be repopulated by donor cells.
[b-f] See footnotes of Table 2.1.

Effect of Aging on the Frequency of Murine Hematopoietic Stem Cells

In the series of LDCRAs presented in this paragraph, it is shown that multi-cell Poisson modeling can provide more dramatic changes on the conclusions previously reported by the authors and based on the SHPM hypothesis. Although hematopoiesis is maintained throughout life by self-renewing stem cells with a high potential for proliferation and multilineage, there is accumulating evidence, via animals models, that as animals age, the number and the functional properties of HSCs become altered (Geiger and Van Zant, 2002). In their study based on LDCRAs, Liang et al. (2005) investigated the effect of aging on engraftment of murine hematopoietic stem cells by injecting young or old C57BL/6 BMC into old or young Ly5 congenic mice. Limiting dilution assays were performed with young (2 months of age) BMC transplanted into old (2 years of age) recipients, and conversely LDCRAs were performed with old BMC transplanted into young recipients. One of the major conclusions of the paper was that the frequency of HSCs approximately increased 2-fold from 2 months to 2 year of age, indicating that young stem cells have only approximately one-half the competitive repopulating activity of old stem cells. As can be seen in Table 2.3, all 8 reported LDCRAs could be successfully modeled by MCPM, with moderate number of competing models in every LDCRA. In comparison to HSC frequencies based on the SHPM hypothesis, changes in HSC frequencies under the use of MCPM were especially notable (usually, more than 2-fold change) for transplanted BMC from young (6–8 weeks of age) mice, whereas changes were modest for transplanted BMC from old (20–22 months of age) mice (less than 1.5-fold change). It follows that, based on MCPM modeling, HSC frequency estimates are found to be comparable for both young and old mice, challenging the SHPM-based conclusion of Liang et al. (2005) that aging affect the ability of HSCs to engraft into recipients. Finally, it should be emphasized that most of these age-related changes are controversial, and contradictory data have been published for almost every aspect of the behavior of aged HSCs. Based on the evidence that the HSC compartment consists of distinct subsets of HSCs (Roeder et al., 2008), it is probable that aging changes the HSC compartment but not the individual HSC (Cho et al., 2008).

Effect of Prostaglandin E2 on the Frequency of Murine Hematopoietic Stem Cells

In their study, North et al. (2007) illustrate that prostaglandin E2 (PGE2) functions as a potent regulator of HSCs in vertebrates, and may prove useful in treating patients with bone marrow failure or following transplantation. To support this conclusion, LDCRAs were conducted to determine the effects of 16,16-dimethyl-PGE2 (dmPGE2), a derivative of PGE2, on HSC reconstitution. In a mouse system, whole BMC (CD45.1 phenotype) exposed to dmPGE2 ex vivo were injected into congenic recipient mice (CD45.2 phenotype); whole BMC treated with ethanol (EtOH) served as control. Based on the

Table 2.3 Comparison of HSC frequencies estimated by SHPM and MCPM fitting to LDCRAs aimed to examine the impact of aging on short-term and long-term engraftment of HSCs in a mouse model

LDCRA[a]	F_{SHPM}[b]	Number of plausible models (Values of C^c)	$Z = F_{MCPM} / USE(F_{MCPM})$[d]	P-value (Z)	MCPM hypothesis	F_{MCPM}	F_{MCPM} / F_{SHPM}
Young BMC 5 weeks-ptp[e] $n = 55$[f]	1/15,242	5 ($C = 1$ to $C = 5$)	2.5	0.012	Accepted	1/6,320	2.41
Old BMC 5 weeks-ptp $n = 51$	1/7,006	3 ($C = 1$ to $C = 3$)	2.27	0.023	Accepted	1/5,139	1.37
Young BMC 10 weeks-ptp $n = 55$	1/16,814	4 ($C = 1$ to $C = 4$)	2.215	0.027	Accepted	1/8,034	2.09
Old BMC 10 weeks-ptp $n = 51$	1/7,006	3 ($C = 1$ to $C = 3$)	2.27	0.023	Accepted	1/5,139	1.37
Young BMC 17 weeks-ptp $n = 55$	1/23,608	3 ($C = 1$ to $C = 3$)	1.94	0.052	Accepted	1/14,430	1.54
Old BMC 17 weeks-ptp $n = 50$	1/10,019	3 ($C = 1$ to $C = 3$)	2.82	0.048	Accepted	1/8,501	1.18
Young BMC 26 weeks-ptp $n = 54$	1/24,578	5 ($C = 1$ to $C = 5$)	2.22	0.026	Accepted	1/9,942	2.47
Old BMC 26 weeks-ptp $n = 50$	1/11,304	2 ($C = 1$ and $C = 2$)	3.5	0.0005	Accepted	1/10,474	1.08

[a] All statistical reanalyzes of LDCRAs were based on the crude limiting dilution data presented in Tables 1 and 2 of Liang et al. (2005); Young BMC means that HSC frequencies were determined by transplanting graded numbers of whole BMC from young (6–8 weeks of age) Ly-5.2 donors into lethally irradiated old (20–22 months of age) Ly-5.1 recipients; conversely, old BMC means that HSC frequencies were determined by transplanting graded numbers of whole BMC from old (20–22 months of age) Ly-5.2 donors into lethally irradiated young (6–8 weeks of age) Ly-5.1 recipients; negative mice were defined as animals in which less than 5% of the circulating B or T lymphocytes or myeloid cells, or any combination of them, were derived from donor as estimated by flow cytometry.
[b–d] See footnotes of Table 2.1.
[e] Post transplantation time point of engraftment analysis.
[f] n, is the total number of recipients in the LDCRA.

SHPM hypothesis, the calculated frequency of repopulating HSCs was enhanced 3.3-fold in dmPGE2-treated BMC recipients in comparison to EtOH-treated BMC recipients at 6 weeks post transplantation (exploring short-term HSCs), and enhanced 2.5-fold at 12 weeks post transplantation (exploring long-term HSCs). At 24 weeks post transplantation, the frequency of long-term repopulating HSCs was enhanced 2.3-fold in dmPGE2-treated BMC recipients in comparison to EtOH-treated BMC recipients. Therefore, there is little doubt that PGE2 enhances the number of HSCs in this mouse model. As presented in Table 2.4, the MCPM assumption was found to be receivable in 3 out the 6 LDCRAs. In the LDCRA performed with EtOH-treated BMC recipients and analyzed at 6 weeks post transplantation, the increase of model-averaged HSC frequency in comparison to SHPM-based frequency was modest (1.075-fold change). Such a small change does not meaningfully impact the previous SHPM-based conclusion reported by the authors that dmPGE2 significantly stimulates short-term stem cell engraftment. More substantial, in the 2 LDCRAs performed with dmPGE2-treated BMC and analyzed at 12 and 24 weeks post transplantation, both HSC frequency estimates provided by multi-cell Poisson model averaging were approximately 1.5-fold increased in comparison to the frequencies obtained under the fitted SHPM. It turns out that the calculated frequency of repopulating HSCs was enhanced 3.9-fold (instead of 2.5-fold based on SHPM fitting) in dmPGE2-treated BMC

Table 2.4 Comparison of HSC frequencies estimated by SHPM and MCPM fitting to LDCRAs aimed to examine the effect of a long-acting derivative of PGE2, 16,16-dimethyl-PGE2 (dmPGE2) on short-term (6 weeks post transplantation) and long-term (12–24 weeks post transplantation) engraftment of murine HSCs

LDCRA[a]	F_{SHPM}[b]	Number of plausible models (Values of C[c])	$Z = F_{MCPM}$ / $USE(F_{MCPM})$[d]	P-value (Z)	MCPM hypothesis	F_{MCPM}	F_{MCPM} / F_{SHPM}
EtOH-BMC 6 weeks-ptp[e] $n = 37$[f]	1/71,300	2 (C = 1 and C = 2)	2.985	0.0028	Accepted	1/66,300	1.075
dmPGE2-BMC 6 weeks-ptp $n = 40$	1/21,200	1[g]	NA	NA	Rejected	NA	NA
EtOH-BMC 12 weeks-ptp $n = 37$	1/66,400	7 (C = 1 to C = 7)	1.692	0.09	Rejected	NA	NA
dmPGE2-BMC 12 weeks-ptp $n = 40$	1/26,852	4 (C = 1 to C = 4)	1.975	0.048	Accepted	1/17,624	1.52
EtOH-BMC 24 weeks-ptp $n = 35$	1/80,385	11 (C = 1 to C = 11)	1.69	0.09	Rejected	NA	NA
dmPGE2-BMC 24 weeks-ptp $n = 39$	1/34,626	4 (C = 1 to C = 4)	1.922	0.055	Accepted	1/22,841	1.515

[a] All statistical reanalyzes of LDCRAs were based on the crude limiting dilution data presented in Supplementary Tables 7–9 of North et al. (2007); whole BMC (CD45.1 phenotype) were treated ex vivo with ethanol control vehicle (EtOH; BMC-EtOH) or dmPGE2 (BMC-dmPGE2) at 1 μM per 10^6 cells, and transplanted into sublethally irradiated recipients (CD45.2 phenotype); peripheral blood obtained at 6, 12 and 24 weeks post transplantation was examined by flow cytometry and positive reconstitution was defined as more than 5% CD45.1 multilineage chimerism.
[b–d] See footnotes of Table 2.1.
[e] Post transplantation time point of engraftment analysis.
[f] n, is the total number of recipients in the LDCRA.
[g] The traditional SHPM (featured by C = 1) is the most plausible model, i.e. no other candidate Poisson model from the MCPM series can plausibly compete with the SHPM, as outlined by unacceptably large likelihood and AIC values of every candidate model with C superior to 1. See Boxes 2.1, 2.2, and 2.3 and Bonnefoix and Callanan (2010) for further details regarding the methodology, especially the selection of plausible (competing) models and the computation of $USE(F_{MCPM})$. NA: not applicable due to rejection of the MCPM assumption.

recipients in comparison to EtOH-treated BMC recipients at 12 weeks post transplantation, and enhanced 3.5-fold (instead of 2.3-fold based on SHPM fitting) at 24 weeks post transplantation. These findings reinforce the view that dmPGE2 increases the frequency of both short-term and long-term repopulating HSCs.

Effect of Aldehyde Dehydrogenase on the Frequency of Murine Hematopoietic Stem Cells

There is accumulating evidence in the literature that HSCs are enriched for aldehyde dehydrogenase (ALDH) activity, and that ALDH is a selectable marker for human HSCs (Hess et al., 2004; Storms et al., 2005). However, the function of ALDH in HSC biology is not well understood, although ALDH probably plays a role in regulating HSC differentiation In this regard, it has been recently shown that inhibition of ALDH facilitated the expansion of human hematopoietic cells capable of repopulation in NOD/SCID mice, suggesting that ALDH promotes HSC differentiation (Chute et al., 2006). In their recent study, Muramoto et al. (2010) sought to more precisely determine which cell types within the HSC hierarchy are regulated by ALDH. Based on a series of 4 LDCRAs performed in congenic mice, the authors reported that pharmacologic inhibition of ALDH with diethylaminobenzaldehyde (DEAB) impeded the differentiation of murine CD34$^+$c-kit$^+$Sca-1$^-$lineage$^-$

Table 2.5 Comparison of HSC frequencies estimated by SHPM and MCPM fitting to LDCRAs aimed to examine the effect of diethylaminobenzaldehyde (DEAB), an inhibitor of ALDH, on short-term (4 weeks post transplantation) and long-term (12 weeks post transplantation) engraftment of murine HSCs

LDCRA[a]	F_{SHPM}[b]	Number of plausible models (Values of C^c)	$Z = F_{MCPM}$ / $USE(F_{MCPM})^d$	P-value (Z)	MCPM hypothesis	F_{MCPM}	F_{MCPM} / F_{SHPM}
34⁻KSL-BMC[e] 4 weeks-ptp[f] $n = 49$[g]	1/147	11 (C = 1 to C = 11)	2.28	0.023	Accepted	1/29	5.11
DEAB 4 weeks-ptp $n = 47$	1/39	32 (C = 1 to C = 32)	2.18	0.03	Accepted	1/4	9.6
34⁻KSL 12 weeks-ptp $n = 28$	1/17	11 (C = 1 to C = 11)	1.878	0.06	Accepted	1/4.5	3.78
DEAB 12 weeks-ptp $n = 26$	1/56	10 (C = 1 to C = 10)	2.125	0.033	Accepted	1/15	3.81

[a] All statistical reanalyzes of LDCRAs were based on the crude limiting dilution data presented in Supplementary Tables 1–2 of Muramoto et al. (2010); purified CD34⁻c-kit⁺Sca-1⁻lineage⁻ (34⁻KSL) BMC from B6.SJL mice (CD45.1 phenotype) were cultured with or without 100 μM diethylaminobenzaldehyde (DEAB) for 7 days in the presence of murine thrombopoietin at 20 ng/ml, then transplanted into sublethally irradiated congenic C57BL6 recipients (CD45.2 phenotype); peripheral blood was obtained at 4 and 12 weeks post transplantation and animals were considered to be engrafted if donor CD45.1 cells were present at more than 1% for all lineages as estimated by flow cytometry.
[b–d] See footnotes of Table 2.1.
[f] Post transplantation time point of engraftment analysis.
[e] CD34⁻c-kit⁺Sca-1⁺lineage⁻ BMC.
[g] n, is the total number of recipients in the LDCRA.

(34⁻KSL) HSCs, causing a fourfold increase of the short-term repopulating stem cells among 34⁻KSL BMC (4 weeks post transplantation) in comparison to control (untreated) 34⁻KSL BMC. By contrast, at 12 weeks post transplantation (exploring long-term HSCs) inhibition of ALDH activity does not amplify HSCs among 34⁻KSL BMC compared to control 34⁻KSL BMC. As can be seen in Table 2.5, all 4 LDCRAs can be efficiently modeled by MCPM. The observed increase of model-averaged HSC frequency in comparison to SHPM-based frequency was substantial for all 4 LDCRAs and even remarkably prominent for the LDCRA achieved with DEAB and evaluated at 4 weeks post transplantation (9.6-fold change). Of note, this LDCRA exhibited considerable model selection uncertainty, with 32 competing models. At 4 weeks post transplantation, the ratio of HSC frequencies between DEAB-LDCRA and control-LDCRA is 3.77 based on single-hit Poisson modeling, and switches to 7.5 according to multi-cell Poisson modeling, strongly reinforcing the statement that DEAB stimulates engraftment of short-term 34⁻KSL HSCs. At 12 weeks post transplantation, the ratio of HSC frequencies between control-LDCRA and DEAB-LDCRA is comparable for both SHPM and MCPM statistical approaches (3.29 versus 3.33, respectively), confirming that DEAB does not affect engraftment of long-term 34⁻KSL HSCs. Interestingly, MPCM emphasize the outstanding enrichment of HSCs among 34⁻KSL BMC. Myeloablative conditioning prior to HSC transplantation results in a period of pancytopenia during which patients are highly susceptible to infectious complications. This is particularly true in the setting of adult cord blood transplantation in which hematologic recovery can be delayed for up to 2 months (Laughlin et al., 2004). Previous studies have demonstrated that long-term HSCs are inefficient in providing the rapid hematologic recovery that is required for radioprotection of lethally irradiated recipients (Osawa et al., 1996). The above findings suggest that ALDH inhibition represents a translatable strategy to expand short-term HSCs to augment hematopoietic engraftment in patients undergoing stem cell transplantation.

Effect of Direct Injection into NOD/SCID Mice Bone Marrow on the Frequency of Human Hematopoietic Stem Cells

To conclude this presentation of examples illustrating the usefulness of fitting the MCPM to LDCRAs, it is presented 2 LDCRAs in which detection of the progeny of human cord blood CD34$^+$ CD38$^-$ HSCs transplanted in NOD-SCID mice was investigated by using a human chromosome 17 α-satellite specific primer, in conjunction with conventional flow cytometry (Yahata et al., 2003). The prime goal of the authors was to introduce transplanted CD34$^+$ CD38$^-$ cells into mouse bone marrow directly (intrabone marrow, iBM) to minimize the effect of factors that may interfere with the homing of HSCs, then to compare results of engraftment obtained by conventional intravenous injection of HSCs. When cord blood CD34$^+$ CD38$^-$ cells were transplanted in NOD-SCID mice by iBM, a 15-fold higher HSC frequency was achieved compared with the intravenous method. The authors concluded that the iBM injection strategy is a more sensitive and direct way to measure the capability of human HSCs. In relationship to the topic of a new modeling approach of LDCRAs developed in this chapter, the main point of interest of the study of Yahata et al. (2003) refers to the analysis of human cell engraftment in mice by polymerase chain reaction (PCR) to detect a 1171-bp fragment of human chromosome 17, with detection limit assumed by the authors to be 0.01% human cells in human/mouse mixture. This technique is thought to be more reliable than standard flow cytometry in detecting very low levels of human cell engraftment (Chute et al., 2006) although no direct comparison of the two methods has been presented by the authors in their studies (Yahata et al., 2003; Chute et al., 2006). As can be seen in Table 2.6, no multi-cell Poisson model can plausibly compete with the SHPM for both LDCRAs. This finding suggests that the use of a highly sensitive engraftment detection method, like PCR analysis, or the use of both flow cytometry and chromosome-specific PCR methods in conjunction (Yahata et al., 2003) should avoid the occurrence of false negative outcomes, ensuring maximum accuracy of HSC frequency estimate based on traditional SHPM fitting, provided that it has been carefully checked that no MCPM can compete with the SHPM regarding the limiting dilution data at hand.

Conclusion and Perspectives

A quantitative assay for HSCs is essential for the study of the biologic properties of these cells. In the human system, such an assay would also allow a more rational approach to the development of clinical treatments involving transplantation, ex vivo stem cell expansion, and gene therapy (Weissman and Shizuru, 2008). Currently, repopulation of immunodeficient (NOD-SCID) mice remains the primary method to assay HSCs. Interestingly, it has been shown recently that NOD-SCID-IL2Rγ^{null} mice, which have deletion of the IL2Rγ gene, improved HSC engraftment compared with NOD-SCID mice (McDermott et al., 2010). For many years it seemed logical to use the SHPM as *a priori* the best model to analyze LDCRAs, and to

Table 2.6 Comparison of HSC frequencies estimated by SHPM and MCPM fitting to LDCRAs aimed to examine the effect on HSC engraftment of direct intrabone marrow (iBM) injection of human CD34$^+$ CD38$^-$ cells in comparison to conventional intravenous method

LDCRA[a]	FSHPM[b]	Number of plausible models (Values of C[c])	Z = F$_{MCPM}$ / USE(F$_{MCPM}$)[d]	P-value (Z)	MCPM hypothesis	F$_{MCPM}$	F$_{MCPM}$ / F$_{SHPM}$
iBM n = 58[e]	1/43	1[f]	NA	NA	NA	NA	NA
Intravenous n = 26	1/660	1[f]	NA	NA	NA	NA	NA

[a] Statistical reanalyzes of the 2 LDCRAs were based on the crude limiting dilution data presented in Table 1 of Yahata et al. (2003); NOD-SCID mice were injected intravenously or by iBM with purified, Lin$^{-/low}$ human CD34$^+$ CD38$^-$ cord blood cells; mice were scored positive for engraftment when more than 0.01% human DNA was detected in the murine bone marrow at 8 weeks post transplantation (detection limit of human DNA is given as 0.001%); in flow cytometry analysis, more than 0.01% of human CD45 positive cells was considered positive.
[b-f] See footnotes of Table 2.1.

get HSC frequencies from that best model. As illustrated here with examples dealing with various issues of HSC biology, it follows that a better approach is to compute HSC frequencies from a set of plausible Poisson models, including the SHPM but also models alternative to the traditional SHPM, because these models, collectively called MCPM, can grasp a substantial amount of relevant information from LDCRAs which remains ignored by the SHPM used alone. Multi-cell Poisson modeling captures the presence of false negative recipients, a frequently encountered situation that can significantly hamper effective stem cell quantitation exclusively based on the statistical single-hit Poisson modeling method. Although the SHPM has expected to be most accurate thus far, it is hoped that biologists working in the field of HSCs now realize that the sole use of the SHPM to model their LDCRAs is often inappropriate and can result in inaccurate HSC frequency estimates. It must be bear in mind that the underlying hypothesis of MCPM is that one HSC may not be sufficient to generate detectable hematopoietic reconstitution in recipients. In this view, results of single-cell transplantation experiments performed with various HSC-enriched populations as in the report of Kent et al. (2009) should be regarded cautiously, because they may have chronically underestimated the total HSC frequencies based on the ratio of recipients apparently negative for hematopoietic reconstitution to the total number of recipients. In this regard, using single-cell transplantation studies, Morita et al. (2010) have recently found that a fraction of $CD150^{high}$ cells among $CD34^{-/low}$c-Kit^+Sca-1^+Lin^- (34$^-$KSL) mouse BMC displayed virtually undetectable, or barely detectable myeloid engraftment in primary recipient mice (based on a percentage of donor chimerism of 0.3% or more as detected by flow cytometric analysis) but progressive and robust multilineage repopulating activity in secondary-recipient mice. This study challenges received ideas on the prospective isolation and identification of HSC subsets, and strongly supports the hypothesis underlying MCPM, i.e. the widely criteria for HSC activity, which set the bar at more than 0.1–1% contribution to myeloid and lymphoid progeny in the peripheral blood, is in fact not always operational. However, definition of such newly identified HSC subsets (termed "latent" HSCs, which are undoubtedly very potent HSCs) requires time-consuming successive transplantation experiments. The authors (Morita et al., 2010) concluded that novel assays that permit rapid and efficient detection of all sorts of HSCs need to be developed. We suggest that, provided that the data are analyzed by using multi-cell Poisson modeling, LDCRAs performed in the context of primary transplantation should be efficient to detect and to quantify such HSCs for which it is reasonable to assume that they are unable to generate detectable hematopoietic reconstitution in single-cell transplantation studies.

In conclusion, multi-cell Poisson models represent a significant advance over the exclusive use of the SHPM in the art of modeling limiting dilution assays, and therefore we strongly encourage the routine use of the MCPM instead of the sole SHPM to analyze LDCRAs. Noteworthy is that MCPM can also favorably compete with the SHPM to more accurately quantitate normal and cancer stem cells from solid tissues (Bonnefoix and Callanan; unpublished results); moreover, Poisson models alternative to the SHPM can handle more complicated situations than the presence of false negative outcomes, such as simultaneously assessing the frequency of effector and regulatory cells in the field of Immunology (Bonnefoix et al., 2005). Taken collectively, these findings pave new avenues to statistical and mathematical modeling of limiting dilution assays.

Acknowledgment The authors would like to thank Philippe Carbonnel for expert design of Fig. 2.1.

References

Akala OO, Park IK, Qian D, Pihalja M, Becker MW, Clarke MF (2008) Long-term haematopoietic reconstitution by $Trp53^{-/-}$ $p16^{Ink4a-/-}$ $p19^{Arf-/-}$ multipotent progenitors. Nature 453: 228–232

Anderson DR (2008) Model based inference in the life sciences: a primer on evidence. Springer, New York, NY

Bonnefoix T, Callanan M (2010) Accurate hematopoietic stem cell frequency estimates by fitting multicell Poisson models substituting to the single-hit Poisson model in limiting dilution transplantation assays. Blood 116:2472–2475

Bonnefoix T, Bonnefoix P, Perron P, Mi JQ, Ng WF, Lechler R, Bensa JC, Cahn JY, Leroux D (2005) Quantitating effector and regulatory T lymphocytes in immune responses by limiting dilution analysis modeling. J Immunol 174:3421–3431

Burnham KP, Anderson DR (2002) Model selection and multimodel inference: a practical information – Theoretic approach, 2nd edn. Springer, New York, NY

Buske C, Feuring-Buske M, Abramovich C, Spiekermann K, Eaves CJ, Coulombel L, Sauvageau G, Hogge DE, Humphries RK (2002) Deregulated expression of HOXB4 enhances the primitive growth activity of human hematopoietic cells. Blood 100:862–868

Cho RH, Sieburg HB, Muller-Sieburg CE (2008) A new mechanism for the aging of hematopoietic stem cells: aging changes the clonal composition of the stem cell compartment but not individual stem cells. Blood 111:5553–5561

Chute JP, Muramoto GG, Whitesides J, Colvin M, Safi R, Chao NJ, McDonnell DP (2006) Inhibition of aldehyde dehydrogenase and retinoid signaling induces the expansion of human hematopoietic stem cells. Proc Natl Acad Sci USA 103:11707–11712

Geiger H, Van Zant G (2002) The aging of lymphohematopoietic stem cells. Nat Immunol 3:329–333

Hess DA, Meyerrose TE, Wirthlin L, Craft TP, Herrbrich PE, Creer MH, Nolta JA (2004) Functional characterization of highly purified human hematopoietic repopulating cells isolated according to aldehyde dehydrogenase activity. Blood 104:1648–1655

Himburg HA, Muramoto GG, Daher P, Meadows SK, Lauren Russell J, Doan P, Chi JT, Salter AB, Lento WE, Reya T, Chao NJ, Chute JP (2010) Pleiotrophin regulates the expansion and regeneration of hematopoietic stem cells. Nat Med 16:475–482

Hu Y, Smyth GK (2009) ELDA: Extreme limiting dilution analysis for comparing depleted and enriched populations in stem cell and other assays. J Immunol Methods 347:70–78

Kent DG, Copley MR, Benz C, Wöhrer S, Dykstra BJ, Ma E, Cheyne J, Zhao Y, Bowie MB, Zhao Y, Gasparetto M, Delaney A, Smith C, Marra M, Eaves CJ (2009) Prospective isolation and molecular characterization of hematopoietic stem cells with durable self-renewal potential. Blood 113:6342–6350

Laughlin MJ, Eapen M, Rubinstein P, Wagner JE, Zhang MJ, Champlin RE, Stevens C, Barker JN, Gale RP, Lazarus HM, Marks DI, van Rood JJ, Scaradavou A, Horowitz MM (2004) Outcomes after transplantation of cord blood or bone marrow from unrelated donors in adults with leukemia. N Engl J Med 351:2265–2275

Liang Y, Van Zant G, Szilvassy SJ (2005) Effects of aging on the homing and engraftment of murine hematopoietic stem and progenitor cells. Blood 106:1479–1487

McDermott SP, Eppert K, Lechman ER, Doedens M, Dick JE (2010) Comparison of human cord blood engraftment between immunocompromised mouse strains. Blood 116:193–200

Morita Y, Ema H, Nakauchi H (2010) Heterogeneity and hierarchy within the most primitive hematopoietic stem cell compartment. J Exp Med 207:1173–1182

Muramoto GG, Russell JL, Safi R, Salter AB, Himburg HA, Daher P, Meadows SK, Doan P, Storms RW, Chao NJ, McDonnell DP, Chute JP (2010) Inhibition of aldehyde dehydrogenase expands hematopoietic stem cells with radioprotective capacity. Stem Cells 28:523–534

North TE, Goessling W, Walkley CR, Lengerke C, Kopani KR, Lord AM, Weber GJ, Bowman TV, Jang IH, Grosser T, Fitzgerald GA, Daley GQ, Orkin SH, Zon LI (2007) Prostaglandin E2 regulates vertebrate haematopoietic stem cell homeostasis. Nature 447:1007–1011

Osawa M, Hanada K, Hamada H, Nakauchi H (1996) Long-term lymphohematopoietic reconstitution by a single CD34-low/negative hematopoietic stem cell. Science 273:242–245

Purton LE, Scadden DT (2007) Limiting factors in murine hematopoietic stem cell assays. Cell Stem Cell 1:263–270

Rawat VPS, Arsenib N, Ahmedb F, Mulawb MA, Thoenea S, Heilmeierb B, Sadlond T, D'Andread RJ, Hiddemannb W, Bohlanderb SK, Buske C, Feuring-Buske M (2010) The vent-like homeobox gene *VENTX* promotes human myeloid differentiation and is highly expressed in acute myeloid leukemia. Proc Natl Acad Sci USA 107:16946–16951

Roeder I, Horn K, Sieburg HB, Cho R, Muller-Sieberg C, Loeffler M (2008) Characterization and quantification of clonal heterogeneity among hematopoietic stem cells: A model-based approach. Blood 112:4874–4883

Storms RW, Green PD, Safford KM, Niedzwiecki D, Cogle CR, Colvin OM, Chao NJ, Rice HE, Smith CA (2005) Distinct hematopoietic progenitor compartments are delineated by the expression of aldehyde dehydrogenase and CD34. Blood 106:95–102

Szilvassy SJ, Humphries RK, Lansdorp PM, Eaves AC, Eaves CJ (1990) Quantitative assay for totipotent reconstituting hematopoietic stem cells by a competitive repopulation strategy. Proc Natl Acad Sci USA 87:8736–8740

Taswell C (1981) Limiting dilution assays for the determination of immunocompetent cell frequencies. I. Data analysis. J Immunol 126:1614–1649

Weissman IL, Shizuru JA (2008) The origins of the identification and isolation of hematopoietic stem cells, and their capability to induce donor-specific transplantation tolerance and treat autoimmune diseases. Blood 112:3543–3553

Wilson A, Laurenti E, Oser G, van der Wath RC, Blanco-Bose W, Jaworski M, Offner S, Dunant CF, Eshkind L, Bockamp E, Lió P, Macdonald HR, Trumpp A (2008) Hematopoietic stem cells reversibly switch from dormancy to self-renewal during homeostasis and repair. Cell 135:1118–1129

Yahata T, Ando K, Sato T, Miyatake H, Nakamura Y, Muguruma Y, Kato S, Hotta T (2003) A highly sensitive strategy for SCID-repopulating cell assay by direct injection of primitive human hematopoietic cells into NOD/SCID mice bone marrow. Blood 101:2905–2913

Zon LI (2008) Intrinsic and extrinsic control of haematopoietic stem-cell self-renewal. Nature 453:306–313

Chapter 3

Characteristics of Cord Blood Stem Cells: Role of Substance P (SP) and Calcitonin Gene-Related Peptide (CGRP)

Massoumeh Ebtekar, Somayeh Shahrokhi, and Kamran Alimoghaddam

Abstract Cord blood (CB) stem cell transplantation has developed into a safe, efficient and affordable method in the clinic. However there are yet important issues that need to be resolved to enable the widespread use of this valuable source of stem cells. The most important limitation of CB transplantation is inadequate number of hematopoietic stem/progenitor cells especially for adults. One of the methods for solving this problem is expansion of CB stem cells without losing their engraftment potential. Importantly, improving expansion and expression of cell adhesion molecules would improve CB stem cell transplantation. Several studies have been performed on interactions of various biological mediators with the objective of improving the expansion and homing properties of these cells. Researchers have applied cytokines and growth factors as well as, recently neuropeptides. This review will focus on recent works designed to achieve more effective regimens for CB transplantation by employing neuropeptides.

Keywords Cord blood · Hematopoietic stem cells · Expansion · Neuropeptide · Adhesion molecule expression

M. Ebtekar (✉)
Department of Immunology, Faculty of Medical Sciences,
Tarbiat Modares University, Tehran, Iran
e-mail: ebtekarm@modares.ac.ir

Introduction

Application of cord blood (CB) hematopoietic stem cells (HSC) for transplantation encounters two major challenging issues; low cell count and delayed engraftment (Robinson et al., 2005). To achieve an ideal growth factor cocktail for expansion of CB-HSC, scientists need to focus on designing a growth factor cocktail that mimics the in vivo hematopoetic microenvironment. Thus, inclusion of biological mediators other than cytokines, such as neuropeptides would be valuable. There are few studies that consider the role of mediators other than cytokines in HSC cultures. Previous studies regarding neuropeptides and stem cells interactions focused on bone marrow (BM) stem cells (Rameshwar et al., 1993). However, based on the beneficial features of CB stem cells, researchers have assessed a combination of cytokine and neuropeptide impacts on CB characteristics (Shahrokhi et al., 2010a, b, c).

Several studies on cytokines and neuropeptides point to the importance of obtaining an optimum and efficient cocktail medium for attaining the ideal conditions for transplantation. Some groups have reported the effect of neuropeptides on CB stem cell (Harzenetter et al., 2002). However, until recently there was no direct evidence regarding the effects of SP and CGRP on the proliferative capacity of CB CD34$^+$cells and their adhesion molecule expression. Researchers have reported, the potential effect of these two neuropeptides – as a non hematopoietic growth factor – in addition to a conventional cytokine cocktail to induce expansion (Shahrokhi et al., 2010c) and adhesion molecules expression on CB stem cells (Shahrokhi et al., 2010a). This review will discuss challenges in

CB-HSC transplantation and explain how neuropeptides may be involved in cell expansion and adhesion molecules expression.

Cord Blood Stem Cells

Hematopoietic stem cell transplantation is a modern approach of treating non/malignant haematological disorders. There are three major sources of HSCs, including: BM, peripheral blood (PB) and CB stem cells. Although, both patient and disease characteristics designate selection of HSC sources, the availability of stem cells is a very important limiting criteria. Transplantation of CB-HSC is an alternative and efficient approach, especially for racial and ethnic minorities. Some advantages of CB-HSC include the "off-shelf" HLA matching which is a great advantage of this source of stem cell. Additionally, disparity at one or two loci, cause no significant increase in graft vs host disease (GVHD) (Robinson et al., 2005). So this would beneficial for emergency cases of transplantation or when there is no matched HLA. Furthermore, there is no risk at CB harvesting for either mother or infant. None or rare viral pathogenesis is another asset of CB transplantation.

The major disadvantage of CB stem cell is a delay in hematopoietic reconstitution; neutropenia and thrombocytopenia –as two major observed consequences. Most studies have reported 20–30 days of neutrophil recovery which makes the patient susceptible to infection. Low frequency of cell number is one of the major causes of this phenomenon and most studies have focused in this area. Recently, in comparison to degree of HLA mismatch, the number of infused nucleated cells has been considered as a predictor factor of successful CB transplantation (Gluckman et al., 2005). So, adequate cell dose is more important in cases of urgent transplantation or no match HLA. To date, the most successful CB transplantations have been performed on children.

Noticeably, less maturation of CB-HSC is beneficial for less GVHD reactions, while this matter affects phenotypic and functional characteristics such as adhesion molecule expression which leads to lower homing capacity. Interestingly, reduced adhesion molecule expression might be another explanation for delay in homing and immune reconstitution after CB transplantation. To circumvent delay in immune reconstitution (due to cell dose or immature cell) scientists have investigated different approaches (Denning-Kendall et al., 2003; Robinson et al., 2005), such as expansion of nucleated or enriched HSCs by different growth factors, infusion of multi CB unit, intra BM cell infusion, stromal co-transplantation and dynamic cultivation in bioreactors, or stimulation of cell adhesion molecules expression. Long term cultivation is another approach to optimize HSC expansion, however, altered nature of primary stem cell, decreased expression of cell adhesion molecules and risk of contamination compromise the integrity of this approach. This review will focus on the role of growth factor cocktails and specifically neuropeptides in CB-HSC expansion and cell adhesion molecule expression.

Growth Factor Cocktail for Expansion

Expansion of CB-HSC is an approach to increase cell dose and make CB-HSC applicable for adult transplantation. Furthermore, optimum growth factor cocktail for expansion facilitates gene transduction which is useful for gene therapy applications. Importantly, diverse range of biological mediators such as cytokines, chemokines, and neuropeptides as well as other microenvironment components control hematopoesis. There are many unknown aspects about the interaction of this complex network. However, designing ex vivo experiments based on in vivo interactions will provide shed light on the dimensions involved and this has encouraged scientists to design such research. Therefore formulating an optimum growth factor cocktail is vital for achieving a practical reasonable expansion.

Cytokines are main considered growth factors in expansion protocols of CB-HSCs. However, the priority is how to choose the vital ones that lead to preserve stem cell capacity and reasonable expansion. Various combination and dose of cytokines have been studied in experiments. However, some cytokines have received more attention particularly those with known roles in stem cell expansion. For instance, the synergistic effect of IL3, alongside SCF, FL and TPO, as an indispensable early acting cytokine, and IL6 as "non-specific early acting cytokine" has been clarified (Alimoghaddam et al., 2006). Cytokines such as SCF and IL6 increase the proliferative capacity of HSC subsets while FL and TPO preserve self renewal ability of primitive stem cells (Robinson et al., 2005).

Interestingly, serum free media leads to less maturation of CD34+cells and more increase in colony forming count (CFC). Additionally, serum free media condition is applicable in the clinic and considering this application is important in protocol design. Researchers report that cytokine cocktail containing SCF, FL, TPO (100 ng/ml) and GSCF (10 ng/ml) leads to 52 and 152 fold increases in nucleated CB cells in serum free media. Expansion rate of 13 and 16 fold was observed at day 7 and 10 in CD34+ cells cultivation (Denning-Kendall et al., 2003).

Additionally, it has been reported (Dravid and Rao, 2002) that combination of FL, SCF and TPO results in 5.67 and 7.21 fold increase in absolute number of CD34+ and CD34+CD38−cells, respectively. Also, most experiments reported that cultures expanded for 7 days were better than longer cultivations systems. This is due to insignificant increase of CD34+cells, increased apoptotic cells and stem cell differentiation and loss of HSC potential (Zhai et al., 2004; Shahrokhi et al., 2010c).

Regarding growth factors other than cytokines there is little evidence. Recently it has been reported that nanofiber in combination with growth factors improves expansion (Lu et al., 2010). Additionally, some non-haematopoietic growth factors involved in pathways of mesodermal induction and stroma derived mediators have been reported in CB-HSC expansion (Hutton et al., 2007).

Based on recent findings, scientists have focused on optimization of a growth factor cocktail for CB-HSC that preserves and expands primary stem cell with reasonable expansion fold. However; heterogeneity of CB samples and experimental conditions leads to inconsistency among results and there is no unique growth factor cocktail that is universally applicable. In spite of many efforts in this way, achieving the optimal culture condition for expansion of CB CD34+cell and its practical applications, particularly for adult transplantation, is still the unachievable ambition of most clinicians.

Modulation of Cell Adhesion Molecule Expression

Communication between extracellular matrix components and adhesion molecules regulates stem cell homing. One of the reasons for delayed engraftment of CB-HSCs is considered to be the immaturity of CB-HSCs, and consequently, low expression of certain adhesion molecules. Modulation of adhesion molecules expression on the surface of CB-CD34+cells may be a helpful approach to overcome the delay in CB engraftment. Importantly, adhesion molecules regulate survival, proliferation and differentiation of progenitors cells via interaction with microenvironment components and biological mediators such as cytokines, chemokines and neuropeptides (Verfaillie, 1998).

Homing processes involve a variety of integrin, selectins and chemokines families. Furthermore, mediators derived from the microenvironment regulate expression of adhesion molecules and matrix metalloproteinase. There are controversial reports regarding the expression levels of adhesion molecules on CB stem cells. However, most agree that higher expression of adhesion molecules correlates with shorter engraftment time. Cytokines such as SCF, upregulate adhesion molecule expression (Zheng et al., 2003). There is supportive evidence that cytokine cocktail SCF, FL, TPO and GSF cause three to nine fold increased expression of cell adhesion molecules on CB stem cells (Denning-Kendall et al., 2003). However, there are reports that adhesion molecules expression has not been affected by cytokine culture (Dravid and Rao, 2002). It is likely that various microenvironment mediators and cytokines affect cell adhesion molecule expression.

Interestingly, there is an association between neutrophil synthesis and CXCR4 as well as platelet synthesis with both CD62L and CXCR4 (Liu et al., 2003). So, increased expression of these molecules could shorten engraftment time and consequently decrease thrombocytopenia and neutropenia as two major side effects of CB transplantation. To assess the importance of the level of adhesion molecule expression, transplantation into NOD/SCID mice can be performed. Additionally, the final stage of these experiments should be optimization of adhesion molecule expression for clinical purposes.

Neuropeptides

The nervous system is one of the main control systems of the body. Innervation and release of neurotransmitters regulates biological actions and they have a close interaction with nonnoeuronal cells/mediators. Interestingly release of neurotransmitters and existence of their receptors in non-neuronal cells add another complexity to this network. The classical neurotransmitters in sympathetic and parasympathetic nerves are noradrenalin and acetylcholine, respectively. The other category of neurotransmitters released from nonadrenergic and noncolinergic nerves are neuropeptides. Neuropeptides are mediators of nervous system that are released from nerves found in the central and peripheral nervous system and mediate a range of biological responses (Brain and Cox, 2006).

The sensory nerves that contain and release neuropeptides are primarily unmyelinated sensory C-fibres. In contrast to classical neurotransmitters, they are derived from large precursor proteins. Alternative and differential splicing leads to their specific tissue expression. Neuropeptides are packaged and formed in Golgi, then stored in secretory granules upon their release. Most organs are innervated and these mediators are released in the parenchyma following stimulation. Neuropeptides have a close cross talk with other biological mediators and thereby regulate each other. Hematopoietic involvement of neuropeptides is the focus of this review and will be discussed in detail.

Neuropeptides in Hematopoesis

Apart from cytokines, which are the main growth factor in most experiments, existence of neuropeptides and their receptors on HSC suggest their involvement in hematopoesis. Evidence indicating a bidirectional communication between nervous and immuno hematopoietic systems, through their secreted mediators such as neuropeptides and cytokines is overwhelming. This communication is performed via receptor specific interactions. Some neuropeptide receptors reported on HSCs such as nerve growth factor (NGF), vasoactive intestinal peptide (VIP), somatostatin, neuropeptide Y, substance p (SP), neurokinin 1(which is a receptor for SP) and calcitonin gene-related peptide (CGRP) (Broome and Miyan, 2000).

There is evidence indicating that granulopesis and particularly neutrophil production in BM is under the control of the neuropeptide network and any abrogation in innervation of SP and CGRP can cause serious consequences for blood cell production. Nerve growth factor, SP, neurokinin 1, and CGRP have positive impacts on CFU-GM (Broome and Miyan, 2000). In contrast to direct stimulatory role of CGRP on myeloid progenitor cells, SP shows indirect effects via inducing mediator release from BM stromal cell or modulating the interaction of BM HSC and stromal cells (Harzenetter et al., 2002).

Additionally, there is evidence showing the expression of VIP receptor in CB-derived $CD34^+CD38^-$ cells, and suggesting VIP as growth factor for this subpopulation. The results showed positive stimulatory effect in synergy with FL, SCF and TPO in serum free media, and effective roles on CFU-GM and CFU-Mix colony formations (Kawakami et al., 2004). Although it was reported that VIP display a suppressive effect on colonogenic assay with BM progenitor cells (Rameshwar et al., 2002), this may relate to different behaviour of various sources of $CD34^+$ cells.

Studies indicate that adherent BM cells play a critical role in the hematopoietic effects of SP. Also, a mitogenic effect of SP on fibroblasts and endothelial cells has been reported. Stromal cells such as fibroblasts, endothelial cells, macrophages, reticular cells, and adipocytes interact with stem cells via a complex network of cytokines and neuropeptides. The expression of SP receptor and its production has been identified on macrophage, T and B lymphocyte, $CD34^+$ cells, fibroblasts and endothelial cells. Cooperation of these cells in hematopoesis is dependent on the role of SP. Additionally, stem cell niches and osteoblasts regulate HSC characteristics via their interaction with HSC and mediators such as signalling molecules, extracellular matrix and cell adhesion molecules. The presence of neuropeptide receptors on osteoblast and their role on osteoblastic functions add another level of neuropeptide involvement in hematopoesis process (Lerner, 2002). However, this is yet a novel research area and there are many unknown aspects which require further research and investigation.

Substance P

The Tachykinin family regulates immune-hematopoietic reconstitution. The neuropeptide SP is a member of tachykinin family produced from the preprotachykinin-I gene (PPT-I). The other derived neuropeptide is neurokinin-A (NK-A) which functions are an opposite to SP. Neuropeptide SP is released from sensory nerve endings of C type nerve fibres and widely exists in the central and peripheral nervous system as well as hematopoetic system which is a sign of its non-neural roles. Members of the tachykinin family, particularly SP perform their effects through interactions with G protein-coupled receptors. Three types of SP receptors include neurokinin-1R (NKlR), NK-2R, and NK-3R. Existence of NK-1R has been shown in peripheral nervous system such as immune cells.

Importantly, SP displays proinflammatory characteristics and acts mainly by activation of immune cells and secretion of inflammatory cytokines. The neuro-immumodulatory role of SP has been studied. Neuronal and non neural sources such as stroma cells possess the repertoire of SP and its receptors, which indicate the hematopoetic role of SP. Interestingly, cytokines produced by HSCs and stromal cells stimulate both cell subsets and PPT-1 is expressed following these interactions. Researchers have demonstrated that SP and cytokines regulate synthesis of each other and even their receptors (Greco et al., 2004). In comparison to other neuropeptides, the role of SP in hematopoesis of BM–HSC has been almost identified.

Depending on the interacting receptor and crosstalk between NK-1 and NK-2, SP displays both inhibitory and stimulatory effects on hematopoesis. Noticeably, SP shows a preference in affinity for NK-1 which leads to stimulatory effects of SP on hematopoesis, while studies indicate that a suppression of hematopoesis occurs during NK2 involvement. Additionally, role of microenvironment and the particular ligand that binds NK receptor determines the outcome of the response. For instance, during digestion of SP by endogenous endopeptidase, a small fragment – called SP (1–4) – is generated that binds to NK1 and exerts inhibition on hematopoesis (Bandari et al., 2003). Other works have demonstrated that there is negative feedback between SCF and SP. Following hematopoietic stimulation by SCF, SP degrades to SP (1–4) which is capable of inducing transforming growth factor (TGF)–β and tumor necrosis factor (TNF)–α in BM stroma and inhibit proliferative responses caused by SCF. This indicates a network communication between cytokine and neuropeptide in hematopoesis (Joshi et al., 2001).

Rameshwar has extensively investigated various effect of SP, as an important mediator in neuro-immuno-hematopoetic network, on CD34$^+$ cells of BM. Certain hematopoetic impacts of SP are exerted by growth factors. Stimulation of interleukin-1 (IL-1), IL-3, IL-6 and GM-CSF has been reported in BM mononuclear cells following SP induction. Noticeably, stimulation of SCF and IL-1 in BM stroma can regulate hematopoesis via autoregulation of NK-R and synergy with other cytokines. Interestingly, IL-1 is involved in IL-3, GM-CSF secretion and also SP-mediated activation of T cells (Rameshwar et al., 1993; Greco et al., 2004).

Also, there is evidence shows that SP alone – without exogenous growth factors – can maintain hematopoiesis in vitro. This occurs via induction of IL-3 and GM-CSF (at 10^{-11} M) from the adhesive cells of BM. Therefore, SP neuropeptide displays a distinct role in hematopoesis regulation. The concentration range of 10^{-8} M to 10^{-11} M is optimum for in vitro assays of SP (Rameshwar et al., 1993) and the optimum concentration for SCF and IL1 induction was observed at 10^{-9} M. On the basis of research performed, SP seems to play the role of several cytokines alone, in hematopoiesis.

Interestingly, human CB stem cells express SP and its receptor (Li et al., 2000), supporting the critical role of SP on HSC characteristics. Based on the evidence provided concerning BM-CD34$^+$cells, researchers have assessed the role of SP on expansion and cell adhesion molecules of CB-CD34$^+$cells.

Calcitonin Gene-Related Peptide

CGRP is a 37-amino acid residue neuropeptide of the calcitonin family. There are two isoforms, α and β, which quite have similar biological activities. They are stored and released from C-fibers sensory nerves. Neuropeptide CGRP is synthesised at dorsal root ganglion which posses the cell bodies of capsaicin-sensitive sensory neurons. In the absence of afferent nerve stimulation, CGRP may be released from capsaicin-sensitive sensory nerve terminals. The neuropeptide, CGRP acts as neurotransmitter, vasodilator, and neurotrophic effector. The major physiologic effect of CGRP is vasodilation (Wang et al., 2002).

Importantly, CGRP regulates growth factor production by BM cells. The existence of CGRP containing nerves in lymphoid organs and BM has been reported. In addition to physiologic actions of CGRP, its regulatory role in immunologic and hematopoesis processes have been demonstrated. High affinity receptors of CGRP exist on lymphocytes, macrophages and BM cells. Modulation of adhesion and migration of immune cells as well as haematopoiesis regulation in BM has been demonstrated. Murine studies show that capsaicin dependent denervation leads to decreased cell production especially negative effect on granulomonocytic progenitors. Importantly direct stimulatory role of CGRP was obvious on myeloid progenitors (Broome and Miyan, 2000). Inhibition of T cell proliferation and secretion of IL-2 and IFN-γ in vitro and suppressive effects on antigen-presenting cells has been reported by CGRP (Wang et al., 2002).

Noticeably, the CGRP receptor is expressed on CB CD34+cells and CGRP has a direct stimulatory impact on immature CD34+cells. Increased formation of granulomonocytic colonies is correlated with receptor downregulation in these cells (Harzenetter et al., 2002). Neuropeptide CGRP seems to display both stimulatory and inhibitory behaviour depending on target cells and receptors involved. Taken together, modulated expression of CGRP receptors on HSC and innervation and functional behaviour in BM suggest hematopoetic involvement of CGRP. These preliminary findings demand further investigation on the role of CGRP on CB CD34+cells function and characteristics.

Why SP and CGRP Together?

Neuropeptides SP and CGRP are co-localized at the same C-fiber nerve endings (Fig. 3.1). Similar stimuli cause their release and they display cooperative physiological effects. Neuropeptides SP and CGRP are involved, mainly, in proinflammatory responses, however, occasionally they represent antagonist actions and CGRP shows anti inflammatory properties, in contrast to SP. They play synergistic or antagonistic effects in different conditions together. There is a cross-talk

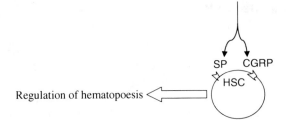

Fig. 3.1 Co release of SP and CGRP

between CGRP and SP function, for instance CGRP induces the increased level of cAMP. This consequently, leads to NK1 receptor mRNA induction and sensitizes target cells to SP (Wu et al., 2007). So, evaluating their actions on specified cell populations, at the same time, could be informative and instrumental in understanding the mechanisms involved. Next sections will discuss role of SP and CGRP individually or combined on CB stem cells characteristics.

SP and CGRP on Expansion

According to scientific evidence provided, recently the authors of this review embarked on a research project to shed light on the role of SP and CGRP on expansion of CB CD34+cells for the first time and thus considered SP and CGRP as growth factors involved. To analyze this hypothesis, total expansion fold of nucleated cells, subsets of primitive CD34+cells such as CD34+CD133+, CD3+CD38− and CED34+CD45dim were evaluated (Shahrokhi et al., 2010c).

Research data showed substantial increase in growth from day 0 to day 11 of total expanded cells. In most neuropeptide-cytokine cocktails at day 7 and 11 maximum expansion was observed in the order of 10^{-9} M > 10^{-11} M > 10^{-7} M of neuropeptides. Synergistic and antagonistic effects of SP+CGRP (SG) were dominant at 10^{-9} M and 10^{-7} M dose on total nucleated cells and immature subsets of CD34+CD38−cells, respectively (Shahrokhi et al., 2010c). These results are in agreement with stimulatory dose of SP on BM-CD34+cells. Interestingly, concentration 10^{-9} M of SP leads to optimal production of SCF and IL1 in BM stroma (Rameshwar et al., 1993). Consequently, induction of the proinflammatory responses such as a NFK-B activation in immune cells has been reported to be maximal in this concentration. It seems that the proliferation of immuo-hematopoetic cells is a consequence of these interactions.

These researchers show a significant two-fold increase in total count of neuropeptide treated vs. untreated expanded cells on 7 days. The ideal scenario would be to achieve a reasonable expansion at short time, since due to less differentiation of HSCs and existence of more primary cells engraftment will be facilitated. Also, these results show that extension of cultivation period has negative impact on expansion and minimizes the distinct proliferative capacity of neuropeptide treated or untreated cells. This occurrence might be due to cell differentiation or neuropeptide receptor desensitization on cell surface following extended culture (Shahrokhi et al., 2010c).

Accordingly, CGRP treated cells lead to 1.5–4 fold expansion of another primitive subpopulation of CB- HSCs, – $CD34^+CD133^+$cells, in comparison to conventional cytokine cocktail at 7 days of culture. This preferential expansion capacity was observed for CGRP, while SP alone didn't represent any significant changes on this subpopulation. Further studies are required to reveal underlying mechanisms and differences in signaling pathways.

Also, authors have investigated the expansion capacity of CD34 CD45dim cells, the results of which show the superior role of SP in this case. Neuropeptide CGRP alone, or in combination with SP did not cause any significant changes (Shahrokhi et al., 2010c) indicating a potential blocking or inhibitory role for CGRP. This finding has been supported by previous experiments which show binding sites for SP on CD34 CD45dim cells.

To determine whether expansion affects the colonogenic capacity of CB stem cells, authors analyzed non/expanded cells with CFU and the results show a preferential induction of myeloid lineage (i.e, CFU-GM, -M, and -G colonies) in CGRP treated cells. Previous reports have shown positive effects for SP (at 10^{-7} M) and CGRP (at 10^{-12} M) on CFU-GM formation in BM and a critical role in granulopoesis (Broome and Miyan, 2000). In agreement to previous reports, this recent data show that SP induces erythroid (CFU-E and BFU E) colony formation. In accordance to total nucleated cell expansion, dose dependency of each colony's type represents distinctive role of these neuropeptides (Shahrokhi et al., 2010c). In agreement to expansion results, antagonistic effects of SG was obvious on 10^{-7} M and individual addition of neuropeptides tends to more mature colony type such as CFU-M, CFU-G. However, individual or combined addition of these neuropeptides leads to existence of more primary cells (CFU-GEM) as well as higher total fold of CFU. Interestingly, short time culture with neuropeptides (7 days) shows positive effects on presence of primary cells with reasonable expansion fold compare to conventional cytokine treated cells (Shahrokhi et al., 2010c).

This research constituted the first report considering SP and CGRP as growth factor for expansion of CB-HSC and their preferential impact in a dose and time dependent manner for CB stem cell expansion. Heterogenicity of CB-HSC makes it difficult to obtain a universal growth factor cocktail and cultivation conditions to achieve an ideal expansion. Based on these preliminary findings, identifying neuropeptide receptors on CB-HSC subsets and signaling pathways involved in expansion would be informative. This implies that, the design of a new generation of growth factor cocktails for expansion of CB stem cells would be achievable.

Role of SP/CGRP on Cell Adhesion Molecule Expression

Based on the evidence showing the role of adhesion molecules in CB $CD34^+$ cells, authors of this review have evaluated the modulation of adhesion molecule expression by neuropeptides SP and/or CGRP. Importantly, $CD34^+CXCR4^+$ cells are critical subpopulation involved in stem cell homing. Noticeably, CXCR4 can activate other homing molecules like integrins, especially, very late antigen 4 (VLA-4) and VLA-5 integrin on human $CD34^+$cells. Consequently, overexpression and activation of homing associate molecules leads to HSC mobilization and engraftment. Previous studies focused on the role of cytokines and other culture conditions and researchers reported for the first time, have reported the effect of SP and CGRP either individually or combined on genomic and protein level of CXCR4 molecule on CB stem cells. In accordance to optimal expansion of neuropeptide treated cells at 7 days culture (Shahrokhi et al., 2010c), flowcytometric results of adhesion molecules show enhanced frequency at this time period. The structural similarity of CXCR4 to SP receptor –transmembrane G protein coupled receptors – may explain increased CXCR4 (Watt and Forde, 2008). Analysis of genomic expression of CXCR4, showed an increased expression at 11 days culture in 10^{-9} M of SP and CGRP treatment. However, no changes occurred at protein levels. This discrepancy might be due to short half life of CXCR4 mRNA or inefficient transition from mRNA to protein (Shahrokhi et al., 2010d).

Overexpression of CXCR4 protein leads to extensive proliferation and migration of $CD34^+CXCR4^+$-cells to its ligand – SDF1 – and consequently enhances Tac-1 (SP producer gene) expression. Then, SP causes hematopoetic stimulation via its interaction with its stimulatory receptor NK1. Since G protein-coupled receptors, such as neuropeptide and chemokine receptors have critical role in a variety of biological processes, they act for a brief period and are quickly down regulated. Findings of certain studies show that SP enhances GM-CSF and HSC mobilization (Corcoran et al., 2007). Also, antagonists to SDF and SP such as dipeptidylpeptidase IV/CD26 and MMP-2/9 increase CXCR4 expression and HSCs mobilization (Watt and Forde, 2008). There is no direct report for CGRP actions however, the authors findings support the stimulatory role of CGRP – alone or in combination to SP – on protein expression of CXCR4 (Shahrokhi et al., 2010d). To understand the basic mechanisms underlying these processes and the consequent in vivo responses more research on involved signaling and biochemical pathways are required.

In this research, the expression of CD49e and CD44 was analyzed on $CD34^+$ cells. The percentage of $CD34^+CD44^+/CD49e^+$ cells in neuropeptide–cytokine treated cells was more than cytokine treated cells in short time culture and they exhibited a resistance to percentage decline. Concentration of 10^{-11} M SP alone or in combination to CGRP represents dose responsiveness and synergistic effects on $CD34^+$ $CD49e^+$ cells. Flowcytometric analysis of another homing associated subpopulation, $CD34^+$ $CD62L^+$ cells, show a resistance to frequency among SG-treated cells (at 10^{-9} M and 10^{-11} M) compared with control group in 7 days culture. However existence of low and high frequency of $CD34^+$ $CD62L^+$ cells in CB samples caused high variation and consequently insignificant changes (Shahrokhi et al., 2010a).

Noticeably, there are interactions between SP and cytokines concerning adhesion molecule expression. Evidence indicates that SP reduces matrix metalloproteinase MMP activity (Cohen et al., 2007) while cytokines such as SCF (Zheng et al., 2003) play a stimulatory role. Therefore, this might be considered as the mechanism responsible for resistance to frequency decline in neuropeptide treated cells. Even though there is no direct mechanism for CGRP, however, their physiological collocation and cooperative effects observed in research findings suggest CGRP involvement.

In accordance to previous reports, extension of incubation time shows negative effects on adhesion molecule expression. Interestingly, there was a reverse correlation between percentage of adhesion molecule and mean fluorescence intensity (MFI) of studied adhesion molecules, which seems to act as a compensating mechanism. Conclusively, these data provide the first evidence of modulatory actions of neuropeptide SP and CGRP on expression of adhesion molecules on CB $CD34^+$ cells (Shahrokhi et al., 2010a, d). Although, the neurological role of these neuropeptides is the focus of most experiments, however, other biological actions such as regulation of adhesion molecules expression would be a new area which demands more investigation to clarify underlying mechanisms. This work and other research in this line serves as a novel step towards that goal. Additional specific characterization and functional experiments in the future will shed light on the ambiguous aspects of these interactions.

Clinical Importance of Optimum Growth Factor Cocktail

The most important limitation for successful CB transplantation (especially in an adult patient) is cell dose. Usually more than 2.5×10^7 total nucleated cell /kg weight of recipient are necessary to have a good engraftment. This goal is not achievable for most of adults with current CB in CB banks. Despite of success in laboratory research and expansion of CB stem/progenitor cells, there is a long way ahead in the clinical application of these expanded cells in patients. There are many concerns for clinical application of these ex-vivo expanded CB cells.

The first concern is the safety of CB, possible risk of contamination when these cells remain outside of body for a long time. Although this concern would be solved by meticulous attention to culture environment and applying strict standards (Patah et al., 2007). Another concern is loss of stemness during ex-vivo manipulation of cells. It seems that ex vivo expansion can multiply short term repopulating cells instead of long term repopulating cells (Mcniece et al., 2002). Advantage of this expansion is that it provides a source for rapid engraftment of hematopoietic cells after transplantation and reducing rate of complication of delayed engraftment (that usually CB transplanted patients expose) but it may be increase late graft failure risk (Williams, 1993).

One of the methods to preserve long term and short term repopulating cells in graft is to expand a part of the CB and transplant another part un-manipulated. Another issue in CB expansion is timing of transplantation. Most of CB expansion protocols need at least two weeks in culture and timing of these procedures with transplantation time is not easy (especially if we consider the possibility that the expansion procedure my fail and expose patients to the risk of losing the possibility of successful transplantation). So choosing the optimum growth factor cocktail and applying it at right time with standard and supervised procedures has paramount importance for successful transplantation.

Conclusions and Future Perspectives

The various neuropeptide receptors expressed on CB-HSC implicate their hematological involvement although there are few studies to determine their role. This review appraised the potential role of SP and CGRP as novel growth factors for the expansion and modulation of cell adhesion molecules on CB CD34$^+$ cells. Recent research indicates that expansion and modulating the expression of adhesion molecules on HSCs could enhance the homing process and thereby help to overcome difficulties regarding CB stem cell transplantation. This field deserves more attention from both clinicians and researchers who hope to develop more effective methods for efficient transplantation. Further research on the role of neuropeptides and the interrelationship between stem cells and the neuro-immune network may prove to shed light on unrevealed dimensions in this emerging field.

References

Alimoghaddam K, Khalili M, Soleimani M, Moezi L, Ghodsi P, Arjmand A, Ghavamzadeh A (2006) Evaluation of the effects of MIP1-α on ex vitro expansion of hematopoietic progenitor cells in different culture media for the purpose of cord blood transplantation. Molecular Therapy 13(S1):S138–S

Bandari PS, Qian J, Oh HS, Potian JA, Yehia G, Harrison JS, Rameshwar P (2003) Crosstalk between neurokinin receptors is relevant to hematopoietic regulation: cloning and characterization of neurokinin-2 promoter. J Neuroimmunol 138:65–75

Brain SD, Cox HM (2006) Neuropeptides and their receptors: innovative science providing novel therapeutic targets. Br J Pharmacol 147(Suppl 1):S202–S211

Broome CS, Miyan JA (2000) Neuropeptide control of bone marrow neutrophil production. A key axis for neuroimmunomodulation. Ann N Y Acad Sci 917:424–434

Cohen PA, Gower AC, Stucchi AF, Leeman SE, Becker JM, Reed KL (2007) A neurokinin-1 receptor antagonist that reduces intraabdominal adhesion formation increases peritoneal matrix metalloproteinase activity. Wound Repair Regen 15:800–808

Corcoran KE, Patel N, Rameshwar P (2007) Stromal derived growth factor-1 alpha: another mediator in neural-emerging immune system through Tac1 expression in bone marrow stromal cells. J Immunol 178:2075–2082

Denning-Kendall P, Singha S, Bradley B, Hows J (2003) Cytokine expansion culture of cord blood CD34+ cells induces marked and sustained changes in adhesion receptor and CXCR4 expressions. Stem Cells 21:61–70

Dravid G, Rao SG (2002) Ex vivo expansion of stem cells from umbilical cord blood: expression of cell adhesion molecules. Stem Cells 20:183–189

Gluckman E, Koegler G, Rocha V (2005) Human leukocyte antigen matching in cord blood transplantation. Semin Hematol 42:85–90

Greco SJ, Corcoran KE, Cho KJ, Rameshwar P (2004) Tachykinins in the emerging immune system: relevance to bone marrow homeostasis and maintenance of hematopoietic stem cells. Front Biosci 9:1782–1793

Harzenetter MD, Keller U, Beer S, Riedl C, Peschel C, Holzmann B (2002) Regulation and function of the CGRP receptor complex in human granulopoiesis. Exp Hematol 30:306–312

Hutton JF, D'andrea RJ, Lewis ID (2007) Potential for clinical ex vivo expansion of cord blood haemopoietic stem cells using non-haemopoietic factor supplements. Curr Stem Cell Res Ther 2:229–237

Joshi DD, Dang A, Yadav P, Qian J, Bandari PS, Chen K, Donnelly R, Castro T, Gascon P, Haider A, Rameshwar P (2001) Negative feedback on the effects of stem cell factor on hematopoiesis is partly mediated through neutral endopeptidase activity on substance P: a combined functional and proteomic study. Blood 98:2697–2706

Kawakami M, Kimura T, Kishimoto Y, Tatekawa T, Baba Y, Nishizaki T, Matsuzaki N, Taniguchi Y, Yoshihara S, Ikegame K, Shirakata T, Nishida S, Masuda T, Hosen N, Tsuboi A, Oji Y, Oka Y, Ogawa H, Sonoda Y, Sugiyama H, Kawase I, Soma T (2004) Preferential expression of the vasoactive intestinal peptide (VIP) receptor VPAC1 in human cord blood-derived CD34+CD38- cells: possible role of VIP as a growth-promoting factor for hematopoietic stem/progenitor cells. Leukemia 18:912–921

Lerner UH (2002) Neuropeptidergic regulation of bone resorption and bone formation. J Musculoskelet Neuronal Interact 2:440–447

Li Y, Douglas SD, Ho W (2000) Human stem cells express substance P gene and its receptor. J Hematother Stem Cell Res 9:445–452

Liu B, Liao C, Chen J, Gu S, Wu S, Xu Z (2003) Significance of increasing adhesion of cord blood hematopoietic cells and a new method: platelet microparticles. Am J Hematol 74:216–217

Lu J, Aggarwal R, Pompili VJ, Das H (2010) A novel technology for hematopoietic stem cell expansion using combination of nanofiber and growth factors. Recent Pat Nanotechnol 4:125–135

Mcniece IK, Almeida-Porada G, Shpall EJ, Zanjani E (2002) Ex vivo expanded cord blood cells provide rapid engraftment in fetal sheep but lack long-term engrafting potential. Exp Hematol 30:612–616

Patah PA, Parmar S, Mcmannis J, Sadeghi T, Karandish S, Rondon G, Tarrand J, Champlin R, De Lima M, Shpall EJ (2007) Microbial contamination of hematopoietic progenitor cell products: clinical outcome. Bone Marrow Transplant 40:365–368

Rameshwar P, Ganea D, Gascon P (1993) In vitro stimulatory effect of substance P on hematopoiesis. Blood 81:391–398

Rameshwar P, Gascon P, Oh HS, Denny TN, Zhu G, Ganea D (2002) Vasoactive intestinal peptide (VIP) inhibits the proliferation of bone marrow progenitors through the VPAC1 receptor. Exp Hematol 30:1001–1009

Robinson S, Niu T, De Lima M, Ng J, Yang H, Mcmannis J, Karandish S, Sadeghi T, Fu P, Del Angel M, O'connor S, Champlin R, Shpall E (2005) Ex vivo expansion of umbilical cord blood. Cytotherapy 7:243–250

Shahrokhi S, Alimoghaddam K, Ebtekar M, Pourfathollah AA, Kheirandish M, Ardjmand A, Ghavamzadeh A (2010a) Effects of neuropeptide substance P on the expression of adhesion molecules in cord blood hematopoietic stem cells. Ann Hematol 89:1197–1205

Shahrokhi S, Alimoghaddam K, Ghavamzadeh A (2010b) Role of substance P (SP) and calcitonin gene-related peptide (CGRP) in gibbon-ape-leukemia virus (GALV) transduction of CD34+ cells. Neuropeptides 44:491–494

Shahrokhi S, Ebtekar M, Alimoghaddam K, Pourfathollah AA, Kheirandish M, Ardjmand A, Shamshiri AR, Ghavamzadeh A (2010c) Substance P and calcitonin gene-related neuropeptides as novel growth factors for ex vivo expansion of cord blood CD34(+) hematopoietic stem cells. Growth Factors 28:66–73

Shahrokhi S, Ebtekar M, Alimoghaddam K, Sharifi Z, Ghaffari SH, Pourfathollah AA, Kheirandish M, Mohseni M, Ghavamzadeh A (2010d) Communication of substance P, calcitonin-gene-related neuropeptides and chemokine receptor 4 (CXCR4) in cord blood hematopoietic stem cells. Neuropeptides 44:385–389

Verfaillie CM (1998) Adhesion receptors as regulators of the hematopoietic process. Blood 92:2609–2612

Wang H, Xing L, Li W, Hou L, Guo J, Wang X (2002) Production and secretion of calcitonin gene-related peptide from human lymphocytes. J Neuroimmunol 130:155–162

Watt SM, Forde SP (2008) The central role of the chemokine receptor, CXCR4, in haemopoietic stem cell transplantation: will CXCR4 antagonists contribute to the treatment of blood disorders? Vox Sang 94:18–32

Williams DA (1993) Ex vivo expansion of hematopoietic stem and progenitor cells—Robbing Peter to pay Paul? Blood 81:3169–3172

Wu H, Guan C, Qin X, Xiang Y, Qi M, Luo Z, Zhang C (2007) Upregulation of substance P receptor expression by calcitonin gene-related peptide, a possible cooperative action of two neuropeptides involved in airway inflammation. Pulm Pharmacol Ther 20:513–524

Zhai QL, Qiu LG, Li Q, Meng HX, Han JL, Herzig RH, Han ZC (2004) Short-term ex vivo expansion sustains the homing-related properties of umbilical cord blood hematopoietic stem and progenitor cells. Haematologica 89:265–273

Zheng Y, Watanabe N, Nagamura-Inoue T, Igura K, Nagayama H, Tojo A, Tanosaki R, Takaue Y, Okamoto S, Takahashi TA (2003) Ex vivo manipulation of umbilical cord blood-derived hematopoietic stem/progenitor cells with recombinant human stem cell factor can up-regulate levels of homing-essential molecules to increase their transmigratory potential. Exp Hematol 31:1237–1246

Chapter 4

A New Concept of Stem Cell Disorders, and the Rationale for Transplantation of Normal Stem Cells

Susumu Ikehara

Abstract There are at least two types of stem cells in the bone marrow of mice and humans: hemopoietic stem cells (HSCs) and mesenchymal stem cells (MSCs). As all cells in the body are differentiated from HSCs or MSCs, it is conceivable that all diseases originate from disorders in these cells. We here provide evidence that most diseases are, in fact, stem cell disorders, and that a newly developed method of bone marrow transplantation (BMT) can be used to prevent and treat most intractable diseases, since it permits the recipient's abnormal HSCs and MSCs to be replaced with the donor's normal HSCs and MSCs.

Keywords Hemopoietic stem cells · Mesenchymal stem cells · Bone marrow transplantation · Major histocompatibility complex · Aspiration method · Perfusion method

Introduction

Various mouse strains that spontaneously develop autoimmune diseases have contributed not only to a better understanding of the fundamental nature of autoimmune diseases but also to the analysis of their etiopathogenesis. In 1985, we found that allogeneic (but not syngeneic or autologous) bone marrow transplantation (BMT) could be used to treat autoimmune diseases in autoimmune-prone mice (Ikehara et al.,

S. Ikehara (✉)
First Department of Pathology, Kansai Medical University, Moriguchi City, Osaka 570-8506, Japan
e-mail: ikehara@takii.kmu.ac.jp

1985a, b). Since then, using various autoimmune-prone mice, we have confirmed that allogeneic BMT can indeed be used to treat autoimmune diseases (Oyaizu et al., 1988; Than et al., 1992; Nishimura et al., 1994). Conversely, we have succeeded in inducing autoimmune diseases in normal mice by the transplantation of T cell-depleted bone marrow cells (BMCs) or partially purified hemopoietic stem cells (HSCs) from autoimmune-prone mice (Ikehara et al., 1990; Kawamura et al., 1997). Based on these findings, we have proposed that autoimmune diseases are "stem cell disorders (SCDs)" (Ikehara et al., 1990; Kawamura et al., 1997; Ikehara, 2003).

Our findings were also confirmed in humans: patients with autoimmune diseases were cured after allogeneic BMT, while autoimmune diseases were transferred to recipients after BMT from donors who were suffering from autoimmune diseases (Marmont, 1994).

In this article, we show that various otherwise intractable diseases (including SCDs) can be cured by our novel BMT method (intra-bone marrow [IBM]-BMT).

Qualitative Differences Between Normal and Abnormal HSCs

We first examined whether there were any qualitative differences between normal and abnormal HSCs. We carried out BMT between normal and autoimmune-prone mice using partially purified HSCs. The transplantation of partial purified abnormal HSCs obtained from autoimmune-prone mice induced autoimmune diseases in normal mice, as did the transplantation of whole BMCs. However, the transplantation of partial purified normal HSCs could not reconstruct hemopoiesis in autoimmune-prone mice, due to graft rejection (Kawamura et al., 1997), although the transplantation of T cell-depleted BMCs from normal mice could be used to prevent and treat autoimmune diseases in autoimmune-prone mice (Ikehara et al., 1985a, b, 1989). This finding suggests that abnormal HSCs are more resilient than normal HSCs; the former can proliferate in major histocompatibility complex (MHC)-mismatched microenvironments, while the latter cannot. This was also confirmed in in vitro experiments. Abnormal HSCs can proliferate in collaboration with MHC-incompatible MSCs, although normal HSCs can do so only in collaboration with MHC-compatible (not MHC-incompatible) MSCs.

MHC Restriction Between HSCs and MSCs

We have thus found that donor-derived MSCs play a crucial role in successful BMT across MHC barriers. This finding prompted us to examine whether there is an MHC restriction between HSCs and MSCs. Hemopoiesis was observed only in the bone marrow (BM) engrafted with the BALB/c bone when BALB/c BMCs (T cell-depleted and adherent cell-depleted BMCs) were i.v. injected into irradiated C3H/HeN mice that had been engrafted with bones of C3H/HeN, B6 and BALB/c mice or with a teflon tube as a control. This finding strongly suggests that an MHC restriction exists between HSCs and MSCs in vivo. This was confirmed in in vitro experiments; when B10 (H-2^b) HSCs were cocultured with B10 MSCs, the HSCs proliferated, whereas, when B10 HSCs were cocultured with B10D2 (H-2^d) MSCs, the HSCs showed poor proliferative responses (Ikehara, 1998).

Strategies for Recruitment of Donor MSCs

Using radiosensitive and chimeric-resistant MRL/lpr mice, we have found that the recruitment of donor MSCs is essential for successful allogeneic BMT (Kushida et al., 2000). We have found that the following three methods are effective in replacing recipient MSCs with donor-derived MSCs: (1) conventional intravenous BMT (IV-BMT) plus bone graft (Ishida et al., 1994); (2) BMT from the portal vein (PV-BMT) because tolerance can be easily induced in the liver (Kushida et al., 2000); and finally (3) IBM-BMT (Kushida et al., 2001): IBM-BMT was found to be the most effective approach, since IBM-BMT allows both HSCs and MSCs to be recruited, thereby preventing the risk of graft rejection and allowing us to use a mild conditioning regimen (5Gyx2). We therefore used IBM-BMT instead of the conventional IV-BMT in subsequent experiments.

IBM-BMT for Organ Transplantation

We previously found that the combination of organ allografts and conventional IV-BMT from the same donors prevented the rejection of organ allografts (Nakamura et al., 1986), so we attempted to apply IBM-BMT to organ allografts. IBM-BMT was the most effective strategy, since the radiation dose could be reduced to 4 Gy × 2 in skin allografts (Nakamura et al., 1986; Ikehara, 2008). In addition, we have found that IBM-BMT is applicable to allografts of other organs and tissues in rats, such as pancreas islets legs, lungs, and heart (Esumi et al., 2003; Kaneda et al., 2005; Ikebukuro et al., 2006; Guo et al., 2008).

IBM-BMT for Regeneration Therapy

As it was apparent that donor MSCs could be effectively recruited by "IBM-BMT", we next attempted to treat osteoporosis in SAMP6 mice; the SAMP6 mouse (a substrain of senescence-accelerated mice) spontaneously develops osteoporosis early in life and is therefore a useful model for examining the mechanisms underlying osteoporosis. After IBM-BMT, the hematolymphoid system was completely reconstituted with donor-type cells. Thus-treated SAMP6 mice (8 months after IBM-BMT) showed marked increases in trabecular bone even at 20 months of age, and the bone mineral density (BMD) remained similar to that of normal B6 mice. BM MSCs in "IBM-BMT"-treated SAMP6 mice were replaced with donor MSCs (Ichioka et al., 2002; Takada et al., 2006). We thus succeeded in curing osteoporosis in SAMP6 mice by IBM-BMT, which can recruit both HSCs and MSCs from the donor.

Since IBM-BMT appeared to be a powerful strategy in regeneration therapy, we next used tight-skin (Tsk) mice (an animal model for emphysema) to examine whether emphysema could be cured by IBM-BMT. IBM-BMT was carried out from C3H (H-2^k) mice into Tsk (H-2^b) mice (8–10 weeks old) that had already shown emphysema. Eight months after the transplantation, the lungs of all the Tsk mice treated with IBM-BMT [C3H→Tsk] showed structures similar to those of normal mice, whereas the [Tsk→Tsk] mice showed emphysema, as seen in age-matched Tsk mice. Next, we attempted to transfer emphysema from Tsk mice to C3H mice by IBM-BMT. Six months after IBM-BMT, the [Tsk→C3H] mice showed emphysema (Adachi et al., 2006). These results strongly suggested that emphysema in Tsk mice originates from defects in the stem cells (probably MSCs and/or HSCs) in the BM.

IBM-BMT + Donor Lymphocyte Infusion (DLI) for Treatment of Malignant Tumors

It is well known that the graft-versus-leukemia reaction (GvLR) can cure patients of a variety of hematological malignancies (Thomas and Blume, 1999). Recently, it has been reported that graft-versus-tumor (GvT) effects can induce partial (complete in some) remission of metastatic solid tumors such as breast cancer (Ueno et al., 1998) and renal cell carcinoma (Childs et al., 2000; Appelbaum and Sandmaier, 2002; Bregni et al., 2002). Based on these findings, donor lymphocyte infusion (DLI) has recently been used for the treatment of malignant solid tumors even in humans. However, it is very difficult to completely eradicate the tumors, since extensive DLI induces graft-versus-host disease (GvHD). We therefore attempted to establish a new method for the treatment of malignant tumors, this method consisting of IBM-BMT plus DLI, since we have recently found that IBM-BMT can allow a reduction in radiation doses as a conditioning regimen and prevent GvHD (Kushida et al., 2001). Using the Meth-A cell line (BALB/c-derived fibrosarcoma), we found that IBM-BMT plus the injection of $CD4^+$ T-cell-depleted C57BL/6 spleen cells (as DLI) can prevent GvHD while suppressing tumor growth (Suzuki et al., 2005). In addition, we have found that IBM-BMT plus extensive DLI (3 times every 2 weeks) can lead to the complete rejection of the tumor, although the success rate (3/50) has so far not been very high (Suzuki et al., 2005). In addition, we have examined whether this strategy (IBM-BMT plus DLI) could be applicable to other tumors in other animals: We have obtained similar results in another system (colon cancer: ACL-15 in rats) (Koike et al., 2007). We are now establishing more efficient strategies to eradicate malignant tumors.

Novel BMT (PM+IBM-BMT) Is Superior to Conventional BMT

Conventional BMT is carried out as follows: BM needles are inserted into the iliac bones more than 100 times, and the BMCs are collected by the aspiration method (AM). Therefore, contamination with peripheral blood (particularly T cells) is inevitable. When cells collected in this manner are intravenously injected (IV-BMT), most become trapped in the lung and only a few migrate into the BM.

To apply our new BMT methods to humans, we established, using cynomolgus monkeys, a perfusion method (PM), which minimizes the contamination of BMCs with T cells. Two needles are inserted into a iliac bone or a long bone such as the humerus, femur, or tibia. The end of the extension tube is connected to a needle. The other end is placed in a syringe containing 0.5 ml heparin. The other needle is connected to a syringe containing 30 ml of saline, and the saline is then pushed gently from the syringe into the medullary cavity to flush out the BM. The saline containing the BM fluid is then collected.

There is significantly less contamination with T cells when using the PM (<10%) than with the conventional AM (>20%) (Kushida et al., 2002; Inaba et al., 2007). Therefore, T cell-depletion is unnecessary with the PM, and whole BMCs can be used. However, in the case of the conventional AM, T cell-depletion is necessary, and the loss of some important cells such as MSCs during the process of T cell-depletion is inevitable. Furthermore, the number and progenitor activities of the cells harvested using the PM are greater than when using the conventional AM (Kushida et al., 2002; Inaba et al., 2007).

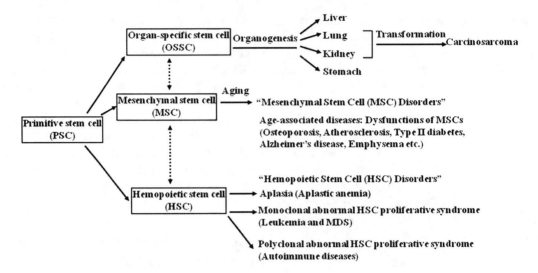

Fig. 4.1 A novel concept of stem cell disorders

We have also found that the PM is applicable to the iliac bones as well as the long bones not only in monkeys but also in humans.

A New Concept of Stem Cell Disorders and Future Directions

Finally, I would like to present a new concept of SCDs after a minor modification of my previous proposal (Ikehara, 2003, 2008). As shown in Fig. 4.1, various types of stem cells exist. In the BM, HSCs, MSCs, and organ-specific stem cells (OSSCs) should be differentiated from embryonic stem (ES)-like cells. We have recently found that ES-like cells are present in the BM of even human adults (Petrini et al., 2009). HSC disorders are recognized as falling into the following categories: (1) aplasia of HSCs (aplastic anemia), (2) monoclonal or oligoclonal abnormal HSC proliferative syndromes (leukemias and myelodysplastic syndrome), and (3) polyclonal abnormal HSC proliferative syndromes (autoimmune diseases) (Ikehara, 2003).

On the other hand, there are MSC disorders, which include age-associated diseases, such as osteoporosis (Ueda et al., 2007) and emphysema (Adachi et al., 2006). It has also been proposed that autoimmune mechanisms are involved in the development of atherosclerosis (Fernandes et al., 1983; Ikehara, 2003; Rose and Afanasyeva, 2003) and Alzheimer's disease (Baron et al., 2007). Recently, the existence of OSSCs or tissue-committed stem cells has been proposed (Ikehara, 2003; Ratajczak et al., 2004), and we would also like to propose that carcinosarcoma (in the liver, lung, and kidney) is a result of the malignant transformation of OSSCs. From the findings to date, it is conceivable that all the body's cells originate in the BM, and that all diseases might therefore originate from BM-derived cells (Houghton et al., 2004). Because most intractable diseases are not only HSC disorders but also MSC disorders, we believe that the use of our new BMT method (PM+IBM-BMT), which can efficiently collect both HSCs and MSCs and transplant both, will become a valuable strategy for the treatment of various intractable diseases. In conclusion, this discovery is, in many respects, an "Egg of Columbus;" the combination of PM+IBM-BMT is a simple solution that seems obvious in retrospect. It is also a solution that heralds a revolution in the field of transplantation (BMT and organ transplantation) and regeneration therapy.

References

Adachi Y, Oyaizu H, Taketani S, Minamino K, Yamaguchi K, Shultz LD, Iwasaki M, Tomita M, Suzuki Y, Nakano K, Koike Y, Yasumizu R, Sata M, Hirama N, Kubota I, Fukuhara S, Ikehara S (2006) Treatment and transfer of emphysema by a new bone marrow transplantation method from normal mice to Tsk mice and vice versa. Stem Cells 24:2071–2077

Appelbaum FR, Sandmaier B (2002) Sensitivity of renal cell cancer to nonmyeloablative allogeneic hematopoietic cell transplantations: unusual or unusually important? J ClinOncol 20:1965–1967

Baron R, Harpaz I, Nemirovsky A, Cohen H, Monsonego A (2007) Immunity and neuronal repair in the progression of Alzheimer's disease: a brief overview. Exp Gerontol 42: 64–69

Bregni M, Dodero A, Peccatori J, Pescarollo A, Bernardi M, Sassi I, Voena C, Zaniboni A, Bordignon C, Corradini P (2002) Nonmyeloablative conditioning followed by hematopoietic cell allografting and donor lymphocyte infusions for patients with metastatic renal and breast cancer. Blood 99:4234–4236

Childs R, Chernoff A, Contentin N, Bahceci E, Schrump D, Leitman S, Read EJ, Tisdale J, Dunbar C, Linehan WM, Young NS, Barrett AJ (2000) Regression of metastatic renal-cell carcinoma after nonmyeloablative allogeneic peripheral-blood stem-cell transplantation. N Engl J Med 343:750–758

Esumi T, Inaba M, Ichioka N, Kushida T, Iida H, Ikehara S (2003) Successful allogeneic leg transplantation in rats in conjunction with intra-bone marrow injection of donor bone marrow cells. Transplantation 76:1543–1548

Fernandes G, Alonso DR, Tanaka T, Thaler HT, Yunis EJ, Good RA (1983) Influence of diet on vascular lesions in autoimmune-prone B/W mice. Proc Natl Acad Sci USA 80:874–877

Guo K, Inaba M, Li M, An J, Cui W, Song C, Wang J, Cui Y, Sakaguchi Y, Tsuda M, Omae M, Ando Y, Li Q, Wang X, Feng W, Ikehara S (2008) Long-term donor-specific tolerance in rat cardiac allografts by intrabone marrow injection of donor bone marrow cells. Transplantation 85:93–101

Houghton J, Stoicov C, Nomura S, Rogers AB, Carlson J, Li H, Cai X, Fox JG, Goldenring JR, Wang TC (2004) Gastric cancer originating from bone marrow-derived cells. Science 306:1568–1571

Ichioka N, Inaba M, Kushida T, Esumi T, Takahara K, Inaba K, Ogawa R, Iida H, Ikehara S (2002) Prevention of senile osteoporosis in SAMP6 mice by intrabone marrow injection of allogeneic bone marrow cells. Stem Cells 20:542–551

Ikebukuro K, Adachi Y, Suzuki Y, Iwasaki M, Nakano K, Koike Y, Mukaide H, Yamada Y, Fujimoto S, Seino Y, Oyaizu H, Shigematsu A, Kiriyama N, Hamada Y, Kamiyama Y, Ikehara S (2006) Synergistic effects of injection of bone marrow cells into both portal vein and bone marrow on tolerance induction in transplantation of allogeneic pancreatic islets. Bone Marrow Transplant 38:657–664

Ikehara S (1998) Autoimmune diseases as stem cell disorders: normal stem cell transplant for their treatment (review). Int J Mol Med 1:5–16

Ikehara S (2003) A new concept of stem cell disorders and their new therapy. J Hematother Stem Cell Res 12:643–653

Ikehara S (2008) A novel method of bone marrow transplantation (BMT) for intractable autoimmune diseases. J Autoimmun 30:108–115

Ikehara S, Good RA, Nakamura T, Sekita K, Inoue S, Oo MM, Muso E, Ogawa K, Hamashima Y (1985a) Rationale for bone marrow transplantation in the treatment of autoimmune diseases. Proc Natl Acad Sci USA 82:2483–2487

Ikehara S, Ohtsuki H, Good RA, Asamoto H, Nakamura T, Sekita K, Muso E, Tochino Y, Ida T, Kuzuya H et al (1985b) Prevention of type I diabetes in nonobese diabetic mice by allogenic bone marrow transplantation. Proc Natl Acad Sci USA 82:7743–7747

Ikehara S, Yasumizu R, Inaba M, Izui S, Hayakawa K, Sekita K, Toki J, Sugiura K, Iwai H, Nakamura T et al (1989) Long-term observations of autoimmune-prone mice treated for autoimmune disease by allogeneic bone marrow transplantation. Proc Natl Acad Sci USA 86:3306–3310

Ikehara S, Kawamura M, Takao F, Inaba M, Yasumizu R, Than S, Hisha H, Sugiura K, Koide Y, Yoshida TO et al (1990) Organ-specific and systemic autoimmune diseases originate from defects in hematopoietic stem cells. Proc Natl Acad Sci USA 87:8341–8344

Inaba M, Adachi Y, Hisha H, Hosaka N, Maki M, Ueda Y, Koike Y, Miyake T, Fukui J, Cui Y, Mukaide H, Koike N, Omae M, Mizokami T, Shigematsu A, Sakaguchi Y, Tsuda M, Okazaki S, Wang X, Li Q, Nishida A, Ando Y, Guo K, Song C, Cui W, Feng W, Katou J, Sado K, Nakamura S, Ikehara S (2007) Extensive studies on perfusion method plus intra-bone marrow–bone marrow transplantation using cynomolgus monkeys. Stem Cells 25:2098–2103

Ishida T, Inaba M, Hisha H, Sugiura K, Adachi Y, Nagata N, Ogawa R, Good RA, Ikehara S (1994) Requirement of donor-derived stromal cells in the bone marrow for successful allogeneic bone marrow transplantation. Complete prevention of recurrence of autoimmune diseases in MRL/MP-lpr/lpr mice by transplantation of bone marrow plus bones (stromal cells) from the same donor. J Immunol 152:3119–3127

Kaneda H, Adachi Y, Saito Y, Ikebukuro K, Machida H, Suzuki Y, Minamino K, Zhang Y, Iwasaki M, Nakano K, Koike Y, Wang J, Imamura H, Ikehara S (2005) Long-term observation after simultaneous lung and intra-bone marrow–bone marrow transplantation. J Heart Lung Transplant 24: 1415–1423

Kawamura M, Hisha H, Li Y, Fukuhara S, Ikehara S (1997) Distinct qualitative differences between normal and abnormal hemopoietic stem cells in vivo and in vitro. Stem Cells 15:56–62

Koike Y, Adachi Y, Suzuki Y, Iwasaki M, Koike-Kiriyama N, Minamino K, Nakano K, Mukaide H, Shigematsu A, Kiyozuka Y, Tubura A, Kamiyama Y, Ikehara S (2007) Allogeneic intrabone marrow–bone marrow transplantation plus donor lymphocyte infusion suppresses growth of colon cancer cells implanted in skin and liver of rats. Stem Cells 25:385–391

Kushida T, Inaba M, Takeuchi K, Sugiura K, Ogawa R, Ikehara S (2000) Treatment of intractable autoimmune diseases in MRL/lpr mice using a new strategy for allogeneic bone marrow transplantation. Blood 95:1862–1868

Kushida T, Inaba M, Hisha H, Ichioka N, Esumi T, Ogawa R, Iida H, Ikehara S (2001) Intra-bone marrow injection of allogeneic bone marrow cells: a powerful new strategy for treatment of intractable autoimmune diseases in MRL/lpr mice. Blood 97:3292–3299

Kushida T, Inaba M, Ikebukuro K, Ichioka N, Esumi T, Oyaizu H, Yoshimura T, Nagahama T, Nakamura K, Ito T, Hisha H, Sugiura K, Yasumizu R, Iida H, Ikehara S (2002) Comparison of bone marrow cells harvested from various bones of cynomolgus monkeys at various ages by perfusion or aspiration methods: a preclinical study for human BMT. Stem Cells 20:155–162

Marmont AM (1994) Immune ablation followed by allogeneic or autologous bone marrow transplantation: a new treatment for severe autoimmune diseases? Stem Cells 12:125–135

Nakamura T, Good RA, Yasumizu R, Inouc S, Oo MM, Hamashima Y, Ikehara S (1986) Successful liver allografts in mice by combination with allogeneic bone marrow transplantation. Proc Natl Acad Sci USA 83:4529–4532

Nishimura M, Toki J, Sugiura K, Hashimoto F, Tomita T, Fujishima H, Hiramatsu Y, Nishioka N, Nagata N, Takahashi Y et al (1994) Focal segmental glomerular sclerosis, a type of intractable chronic glomerulonephritis, is a stem cell disorder. J Exp Med 179:1053–1058

Oyaizu N, Yasumizu R, Miyama-Inaba M, Nomura S, Yoshida H, Miyawaki S, Shibata Y, Mitsuoka S, Yasunaga K, Morii S et al (1988) (NZW x BXSB)F1 mouse. A new animal model of idiopathic thrombocytopenic purpura. J Exp Med 167:2017–2022

Petrini M, Pacini S, Trombi L, Fazzi R, Montali M, Ikehara S, Abraham NG (2009) Identification and purification of mesodermal progenitor cells from human adult bone marrow. Stem Cells Dev 18:857–866

Ratajczak MZ, Kucia M, Reca R, Majka M, Janowska-Wieczorek A, Ratajczak J (2004) Stem cell plasticity revisited: CXCR4-positive cells expressing mRNA for early muscle, liver and neural cells 'hide out' in the bone marrow. Leukemia 18:29–40

Rose N, Afanasyeva M (2003) Autoimmunity: busting the atherosclerotic plaque. Nat Med 9:641–642

Suzuki Y, Adachi Y, Minamino K, Zhang Y, Iwasaki M, Nakano K, Koike Y, Ikehara S (2005) A new strategy for treatment of malignant tumor: intra-bone marrow–bone marrow transplantation plus CD4- donor lymphocyte infusion. Stem Cells 23:365–370

Takada K, Inaba M, Ichioka N, Ueda Y, Taira M, Baba S, Mizokami T, Wang X, Hisha H, Iida H, Ikehara S (2006) Treatment of senile osteoporosis in SAMP6 mice by intra-bone marrow injection of allogeneic bone marrow cells. Stem Cells 24:399–405

Than S, Ishida H, Inaba M, Fukuba Y, Seino Y, Adachi M, Imura H, Ikehara S (1992) Bone marrow transplantation as a strategy for treatment of non-insulin-dependent diabetes mellitus in KK-Ay mice. J Exp Med 176:1233–1238

Thomas ED, Blume KG (1999) Historical markers in the development of allogeneic hematopoietic cell transplantation. Biol Blood Marrow Transplant 5:341–346

Ueda Y, Inaba M, Takada K, Fukui J, Sakaguchi Y, Tsuda M, Omae M, Kushida T, Iida H, Ikehara S (2007) Induction of senile osteoporosis in normal mice by intra-bone marrow–bone marrow transplantation from osteoporosis-prone mice. Stem Cells 25:1356–1363

Ueno NT, Rondon G, Mirza NQ, Geisler DK, Anderlini P, Giralt SA, Andersson BS, Claxton DF, Gajewski JL, Khouri IF, Korbling M, Mehra RC, Przepiorka D, Rahman Z, Samuels BI, Van Besien K, Hortobagyi GN, Champlin RE (1998) Allogeneic peripheral-blood progenitor-cell transplantation for poor-risk patients with metastatic breast cancer. J Clin Oncol 16:986–993

Chapter 5

Differentiation of Human Embryonic Stem Cells into Functional Hepatocyte-Like Cells (Method)

Takamichi Ishii

Abstract Hepatocytes derived from human embryonic stem cells (ESCs) are a potential cell source for regenerative medicine. However, the successful differentiation of human ESCs into mature hepatocytes has been difficult to achieve because the definitive mechanisms governing hepatocyte differentiation have not yet been well defined. The CD45$^-$CD49f±Thy1$^+$gp38$^+$ mesenchymal cells that reside in murine fetal livers induce hepatic progenitor cells to differentiate into mature hepatocytes by direct cell-cell contact. A cell line named MLSgt20 was also successively established from these mesenchymal cells. These MLSgt20 cells possess the ability to promote the hepatic maturation of not only murine ESCs, but also human ESC-derived endodermal cells. To promote this maturation, human ESCs are treated with a two-step procedure for hepatic maturation; first, human ESCs are differentiated into endodermal cells, then human ESC-derived endodermal cells are matured into functional hepatocytes by co-culture with the MLSgt20 cells, thereby forming cell aggregates. These human ESC-derived hepatocyte-like cells possess hepatic functions.

Keywords Embryonic stem cells · Alpha-fetoprotein · Enhanced green fluorescent protein · Hepatocyte growth factor · Dulbecco's modified Eagle's medium · Hepatocyte-like cells

T. Ishii (✉)
Department of Surgery, Graduate School of Medicine Kyoto University, 54 Kawahara-cho Shogoin Sakyo-ku, Kyoto, 606-8507, Japan
e-mail: taishii@kuhp.kyoto-u.ac.jp

Introduction

Embryonic stem cells (ESCs) are established from inner cell masses and possess pluripotency, thus allowing them to differentiate into all three germ layers. Hepatocytes derived from ESCs are anticipated to provide a cell source of cell transplantation, hybrid-artificial livers, and drug discovery support systems (Ishii et al., 2007). However, there have been difficulties in differentiating ESCs into mature functional hepatocytes because the molecular mechanisms that underlie hepatic development are still largely unknown.

Our previous study revealed the hepatic maturation of fetal hepatic progenitor cells to be greatly facilitated by mesenchymal cells that reside in murine fetal livers (Hoppo et al., 2004). These mesenchymal cells are fractionized as CD45$^-$CD49f±Thy1$^+$gp38$^+$ cells (Kamo et al., 2007). In addition, our further experiments demonstrated the ability of these cells to induce the maturation of murine and human ESCs into functional hepatocytes (Ishii et al., 2005, 2010). Moreover, a cell line (MLSgt20) was successfully established from the CD45$^-$CD49f±Thy1$^+$gp38$^+$ murine fetal liver mesenchymal cells by the transfection of the cells with the immortalizing SV40 large T antigen gene (Fukumitsu et al., 2009). The MLSgt20 cells promoted the maturation of murine hepatic progenitor cells and murine ESC-derived alpha-fetoprotein (AFP)-producing cells, as well as human ESC-derived AFP-producing cells, into functional hepatocyte-like cells (Ishii et al., 2010). The effects of the MLSgt20 cells on hepatic maturation are achieved by direct cell-cell contact (Fukumitsu et al., 2009). They do not induce the hepatic maturation of undifferentiated

ESCs, thus suggesting that the MLSgt20 cells are relatively ineffective at hepatic specification and differentiation of undifferentiated ESCs (Ishii et al., 2010).

This chapter describes the two-step procedure for inducing the hepatic maturation of human ESCs utilizing the MLSgt20 cells (Ishii et al., 2010). In this protocol, a human ESC line expressing enhanced green fluorescent protein (EGFP) under the control of the human AFP enhancer/promoter is used (Ishii et al., 2008). First, undifferentiated human ESCs are differentiated into AFP-producing endodermal cells using sequential addition of activin A and hepatocyte growth factor (HGF) on Matrigel-coated culture dishes. Next, the AFP-producing cells are isolated as the EGFP-positive cells using flow cytometry. Second, the human ESC-derived AFP-producing cells are matured into functional hepatocyte-like cells by co-culture and forming cell aggregates with the MLSgt20 cells. A key step in this procedure is to obtain a viable cell fraction of the isolated AFP-producing cells from human ESCs, and to form cell aggregates with the MLSgt20 cells. These procedures are summarized in Fig. 5.1. We also describe how to isolate and culture the CD45$^-$CD49f$\pm$Thy1$^+$gp38$^+$ murine fetal liver mesenchymal cells.

Composition of Culture Media and Solutions

1. ESC medium: A 1:1 mixture of Dulbecco's modified Eagle's medium (DMEM) and Ham's nutrient mixture F12 (Sigma-Aldrich, St. Louis,

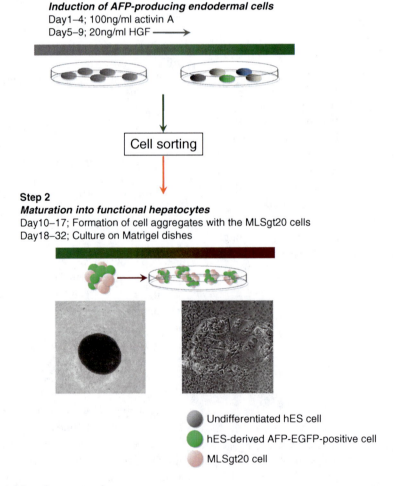

Fig. 5.1 A summary of the culture protocol

MO) supplemented with 20% Knockout SR (KSR, Gibco, Grand Island, NY), 0.1 mM 2-mercaptoethanol (Sigma-Aldrich), and MEM nonessential amino acids (Gibco).

2. ED medium: RPMI1640 (Gibco) with 0.5% fetal bovine serum (FBS), (HyClone, Logan, UT), 1 mM sodium pyruvate (Sigma-Aldrich), 10 mM nicotinamide (Sigma-Aldrich), 2 mM L-ascorbic acid phosphate (Wako Pure Chemical, Osaka, Japan), insulin-transferrin-selenium supplement (Gibco), and 0.1 μM dexamethasone (Sigma-Aldrich).

3. HD medium: DMEM supplemented with 10% FBS, 1 mM sodium pyruvate (Sigma-Aldrich), 10 mM nicotinamide, 2 mM L-ascorbic acid phosphate, insulin-transferrin-selenium supplement, 0.1 μM dexamethasone, and 20 ng/ml HGF (R&D System, Inc., Minneapolis, MN).

4. CTK solution; A solution of 0.05% collagenase IV (Gibco), 0.25% trypsin (Gibco), and 20% KSR.

5. A solution of 0.25% trypsin (Gibco) and 1 mM ethylenediaminetetraacetic acid (EDTA; Dojindo laboratories, Kumamoto, Japan; 0.25% trypsin-EDTA solution).

6. A solution of 0.05% trypsin and 1 mM EDTA (0.05% trypsin-EDTA solution).

7. Hank's balanced salt solution (HBSS; 30 ml) with 3% FBS (1 ml; 3% FBS/HBSS).

8. HBSS-based buffer: Ca^{2+}-free Mg^{+}-free Hank's balanced salt solution with phenol red (HBSS (−), Gibco) with 10 mM HEPES (Sigma-Aldrich) and 0.5 mM EDTA.

9. Irrigation solution 1 (50 ml): HBSS-based buffer (45 ml) supplemented with 10% FBS (5 ml), and 2 U/ml heparin sodium solution (0.1 ml). Heparin sodium solution at 1000 U/ml is readily purchased from several pharmaceutical companies. This solution is prepared as required and then is kept at 4°C. Heparin is added in order to prevent clot formation.

10. Irrigation solution 2 (50 ml): HBSS-based buffer (45 ml) supplemented with 50 mg/ml DNase I (Roche) (1 ml of stock solution), and 2 U/ml heparin sodium (0.1 ml). DNase I is dissolved at 25 mg/ml in distilled water, and stored in single use aliquots at −20°C. This solution is prepared as required, and kept at 4°C. DNase is added in order to reduce the viscosity caused by DNA that is released from damaged cells.

11. Digestion medium (30 ml): 0.5% (w/v) collagenase type II (150 mg, Gibco) is dissolved in 30 ml collagenase buffer and 0.1 ml heparin sodium. This medium is kept at 37°C prior to use. Collagenase buffer contains 0.2 g $MgSO_4 \cdot 7H_2O$, 0.735 g $CaCl_2 \cdot 2H_2O$, 2.383 g HEPES, and 0.05 g trypsin inhibitor in 1 l HBSS (−). All chemicals can be purchased from either Wako Pure Chemical or Sigma-Aldrich.

Differentiation of Human ESCs into Endodermal Cells (Step 1)

Human ESCs are cultured in the undifferentiated state on mouse embryonic fibroblast (MEF) feeder layers. They are sub-cultured using CTK solution. MEFs are prepared according to the standard protocols. In this study, a human ESC line that expresses EGFP under the control of the AFP enhancer/promoter was used. The parental human ESC line used was KhES3, which was established by Suemori et al. (2006).

1. A confluent culture of undifferentiated human ESCs on a 60 mm dish is dissociated by CTK solution. The dissociated cells are transferred into a 15 ml plastic tube in the ESC medium and left for 5 min at room temperature to deplete MEFs. The CTK solution dissociates the human ESC colonies into cell clusters that contain several dozen human ESCs, so that the human ESC clusters settle to the bottom of tubes. The supernatant fluid is then discarded by decantation.

2. The cell suspension is harvested and centrifuged at 1000 rpm for 3 min. The cell pellet is mildly resuspended and replated on a 60 mm culture dish coated with 1:80 Matrigel (BD Biosciences, Franklin Lakes, NJ) in ESC medium (day 0). Human ESCs can be damaged by mechanical manipulation; therefore, all processes dealing with human ESCs have to be performed carefully and with very mild and gentle movements. The undifferentiated human ESCs on one 60 mm dish can be transferred onto one 60 mm Matrigel-coated dish.

3. The culture medium is changed from ESC medium to ED medium on day 1. One hundred ng/ml activin

A is added to the ED medium for the first 4 days (days 1–4), and 20 ng/ml HGF is added for the next 5 days (days 5–9).
4. A total of 2 ml of 0.05% trypsin-EDTA solution are added into the 60 mm culture dishes on day 10 to dissociate the differentiated cells, and they are incubated at 37°C for 5 min. The cultured cells are well dissociated into a single cell suspension and then are resuspended in cold 3% FBS/HBSS solution for flow cytometric sorting. Because human ESCs are vulnerable to enzymatic and mechanical damage, the trypsin reaction time should be minimal, and the flow cytometric procedures should be done as quickly as possible.
5. The EGFP-positive cell fraction is isolated by flow cytometry. Approximately 20% of the differentiated human ESCs are positive for EGFP (Ishii et al., 2008). The harvested cells are resuspended in HD medium supplemented with oncostatin M (R&D System, Inc.) at a concentration of 1×10^5 cells/ml for further experiments.

Preparation of the MLSGT20 Cells

1. The MLSgt20 cells are cultured in HD medium on collagen type I-coated dishes (BD Biosciences) at 33°C, because they have been transfected with a temperature-sensitive SV40 large T antigen. The cells are then sub-cultured using 0.25% trypsin-EDTA solution.
2. The MLSgt20 cells are dissociated using a 0.25%-EDTA solution into a single cell suspension, centrifuged at 1000 rpm for 3 min, and then resuspended in HD medium supplemented with oncostatin M at a concentration of 1×10^5 cells/ml for further experiments.

Maturation of the Human ESC-Derived Endodermal Cells (Step 2)

1. The isolated AFP-producing EGFP-positive endodermal cell suspension is combined (1:1) with the dissociated MLSgt20 cell suspension so that the cell mixture contains the same number of human ESC-derived AFP-producing cells and MLSgt20 cells.
2. One hundred μl of the cell mixture is added into the each well of the Sumilon Celltight Spheroid 96-well plates (Sumitomo Bakelite Co., Ltd., Tokyo, Japan), thus allowing for the formation of cell aggregates. One well should contain 5,000 MLSgt20 cells and 5,000 human ESC-derived AFP-producing cells. Only one spheroid is formed per well by using Sumilon Celltight Spheroid 96-well plates. Other devices do not allow the formation of a single spheroid in one well. The culture plates are incubated at 37°C.
3. Add 10–20 μl of the fresh HD medium with oncostatin M into each well every 2 days. The culture is continued for 7 days (day 10–17).
4. The cell aggregates are harvested from individual wells after the 7-day period using a 500 μl micropipette. Approximately 12–16 cell aggregates can be transferred onto one well of 24-well Matrigel-coated culture plates.
5. The culture is maintained for an additional 14 days, and the medium is exchanged for fresh HD medium with oncostatin M each day (day 18–32). The differentiated cells possess an ammonia removal activity, and also the ability to store and synthesize glycogen, and cytochrome P450 enzyme activity at day 32.

Primary Culture of Murine CD45⁻CD49F±Thy1⁺gp38⁺ Mesenchymal Cells

1. Two pregnant mice are sacrificed and subjected to cesarean section. All uteri are removed and placed into a 100 mm Petri dish with cold irrigation solution 1. The amniotic membranes and placentae are removed, and fetal mice are transferred to a new 100 mm Petri dish with cold irrigation solution 1.
2. The liver tissues are then dissected under a stereomicroscope (Fig. 5.2), and placed into a new 100 mm Petri dish with cold irrigation solution 1. The harvested livers are then minced into pieces with a surgical knife into segments no larger than 1 mm in diameter.
3. A nylon mesh (50 μm pore size) is placed on a 50 ml centrifuge tube. The minced liver

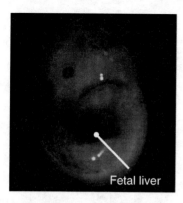

Fig. 5.2 This photograph shows a mouse fetus after removal of the amniotic membrane and placenta. The fetal liver is the *red* organ that is located in the middle of the fetus. Under a stereomicroscope, the liver is dissected using microforceps. The gallbladder and intestinal tract should be removed from the liver

tissues are filtered through this mesh. The mesh is inverted and carefully transferred onto a new 50 ml centrifuge tube. This procedure is necessary in order to eliminate hematopoietic cells. The flow-through, which contains hematopoietic cells, can be discarded.

4. Warm digestion medium (30 ml) is added through the inverted mesh into the 50 ml centrifuge tube, collecting the liver tissues into the tube, together with the digestion medium. The tube is incubated in a water bath at 37°C for 12–15 min with agitation.

5. Four nylon meshes (100 μm pore size) are placed onto four 15 ml centrifuge tubes. The digested tissues are divided into four equal aliquots, filtered through meshes, collected in the centrifuge tubes, and then centrifuged at 300 rpm for 5 min. This procedure is performed to eliminate undigested liver tissues.

6. The cell pellet is re-suspended in 25 ml of irrigation solution 2, collected in a 15 ml centrifuge tube, and then is centrifuged at 300 rpm for 5 min. This procedure is repeated twice.

7. The cell pellet is suspended in HD medium at a density of 5×10^5 cells/ml to 1×10^6 cells/ml, and inoculated onto 35 mm Petri dishes to allow the formation of cell aggregates. The harvested liver cells obtained from one pregnant mouse can usually be seeded onto three 35 mm Petri dishes, although the yield depends on the number of fetuses. The cell aggregates contain not only mesenchymal cells, but also hepatic progenitor cells and hematopoietic cells (Yasuchika et al., 2002).

8. The dissociated cells are incubated at 37°C overnight. The cell aggregates are collected in a 15 ml tube and subjected to gravity sedimentation for 10 min.

9. After the supernatant is removed, the sedimented cell aggregates are re-suspended in new HD media and plated on 6-well culture plates coated with type I collagen. The cell aggregates cultured in one 35 mm Petri dish can usually be transferred to one well of a 6-well culture plate.

10. The cell aggregates are cultured at 37°C for 1–2 days. The culture media are changed every day. The cell aggregates adhere to the culture plates and grow as monolayer colonies.

11. After being washed twice with HBSS, the adherent cells are incubated with 0.25% trypsin/EDTA for 10 min. HD medium is added to stop the trypsin activity, and the cell suspension is collected in a 15 ml tube.

12. The collected cells are centrifuged at 1,000 rpm for 3 min, and then washed twice in 3% FBS/HBSS.

13. The cell pellet is re-suspended in 200 μl 3% FBS/HBSS, and transferred to a 1.5 ml tube. The dissociated cells are incubated with 2 μl CD45-PE (1:100 dilution), 6 μl CD49f-PE (3:100), 2 μl Thy1-FITC (1:100), and 2 μl gp38-APC (1:100) antibodies on ice in the dark for 30 min. All antibodies can be purchased from BD Biosciences.

14. The cells are centrifuged at 2,800 rpm for 2 min, and then the supernatant is discarded.

15. The cells are washed with 3% FBS/HBSS three times.

16. The cells are resuspended in 2–4 ml 3% FBS/HBBS and collected in a 5 ml round-bottom tube through a nylon mesh.

17. The $CD45^-CD49f\pm Thy1^+gp38^+$ cell fraction is separated using a flow cytometer. Density plots using CD45, CD49f, Thy1, and gp38 antibodies are shown in Fig. 5.3. The separated $CD45^-CD49f\pm Thy1^+gp38^+$ mesenchymal cells are collected in HD medium. The combination of the fluorescent dyes is actually atypical, because PE labels both anti-CD45 and anti-CD49f antibodies. However, as shown in Fig. 5.3, the CD45-positive cell fraction is clearly distinguishable

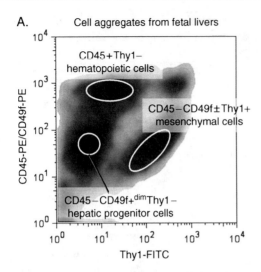
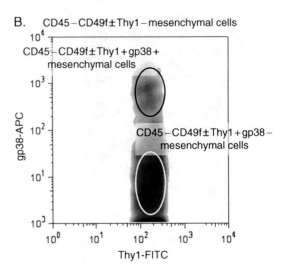

Fig. 5.3 Density plots from the flow cytometric analyses. (**a**) Cell aggregates derived from murine fetal livers are mainly divided by CD45, CD49f, and Thy1 into three cell fractions. The CD45$^+$Thy1$^-$ fraction corresponds to hematopoietic cells, the CD45$^-$CD49f+^{dim}Thy1$^-$ cell fraction corresponds to hepatic progenitor cells, and the CD45$^-$CD49f±Thy1$^+$ cell fraction is the mesenchymal cells. (**b**) The CD45$^-$CD49f±Thy1$^+$ mesenchymal cells are further fractionated by gp38 into two groups. The gp38-positive cells account for approximately 16% of the CD45$^-$CD49f±Thy1$^+$ mesenchymal cells

from the CD49f-positive cell fractions based on their fluorescence intensities. This may result from differences in the expression levels between CD45 and CD49f antigens.

18. The collected cells are resuspended in HD medium and seeded onto 24-well culture plates coated with collagen type I at a density of 1×10^4 cells per well. Cell viability generally shows a marked decrease at a lower density of cultured cells. Eventually, 1.5×10^4 to 2.0×10^4 CD45$^-$CD49f±Thy1$^+$gp38$^+$ mesenchymal cells can be isolated from one pregnant mouse.

Acknowledgements The author would like to thank Prof. Norio Nakatsuji (Institute for Integrated Cell-Material Science, Kyoto University), Dr. Hirofumi Suemori (Institute for Frontier Medical Sciences, Kyoto University), Dr. Yuji Amagai (Stem Cell and Drug Discovery Institute), Dr. Iwao Ikai (Kyoto Medical Center, National Hospital Organization), Dr. Kentaro Yasuchika (Graduate School of Medicine Kyoto University), and Prof. Shinji Uemoto (Graduate School of Medicine Kyoto University) for their valuable support in carrying out this study. This work was supported in part by grants from the Scientific Research Fund of the Ministry of Education, Culture, Sports, Science, and Technology of Japan.

References

Fukumitsu K, Ishii T, Yasuchika K, Amagai Y, Kawamura-Saito M, Kawamoto T, Kawase E, Suemori H, Nakatsuji N, Ikai I, Uemoto S (2009) Establishment of a cell line derived from a mouse fetal liver that has the characteristic to promote the hepatic maturation of mouse embryonic stem cells by a coculture method. Tissue Eng Part A 15:3847–3856

Hoppo T, Fujii H, Hirose T, Yasuchika K, Azuma H, Baba S, Naito M, Machimoto T, Ikai I (2004) Thy1-positive mesenchymal cells promote the maturation of CD49f-positive hepatic progenitor cells in the mouse fetal liver. Hepatology 39:1362–1370

Ishii T, Yasuchika K, Fujii H, Hoppo T, Baba S, Naito M, Machimoto T, Kamo N, Suemori H, Nakatsuji N, Ikai I (2005) In vitro differentiation and maturation of mouse embryonic stem cells into hepatocytes. Exp Cell Res 309:68–77

Ishii T, Yasuchika K, Machimoto T, Kamo N, Komori J, Konishi S, Suemori H, Nakatsuji N, Saito M, Kohno K, Uemoto S, Ikai I (2007) Transplantation of embryonic stem cell-derived endodermal cells into mice with induced lethal liver damage. Stem Cells 25:3252–3260

Ishii T, Fukumitsu K, Yasuchika K, Adachi K, Kawase E, Suemori H, Nakatsuji N, Ikai I, Uemoto S (2008) Effects of extracellular matrixes and growth factors on the hepatic differentiation of human embryonic stem cells. Am J Physiol Gastrointest Liver Physiol 295:G313–G321

Ishii T, Yasuchika K, Fukumitsu K, Kawamoto T, Kawamura-Saitoh M, Amagai Y, Ikai I, Uemoto S, Kawase E, Suemori H, Nakatsuji N (2010) In vitro hepatic maturation of human embryonic stem cells by using a mesenchymal cell line derived from murine fetal livers. Cell Tissue Res 339:505–512

Kamo N, Yasuchika K, Fujii H, Hoppo T, Machimoto T, Ishii T, Fujita N, Tsuruo T, Yamashita JK, Kubo H, Ikai I (2007) Two populations of Thy1-positive mesenchymal cells regulate in vitro maturation of hepatic progenitor cells. Am J Physiol Gastrointest Liver Physiol 292:G526–G534

Suemori H, Yasuchika K, Hasegawa K, Fujioka T, Tsuneyoshi N, Nakatsuji N (2006) Efficient establishment of human embryonic stem cell lines and long-term maintenance with stable karyotype by enzymatic bulk passage. Biochem Biophys Res Commun 345:926–932

Yasuchika K, Hirose T, Fujii H, Oe S, Hasegawa K, Fujikawa T, Azuma H, Yamaoka Y (2002) Establishment of a highly efficient gene transfer system for mouse fetal hepatic progenitor cells. Hepatology 36:1488–1497

Chapter 6

Stem Cell Mobilization: An Overview

Alessandro Isidori and Giuseppe Visani

Abstract Recruitment of hematopoietic stem and progenitor cells (HSCs/HPCs) from the bone marrow to the blood following treatment with chemotherapy, or cytokines, is a clinical process termed *mobilization*. At present, granulocyte colony-stimulating factor-mobilized peripheral blood stem cells are the primary source of hematopoietic cells used to reconstitute hematopoiesis after myeloablative chemotherapies. However, preclinical and clinical studies on alternative molecules, namely chemokines and small chemoattractans, demonstrate that improvements, either quantitative or qualitative, to this mobilization can be reached. It is becoming clear that different agents mobilize HSCs/HPCs with common stem cell function, but also mobilize stem cells with unique intrinsic characteristics. The continuous evaluation of the unexplored corners of the molecular mechanisms responsible for the HSCs/HPCs mobilization will be critical for the development of strategies targeted to mobilize a unique stem cell, with a consequent increase in the use of stem cell transplantation for regenerative aims.

Keywords Hematopoietic stem cells · Hematopoietic progenitor cells · Granulocyte colony-stimulating factor · Bone marrow · Parathyroid hormone · Transforming growth factor

A. Isidori (✉)
Hematology and Stem Cell Transplant Center, San Salvatore Hospital, Pesaro, Italy
e-mail: aisidori@gmail.com

Introduction

The movement of haematopoietic stem/progenitor cells (HSCs/HPCs) between bone marrow (their main site of production) and blood is a physiological process (Wright et al., 2001); few HSCs/HPCs circulate in blood. Early studies (McCredie et al., 1971) showed that HPCs were elevated in blood of patients recovering from chemotherapy. This observation led to the understanding that HSCs and HPCs could be induced to exit bone marrow in response to external *stimuli*, a phenomenon termed "mobilization", and that these mobilized HSCs/HPCs can be collected and will re-home to marrow and repopulate haematopoiesis. Although a variety of agents can mobilize stem cells with different kinetics and efficiencies (Lemoli and D'Addio, 2008; Gertz, 2010) and these agents can be additive or synergistic when used in combination, currently granulocyte colony-stimulating factor (G-CSF) is considered the gold standard to mobilize HSCs/HPCs for transplantation, based upon potency, predictability and safety (Gertz, 2010). However, multiple dosing, graft composition, poor mobilization in some patients, number of aphaeresis and inability to predict optimal mobilization times are still important burning questions on the everyday use of G-CSF. Furthermore, the better comprehension of the molecular pathways leading to the egress of HSCs from the bone marrow or the homing of these cells to the marrow has prompted the development of new drugs, namely chemokines and small chemoattractans regulating HSCs migration, with the aim of improving stem cell collection. Several studies give us the proof of evidence that chemokine-mobilized HSCs/HPCs are different from G-CSF-mobilized HSCs/HPCs (Pelus and Fukuda, 2008), introducing a new scenario in stem cell mobilization. This review will focus on the hot topics of stem cell mobilization in 2011, with an outlook not only on autologous or allogeneic transplantation but also on regenerative medicine.

The Hematopoietic Niche

HSCs and HPCs reside in specific areas of the bone marrow, which provide the necessary signals to determine HSC fate; that is survival, quiescence, self-renewal or commitment and differentiation. These regions are called "niches". Sophisticated live microscopy techniques and genetic manipulations have identified the endosteal region of the bone marrow (BM) as a preferential site of residence for the most potent HSC – able to reconstitute in serial transplants – with osteoblasts and their progenitors as critical cellular elements of these endosteal niches (Lévesque et al., 2010). In fact, proliferation and release of HPCs/HSCs require dynamic cycles of BM destruction/restructuring, which seem to be strictly linked to bone remodelling by osteoclast/osteoblast interactions. Recent studies confirmed that HSC number is higher in mice carrying transgenes that enhance bone-formation (Calvi et al., 2003). Moreover, new experiments on mice demonstrated that HSC mobilization could be doubled with the administration to mice of the bisphosphonate pamidronate or parathyroid hormone (PTH) in conjunction with G-CSF. Consequently, a phase I clinical trials was performed on 20 poor-mobilizing patients; following 14 days of PTH administration, 40% of these patients mobilized acceptable levels of CD34 cells in response to G-CSF (Ballen et al., 2007).

The second type of niche reported in mouse bone marrow is the endothelial niche. A significant proportion of HSC are, in fact, intimately associated with sinusoidal endothelial cells in the endothelial niche, where they are ready to enter peripheral blood and start differentiation (Adams and Scadden, 2006). Rather than comprising a static compartment, niches act as dynamic environment and, thus, may support rapid increases in hematopoietic cell production depending on the physiological requirements. Detachment of HSCs from these niches is believed to be associated with their entry into the cell cycle, proliferation, and differentiation, which is also accompanied by increased migration and recruitment to the circulation (Lapidot and Kollet, 2010). In addition, growth factors and cytokines, including stromal cell-derived factor (SDF)-1α and transforming growth factor (TGF)-β, modulate HSC/HPC proliferation within BM niches. For example, TGF-β, which is well-known to exert several effects on cells including proliferation, differentiation and apoptosis, regulates the cell cycle entry of HSCs/HPCs and in this manner modulates their quiescence (Yamazaki et al., 2009). In addition to TGF-β, SDF-1α (CXCL-12) regulates HSC/HPC function and maintains these cells in a quiescent state, which is critical to sustain a pool of highly regenerative stem cells. Recent evidences suggest that activated HSCs/HPCs reversibly switch from dormancy to self-renewal during homeostasis and repair (Wilson et al., 2008). All these data represent the body of evidence that the fate of a HSC/HPC is largely regulated by its immediate environment, and that several common pathways able to trigger HSC/HPC mobilization involve changes in the bone marrow environment.

The Biology of Stem Cell Mobilization

Chemo-attractant cytokines, growth factors, and hormones are modulators that control the egress of HSCs/HPCs from BM. HSC/HPC mobilization from BM enables migration to peripheral blood and homing to peripheral tissues. This process is tightly controlled by specialized signals. HSCs/HPCs express a broad array of cell surface receptors, namely the adhesion molecules lymphocyte function-associated Ag-1 (LFA-1), very late Ag-4 (VLA-4) and Mac-1; the chemokine receptors CXCR4 and CXCR2; the cell surface glycoproteins CD44 and CD62L; and the tyrosine kinase receptor c-kit (Bensinger et al., 2009). The BM stroma contains stromal cell-derived factor-1 (SDF-1), CXC chemokine GRO-β, vascular cell adhesion molecule-1, kit ligand, P-selectin glycoprotein ligand-1 and hyaluronic acid, all of these are cognate ligands for the stem cell adhesion molecules (Bensinger et al., 2009). Data from a number of preclinical models showed that inhibition of these receptor-ligand interactions resulted in enhanced progenitor cell mobilization (Bensinger et al., 2009).

Stress-induced signals activate neutrophils and osteoclasts which, in turn, cause shedding and release of membrane-bound stem cell factor (SCF), proliferation of HSC, activation and/or degradation of adhesion molecules such as VLA-4 and P/E selectins (Lemoli and D'Addio, 2008). Furthermore, a pivotal role in stem cell mobilization is played by the inactivation of the chemokine stromal cell derived factor-1 (SDF-1)/CXCL12, interleukin-8 (IL-8)/CXCL8 along with the proteolytic activity of elastase, cathepsin G, proteinase 3, CD26 and metalloproteinase (MMP)-2 and MMP-9 which disrupt the SDF-1/CXCR4 axis resulting in HSC/HPC release in the bloodstream (Lemoli and D'Addio, 2010). SDF-1 also mediates a variety of other cellular function such as engraftment in peripheral tissues. Binding of GRO-β to its receptor CXCR2 also induces mobilization of HSCs/HPCs. Mobilization by repeated G-CSF stimulation requires awakening the quiescent HSCs/HPCs, generating guiding signals, locally repressing the inhibitory attachment apparatus, and gaining motility (Lapidot and Kollet, 2010). Furthermore, G-CSF activates in HSC/HPC the reactive oxygen species (ROS) signaling. By turning on the c-Met/HGF (hepatocyte growth factor) axis, G-CSF augments the production of ROS, which determines HPC/HSC mobilization (Tesio et al., 2011). Accordingly, ROS inhibition decreases both G-CSF-induced mobilization and the increased HSC motility, showing the key role of ROS as a regulator of enhanced HPC/HSC migration, proliferation and differentiation, leading to reduced long-term stem cell population (Tesio et al., 2011). On the other hand, this transitory increase in ROS is reversible, and the long-term repopulation potential can be re-established by in vitro ROS inhibition (Tesio et al., 2011).

In addition to neutrophil activation, it has recently emerged that a number of non-specific inflammatory/immune responses may play a role in HCS/HPC mobilization (Winkler and Levesque, 2006). The complement system, critical in inflammation and innate immunity, seems also to be involved in BM retention and mobilization of HSCs/HPCs. The plasminogen/plasmin system seems also to be involved. In fact, the administration of G-CSF results in an increase in blood concentration of soluble urokinase-type plasminogen activator receptor (suPAR), upregulation of urokinase-type plasminogen activator receptor (uPAR) on CD33$^+$ myeloid and CD14$^+$ monocytic cells, and release of a cleaved formed of suPAR that inhibits CD34$^+$ cell migration in response to CXCL12,

suggesting that uPAR shedding may have an important role in HSC/HPC mobilization (Selleri et al., 2005).

Finally, the treatment with G-CSF enhances the number of bone-resorbing osteoclasts secreting elevated levels of the proteolytic enzymes MMP-9, the mobilizing chemokine IL-8, and cathepsins that cleave SDF-1. SDF-1 expressed by endosteal osteoblasts recruits osteoclast precursors from the peripheral blood to the bone marrow. Fascinatingly, G-CSF represses the expression of SDF-1 on osteoblasts, hence inducing stem cell delivery in the circulation by the stimulation of the peripheral nervous system. The bone remodelling process, niche alterations, HSC activation and mobilization are, therefore, partially determined by the same pathways (Lemoli and D'Addio, 2008).

Mobilization Agents Available

Filgrastim (Neupogen, Amgen Inc., Thousand Oaks, CA, USA) is a granulocyte colony-stimulating factor analog used to stimulate the proliferation and differentiation of granulocytes. It is produced by recombinant DNA technology. The gene for human G-CSF is inserted into *Escherichia coli* and the G-CSF produced looks like naturally produced G-CSF in humans. One of the major problems with recombinant G-CSF, produced in bacteria and, therefore, unglycosylated, is the relatively short half-life of 4–6 hours consequent to the rapid plasma clearance necessitating multiple dosing by daily injection. The most common adverse effects observed are mild to moderate bone pain after repeated daily injection and local skin reactions at the site of injection. Splenic rupture, alveolar hemorrage, acute respiratory distress and hemoptysis, although rare, were also reported as possible adverse effects of unglycosylated G-CSF.

Sarmograstim (GM-CSF, Leukine, Bayer Healthcare Pharmaceuticals, Seattle, WA, USA) is a recombinant granulocyte macrophage colony-stimulating factor that functions as an immunostimulator and is produced in yeast. These two agent, that were developed concurrently 20 years ago, are currently the only FDA-approved colony-stimulating factors (CSFs) for stem cell mobilization. G-CSF stimulates the production and maturation of neutrophils, eosinophils, basophils, monocytes and dendritic cells. In addition to stimulating myelopoiesis, CSFs also cause the release of proteases that diminish the anchoring of stem cells to the bone marrow stroma, releasing progenitor cells into the circulation. Although historically approved for mobilization, GM-CSF is little used for this purpose today. On the other side, G-CSF, alone or in combination with chemotherapy, is widely considered the gold standard to mobilize peripheral blood stem cell for transplantation.

Pegfilgrastim (Neulasta, Amgen Inc, Thousand Oaks, CA, USA) is a longer lasting variant of G-CSF, resulting from the conjugation of recombinant G-CSF to polyethylene glycol. Its plasma half-life of 33 hours is considerably longer than G-CSF. A slow rate of renal elimination allows a single injection to result in clinically effective serum levels from administration until neutrophil recovery (Isidori et al., 2005). This agent got the FDA approval for the prevention of prolonged neutropenia after chemotherapy in solid tumors. However, several studies on haematological patients demonstrated the safety and the efficacy of Pegfilgrastim as a mobilizing agent after a single injection of 6–12 mg in haematological malignancies. Adverse effects occurs with similar frequency to G-CSF.

Lenograstim is a recombinant granulocyte colony-stimulating factor and is glycosylated as opposed to pegylated. Clinical trials have proven its efficacy for preventing chemotherapy-induced neutropenia and for progenitor-cell transplantation, almost similar to filgrastim. Its benefit is compelling in some well-defined settings (highly myelosuppressive chemotherapy, advanced cancer, high-risk patients) (Gunzer et al., 2010).

Plerixafor (AMD 3100, Genzyme Corporation, Cambridge, MA, USA) was initially evaluated as an antiviral treatment for HIV-infected patients. Plerixafor is a selective and reversible antagonist of CXCR4 and disrupts its interaction with SDF-1, thereby releasing hematopoietic stem cells into the circulation (Broxmeyer et al., 2005). Plerixafor was found to be a strong inducer of mobilization of hematopoietic stem cells from the bone marrow to the blood stream. In December 2008, the FDA approved Plerixafor 0.24 mg/kg/day, administered the night prior to each apheresis session up to 4 doses, in combination with G-CSF for stem cell mobilization and subsequent autologous stem cell transplantation (ASCT) in patients with multiple myeloma (MM) or non-Hodgkin Lymphoma (NHL). In pharmacokinetics studies of healthy volunteers, as well as patients with haematological malignancies, plerixafor demonstrated a 3-compartment model with linear kinetics. Peak plasma concentration occur 30 min after administration, and have a terminal half-life of 4.6 h. The maximum increase in circulating CD-34 cells occurs approximately 10 h after injection (Broxmeyer et al., 2005).

Ancestim is a recombinant human stem cell factor (rhSCF) and is a 166 amino acid polypeptide produced in *Escherichia coli*, carrying the human gene for soluble human stem cell factor. Ancestim showed promising synergy in combination with G-CSF for stem cell mobilization (Herbert et al., 2010). On the other hand, the traditional cytokine stem cell factor (SCF) was withdrawn from clinical development in the United States due to toxicity concerns in early 2000s. Other cytokines that are no longer or rarely used to mobilize HSCs/HPCs are Interleukin-3, Interleukin-1, Interleukin-6, Interleukin-8 and ligands of tyrosine kinase receptors such as KIT ligand. Preclinical studies on the use of antibodies for VLA-4 (natalizumab, used for the treatment of multiple sclerosis and Chron's disease) demonstrated the efficacy of this agent in primates, with a 200-fold increase in CD34$^+$ cells over baseline after 24 h from treatment. However, the FDA withdrawn the drug due to important safety concerns regarding the development of 3 cases of progressive multifocal leucoencephalopathy in multiple sclerosis/Chron's disease patients in 2004, and its clinical application in stem cell mobilization seems to be very far from reality.

Highly negative charged polymers (polyanions) such as polymethacrylic acid, sulphogalactosylceramide, dextran sulphate, sulphated fucosoidan or defibrotide induce rapid mobilization within the first 2 h of administration. Apart from sulphated fucoidan, the mechanism of action of mobilizing polyanions is unclear (Winkler and Levesque, 2006).

Finally, as reported elsewhere in this review, alterations in bone turnover are expected to affect HPC/HSC mobilization, especially when these changes involve the endosteal region, close to the HSC niche. Therefore, strategies to either boost the number of functional HSC endosteal niches or to reduce osteoclast function should improve mobilization.

Factors Affecting Stem Cell Mobilization

High-dose chemotherapy, in conjunction with autologous stem cell transplantation (ASCT), emerged as preferred treatment for a variety of hematological malignancies including multiple myeloma, non-Hodgkin's lymphoma and Hodgkin disease (HD). Traditionally, HSCs were collected by multiple bone marrow aspirations. However, the serendipitous discovery that HSCs could be forced to egress in large numbers from the BM into the peripheral blood, from where they could be easily collected, dramatically changed clinical practice. Furthermore, several randomized studies demonstrated the superiority in terms of faster engraftment, decrease of morbidity and reduction of supportive measures (e.g.: hospitalization, administration of intravenous antibiotics, low transfusion requirement) of mobilized HSCs over the bone marrow for ASCT (Beyer et al., 1995; Schmitz et al., 1996).

Administration of G-CSF, alone or in combination with chemotherapy, is widely considered the most effective treatment to increase the number of circulating $CD34^+$ stem cells. The collection of an adequate number of $CD34^+$ cells, a surrogate marker for HSCs, is paramount because the number of infused $CD34^+$ cells influences the success and rate of hematopoietic recovery (Haas et al., 1994). Thus, patients receiving at least 2×10^6 $CD34^+$ cells/kg show a rapid neutrophil recovery, and patients transplanted with $\geq 5 \times 10^6$ $CD34^+$ cells/kg have faster multilineage engraftment. Conversely, below the minimum threshold level of 1×10^6 $CD34^+$ cells/kg reinfused, the risk of delayed hematopoietic recovery and increased transplantation mortality is high (Haas et al., 1994). Optimizing HSC/HPC collection is dependent also on when to start collection. At present, the best available predictor of adequate collection is the number of $CD34^+$ cells/μl in the blood on the morning of collection. Collection should start when 8–20 $CD34^+$ cells/μl are present in peripheral blood to increase the likelihood of collecting at least 2×10^6 $CD34^+$ cells/kg in a single apheresis.

In addition, factors that can affect the success of a mobilization strategy include the underlying disease, previous chemo-radiotherapy, the interval between last therapy and mobilization and marrow fibrosis (Haas et al., 1994). Moreover, there is a negative correlation between age and the yield of $CD34^+$ cells (Gertz, 2010). Although there is no specific age after which it is difficult or impossible to mobilize stem cells, the older the patient, the more difficult it is to mobilize an adequate yield of stem cells. Other predictors of low-yield in patients include elevation of LDH, previous interferon use, higher creatinine, low albumin level and transfusion-associated iron overload (Gertz, 2010). Last but not least, previous chemotherapy exposure has a relevant effect on the successful mobilization of HSCs/HPCs. In particular, drugs known to act as stem cell poison, such as chlorambucil, melphalan and fludarabine should be avoided in patients who have other possible factors that negatively influence HSC mobilization. On the other hand, most important predictors of successful mobilization are the number of months since last chemotherapy or radiation and peripheral blood platelet count at the time of mobilization (Gertz, 2010).

Stem Cell Mobilization with Cytokines Plus Chemotherapy

The main objectives of combining chemotherapy to growth factors for HSCs mobilization are the reduction of tumor burden coupled with purging of hematopoietic graft, and the increase in the $CD34^+$ cells yield. Prior to the development of hematopoietic cytokines as mobilization agents, transitory increases in the number of HSCs in peripheral blood had been observed after the administration of myelotoxic chemotherapy. Accordingly, the first protocols to mobilize HSCs into the peripheral blood used chemotherapy alone. Bensinger et al. (1995) originally administered chemotherapy to patients with advanced disease who could benefit from the reduction of the tumor burden before ASCT. Chemotherapy administered to patients included cyclophosphamide (CY), either alone either in combination with etoposide or etoposide and cysplatin or paclitaxel. G-CSF or GM-CSF were administered following chemotherapy and peripheral blood collection began 24 hours after the white blood cell count was greater than 1×10^9/l. Chemotherapy plus cytokine collection resulted in a median collection of 10.75×10^6 $CD34^+$/kg in 124 patients.

After that study, a variety of chemotherapeutic agents were used in combination with cytokines with the aim of mobilizing HSCs for autologous transplantation. The kind of mobilizing chemotherapy utilized is usually disease specific. Cyclophosphamide is the most common chemotherapy regimen used together with G-CSF to mobilize HSCs, and is highly active against tumor cells. Even if a consensus on the dosage of CY, ranging in literature from 1.5 to 7 g/m^2, is missing, the vast majority of Clinicians worldwide use CY at 4 g/m^2, both in MM and NHL patients. When 7 g/m^2 was compared to 4 g/m^2 in a retrospective study, the 4 g/m^2 dose decreased hematological and extra-hematological toxicity with superimposable CD34$^+$ cell collection efficiency compared to the higher dose suggesting that extremely high dose of CY are not required (Gertz, 2010). In fact, the dark side of mobilization chemotherapy is the increased morbidity. Although treatment-related mortality is rare, significant morbidity related to neutropenia has been described, and many reports point to greater resource utilization with chemomobilization than with cytokine-alone mobilization. In one study of chemotherapy-induced mobilization, the total duration of neutropenia was 6 days (Gertz, 2010). Bacteremia was observed in 22% of patients, with 40% of patients developing a gastrointestinal colonization with yeast, which is a risk factor for invasive fungal infection with myeloablative therapy and ASCT (Gertz, 2010). Nevertheless, mobilization with CY and G-CSF requires fewer apheresis session to collect sufficient number of HSCs for ASCT than does mobilization alone.

Another important point to keep in mind is that chemotherapy may exert long-term detrimental effects on the BM or the marrow microenvironment. Several lines of evidence suggest that cytotoxic chemotherapy and radiotherapy administered before ASCT contributes to the subsequent development of treatment-related myelodysplastic syndrome (t-MDS) and acute myelogenous leukemia (AML) after ASCT (Kalaycio et al., 2006). The approximate 10% risk of t-MDS/AML after standard chemotherapy with or without radiotherapy is similar to the risk after ASCT. The latency period for the development of t-MDS/AML is approximately 6 years after initial cytotoxic exposure, whether or not ASCT is used (Kalaycio et al., 2006). Many patients have documented clonal cytogenetic abnormalities detectable before ASCT. Kalaycio et al. reported an increased long-term risk of t−MDS or AML after ASCT in patients whose marrow had been damaged by prior chemotherapy and radiation (Kalaycio et al., 2006). Pre-transplantation characteristics, including age, diagnosis of NHL or HD, bone marrow involvement, prior radiation therapy, prior exposure to chemotherapy, lactate dehydrogenase at the time of ASCT, disease status, and method of stem-cell mobilization, were then analyzed with respect to the subsequent development of t-MDS/AML (Kalaycio et al., 2006). By multivariable analysis, prior exposure to radiation therapy, four or more chemotherapy regimens, and more than 5 days of apheresis needed to harvest enough stem cells were identified as independent risk factors for t-MDS/AML (Kalaycio et al., 2006).

Finally, how to approach patients who failed to mobilize adequate number of stem cells (2 × 10^6/kg) on the first attempt is complex and is still a matter of debate. Chemotherapy in conjunction with G-CSF is frequently used to mobilize patients who had previously failed to collect sufficient CD34$^+$ cells for ASCT. Although this combination is usually more effective than the use of G-CSF alone for second mobilization challenges, the repeated administration of chemotherapeutic drugs for HSC/HPC mobilization causes additional toxicity and may be not the best approach for patients in whom chemomobilization has already failed, specially after the discovery of chemokine as potent HSC/HPC mobilization agents.

In conclusion, the literature shows that the use of chemotherapy in addition to G-CSF for mobilization of stem cells carries no benefit for patient survival over use of G-CSF alone. A recent randomized trial comparing these two strategies found no differences in overall survival and progression-free survival after 21 months (Narayanasami et al., 2001). In addition, increased CD34$^+$ cells/kg obtained after chemotherapy plus G-CSF has not resulted in any significant enhancement of neutrophil or platelet engraftment after ASCT. A recent pilot study explored the safety of plerixafor mobilization when incorporated into a conventional stem cell mobilization regimen of chemotherapy and G-CSF (Dugan et al., 2010). Plerixafor was well tolerated and its addition to a chemo-mobilization regimen resulted in an increase in the peripheral blood CD34$^+$ cells (Dugan et al., 2010). The mean rate of increase in the peripheral blood CD34$^+$ cells was 2.8 cells/μl/h pre- and 13.3 cells/μl/h post-plerixafor administration. Even if promising, these results need to be confirmed by further studies in order to evaluate the effect of plerixafor in combination with chemomobilization on stem cell mobilization and collection on the first and subsequent days of apheresis, and its impact on resource utilization.

Stem Cell Mobilization with Cytokines Alone

G-CSF is the most frequently used stem cell mobilizing agent. When G-CSF alone is used for autologous stem cell mobilization, it is administered subcutaneously at dosages ranging from 10 to 32 μg/kg/day, beginning at least 4 days before the first apheresis and continued until the last apheresis session. In a dose-response study on 50 patients with hematological malignancies and solid tumors who received non-myeloablative chemotherapy, Demirer et al. found no clinical benefit to administering G-SCF 8 μg/kg/day versus 16 μg/kg/day (Demirer et al., 2002). The higher-dose arm collected a median number of 8.18 × 10^6 CD34$^+$/kg versus 4.7 × 10^6 CD34$^+$/kg in the lower-dose arm ($p<0.001$). Time to neutrophil engraftment was significantly faster (12 days versus 9 days; $p<0.001$); however, parameters of peritransplant morbidity were similar between the two arms. Because of the short half-life of G-CSF, many physicians prefer a twice-daily schedule over a single injection of G-CSF per day, but there is no evidence that any one schedule is superior and donor/patient preference and convenience is a deciding factor.

In many patients with MM or NHL, HSC mobilization with G-CSF as single agent results in suboptimal CD34$^+$ cell yields. These studies showed that CD34$^+$ cell yields are usually lower when a cytokine only mobilization regimen is used than when cytokine is used with chemotherapy. In addition, the percentage of patients not able to achieve an adequate number of CD34$^+$ cells (defined as CD34$^+$ cell yields of < 2 × 10^6/kg) was extremely variable throughout these studies, ranging from 0 to 23%.

Mobilization with G-CSF alone is the treatment of choice for healthy donors for whom peripheral blood stem cell (PBSC) are used as a source of stem cells in allogeneic settings. G-CSF mobilized, allogeneic PBSC grafts contain 3–4 fold more CD34$^+$ cells compared to allogeneic BM grafts and are associated with faster engraftment and a shorter time to achieve complete donor chimerism when compared to BM. When G-CSF is used for allogeneic stem cell mobilization, it is administered subcutaneously at doses between 5 and 16 μg/kg/day given for 4 or 5 consecutive days. Similarly to ASCT, the dose of CD34$^+$ cells infused correlates well with faster engraftment. However, several studies have suggested that the higher doses of CD34$^+$ cells in the graft might increase the risk for developing chronic GVHD. Even if transplant-related mortality tend to be significantly lower with PBSC with respect to BM, survival does not seem to be significantly modified by the source of stem cells in the allogeneic setting.

Stem Cell Mobilization with Chemokines

The better comprehension of the molecular pathways leading to the exit of HSCs from the bone marrow or the homing of these cells to the marrow has prompted the development of new drugs, namely chemokines and small chemoattractans regulating HSCs migration, with the aim of improving stem cell collection. Macrophage inflammatory protein 1α (MIP1α/CCL3), the CXCR-2 ligands GROβ, the CXCR4 antagonist AMD 3100, the SDF-1α peptide analogs CTCE-0021 and CTCE 0214 and the SDF1 analog Met-SDF-1β are all capable of mobilizing HPCs/HSCs, and all of them seem to have additive or synergistic effect with G-CSF and with each other (Pelus and Fukuda, 2008). In contrast to G-CSF, chemokine mobilization occurs rapidly. In mice, peripheral blood stem cell mobilization by MIP1α, CTCE0021 and AMD 3100 is maximal within 60 min, while mobilization by GROβ is maximal at 15 min (Pelus and Fukuda, 2008). Synergistic HSC/HPC mobilization is seen when MIP1α, CTCE0021, AMD 3100 or GROβ are combined with G-CSF, and even more dramatic synergy is seen using combination of different chemokines (Pelus and Fukuda, 2008). Furthermore, in mice, chemokine-mobilized cells produced significantly higher chimerism than G-CSF-mobilized cells, with chemokine-mobilized grafts containing twice the number of Sca-1+, c-Kit+ and lineage neg (SKL) cells

(Pelus and Fukuda, 2008). These observations clearly demonstrated that not only the quantity of stem cells impact on the function of HSC graft, but also the quality of stem cells matters, intended as cell cycle status, facilitating or accessory cell content or intrinsic differences in proliferative or homing properties.

To date, few studies have evaluated the use of plerixafor in combination with G-CSF for stem cell mobilization. Flomenberg et al. compared G-CSF and G-CSF plus AMD3100 for mobilization of stem cells in patients with MM and NHL (Flomenberg et al., 2005). All the patients underwent two mobilizations, one using G-CSF as a single agent and another using G-CFS plus AMD3100. Patients receiving combination of two agents mobilized more CD34$^+$ cells per leukapheresis, underwent fewer leukaphereses and had a higher yield of total CD34$^+$ cells collected. Of patients receiving plerixafor plus G-CSF, 80% collected at least a goal 5×10^6 CD34$^+$ cells/kg compared to 32% of those receiving G-CSF alone. Eighty-four percent of patients receiving plerixafor increased CD34$^+$ cell collection by at least 50% compared to those receiving G-CSF. Nine patients who failed to mobilize with G-CSF alone were able to mobilize with plerixafor plus G-CSF. The results of two phase III multicenter randomized placebo-controlled studies indicated that the addition of plerixafor to a G-CSF regimen resulted in greater efficacy than was seen with a regimen of G-SCF alone (DiPersio et al., 2009a, b). All patients in both studies received G-CSF 10 μg/kg/day subcutaneously. On the evening of day 4, patients received either placebo or plerixafor (240 μg/kg) subcutaneously followed by morning dose of G-CSF for up to a total of four apheresis sessions or until $\geq 5 \times 10^6$ CD34$^+$ cells/kg were collected. In the myeloma study (DiPersio et al., 2009a) 106 of 148 (71.6%) patients in the plerixafor group and 53 of 154 (34.4%) patients in the placebo group collected more than or equal to 6×10^6 CD34$^+$ cells/kg in less than or equal to 2 aphereses and met the primary end-point of the study ($P < 0.001$). A total of 54% of plerixafor-treated patients reached target after one apheresis, whereas 56% of the placebo-treated patients required 4 aphereses to reach target. The most common adverse events related to plerixafor were gastrointestinal disorders and injection site reaction. In the lymphoma study (DiPersio et al., 2009b) 89 out of 150 (59%) patients in the plerixafor group and 29 out of 148 patients (20%) in the placebo group collected $\geq 5 \times 10^6$ CD34$^+$ cells/kg and met the primary end point of the study ($P < 0.001$). One hundred thirty-five patients (90%) in plerixafor group and 82 patients (55%) in placebo group underwent transplantation after initial mobilization. Median time to engraftment was similar in both groups. The most common plerixafor-associated adverse events were GI disorders and injection site reaction.

The conclusions of the phase III trials indicates that plerixafor and G-CSF were well tolerated and resulted in a significantly higher proportion of patients with myeloma and lymphoma achieving the optimal CD34$^+$ cell target for transplantation in fewer apheresis days, compared with G-CSF alone. More patients receiving plerixafor and G-CSF were able to proceed to transplantation with respect to G-CSF alone. The success of plerixafor and G-CSF extensively addresses a number of areas of improvement in HSCs/HPCs mobilization; however, it still requires multiple dosing. At present, several studies are testing the capacity of plerixafor as a stand-alone mobilizing agent.

Mobilization and Regenerative Medicine

The rising role of marrow as a site of adult stem cells that play a part in regenerative medicine raise the question of whether chemokines can mobilize stem cells other than HSCs or whether new drugs can be developed that differentially mobilize adult stem cell. It is well established that G-CSF administration mobilizes endothelial progenitor cells (EPCs) with high proliferative activity (Rafii and Lyden, 2003). However, going from the bench to the bedside, no significant improvement was observed in patients with acute myocardial infarction who received mobilizing dosages of G-CSF (Kang et al., 2007), and no significant improvement of hepatic function was observed in end-stage liver disease patients treated with 2–15 mg/kg of G-CSF (Lorenzini et al., 2008). Nonetheless, in other recent studies, intracoronary infusion of G-CSF mobilized HSC showed a trend towards efficacy over systemic G-CSF administration in patients with myocardial infarction, and intracardiac injection of autologous G-CSF-mobilized CD34$^+$ cells in patients with intractable angina provided evidence for feasibility, safety and efficacy. Furthermore, it was recently reported the successful use of human circulating CD133$^+$ cells to treat severe skeletal muscle injury in rats, and in a report on patients with critical limb ischemia whose only other option was amputation, the reinfusion of G-CSF mobilized and highly purified CD133+ cells was induced lower extremity limb salvage in 7 out of 9 treated patients.

Regarding chemokines, a recent paper demonstrated that AMD3100 is a potent and rapid mobilizer of EPCs that can be collected by leukaphaeresis after 4 h from its administration (Shepherd et al., 2006). Unfortunately, no clinical data on the use of chemokines for regenerative medicine are, up to now, available. However, what reported by Shepherd et al. open a new scenario for the fast mobilization of cells to sites of vascular injuries in an acute setting and for the collection of cells that can be transplanted directly in to the damaged tissue. Future studies will tell us if chemokine-mobilized HSC are the scientific response to the serendipitous discovery of HSC and if they will become a possible therapeutic option in the changing landscape of regenerative medicine.

References

Adams GB, Scadden DT (2006) The hematopoietic stem cell in its place. Nat Immunol 7:333–337
Ballen KK, Shpall EJ, Avigan D, Yeap BY, Fisher DC, McDermott K, Dey BR, Attar E, McAfee S, Konopleva M, Antin JH, Spitzer TR (2007) Phase I trial of parathyroid hormone to facilitate stem cell mobilization. Biol Blood Marrow Transplant 13(7):838–843
Bensinger W, Appelbaum F, Rowley S, Storb R, Sanders J, Lilleby K, Gooley T, Demirer T, Schiffman K, Weaver C (1995) Factors that influence collection and engraftment of autologous peripheral-blood stem cells. J Clin Oncol 13(10):2547–2555
Bensinger W, Di Persio JF, McCarty JM (2009) Improving stem cell mobilization strategies: future directions. Bone Marrow Transpl 43:181–195
Beyer J, Schwella N, Zingsem J, Strohscheer I, Schwaner I, Oettle H, Serke S, Huhn D, Stieger W (1995) Hematopoietic rescue after high-dose chemotherapy using autologous peripheral-blood progenitor cells or bone marrow: a randomized comparison. J Clin Oncol 13(6):1328–1335
Broxmeyer HE, Orschell CM, Clapp DW, Hangoc G, Cooper S, Plett PA, Liles WC, Li X, Graham-Evans B, Campbell TB, Calandra G, Bridger G, Dale CD, Srour EF (2005) Rapid mobilization of murine and human hematopoietic stem and progenitor cells with AMD 3100, a CXCR4 antagonist. J Exp Med 201(8):1307–1318
Calvi LM, Adams GB, Weibrecht KW, Weber JM, Olson DP, Knight MC, Martin RP, Schipani E, Divieti P, Bringhurst FR, Milner LA, Kronenberg HM, Scadden DT (2003) Osteoblastic cells regulate the haematopoietic stem cell niche. Nature 425(6960):841–846
Demirer T, Ayli M, Ozcan M, Gunel N, Haznedar R, Dagli M, Fen T, Genc Y, Dincer S, Arslan O, Gürman G, Demirer S, Ozet G, Uysal A, Konuk N, Ilhan O, Koc H, Akan H (2002) Mobilization of peripheral blood stem cells with chemotherapy and recombinant human granulocyte colony-stimulating factor (rhG-CSF): a randomized evaluation of different doses of rhG-CSF. Br J Haematol 116(2):468–474
DiPersio JF, Stadtmauer EA, Nademanee A, Micallef IN, Stiff PJ, Kaufman JL, Maziarz RT, Hosing C, Früehauf S, Horwitz M, Cooper D, Bridger G, Calandra G (2009a) Plerixafor and G-CSF versus placebo and G-CSF to mobilize hematopoietic stem cells for autologous stem cell transplantation in patients with multiple myeloma. Blood 113(23):5720–5726
DiPersio JF, Micallef IN, Stiff PJ, Bolwell BJ, Maziarz RT, Jacobsen E, Nademanee A, McCarty J, Bridger G, Calandra G (2009b) Phase III prospective randomized double-blind placebo-controlled trial of plerixafor plus granulocyte colony-stimulating factor compared with placebo plus granulocyte colony-stimulating factor for autologous stem-cell mobilization and transplantation for patients with non-Hodgkin's lymphoma. J Clin Oncol 27(28):4767–4773
Dugan MJ, Maziarz RT, Bensinger WI, Nademanee A, Liesveld J, Badel K, Dehner C, Gibney C, Bridger G, Calandra G (2010) Safety and preliminary efficacy of plerixafor (Mozobil) in combination with chemotherapy and G-CSF: an open-label, multicenter, exploratory trial in patients with multiple myeloma and non-Hodgkin's lymphoma undergoing stem cell mobilization. Bone Marrow Transplant 45(1):39–47
Flomenberg N, Devine SM, Dipersio JF, Liesveld JL, McCarty JM, Rowley SD, Vesole DH, Badel K, Calandra G (2005) The use of AMD3100 plus G-CSF for autologous hematopoietic progenitor cell mobilization is superior to G-CSF alone. Blood 106(5):1867–1874
Gertz M (2010) Current status of stem cell mobilization. Br J Haematol 150(6):647–662
Gunzer K, Clarisse B, Lheureux S, Delcambre C, Joly F (2010) Contribution of glycosylated recombinant human granulocyte colony-stimulating factor (lenograstim) use in current cancer treatment: review of clinical data. Expert Opin Biol Ther 10(4):615–630
Haas R, Möhle R, Frühauf S, Goldschmidt H, Witt B, Flentje M, Wannenmacher M, Hunstein W (1994) Patient characteristics associated with successful mobilizing and autografting of peripheral blood progenitor cells in malignant lymphoma. Blood 83(12):3787–3794
Herbert KE, Prince HM, Ritchie DS, Seymour JF (2010) The role of Ancestim (recombinant human stem-cell factor, rhSCF) in hematopoietic stem cell mobilization and stem cell reconstitution. Expert Opin Biol Ther 10(1):113–125
Isidori A, Tani M, Bonifazi F, Zinzani P, Curti A, Motta MR, Rizzi S, Giudice V, Farese O, Rovito M, Alinari L, Conte R, Baccarani M, Lemoli RM (2005) Phase II study of a single pegfilgrastim injection as an adjunct to chemotherapy to mobilize stem cells into the peripheral blood of pretreated lymphoma patients. Haematologica 90(2):225–231
Kalaycio M, Rybicki L, Pohlman B, Sobecks R, Andresen S, Kuczkowski E, Bolwell B (2006) Risk factors before autologous stem-cell transplantation for lymphoma predict for secondary myelodysplasia and acute myelogenous leukemia. J Clin Oncol 24(22):3604–3610

Kang HJ, Kim HS, Koo BK, Kim YJ, Lee D, Sohn DW, Oh BH, Park YB (2007) Intracoronary infusion of the mobilized peripheral blood stem cell by G-CSF is better than mobilization alone by G-CSF for improvement of cardiac function and remodeling: 2-year follow-up results of the Myocardial Regeneration and Angiogenesis in Myocardial Infarction with G-CSF and Intra-Coronary Stem Cell Infusion (MAGIC Cell) 1 trial. Am Heart J 153(2):237–238

Lapidot T, Kollet O (2010) The brain–bone–blood triad: traffic lights for stem-cell homing and mobilization. Hematology Am Soc Hematol Educ Program 2010:1–6

Lemoli RM, D'Addio A (2008) Hematopoietic stem cell mobilization. Haematologica 93(3):321–324

Lévesque JP, Helwani FM, Winkler IG (2010) The endosteal 'osteoblastic' niche and its role in hematopoietic stem cell homing and mobilization. Leukemia 24(12):1979–1992

Lorenzini S, Isidori A, Catani L, Gramenzi A, Talarico S, Bonifazi F, Giudice V, Conte R, Baccarani M, Bernardi M, Forbes SJ, Lemoli RM, Andreone P (2008) Stem cell mobilization and collection in patients with liver cirrhosis. Aliment Pharmacol Therap 27(10):932–939

McCredie KB, Hersh EM, Freireich EJ (1971) Cells capable of colony formation in the peripheral blood of man. Science 171:293–294

Narayanasami U, Kanteti R, Morelli J, Klekar A, Al-Olama A, Keating C, O'Connor C, Berkman E, Erban JK, Sprague KA, Miller KB, Schenkein DP (2001) Randomized trial of filgrastim versus chemotherapy and filgrastim mobilization of hematopoietic progenitor cells for rescue in autologous transplantation. Blood 98(7):2059–2064

Pelus LM, Fukuda S (2008) Chemokine-mobilized adult stem cells; defining a better hematopoietic graft. Leukemia 22:466–473

Rafii S, Lyden D (2003) Therapeutic stem and progenitor cell transplantation for organ vascularization and regeneration. Nat Med 9:702–712

Schmitz N, Linch DC, Dreger P, Goldstone AH, Boogaerts MA, Ferrant A, Demuynck HM, Link H, Zander A, Barge A (1996) Randomised trial of filgrastim-mobilised peripheral blood progenitor cell transplantation versus autologous bone-marrow transplantation in lymphoma patients. Lancet 347:353–357

Selleri C, Montuori N, Ricci P, Visconte V, Carriero MV, Sidenius N, Serio B, Blasi F, Rotoli B, Rossi G, Ragno P (2005) Involvement of the urokinase-type plasminogen activator receptor in hematopoietic stem cell mobilization. Blood 105(5):2198–2205

Shepherd RM, Capoccia BJ, Devine SM, Dipersio J, Trinkaus KM, Ingram D, Link DC (2006) Angiogenic cells can be rapidly mobilized and efficiently harvested from the blood following treatment with AMD3100. Blood 108(12):3662–3667

Tesio M, Golan K, Corso S, Giordano S, Schajnovitz A, Vagima Y, Shivtiel S, Kalinkovich A, Caione L, Gammaitoni L, Laurenti E, Buss EC, Shezen E, Itkin T, Kollet O, Petit I, Trumpp A, Christensen J, Aglietta M, Piacibello W, Lapidot T (2011). Enhanced c-Met activity promotes G-CSF-induced mobilization of hematopoietic progenitor cells via ROS signaling. Blood 117(2):419–428

Wilson A, Laurenti E, Oser G, van der Wath RC, Blanco-Bose W, Jaworski M, Offner S, Dunant CF, Eshkind L, Bockamp E, Lió P, Macdonald HR, Trumpp A (2008) Hematopoietic stem cells reversibly switch from dormancy to self-renewal during homeostasis and repair. Cell 135(6):1118–1129

Winkler IG, Levesque JP (2006) Mechanisms of hematopoietic stem cell mobilization: when innate immunity assails the cells that make blood and bone. Exp Hematol 34:996–1009

Wright DE, Wagers AJ, Gulati AP, Johnson FL, Weissman LL (2001) Physiological migration of hematopoietic stem and progenitor cells. Science 294:1933–1936

Yamazaki S, Iwama A, Takayanagi S, Eto K, Ema H, Nakauchi H (2009) TGF-beta as a candidate bone marrow niche signal to induce hematopoietic stem cell hybernation. Blood 113(6):1250–1256

Chapter 7

Status and Impact of Research on Human Pluripotent Stem Cells: Cell Lines and Their Use in Published Research

Peter Löser, Anke Guhr, Sabine Kobold, Anna M. Wobus, and Andreas Kurtz

Abstract Research on human pluripotent stem cells is rapidly progressing. In the present chapter the current state of research on human embryonic stem cells (hESCs) and human induced pluripotent stem cells (hiPSCs) is analyzed with respect to the number of publicly disclosed cell lines and to the extent and impact of published scientific work involving these cells. Our data reveal that activities in both research fields have markedly increased over the past years and that there are no indications for a diminished role of hESCs in international research as a consequence of the availableness of hiPSCs. Moreover, recent data presented here confirm the global dominance of only a few hESC lines for research, and preferences for distinct hESCs in different countries. Possible causes for these phenomena are discussed.

Keywords Human embryonic stem cells · Human induced pluripotent stem cells · Pre-implantation genetic diagnosis · Cell lines · Stem cell bank · Pluripotent

Introduction

Since the establishment of the first human embryonic stem cells (hESCs) in 1998 (Thomson et al., 1998), there has been an enormous scientific interest in hESCs because these cells have the capacity to proliferate indefinitely and to differentiate into many, if not all, human cell types. On the other hand, derivation of these cells involves the destruction of human embryos, and therefore research on hESCs has been a matter of debate for more than one decade which resulted in variable national legislations on this research. A novel source for human pluripotent stem cells (hPSCs) was made accessible to the scientific community with the first generation of human induced pluripotent stem cells (hiPSC) in 2007 (Takahashi et al., 2007; Yu et al., 2007). Generation of hiPSCs does not require the destruction of human embryos and is therefore considered as ethically less problematic. It is believed that hiPSCs are highly similar, if not identical, to hESCs, although recent data partially challenged this concept (Lister et al., 2011). However, a public controversy has started with the generation of hiPSCs whether and for which purposes hESC research is still justifiable and if hiPSCs may replace hESCs in the short term.

Currently, applications of hiPSCs come to the fore, such as their use for disease modelling (Ben-Yosef et al., 2008; Saha and Hurlbut, 2011), drug screening (Ebert and Svendsen, 2010) and toxicology research (Wobus and Löser, 2011). In the recent past, the FDA granted several permissions to initiate clinical trials involving hESC-derived cells (Alper, 2009; Connor, 2010; Anon, 2011). Consequently, both hESCs and hiPSCs are in high demand as an object of research and for applications in the short and medium term. The present chapter seeks to substantiate the current discussion by providing a comparative view on the current status of research on pluripotent stem cells. Comprehensive information on the number of existing hESC and hiPSC lines on a global level is presented, and the extent and impact of research on both

P. Löser (✉)
Roberts Koch Institute, DGZ-Ring1, D-13086, Berlin, Germany
e-mail: loeserP@rki.de

hESCs and hiPSCs is analyzed on the basis of about 1400 research papers. Moreover, recent data on the use of specific hESC lines in international research is provided.

Overview of Currently Existing hESC and hiPSC Lines

Several efforts have been undertaken to compile data on existing human embryonic and induced pluripotent stem cell lines and make them available to the scientific community. Accordingly, several registries on human pluripotent stem cells were established, for example in the United States, the United Kingdom or by the European Union (Luong et al., 2008; Borstlap et al., 2010). In contrast to stem cell banks that store biological materials (e. g., human embryonic or adult stem cell lines) and establish procedures for uniform and standardized characterization, cryopreservation, documentation and distribution of the deposited material, stem cell registries aim at the provision of comprehensive scientific and procurement information associated with stem cell lines.

In case of human pluripotent stem cell lines, only partial information on derivation, culture and characterization of many individual cell lines is available from the literature. Therefore, stem cell registries aim at the organization, integration and documentation of *all* data on a pluripotent stem cell line. In case of hESC lines, the registries may also provide important information on the provenance of the cell lines and the circumstances of their derivation. Indeed, one objective of the establishment of registries such as the *hESCreg* and the Registry of the *UK Stem Cell Bank* was to avoid the redundant derivation of hESC lines from human embryos thereby limiting embryo destruction for research purposes. In addition, the installation of hESC registries may also be owed to the necessity to enforce political precepts. The establishment of the NIH registries in 2001 and 2009 falls into this category.

Currently, there are three major stem cell registries worldwide that provide data on a multitude of existing hESC lines. The actual NIH Human Embryonic Stem Cell Registry was established in response to Executive Order 13505, issued on March 9, 2009, and following the principles developed in the NIH Guidelines for Human Stem Cell Research (Taymor and Scott, 2009). In this registry, those hESC lines are listed that are eligible for use in NIH-supported research under the present guidelines, and cell lines listed in this registry must meet all requirements of these guidelines. Additional information, e. g. with respect to characterization data, culture protocols or availability of cell lines is not provided. Currently (February, 2011), 86 hESC lines are eligible for use in NIH-funded projects, 69 hESC lines are under review and 59 cell lines are in a draft status. 53 lines were not approved for the registry.

The Stem Cell Registry of the European Union (hESCreg, Borstlap et al., 2008) was established in 2007 under the 6th European Union Framework Research Programme as a mere hESC registry, but lately also several hiPSCs lines were included. hESCreg seeks to provide information on derivation and culture methods of pluripotent stem cells, on characterisation profiles and availability of cell lines, their banking status, as well as on research projects involving pluripotent stem cells. Currently, hESCreg contains information on 667 hESC lines and 18 additional sub-lines derived from those (Borstlap et al., 2008).

The currently most comprehensive pluripotent stem cell registry is the University of Massachusetts (UMass) International Stem Cell Registry that was initiated in 2008 (Isasi and Knoppers, 2009). Its mission is to provide a searchable, comprehensive database that includes published and validated unpublished information on all hESC and hiPSC cell lines. This registry contains information on cell lines in the format of a specific profile that presents a multitude of data, e. g., on derivation, presence of pluripotency-associated markers, differentiation characteristics and availability of the cell line. For many cell lines, blank informed consent sheets used in the context of deriving the respective cell line are accessible via the registries' web page. Importantly, this registry is also linking scientific publications to specific cell lines via a searchable literature database thereby providing important information on the use of cell lines in research projects. By February 2011, the UMass Stem Cell Registry contained at least some information on 1039 original hESC lines and 13 sub-lines derived from those. A summary of hESC registries, some of which were established in the context of a specific stem cell bank, is given in Table 7.1.

The number of hESC lines is growing steadily, and the derivation frequency of novel hiPSC lines reported

Table 7.1 Summary of several currently existing stem cell registries. Some were installed with the establishment of the respective stem cell bank

European Human Embryonic Stem Cell Registry	http://www.hescreg.eu/
Korean Stem Cell Bank	http://www.koreastemcellbank.org/
NIH Human Embryonic Stem Cell Registry	http://stemcells.nih.gov/research/registry/
Sidney IVF Stem Cell Bank	http://www.sydneyivfstemcells.com/AboutUs/Ourstemcells/tabid/648/Default.aspx
Singapore Stem Cell Bank	http://www.sscc.a-star.edu.sg/stemCellBank.php
Spanish Stem Cell Bank	http://www.isciii.es/htdocs/terapia/terapia_lineas.jsp
Stem Ride International Stem Cell Bank	http://stemride.com/Stem_Cell_Bank.htm
Stem Cell Lines derived in Switzerland	http://www.bag.admin.ch/themen/medizin/03301/03305/index.html
UK Stem Cell Bank	http://www.ukstemcellbank.org.uk/
University of Massachusetts (UMASS) International Stem Cell Registry	http://www.umassmed.edu/iscr/index.aspx
Wisconsin International Stem Cell Bank	http://www.iscr-admin.com/?Action=select%20sc%20for%20view

in the literature is rapidly increasing. In the past, we have undertaken efforts to provide and summarize current information on publically reported hESC lines (Guhr et al., 2006; Löser et al., 2010). While only 171 of 414 known hESC lines were reported in the scientific literature by 2005, 694 of 1071 known hESC lines had been published in peer-reviewed scientific articles in English language journals by the end of 2009. An overview on the number of hESC lines, the number of institutions involved in hESC derivation and the countries of origin as determined by the end of 2009 is given in Table 7.2. At present (February, 2011), the number of original hESC lines has increased to at least 1313. 849 of these (64.6%) have been reported in scientific papers so far, and characterization data for 733 hESC lines are available from the scientific literature. In addition, at least 37 sub-lines derived from original hESC lines have been reported up to now.

Whereas the number and characteristics of hESC lines are well documented both in the literature and in several registries, there is only very limited and less comprehensive information on the scale of currently existing hiPSC lines. For example, only 156 hiPSC lines are listed in the UMASS registry, and hESreg provides information on only 24 of these cell lines. However, data on 777 hiPSC lines were presented in a recent report on the documentation of teratoma formation of human pluripotent stem cell lines (Müller et al., 2010). Our own analysis of papers reporting experimental work involving hiPSCs and published by the end of 2009 revealed the existence of at least 679 hiPSC lines produced at 36 institutions of 9 countries (see Table 7.2).

Several reasons may account for this obvious lack of public documentation of hiPSC lines. First, the documentation of hiPSC characteristics in respective papers is often only fragmentary. This lack of information results in uncertainty about the number of hiPSC lines derived in the respective study and their true pluripotency. Second, although far from being simplistic, the generation of hiPSC lines is not as demanding as hESC derivation since no human embryos are involved. In addition, derivation of hiPSC lines does not require collaboration with IVF clinics to get access to early human embryos. Moreover, whereas the establishment of a single hESC line usually requires the use of several human embryos, multiple hiPSC clones giving rise to several hiPSC lines can be derived in a single reprogramming experiment. Thus, while the derivation of novel hESC lines may be subject to a separate scientific report even 12 years after the first hESC derivation, hiPSC production is now reported as a routine process in many papers in the context of a specific scientific question. Third, ethical and regulatory considerations are fundamentally different. In contrast to the derivation of hESC lines, which is strictly regulated or even prohibited in many countries, there are no special regulations on hiPSC derivation in most countries and only common ethical principles of experimental work involving donated human materials have to be considered.

Consequently, many laboratories are producing their own hiPSC lines. This is documented by the fact that in 73 of 102 studies on hiPSCs (71.6%) published from 2007 to 2009 in each case at least one hiPSC line was produced. In contrast, only 37 of 291

Table 7.2 Overview of publicly reported hESC and hiPSC lines as determined by the end of 2009. Shown are numbers of cell lines derived in a specific country and the number of institutions that reported successful derivation of hESC lines. For hESCs, the number of cell lines reported in peer-reviewed English-language journals is also shown, while all hiPSC lines were published in the scientific literature. Note that hESC lines derived at the Reproductive Genetics Institute (Chicago, IL), which are partially distributed by Stemride International Limited, were assigned to the United States. hESC lines from ES Cell. International Pte Ltd were assigned to Singapore. Stem cell lines derived from parthenogenetic embryos were not included. A detailed list of the hESC lines can be found in Löser et al. (2010)

Country	Number of hESC lines reported	Number of institutions involved in hESC derivation	Number of hESC lines published in peer-reviewed papers	Number of hiPSC lines reported	Number of institutions involved in hiPSC derivation
Australia	19	3	14		
Belgium	29	3	23		
Brazil	1	1	0		
Canada	4	2	2	6	2
China (incl. Taiwan)	236	13	228	57	5
Czech Republic	7	1	4		
Denmark	31	4	14		
Finland	10	2	5		
France	20	4	0		
Germany	0	0	0	13	2
India	15	5	5		
Iran	6	1	6		
Israel	14	3	12	12	1
Japan	3	1	3	79	3
Korea	37	5	35		
Netherlands	4	1	4		
Russia	16	2	5		
Singapore	15	2	15		
Spain	18	3	13	54	2
Sweden	90	3	45		
Switzerland	1	1	1	8	1
Thailand	1	1	1		
Turkey	18	1	7		
UK	42	8	28	84	3
USA	434	17	224	366	17
Total	**1071**	**87**	**694**	**679**	**36**

original hESC research papers (12.7%) published in the first seven years of hESC research (1998–2005) involved the derivation of novel hESC lines. This early diversification in hiPSC lines may be that reason for an apparently lesser need for exchange of hiPSC lines in international research, resulting in a less comprehensive documentation of these cells in national and international registries.

One promising approach of research involving human pluripotent stem cells is the study of disease phenotypes on the molecular and cellular levels to gain a deeper understanding of disease processes, to identify potential drug targets and to develop novel cures. hESC lines derived from embryos diagnosed for monogenetic diseases by pre-implantation genetic diagnosis (PGD) potentially allow investigation of the respective genetic defect and its effects on early embryo development and organogenesis, thereby potentially unrevealing disease mechanisms (Ben-Yosef et al., 2008). Accordingly, the number of such "disease-specific" hESC line increased steadily over the past years. By the end of 2005, only 27 of known 414 hESC lines harboured a disease-specific genetic alteration (Guhr et al., 2006). However, this number increased to at least 56 by 2008 (Sermon et al., 2009) and 116 by November 2009 (Löser et al., 2010, Table 7.3). Currently, there is evidence for at least 166

Table 7.3 Overview of hESC lines with mutations linked to inheritable genetic human disorders as determined by November 2009. For further details, see Löser et al. (2010)

Genetic disorder	Number of hESC lines
Adrenoleukodystrophy	1
Alpha-Thalassaemia	2
Beta-Thalassaemia	7
Charcot-Marie tooth disease 1A (CMT1A)	2
Cystic fibrosis (CF)	15
Dystrophya myotonica type 1 (DM1)	6
Fabry syndrome	1
Facioscapulohumeral (FSH) muscular dystrophy	9
Familial adenomatous polyposis (FAP)	3
Familial breast cancer	1
Fanconi anaemia	1
Fragile X Syndrome (FX)	9
Hemophilia A	1
Huntington's disease (HD)	11
Marfan syndrome (MFS)	4
Multiple endocrine neoplasia, type 1	2
Multiple endocrine neoplasia, type 2	4
Muscular dystrophy, type Becker	1
Muscular dystrophy, type Duchenne	4
Muscular dystrophy, Emery Dreifuss	4
Myotubular myopathy (MTM), cross-linked	2
Neurofibromatosis type 1	7
Ocular albinism	2
Osteogenesis imperfecta type 1	1
Pelizaeus-Merzbacher disease (PMLD)	1
Popliteal Pterygium syndrome (PPS)	1
Sandhoff disease	3
Sickle cell anaemia	3
Spinal muscular atrophy type 1 (SMA1)	2
Spinocerebellar ataxia type 2 (SCA2)	1
Spinocerebellar ataxia type 7 (SCA7)	1
Torsion dystonia (DYT1)	2
Tuberous sclerosis	3
Total	**116**

disease-specific cell lines, which is 12.6% of all hESC lines publically reported so far.

However, disease-specific hESCs are usually derived from embryos diagnosed for monogenetic disorders and, consequently, hESC derived cell models can only mirror a small fraction of human diseases. In contrast, hiPSCs can be derived from patients afflicted by much more diseases that have, for example, polygenic origins and poorly understood or even unknown causes. In the last three years, dozens of disease-specific hiPSC lines were generated and partially shown to model certain aspects of the respective disease. Table 7.4 gives an overview of hiPSC lines that were derived from patients with specific disorders by the end of 2009. Until now (February, 2011), additional disease-specific hiPSC lines have been established, for example from patients affected by Long QT Syndrome (Moretti et al., 2010) or Leopard Syndrome (Carvajal-Vergara et al., 2010). With respect to disease-specific hiPSC lines, the establishment of an international registry and respective stem cell banks would be of major interest since modelling of rare diseases requires access to special patient groups. The generation of hiPSC lines may be difficult in these cases, for example due to older age of patients. While the establishment of a registry for disease-specific hESC lines is under discussion (Sermon et al., 2009), directed efforts to establish registries and stem cells banks with a focus on disease-specific hiPSC lines have not been initiated yet.

Extent of Research on Human Pluripotent Stem Cells

Research on human pluripotent stem cells has been a matter of debate over the last decade. Specifically, reservations with regard to hESC research by fractions of the general public and the policy community as well as funding restrictions may have caused a delay of this research field. On the other hand, research involving hiPSCs is highly welcomed even by those fractions of the public and the policy communities that have regarded hESC research as critical for ethical, religious or ideological reasons, whereas hiPSC research is considered to be "free" of ethical problems. Some researchers and politicians state that hiPSCs would replace hESCs in research in near future. Since the public debate on research on human pluripotent stem cells may have far reaching consequences for national stem cell policies and funding opportunities it is important to substantiate it by data that provide insight in the extent and impact of research on pluripotent stem cells.

Table 7.4 Overview of hiPSC lines derived from diseased patients as determined by the end of 2009

Genetic disorders	Number of hiPSC lines
Beta-Thalassemia	6
Down syndrome (trisomy 21)	5
Dyskeratosis congenita	2
Familial dysautonomia (FD)	4
Gaucher disease type III	2
Huntington's disease (HD)	3
Lesch-Nyhan syndrome (carrier)	12
Muscular dystrophy, type Becker	2
Muscular dystrophy, type Duchenne	2
Rett syndrome	1
Severe combined immunodeficiency (ADA-SCID)	2
Shwachmann-Bodian-Diamond syndrome	3
Sickle Cell Anemia	3
Spinal muscular atrophy type 1 (SMAI)	2
Sub-total	**49**
Other Diseases	
Amyotrophic lateral sclerosis (ALS)	3
Diabetes mellitus type 1	5
Juvenile diabetes mellitus	5
Parkinson's disease	29
Polycythemia vera	9
Primary myelofibrosis (PMF)	2
Sub-total	**53**

Table 7.5 Number of original hESC research papers published 1998–2009 and indexed in the PubMed database. Also shown is the share of papers from a specific country in the total number of research papers. Assignment of papers to a country was according to the address of the corresponding author. Note that 46 hESC research papers published online ahead of print in 2009, but printed in 2010, are not included. For details of search methodology, see Guhr et al. (2006)

Country	Number of hESC research papers	% of total hESC research papers
Australia	52	3.8
Austria	1	0.1
Belgium	17	1.2
Brazil	1	0.1
Canada	40	2.9
China (incl. Taiwan)	69	5.0
Czech Republic	7	0.5
Denmark	10	0.7
Estonia	1	0.1
Finland	15	1.1
France	18	1.3
Germany	23	1.7
Hungary	2	0.1
India	17	1.2
Iran	10	0.7
Israel	81	5.9
Italy	12	0.9
Japan	50	3.6
Korea	70	5.1
Netherlands	16	1.2
Portugal	1	0.1
Romania	1	0.1
Russia	6	0.4
Singapore	71	5.2
Spain	18	1.3
Sweden	54	3.9
Switzerland	8	0.6
Thailand	1	0.1
Turkey	5	0.4
United Kingdom	112	8.1
United States	588	42.7
Total	**1377**	**100**

With regard to hESCs, we and others have undertaken efforts to systematically examine international research activities in this field. In some countries, such as Germany, all ongoing research on hESCs has to be published in a governmental registry. In other countries such as Great Britain, only projects involving destruction of embryos for hESC derivation have to be disclosed to the public. In some cases, information on hESC research is available only due to the obligation to publically disclose funding decisions. Thus, it is impossible to gain insight into all hESC research projects currently performed worldwide and to identify institutions involved in this research. To assess hESC research activities we (Guhr et al., 2006; Löser et al., 2008, 2010) and others (Owen-Smith and McCormick, 2006; Levine, 2008) analyzed research papers in the hESC field. Although this practise only reflects past research activities, it may be suitable to draw conclusion on the impact, for example, of national stem cell and funding policies on research.

Results of a recent analysis of hESC research papers published from 1998 to 2009 in English language peer-reviewed journals are shown in Table 7.5. According to these results, hESC research has been carried out in at least 31 countries. Most of the research papers came from groups based in the United States (42.7%), followed by groups from the United Kingdom (8.1%), Israel (5.9%), Singapore (5.2%), Korea (5.1) and China

7 Status and Impact of Research on Human Pluripotent Stem Cells: Cell Lines and Their Use in Published Research

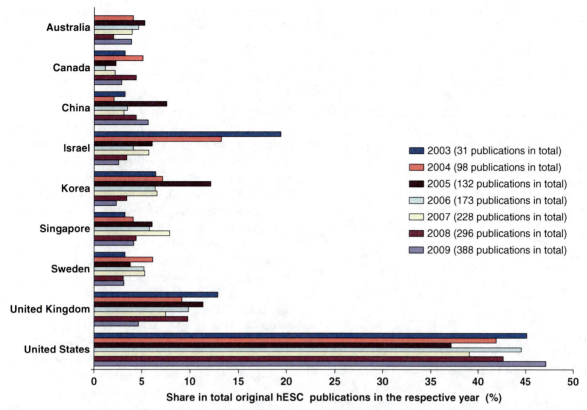

Fig. 7.1 Share of published hESC research from selected countries on the total number of hESC papers published worldwide from 1998 to 2009 in peer reviewed English language journals. Only the 20 countries with at least 10 hESC papers were included, although hESC research is being performed in at least 11 additional countries. Numbers in *brackets* refer to the number of hESC research papers originating from the respective country. Assignment of a paper to a country was done according to the corresponding authors address. Only work involving experimental use of hESCs was included. Reviews, comments and papers reporting previously published methods or legal and ethical aspects of hESC research have not been regarded

(5%) underlining the leading position of US research in the hESC field. Others also reported a leading position of US research in the hESC field, but perceived either a productivity gap (Owen-Smith and McCormick, 2006) or underperformance (Levine, 2008) of US-based hESC research which were assumed to be due partially to the restrictive NIH funding policy.

However, as shown in Table 7.5 and Fig. 7.1, the United States maintained their leading position in hESC research over the last years. Since 2003, approximately 40% of publications in this field originated from US-based groups, although the total extent of hESC research increased dramatically worldwide. In contrast, research from other countries such as Israel, Sweden or the United Kingdom did not increase to the same extent as international research did. It will be interesting to see whether the altered stem cell funding policy will further strengthen the US position in hESC research since its implementation in 2009.

While research on hESCs is being performed for more than a decade, research on hiPSCs only started in 2007 with the first successful derivation of hiPSC lines (Takahashi et al., 2007; Yu et al., 2007). Since then, research on hiPSCs has spread into many laboratories, and the number of publications markedly increased (see Table 7.6). By the end of 2009, there were at least 102 publications involving derivation and/or use of hiPSCs that originated from research groups in 11 countries. Nearly 60% of hiPSC papers came from US-based laboratories, while about 16% of publications resulted from work of Japanese groups. It should be noted that some nations with a relatively strong position in hESC research such as the United Kingdom, Sweden, Australia, Singapore or Korea did

Table 7.6 Number of hiPSC research papers published 2007–2009 and indexed in the PubMed database. Also shown is the share of papers from a specific country on the total number of research papers. Assignment of papers to a country was done according to the address of the corresponding author. For details of search methodology, see Löser et al. (2010)

Country	Number of hiPSC research papers	% of Total hiPSC research papers
Canada	3	2.9
China	7	6.9
France	1	1.0
Germany	3	2.9
Iran	1	1.0
Israel	1	1.0
Japan	16	15.7
Spain	5	4.9
Switzerland	1	1.0
United Kingdom	4	3.9
United States	60	58.8
Total	**102**	**100.0**

not play a similar role in this novel research field until 2009. It is a matter of speculation whether this delay is caused by a relatively small basic stem cell research community in these countries, by funding restrictions, or other reasons. In 2010, research on hiPSCs expanded further. While 86 hiPSC research papers were published in 2009 in peer-reviewed English language journals, this number increased to at least 155 in 2010 (preliminary data), with 23 additional studies published online (but did not yet appear in print). Notably, of the said 155 original research papers, at least 119 (76.7%) also involved the parallel use of hESCs (e.g., for investigating a scientific question in hESCs before studying hiPSCs) or the use of hESC-derived materials (mainly for comparative studies). This shows that both research fields have further expanded, are highly inter-connected, and partially overlap while there is no indication for decline of research on hESCs due to increased research activities in the hiPSC field.

Impact of International Research on Human Pluripotent Stem Cells

Publication numbers do not necessarily present a measure for impact of the respective research on the field. For example, the number of hESC research papers published by Chinese groups now exceeds the number of publications from Australia, Canada or Japan (see Table 7.5). Does this quantitative output of research performed in a specific country reflect the impact of this research? To answer this question, we and others analyzed the average ISI Journal Citation Impact Factors of journals that published experimental hESC work (Owen-Smith and McCormick, 2006; Löser et al., 2008). These analyses revealed that papers from US groups were published in journals with a significantly higher average impact factor than studies from other countries. This phenomenon was confirmed in our more recent study (Löser et al., 2010): While the weighted average 5-year impact factor (2004–2008) of journals that published hESC studies was 7.422, work from US-based groups were printed in journals with an average impact factor of 9.123. Accordingly, work from groups in other countries such as China or Korea was published in less influential journals. An isolated investigation of actual hESC papers (published in print in 2009) revealed that this trend further stabilized. Again, the weighted average impact factor of journals publishing hESC research further increased to 7.880, but studies from the United States were published in journals with an average impact factor of 9.353. In contrast, studies from Singapore, Korea, China or even the United Kingdom appeared in journals with a lower average impact factor (4.889, 5.389, 5.472 and 6.241, respectively).

However, the journal impact factor may not be representative for the quality and impact of *individual* articles published in this journal. Additionally it was argued that the journal selection and publication process reflects publication bias that makes it easier for Western and English-speaking scientists to publish their work in highly influential journals. An alternative measure to estimate the impact of research from a specific country is the actual citation frequency of these studies. Analyzing the citation frequencies of ~950 original hESC research papers published between 2004 and 2008 revealed that papers were cited at an average of 38.5 citations per paper by the end of 2009. Articles published before 2003 were omitted from the analysis to avoid an excessive impact of pioneering hESC work (e. g., the Thomson paper had about 3,400 citations by the end of 2009). With respect to citation frequencies up to 2009, papers from US-based groups overperformed (51.7 citations per paper) while papers from countries such as China, Korea and Singapore were

Table 7.7 Citation frequencies of papers from specific countries reporting experimental use of hESCs and published from 2003 to 2008. Citation analysis was performed in June 2010 for the reference date end of 2009 using the Scopus literature database

Origin country of hESC papers	Number of hESC papers (2003–2008)	Total citations until 2009	Average citations until 2009
United States	395	20402	51.7
Netherlands	13	613	47.2
Israel	57	2682	47.1
Canada	29	1209	41.7
United Kingdom	91	3448	37.9
Italy	7	257	36.7
Japan	30	1048	34.9
Sweden	42	1134	27.0
Singapore	54	1452	26.9
Denmark	6	146	24.3
Australia	34	813	23.9
Iran	7	159	22.7
Korea	61	1369	22.4
Germany	17	368	21.6
Finland	8	171	21.4
Czech Republic	4	80	20.0
China (incl. Taiwan)	43	748	17.4
Belgium	10	165	16.5
France	9	134	14.9
Spain	13	189	14.5
Russia	4	43	10.8
Switzerland	4	41	10.3
Hungary	1	7	7.0
Turkey	4	27	6.8
Estonia	1	6	6.0
India	11	60	5.5
Romania	1	0	0.0
Total	**956**	**36771**	**38.5**

less often cited in the same period (17.4, 22.4 and 26.9 citations, respectively, Table 7.7). Consequently, the publication of hESC research papers in more influential journals is obviously paralleled by their (average) appreciation by the scientific community. However, it should be considered that citation frequency may be also influenced by non-scientific factors such as the prominence of a researcher or the existence of citation networks.

With respect to hiPSC research papers, the investigation of citation frequencies is not yet an appropriate measure to weight the influence of research since the large majority of hiPSC research papers is too new to allow for individual citation analyses. Therefore, only the impact factors of journals publishing hiPSC work was investigated so far. The weighted average impact factor of those journals that published original hiPSC research papers by the end of 2009 was extraordinarily high (15.992). Even when pioneering work (Takahashi et al., 2007; Yu et al., 2007) is omitted, the impact factor remains at 15.672. This might be due to the large interest of the scientific community in this novel research field, but also by the high expectations of the non-scientific public in the potential of hiPSC research. As in the case of hESC research, studies from US-based groups were published in more influential journals (weighted average impact factor 17.555) than studies from other countries with an active hiPSC research, such as Japan and China (9.972 and 8.983, respectively). The strong position of US research in the hiPSC field may be explained by the depth of basic and translational science, the broad and variable funding mechanisms, but also by the leading position of the United States in hESC research. Other, non-scientific factors for the US leadership in hiPSC research such as obstruction of papers from non-US authors by a deliberate delay of publication were also discussed as potential reasons (Aldhous, 2010). However, when analyzing the period from manuscript submission to online publication of 102 hiPSC articles published through 2009, we did not find any sign for a delay in publication of studies from non-US-based groups in the field of hiPSC research. While the average duration from submission of a manuscript to its publication was 99.9 days at average for studies from US groups, the duration was 99.7 days for studies originating from groups outside the United States. Although quantitative and qualitative publication dominance has a trend-setting effect, and thus provides an inherent advantage for continuing high impact publications, it seems unlikely to us that the US leadership in the hiPSC field is substantially caused by other than scientific reasons.

Use of Human Embryonic Stem Cell Lines in International Research

As mentioned above, by the end of 2009 hiPSC lines were derived in many laboratories and generally used in these laboratories without extensive exchange of cell lines. In contrast, although the number of available

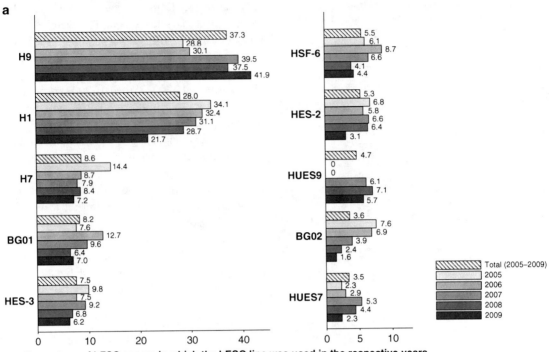
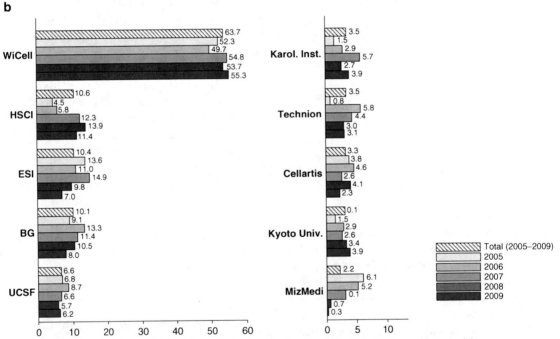

Fig. 7.2 Use of hESC lines in research published from 2005 to 2009. (**a**) Share of hESC research papers in which a specific hESC line was used (in %) on the total number of hESC research papers in the respective year(s). Only data for the 10 most widely used hESC lines were incorporated. Note that in many papers several hESC lines were used. (**b**) Percentage of hESC research papers in which cell lines from the indicated provider were used. WiCell, WiCell Institute, Madison, WI, USA; HSCI, Harvard Stem Cell Institute, Cambridge, MA, USA; ESI, ES Cell International Pte Ltd, Singapore; BG, Bresagen, Division

hESC lines has largely increased over the last decade, international research is dominated by only a few hESC lines. The first study in which the use of hESC lines in international research was investigated on the basis of a comprehensive review of the literature, reported a preferential use of only a few hESC lines, namely those generated by the Thomson group in 1998 and distributed by the WiCell Institute. By the end of 2005, the cell lines H9, H1 and H7 (all of WiCell) were used in 34.9, 29.5 and 11.7%, respectively, of all studies reporting experimental use of hESCs (Guhr et al., 2006).

In the following years, several other studies also analyzed the distribution and/or use of hESC lines. For example, McCormick and co-workers investigated the shipping of cell lines from two providers in the United States (WiCell Institute and Harvard Stem Cell Institute) and found that a total of 1,662 vials of cell lines of these providers had been shipped to groups in 36 nations by the end of 2007, most of them to groups in the United States (McCormick et al., 2009). In a follow-up study the same authors analyzed shipping of the then NIH-approved 21 hESC lines by the then National Stem Cell Bank (NSCB) at WiCell (Scott et al., 2009). According to these data, three cell lines (H1, H7 and H9) accounted for 86.4% of vials distributed by the NSCB. Moreover, these authors reported that the cell line H9 was used in more than 80% of all hESC studies investigated, while H1 and H7 were applied in 60.9 and 24.2% of hESC studies, respectively. Our own study (Löser et al., 2010) principally confirmed the preferential use of WiCell lines, but to a considerably lower extent: H9 was used in 36.7% of all hESC research papers published through 2008, while H1 and H7 were used in 30.8 and 10.2% of these studies, respectively. The difference is most likely due to the broader data basis used in our investigation. Whereas Scott et al. (2009) referred to data from only 534 publications, our analysis included almost 1,000 research papers.

Similarly, the investigation of the use of specific stem cell lines in nearly 1200 original research papers from 2005 through 2009 revealed the sustained predominance of only a few cell lines (Fig. 7.2a). Again, H9 was the most widely used hESC line in 2009, followed by H1 and H7, while other cell lines were used less frequently. Accordingly, when analyzing usage of hESC lines with regard to specific providers it becomes obvious that most studies (53.7%) were performed with at least one cell lines from WiCell, followed by the Harvard Stem Cell Institute (10.8%) and ES Cell International (10.4%; Fig. 7.2b). In contrast, 494 of 733 hESC lines reported in the scientific literature so far (67.4%) have been used only in a single study, and 92 hESC lines (12.6%) have been applied in only two studies. Although there are slight variations in hESC line usage over the last 5 years, there are currently no signs that novel cell lines derived under more appropriate or even animal-free conditions might replace the WiCell lines in international research. A preferential use of WiCell lines was also reported by Scott et al. (2010) who investigated nearly 400 poster abstracts at the 2010 ISSCR meeting for use of hESC lines in the presented research projects (Scott et al., 2010).

However, as reported in our former study (Löser et al., 2010), there are still pronounced regional differences in the usage of hESC lines in certain countries. While groups from the United States, the UK, Canada and Israel preferentially used the WiCell lines, these cell lines were more rarely applied in studies contributed by Australian, Swedish, Japanese and Korean researchers (Fig. 7.3). For example, in most studies from Australia cell lines of ES Cell International Pte Ltd (ESI) were used, while most work of Japanese groups were based on three cell lines of Kyoto University.

It is a matter of debate in how far other than scientific reasons may have contributed to the preferential use of only a few hESC lines in international research, namely of those provided by WiCell. There is no doubt that institutional factors such as assess fees, clauses in Material Transfer Agreements such as use restrictions, or intellectual property rights may influence the

Fig. 7.2 (continued) of Novocell, Athens, GA, USA; UCSF, University of California San Francisco, San Francisco, CA, USA; Karol. Inst., Karolinska Institute, Stockholm, Sweden; Technion, Technion – Israeli Institute of Technology, Haifa, Israel; Cellartis, Cellartis AB, Gothenburg, Sweden; Kyoto Univ., Kyoto University, Kyoto, Japan; MizMedi, MizMedi Hospital – Seoul National University, Seoul, Korea

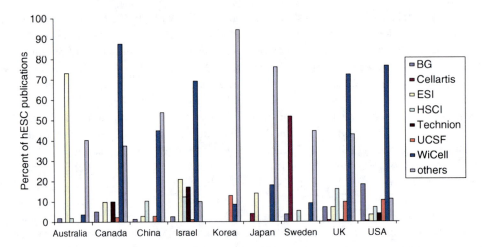

Fig. 7.3 Percentage of hESC papers from selected countries produced with hESC lines of specific providers. Note that in many papers several hESC lines were used. For abbreviations, see Fig. 7.2

decision for or against using a specific cell line. In addition, the federal stem cell policy of the United States and the NIH funding policy of the Bush administration were discussed as possible reasons for the preferential use of just a few cell lines (Scott et al., 2009, 2010). Moreover, uncertainty among scientists as a consequence of frequent changes in US stem cell policy (Levine, 2011) may not only delay hESC projects, but also influence the decision for using specific hESC lines.

Although the United States essentially contributed to hESC research in the last decade and therefore restrictions imposed by federal US stem cell policy will undoubtedly have an impact on the overall use of hESC lines, three phenomena cannot be explained persuasively by the potential impact of the US federal research policy. First, since its installation in 2001, the original NIH registry listed about 20 obtainable cell lines from US and non-US providers, and most of these cell lines were available for nearly a decade. Why were cell lines from other US providers such as the University of San Francisco or Bresagen not used to the same extent as cell lines from WiCell in US-based research? An investigation of NIH funding for hESC studies did not reveal significant differences in the number of NIH-funded studies applying WiCell lines or hESCs from the above-named other two providers (Löser et al., 2010). Second, there is a clear preferential use of WiCell lines also by research groups in countries with un-restricted stem cell policies (such as the UK, Canada and Israel). Why should researchers outside the United States comply with rules for US researchers? One possible reason could be interdependence with US research and, consequently, an indirect transmission of the US federal stem cell policy to other countries via collaborative research of US and non-US groups. However, this turned out to be highly unlikely. Only 22% of the nearly 600 hESC research papers published by US groups by the end of 2009 involved a contribution of a non-US group, and US groups participated, for example, in only 12.5 and 13.6% of studies from the UK and Israel, respectively. Third, an analysis of studies published by US groups in 2008 and 2009 and funded by the California Center for Regenerative Medicine (CIRM), but not by the NIH, revealed that in 54% of these studies the cell line H9 was used. This value is in the range of H9 usage in those studies that obtained NIH funding but no support from CIRM (59.2%) and in the range of all hESC studies from the United States published in the same period (57.1%). One reason for the establishment of CIRM was to allow researchers the use of other hESC lines than those listed in the NIH registry. Why did researchers stick to the use of H9 cells even without the restrictions imposed by NIH funding?

To answers these questions further investigations have to be performed. We are convinced that reasons apart from the US federal stem cell policy account for the worldwide preferential use of less than a handful of hESC lines, especially of just two WiCell lines. We rather believe that factors such as early availability, distribution policy, level of characterization and publicity of a cell line shape a researcher's decision for using a specific cell lines. The favoured use of just a few cell lines undoubtedly is a vicious circle: frequent use and accumulation of data result in further characterization, and extensive characterization and availability of data will cause increased use of the cells. In addition, cultivation of hESCs is still expensive and labour-intensive and, therefore, many laboratories restrict their work to one or two cell lines. Moreover, it cannot be excluded that the H1 and H9 cell lines are now considered as a kind of reference cells, being representative for hESCs in general. This is, for example, supported by the fact, that 53.4% of studies in which hESCs and hiPSCs were compared with respect to specific characteristics also used H9 cells for the intended comparison. Moreover, in a recent study initiated by the International Stem Cell Initiative Consortium and performed in five laboratories to characterize growth of hESCs in defined media, H9 cells were used as "reference cell line" in each of these laboratories in addition to the laboratories' own hESC lines (Akopian et al., 2010). It remains an open question, whether the use of cell lines derived under undefined and suboptimal conditions as a kind of "gold" standards for comparative research is a favourable choice. In any case, differences in the genome, proteome and epigenome of different hESC lines have to be analyzed as extensively and rigorously as, for example, differences between various hiPSC lines (Lister et al., 2011). The current lack of knowledge, deficiencies in the standardization of hESCs and especially the absence of limits for variation from the decreed hESC standard reduce the value not only of this, but more generally of any pluripotent stem cell standard.

Conclusions

The present analysis of research in the area of pluripotent stem cells did not confirm the gradual replacement of hESC by hiPSC that has been predicted in some political statements. In contrast, the field shows the co-evolution of hESC with hiPSC research, their interdependency and steady increase in numbers of cell lines, output of publications and increasing globalization. Although research involving hESCs and hiPSCs is dominated by groups from the United States with respect to output quantity and impact, an increasing number of groups from different countries have contributed to the field.

The available data suggest a continuing high public and scientific interest in hESC and hiPSC research as reflected by the comparatively high average citation impact. Our analysis did not imply dependency of the research output on the availability of an increasing number of different hESC lines, but rather revealed consolidation of dominance of a few hESC lines, namely H1 and H9. This is surprising as it suggests a limited dependence on stem cell policy for the field, but also a rather conservative approach by the research community with potentially problematic consequences: The use of only a few hESC lines unwillingly enforces their standard character without proper justification based on comparative data. A rigorous approach towards the definition of true pluripotent cell characteristics by comparative analyses is needed for hESCs, and in comparison, for hiPSCs (Müller et al., 2008).

Pluripotent stem cell registries may offer a platform for this comparison, and thus it is justified to expand their tasks toward this goal. This includes the registration of hESCs and hiPSCs and especially of variations from the norm, such as pluripotent cell lines derived from subjects with genetic and epigenetic disorders, which would also provide an extremely valuable research resource. The lack of characterization of the majority of established hESC lines and also of many hiPSC lines implied by our analysis, and the limited public access to this information, can only be overcome by a multinational effort that provides the required resources and funds. Clinical and pharmaceutical applications will rather sooner than later require these standards. The cells, the instruments and the public interest are already in place.

References

Akopian V, Andrews PW, Beil S, Benvenisty N, Brehm J, Christie M, Ford A, Fox V, Gokhale PJ (2010) Comparison of defined culture systems for feeder cell free propagation of human embryonic stem cells. In Vitro Cell Dev Biol 46:247–258

Aldhous P (2010) The stem cell wars. New Scientist 2764:12–14

Alper J (2009) Geron gets green light for human trial of ES cell-derived product. Nat Biotechnol 27:213–214

Anon (2011) US approves new trial of embryonic stem cells on blindness. The Independent, 4 Jan 2011, Independent Press Limited, London

Ben-Yosef D, Malcov M, Eiges R (2008) PGD-derived human embryonic stem cell lines as a powerful tool for the study of human genetic disorders. Mol Cell Endocrinol 282:153–158

Borstlap J, Stacey G, Kurtz A, Elstner A, Damaschun A, Aran B, Veiga A (2008) First evaluation of the European hESCreg. Nat Biotechnol 26:859–860

Borstlap J, Luong MX, Rooke HM, Aran B, Damaschun A, Elstner A, Smith KP, Stein GS, Veiga A (2010) International stem cell registries. In Vitro Cell Dev Biol Anim 46:242–246

Carvajal-Vergara X, Sevilla A, D'Souza SL, Ang YS, Schaniel C, Lee DF, Yang L, Kaplan AD, Adler ED, Rozov R, Ge Y, Cohen N, Edelmann LJ, Chang B, Waghray A, Su J, Pardo S, Lichtenbelt KD, Tartaglia M, Gelb BD, Lemischka IR (2010) Patient-specific induced pluripotent stem-cell-derived models of LEOPARD syndrome. Nature 465:808–812

Connor S (2010) Stem cells could help blind patients to see within six weeks. The Independent, 22 Nov 2011, Independent Press Limited, London

Ebert AD, Svendsen CN (2010) Human stem cells and drug screening: opportunities and challenges. Nat Rev Drug Discov 9:367–372

Guhr A, Kurtz A, Friedgen K, Löser P (2006) Current state of human embryonic stem cell research: an overview of cell lines and their use in experimental work. Stem Cells 24:2187–2191

Isasi RM, Knoppers BM (2009) Governing stem cell banks and registries: emerging issues. Stem Cell Res 3:96–105

Levine AD (2008) Identifying under- and overperforming countries in research related to human embryonic stem cells. Cell Stem Cell 2:521–524

Levine AD (2011) Policy uncertainty and the conduct of stem cell research. Cell Stem Cell 8:132–135

Lister R, Pelizzola M, Kida YS, Hawkins RD, Nery JR, Hon G, Antosiewicz-Bourget J, O'Malley R, Castanon R, Klugman S, Downes M, Yu R, Stewart R, Ren B, Thomson JA, Evans RM, Ecker JR (2011) Hotspots of aberrant epigenomic reprogramming in human induced pluripotent stem cells. Nature 471:68–73

Löser P, Guhr A, Kurtz A, Wobus AM (2008) Additional considerations relevant to meta-analyses of hESC publication data. Cell Stem Cell 3:129–130; author reply 131

Löser P, Schirm J, Guhr A, Wobus AM, Kurtz A (2010) Human embryonic stem cell lines and their use in international research. Stem Cells 28:240–246

Luong MX, Smith KP, Stein GS (2008) Human embryonic stem cell registries: value, challenges and opportunities. J Cell Biochem 105:625–632

McCormick JB, Owen-Smith J, Scott CT (2009) Distribution of human embryonic stem cell lines: who, when, and where. Cell Stem Cell 4:107–110

Moretti A, Bellin M, Welling A, Jung CB, Lam JT, Bott-Flugel L, Dorn T, Goedel A, Hohnke C, Hofmann F, Seyfarth M, Sinnecker D, Schomig A, Laugwitz KL (2010) Patient-specific induced pluripotent stem-cell models for long-QT syndrome. N Engl J Med 363:1397–1409

Müller FJ, Laurent LC, Kostka D, Ulitsky I, Williams R, Lu C, Park IH, Rao MS, Shamir R, Schwartz PH, Schmidt NO, Loring JF (2008) Regulatory networks define phenotypic classes of human stem cell lines. Nature 455:401–405

Müller FJ, Goldmann J, Löser P, Loring JF (2010) A call to standardize teratoma assays used to define human pluripotent cell lines. Cell Stem Cell 6:412–414

Owen-Smith J, McCormick J (2006) An international gap in human ES cell research. Nat Biotechnol 24:391–392

Saha K, Hurlbut JB (2011) Disease modeling using pluripotent stem cells: making sense of disease from bench to bedside. Swiss Med Wkly 141:w13144

Scott CT, McCormick JB, Owen-Smith J (2009) And then there were two: use of hESC lines. Nat Biotechnol 27:696–697

Scott CT, McCormick JB, Derouen MC, Owen-Smith J (2010) Federal policy and the use of pluripotent stem cells. Nat Methods 7:866–867

Sermon KD, Simon C, Braude P, Viville S, Borstlap J, Veiga A (2009) Creation of a registry for human embryonic stem cells carrying an inherited defect: joint collaboration between ESHRE and hESCreg. Hum Reprod 24:1556–1560

Takahashi K, Tanabe K, Ohnuki M, Narita M, Ichisaka T, Tomoda K, Yamanaka S (2007) Induction of pluripotent stem cells from adult human fibroblasts by defined factors. Cell 131:861–872

Taymor K, Scott CT (2009) The practical consequences of a national human embryonic stem cell registry. Stem Cell Rev 5:315–318

Thomson JA, Itskovitz-Eldor J, Shapiro SS, Waknitz MA, Swiergiel JJ, Marshall VS, Jones JM (1998) Embryonic stem cell lines derived from human blastocysts. Science 282:1145–1147

Wobus AM, Löser P (2011) Present state and future perspectives of using pluripotent stem cells in toxicology research. Arch Toxicol 85:79–117

Yu J, Vodyanik MA, Smuga-Otto K, Antosiewicz-Bourget J, Frane JL, Tian S, Nie J, Jonsdottir GA, Ruotti V, Stewart R, Slukvin II, Thomson JA (2007) Induced pluripotent stem cell lines derived from human somatic cells. Science 318:1917–1920

Chapter 8

Gliosarcoma Stem Cells: Glial and Mesenchymal Differentiation

Ana C. deCarvalho and Tom Mikkelsen

Abstract Gliosarcoma (GS) is a morphological variant of glioblastoma (GBM), characterized by biphasic glial and sarcomatous compartments. It is not clear whether the mesenchymal metaplasia leading to distinct glial and mesenchymal components in GS is related to the well established mesenchymal gene expression in GBMs, which retain the glial identity. GS stem cells, which preserve the genetic alterations of the original tumors and can differentiate into biphasic mesenchymal and glial components in orthotopic xenografts have been identified. Given the poor prognosis for patients diagnosed with GBM or GS, advances in the understanding of the predictive and prognostic consequences, as well as the mechanisms of activation of mesenchymal programs in these malignancies will likely impact clinical management and outcome.

Keywords Gliosarcoma · Glioblastoma · Cancer stem cells · Glial fibrillary acidic protein · Extracellular matrix · Mesenchymal differentiation

Introduction

Gliosarcoma is one of two histological variants of GBM recognized by the World Health Organization (WHO) classification, the other being giant cell glioblastoma (Louis et al., 2007). GS tumors, characterized by a biphasic composition of glial and sarcomatous components, comprise ~1.8–2.8% of all GBMs (Meis et al., 1991; Lutterbach et al., 2001). GS is one example of the remarkable phenotypic and functional heterogeneity characteristic of GBMs. Integrated analysis of transcriptome, genetic alterations, and signaling pathways from datasets comprising a large number of samples have defined molecularly distinct GBM subtypes, one of which is characterized by the mesenchymal phenotype and associated with poor prognosis (Phillips et al., 2006; Brennan et al., 2009; Verhaak et al., 2010). Thus far, it has not been determined whether GS samples included in the datasets analyzed in these studies belong to the mesenchymal subtype, or whether common pathways drive the mesenchymal phenotype in GBMs and the differentiation of the mesenchymal metaplastic component in GSs.

It has long been proposed that tumor heterogeneity suggests the existence of cancer stem cells (CSCs), defined by the ability of a subgroup of neoplastic cells to self-renew and differentiate into the diverse cell population comprising the tumor. The occurrence and characterization of GBM stem cells is the subject of other chapters in this volume, and numerous publications (Vescovi et al., 2006). This review will address mesenchymal differentiation in GBMs, focusing on the occurrence of metaplasia in GS, the effect of cell culture conditions on mesenchymal and glial differentiation in vitro and in vivo, and the potential of GS stem cells to undergo mesenchymal and glial differentiation, recapitulating the biphasic tumor in orthotopic xenografts.

A.C. deCarvalho (✉)
Hermelin Brain Tumor Center, Neurosurgery Research, E&R 3052, Henry Ford Hospital, Detroit, MI 48202, USA
e-mail: ana@neuro.hfh.edu

Gliosarcoma: Mesenchymal Metaplasia

Gliosarcoma diagnosis relies on the histological identification of two distinct malignant glial and sarcomatous components. The glial portion is identified by the expression of the intermediate filament glial fibrillary acidic protein (GFAP), and display histological features typical of GBMs. The sarcomatous compartment is composed of GFAP-negative spindle cells, and is identified by reticulin staining of the dense extracellular matrix (ECM). The sarcomatous component can display diverse mesenchymal phenotypes, with evidence of differentiation along fibroblastic, osteogenic, chondrogenic, adipogenic, and myogenic lineages, according to the morphological appearance and expression of lineage specific markers (Louis et al., 2007; Miller and Perry, 2007). Evidence of malignant transformation, substantiated by the presence of nuclear atypia, mitotic activity, necrosis, and identical genetic abnormalities in both glial and mesenchymal components, indicates that GS originates from a metaplastic mesenchymal differentiation during the progression of the astrocytic tumor, with both components sharing a common origin (Meis et al., 1990; Biernat et al., 1995; Boerman et al., 1996; Reis et al., 2000; Actor et al., 2002).

Most GSs occur *de novo*, with no previous malignant tumor diagnosis. Primary GS has been considered indistinguishable from primary GBM in relation to median patient age, gender, treatment management, and clinical outcomes (Perry et al., 1995; Galanis et al., 1998; Reis et al., 2000; Lutterbach et al., 2001). A tendency to localize to temporal and frontal lobes has been noted (Galanis et al., 1998; Lutterbach et al., 2001; Han et al., 2010a). The occurrence of certain genetic abnormalities such as TP53 mutations and losses on chromosome 10, which includes the PTEN locus, are similar for GSs and GBMs, while low frequency of EGFR amplification and mutations is a feature more associated with GSs (Reis et al., 2000; Actor et al., 2002; Han et al., 2010a).

Clinical information for GS is limited to case studies and small series, due to the low frequency of this GBM variant. Because GSs are not typically distinguished from GBMs in relation to standard treatment, clinical trial results, and molecular profiling studies, many questions remain, including whether the sarcomatous and glial components have different sensitivities to radiation and/or chemotherapy. Detailed overview of GS treatment modalities will be the subject of another chapter in this volume. As more clinical GS data is systematically analyzed, new patterns are emerging. Previous scattered observations have been substantiated by additional studies showing that primary GSs can be divided into two groups according to observations at the resection surgery, one resembling meningioma and easily separated from the surrounding tissue, and the other similar to GBM, presenting vascular hyperplasia, necrosis, and extensive infiltration into the brain parenchyma (Salvati et al., 2005; Han et al., 2010a). Overall survival and progression-free survival were significantly higher for meningioma-like GS patients (Han et al., 2010a). Molecular signatures distinguishing these two morphological GS groups, cell culture, and experimental models have yet to be developed.

Cases of gliosarcoma developing after radiation treatment of a previously diagnosed GBM, while not frequent, are well recognized, and sometimes referred to as secondary GSs (Perry et al., 1995; Lieberman et al., 2001). These are considered distinct from radiation-induced GSs occurring in patients treated for malignancies other than GBMs (Han et al., 2010b). Conclusive experimental evidence proving a direct causal relationship between radiation and development of gliosarcoma is still missing. Another distinctive feature of GS is the increased incidence of extracranial metastasis, hardly ever observed for GBMs. Some studies suggest a higher frequency of metastasis in GS arising after radiation therapy (Beaumont et al., 2007). With the caveat that asymptomatic metastasis go under-detected, metastasis rate of about 11% for primary GS can be inferred from the literature. However, no metastasis in the series of 20 primary GS cases analyzed recently was identified (Han et al., 2010a).

Mesenchymal Gene Expression in Glioblastoma

Mesenchymal lineage gene expression in GBM cells, which keep their glial identity, has been extensively investigated. Expression of individual markers of differentiated mesenchymal tissues, such as Tenascin-C, have long been characterized in GBMs.

The intermediate filament Vimentin, expressed in both mesenchyma and neural progenitor cells, is prominently expressed in GBMs, as well as in both the glial and the sarcomatous portions of GSs (Meis et al., 1990). Mesenchymal genes, including several ECM components, are highly represented in the list of genes most upregulated in GBMs in relation to non-tumor brain (Tso et al., 2006). Analysis of transcriptome datasets has led to the identification of a pattern of mesenchymal gene expression in GBM, resembling a mesenchymal developmental program, and molecularly defining subgroups associated with poor prognosis (Freije et al., 2004; Phillips et al., 2006). The subclassification of GBMs have been further confirmed by integrative analysis of transcriptome and genomic abnormalities data generated by The Cancer Genome Atlas (TCGA) Network (Verhaak et al., 2010). Gene expression of 200 GBMs and 2 non-tumor brain samples was used to define 4 clusters representing GBM subtypes: classical, mesenchymal, proneural, and neural. A set of 173 "core" representative samples was used to establish 210 gene signatures per subclass (Verhaak et al., 2010). The classical subtype is characterized by genomic amplification, increased expression and gain of function mutations in EGFR, homozygous deletion of CDKN2A, and low frequency of TP53 mutations. Amplification and mutations in the PDGFRA gene, and high mutation rate in the isocitrate dehydrogenase 1 (*IDH1*) gene characterized the proneural subclass. Genes characteristic of differentiated CNS cells are expressed in the neural subtype. The mesenchymal subclass presented a high rate of mutations, deletions, and decreased expression of the tumor suppressor gene NF1, which encodes the Ras-GTPase activating protein neurofibromin. The mesenchymal subtype signature included several transcripts previously associated with the mesenchymal phenotype in GBMs, such as Met receptor and chitinase-3-like-1 (CHI3L1) (Phillips et al., 2006). Histological analysis revealed increased occurrence of necrosis and resulting inflammation for the mesenchymal subtype. Clinically, the mesenchymal and classical subtypes were associated with lower survival, and increased response to intensive therapy relative to the proneural class (Phillips et al., 2006; Verhaak et al., 2010).

An association between GS and the GBM mesenchymal subtype, though expected, has not yet been firmly established. Neuropathology annotation was available for a subset of the 173 core samples used by Verhaak et al. (2010), through the TCGA Neuropathology Group (D. Brat, personal communication), or from the Henry Ford Hospital Neuropathology Dept., leading to the identification of 8 primary GS with subclass assignment identified by Verhaak et al. (2010). The median age at diagnosis for these GS patients, 60.5 years, and the gender distribution, 5 males and 3 females, were within the norm for GBMs. Six of the 8 cases carried point mutations in TP53. The distribution among the molecular subclasses was as follows: 5 mesenchymal, 2 classical, and 1 neural. Thus, the majority of cases with a GS diagnosis belonged to the mesenchymal subclass (62.5%), in agreement with evidence pointing to genomic characteristics shared by GSs and mesenchymal GBMs, such as presence of TP53 mutations and infrequent EGFR amplifications and mutations. The assignment of 3 out of the 8 GS cases to subclasses other than mesenchymal is possibly significant. The results of this preliminary analysis must be expanded and validated when molecular profiling information for a larger number of GS becomes available. It has also been noted that one primary GBM tumor classified as mesenchymal by Verhaak et al. (2010) recurred as a GS (A.C. deCarvalho and T. Mikkelsen, unpublished observations). Additional molecular profiling and patient follow-up data will lead to the determination of the frequency for each of the four primary GBM subtypes to present as gliosarcomas upon recurrence, after various treatment modalities.

Given the poor prognosis for patients diagnosed with GBM or GS, advances in the understanding of the predictive and prognostic consequences, as well as the mechanisms of activation of mesenchymal programs in these malignancies will likely impact clinical management and outcome. The relationship between the mesenchymal gene expression in GBM cells, which retain the glial identity, and the mesenchymal metaplasia leading to distinct glial and mesenchymal components in GS is not understood. Given that the GS mesenchymal component can differentiate along diverse mesenchymal lineages complicates matters, as different sets of regulators are activated during osteogenesis, chondrogenesis, adipogenesis, and myogenesis in adult mesenchymal stem cells (Kolf et al., 2007).

The transcription factors, signal transducer and activator of transcription 3 (STAT3) and CAATT/enhancer binding protein-β (C/EBPβ), have been recently identified as potential master regulators of the GBM mesenchymal differentiation (Carro et al., 2010). STAT3 is expressed in neural stem cells, can function as an oncogene in several tissues, and has been previously implicated in the pathology of GBMs. Testing pharmacological inhibitors for STAT3 in animal models of GS will help elucidate the role of this pathway in the pathology of this malignancy. Because the glial differentiation is repressed in the mesenchymal component of GSs, C/EBPβ, which opposes gliogenesis in neural stem cells, and works in conjunction with STAT3 to reprogram neural stem cells to acquire mesenchymal phenotypes (Carro et al., 2010), is also a plausible candidate for regulation of mesenchymal metaplasia in GS.

Epithelial to mesenchymal transition (EMT) occurs in several phases of development, starting at gastrulation, when cell detachment from epithelial sheets occurs, accompanied by increased motility, and a shift of the differentiation program leading to loss of epithelial characteristics and acquisition of a mesenchymal phenotype by the migrating cells. Not surprisingly, EMT is significantly involved in epithelial cancer progression and metastasis, as mesenchymal cells are non-polarized, loosely associated within the ECM and endowed with mobility potential, as reviewed elsewhere (Thiery et al., 2009). One could speculate that the increase in extracranial metastatic frequency observed for GS, discussed above, is a consequence of the glial to mesenchymal metaplasia, analogous to findings in carcinomas. Numerous signaling and environmental factors are known to induce EMT. Inflammation mediated activation of the NF-κB signalling pathway and hypoxia are examples of microenvironmental factors known to activate the mesenchymal program in carcinomas (Thiery et al., 2009). These stimuli are also involved in the pathology of astrocytic tumors, leading to the speculation that they could be players in the activation of the mesenchymal program during GBM progression. Studies establishing a correlation between EMT miRNA expression signature and the miRNA profiling of GS and GBM subgroups will add crucial information to uncover mechanisms of mesenchymal differentiation in GBMs and GSs. Another area that when further developed will greatly contribute to the design of combination therapies for specific patient subgroups is the activation of the mesenchymal program in GBM and GS, in response to targeted and cytotoxic therapy.

Mesenchymal and Glial Differentiation in Experimental Models

It has been extensively documented that culturing GBM cells as monolayers in serum containing medium results in the down regulation of astrocytic markers expressed in the original tumor, particularly GFAP, while the expression of mesenchymal lineage genes, including collagens and other ECM constituents is upregulated. This phenotypic alteration takes place over time and has been termed "mesenchymal drift" (McKeever et al., 1991). Differentiated serum cultured GBM cell lines have also been shown to transdifferentiate and acquire characteristics of chondrogenic, osteogenic, and lipogenic lineages, upon specific stimulation in vitro (Tso et al., 2006). Gene expression signature of differentiated murine astrocytes cultured in serum correlated with the GBM mesenchymal signature, further substantiating the induction of mesenchymal gene expression in cells of glial origin exposed to serum (Verhaak et al., 2010).

Cancer stem cells (CSCs), whether defined by intrinsic properties or acquired phenotype, are by definition able to self renew and differentiate into the heterogeneous cell population comprising the tumor. It has been shown for several malignancies that neoplastic cells can adopt a CSC phenotype: extensive self-renewing potential, both in vitro and in serial transplantation, and by the ability to differentiate and phenocopy the original tumor in orthotopic xenografts. Long term propagation of glial tumor cells in serum-containing medium results in loss of the CSC population and outgrowth of cells that are genetically and phenotypically quite distinct from their parental tumors (Lee et al., 2006), a possible contribution to the mesenchymal drift described above. On the other hand, culturing dissociated cells from GBM clinical specimens in serum-free medium supplemented with growth factors, formulated for culturing neural stem/progenitor cell, allows for the selection and propagation of multicellular floating cell aggregates, or neurospheres, enriched in cells with CSC phenotype (Lee et al., 2006). While the definition, properties, and clinical significance of central nervous system CSCs are subject of debate, the use of neurosphere culture for selection and long term propagation of a neoplastic cell population containing cells with CSC properties is becoming increasingly popular, particularly for pre-clinical studies. Extensive evidence supports the concept that GBM neurosphere culture allows for long term propagation of cells that preserve the patient specific molecular fingerprint and the ability to reproduce the heterogeneous tumor in animal models (Lee et al., 2006; Vescovi et al., 2006). Another strategy that similarly preserves the genetic and phenotypic heterogeneity characteristic of GBMs is the serial passage of GBM biopsies in the flank of immunocompromised mice (Hodgson et al., 2009). Gene expression patterns for these subcutaneous tumor xenografts were reported to be comparable to the mesenchymal, proneural, and classical GBM subgroups (Verhaak et al., 2010).

Phenotypic drift of neoplastic cells can be attributed to genetic instability, to the action of oncogenic signalling, such as activation of AKT, and to the CSC phenotype. Adult mesenchymal stem cells express embryonic stem cells markers, and can differentiate into multiple lineages (Kolf et al., 2007). Given the proper stimulus, adult mouse neural stem cells differentiate along mesenchymal lineages in vitro and in vivo (Clarke et al., 2000). GBM neurospheres can differentiate along mesenchymal lineages in vitro when the proper stimuli are present (Ricci-Vitiani et al., 2008). Two GBM neurospheres in this study underwent chondroblastic and osteoblastic differentiation in subcutaneous tumor xenografts, but not in orthotopic xenografts (Ricci-Vitiani et al., 2008).

Gliosarcoma Stem Cells

Human GS cell lines cultured in serum containing medium undergo down regulation of glial markers, and upregulation of mesenchymal markers in vitro, as observed for GBMs. This phenomenon is observed when the cells were cultured from tumor sections comprised of both glial and sarcomatous, or predominantly sarcomatous components (McKeever et al., 1984; Rutka et al., 1986; Iwasaki et al., 1992). One of these gliosarcoma cell lines, SF-539, formed orthotopic tumors in immunocompromised mice, which resembled spindle cell sarcoma, with no expression of glial markers (Rutka et al., 1986).

Chemical mutagenesis in Fischer rat resulted in a brain tumor, designated 9L which was cloned and propagated in serum containing medium. Orthotopic xenograft tumors generated from 9L are composed of spindle-shaped cells with a sarcomatous appearance, thus the description as a "gliosarcoma", although evidence of a distinct GFAP positive glial component is lacking (Schmidek et al., 1971). 9L rat gliosarcoma cells form fast growing non-invasive circumscribed tumors in rodents, and have been used in multiple pre-clinical studies. A cell subpopulation with cancer stem cell properties was recovered from long term serum cultured 9L cells, by culturing the cells in neurosphere medium (Ghods et al., 2007). These 9L CSC-like cells exhibited long-term self-renewal in vitro, and expressed the neural stem cell markers Nestin and Sox2, in contrast with the monolayer serum cultured 9L cells. The 9L neurosphere cells presented a lower proliferation rate in vitro, but an increased growth rate in vivo, relative to the parental 9L cells.

Analogous to the GBM stem cell attributes, GS stem cells should display long-term self-renewal, gene expression profiles associated with neural stem/progenitor cells, and the ability to form tumors in orthotopic xenografts with evidence of differentiation into the heterogeneous phenotypes comprising a GS. A comparative study was performed where dissociated cells from a GS (GS1) and several classical GBM surgical specimens were cultured in parallel, in serum and in neurosphere medium. The GS1 tumor was a primary GS removed from an untreated patient, mutant for TP53, and belonged to the mesenchymal molecular subtype. GS1 and GBM neurosphere cultures expressed neural stem cell markers Sox2, Nestin, Musashi-1, as well as the mesenchymal stem cell marker CD105, and formed high grade tumors in orthotopic rat xenografts (deCarvalho et al., 2010). GS stem cells underwent glial and mesenchymal differentiation in immunocompromised rat brain, recapitulating the biphasic parental tumor phenotype. Importantly, CSCs from typical GBMs did not initiate tumors with biphasic expression of GFAP and reticulin (deCarvalho et al., 2010). The GS1 mesenchymal component in the biopsy and xenografts was positive for α-smooth muscle actin (α-SMA) (deCarvalho et al., 2010). Because many mesenchymal lineage genes are associated with GBM/GS host vasculature, the use of human specific antibodies for the detection of mesenchymal markers in GBM/GS xenograft tumors facilitate the identification of mesenchymal phenotype associated with neoplastic cells. A representative histological image demonstrating the

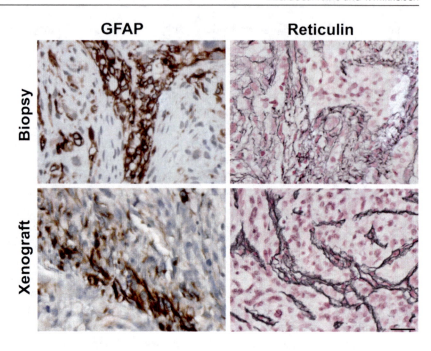

Fig. 8.1 Biphasic glial and mesenchymal differentiation of gliosarcoma stem cells in orthotopic xenograft phenocopy the parental tumor. Cancer stem cells cultured from gliosarcoma GS1 biopsy were implanted intracranially in nude rat. Expression of glial (GFAP) and mesenchymal (reticulin) markers, in a biphasic pattern was observed for the biopsy and paired xenograft tumors. Representative images are shown. Scale, 20 μm

experimental GS phenotype, obtained through implant of GS stem cells in immunocompromised rat, is displayed in Fig. 8.1. This study demonstrated that neoplastic cells from primary GS can adopt CSC properties with intrinsic ability to give rise to the biphasic mesenchymal and glial tumor upon intracranial implantation. This property suggests that epigenetic and gene expression patterns preserved in the neurosphere cultures could distinguish GS stem cells from GBM stem cells, a hypothesis testable by molecular profiling of a statistically significant number of GS and GBM neurosphere lines. No extracranial metastasis was observed for this GS1 rodent model using non invasive bioluminescence imaging (unpublished observation). In light of the wealth of information generated by integrated bioinformatics analysis of clinical specimens, the importance of animal models that preserve the genetic abnormalities and heterogeneous phenotype of high grade astrocytomas for pre-clinical studies cannot be overstated. Validation in appropriate experimental models of findings regarding the mechanisms and consequences of activation of the mesenchymal program, and the predictive value of molecular signatures in GS and GBM, is an important step towards the ultimate goal of improving treatments.

References

Actor B, Cobbers JM, Buschges R, Wolter M, Knobbe CB, Lichter P, Reifenberger G, Weber RG (2002) Comprehensive analysis of genomic alterations in gliosarcoma and its two tissue components. Genes Chromosomes Cancer 34:416–427

Beaumont TL, Kupsky WJ, Barger GR, Sloan AE (2007) Gliosarcoma with multiple extracranial metastases: case report and review of the literature. J Neurooncol 83:39–46

Biernat W, Aguzzi A, Sure U, Grant JW, Kleihues P, Hegi ME (1995) Identical mutations of the p53 tumor suppressor gene in the gliomatous and the sarcomatous components of gliosarcomas suggest a common origin from glial cells. J Neuropathol Exp Neurol 54:651–656

Boerman RH, Anderl K, Herath J, Borell T, Johnson N, Schaeffer-Klein J, Kirchhof A, Raap AK, Scheithauer BW, Jenkins RB (1996) The glial and mesenchymal elements of gliosarcomas share similar genetic alterations. J Neuropathol Exp Neurol 55:973–981

Brennan C, Momota H, Hambardzumyan D, Ozawa T, Tandon A, Pedraza A, Holland E (2009) Glioblastoma subclasses can be defined by activity among signal transduction pathways and associated genomic alterations. PLoS One 4:e7752

Carro MS, Lim WK, Alvarez MJ, Bollo RJ, Zhao X, Snyder EY, Sulman EP, Anne SL, Doetsch F, Colman H, Lasorella A, Aldape K, Califano A, Iavarone A (2010) The transcriptional network for mesenchymal transformation of brain tumours. Nature 463:318–325

Clarke DL, Johansson CB, Wilbertz J, Veress B, Nilsson E, Karlstrom H, Lendahl U, Frisen J (2000) Generalized potential of adult neural stem cells. Science 288:1660–1663 deCarvalho AC, Nelson K, Lemke N, Lehman NL, Arbab AS, Kalkanis S, Mikkelsen T (2010) Gliosarcoma stem cells undergo glial and mesenchymal differentiation in vivo. Stem Cells 28:181–190

Freije WA, Castro-Vargas FE, Fang Z, Horvath S, Cloughesy T, Liau LM, Mischel PS, Nelson SF (2004) Gene expression profiling of gliomas strongly predicts survival. Cancer Res 64:6503–6510

Galanis E, Buckner JC, Dinapoli RP, Scheithauer BW, Jenkins RB, Wang CH, O'Fallon JR, Farr G Jr (1998) Clinical outcome of gliosarcoma compared with glioblastoma multiforme: North Central Cancer Treatment Group results. J Neurosurg 89:425–430

Ghods AJ, Irvin D, Liu G, Yuan X, Abdulkadir IR, Tunici P, Konda B, Wachsmann-Hogiu S, Black KL, Yu JS (2007) Spheres isolated from 9L gliosarcoma rat cell line possess chemoresistant and aggressive cancer stem-like cells. Stem Cells 25:1645–1653

Han SJ, Yang I, Ahn BJ, Otero JJ, Tihan T, McDermott MW, Berger MS, Prados MD, Parsa AT (2010a) Clinical characteristics and outcomes for a modern series of primary gliosarcoma patients. Cancer 116:1358–1366

Han SJ, Yang I, Otero JJ, Ahn BJ, Tihan T, McDermott MW, Berger MS, Chang SM, Parsa AT (2010b) Secondary gliosarcoma after diagnosis of glioblastoma: clinical experience with 30 consecutive patients. J Neurosurg 112: 990–996

Hodgson JG, Yeh RF, Ray A, Wang NJ, Smirnov I, Yu M, Hariono S, Silber J, Feiler HS, Gray JW, Spellman PT, Vandenberg SR, Berger MS, James CD (2009) Comparative analyses of gene copy number and mRNA expression in glioblastoma multiforme tumors and xenografts. Neurol. Oncol. 11:477–487

Iwasaki K, Kikuchi H, Miyatake S, Kondo S, Oda Y (1992) Establishment of a new cell line derived from a human gliosarcoma. Neurosurgery 30:228–235

Kolf CM, Cho E, Tuan RS (2007) Mesenchymal stromal cells. Biology of adult mesenchymal stem cells: regulation of niche, self-renewal and differentiation. Arthritis Res Ther 9:204

Lee J, Kotliarova S, Kotliarov Y, Li A, Su Q, Donin NM, Pastorino S, Purow BW, Christopher N, Zhang W, Park JK, Fine HA (2006) Tumor stem cells derived from glioblastomas cultured in bFGF and EGF more closely mirror the phenotype and genotype of primary tumors than do serum-cultured cell lines. Cancer Cell 9:391–403

Lieberman KA, Fuller CE, Caruso RD, Schelper RL (2001) Postradiation gliosarcoma with osteosarcomatous components. Neuroradiology 43:555–558

Louis DN, Ohgaki H, Weistler OD, Cavenee WK (2007) WHO classification of tumours of the central nervous system. IARC Press, Lyon, France

Lutterbach J, Guttenberger R, Pagenstecher A (2001) Gliosarcoma: a clinical study. Radiother Oncol 61:57–64

McKeever PE, Wichman A, Chronwall B, Thomas C, Howard R (1984) Sarcoma arising from a gliosarcoma. South Med J 77:1027–1032

McKeever PE, Davenport RD, Shakui P (1991) Patterns of antigenic expression of human glioma cells. Crit Rev Neurobiol 6:119–147

Meis JM, Ho KL, Nelson JS (1990) Gliosarcoma: a histologic and immunohistochemical reaffirmation. Mod Pathol 3:19–24

Meis JM, Martz KL, Nelson JS (1991) Mixed glioblastoma multiforme and sarcoma. A clinicopathologic study of 26 radiation therapy oncology group cases. Cancer 67: 2342–2349

Miller CR, Perry A (2007) Glioblastoma. Arch Pathol Lab Med 131:397–406

Perry JR, Ang LC, Bilbao JM, Muller PJ (1995) Clinicopathologic features of primary and postirradiation cerebral gliosarcoma. Cancer 75:2910–2918

Phillips HS, Kharbanda S, Chen R, Forrest WF, Soriano RH, Wu TD, Misra A, Nigro JM, Colman H, Soroceanu L, Williams PM, Modrusan Z, Feuerstein BG, Aldape K (2006) Molecular subclasses of high-grade glioma predict prognosis, delineate a pattern of disease progression, and resemble stages in neurogenesis. Cancer Cell 9:157–173

Reis RM, Konu-Leblebliciogluq D, Lopes JM, Kleihues P, Ohgaki H (2000) Genetic profile of gliosarcomas. Am J Pathol 156:425–432

Ricci-Vitiani L, Pallini R, Larocca LM, Lombardi DG, Signore M, Pierconti F, Petrucci G, Montano N, Maira G, De Maria R (2008) Mesenchymal differentiation of glioblastoma stem cells. Cell Death Differ 15:1491–1498

Rutka JT, Giblin JR, Hoifodt HK, Dougherty DV, Bell CW, McCulloch JR, Davis RL, Wilson CB, Rosenblum ML (1986) Establishment and characterization of a cell line from a human gliosarcoma. Cancer Res 46:5893–5902

Salvati M, Caroli E, Raco A, Giangaspero F, Delfini R, Ferrante L (2005) Gliosarcomas: analysis of 11 cases do two subtypes exist? J Neurooncol 74:59–63

Schmidek HH, Nielsen SL, Schiller AL, Messer J (1971) Morphological studies of rat brain tumors induced by N-nitrosomethylurea. J. Neurosurg 34:335–340

Thiery JP, Acloque H, Huang RY, Nieto MA (2009) Epithelial–mesenchymal transitions in development and disease. Cell 139:871–890

Tso CL, Shintaku P, Chen J, Liu Q, Liu J, Chen Z, Yoshimoto K, Mischel PS, Cloughesy TF, Liau LM, Nelson SF (2006) Primary glioblastomas express mesenchymal stem-like properties. Mol Cancer Res 4:607–619

Verhaak RG, Hoadley KA, Purdom E, Wang V, Qi Y, Wilkerson MD, Miller CR, Ding L, Golub T, Mesirov JP, Alexe G, Lawrence M, O'Kelly M, Tamayo P, Weir BA, Gabriel S, Winckler W, Gupta S, Jakkula L, Feiler HS, Hodgson JG, James CD, Sarkaria JN, Brennan C, Kahn A, Spellman PT, Wilson RK, Speed TP, Gray JW, Meyerson M, Getz G, Perou CM, Hayes DN (2010) Integrated genomic analysis identifies clinically relevant subtypes of glioblastoma characterized by abnormalities in PDGFRA, IDH1, EGFR, and NF1. Cancer Cell 17:98–110

Vescovi AL, Galli R, Reynolds BA (2006) Brain tumour stem cells. Nat. Rev. Cancer 6:425–436

Chapter 9

Generation of Induced Pluripotent Stem Cells from Mesenchymal Stromal Cells Derived from Human Third Molars (Method)

Yasuaki Oda, Hiroe Ohnishi, Shunsuke Yuba, and Hajime Ohgushi

Abstract Generation of induced pluripotent stem (iPS) cells have the potential for investigation of molecular mechanisms of disease, understanding the development of human tissues, and clinical applications. Although it was reported that various kinds of human somatic cells reprogrammed into iPS cells, most of them showed low reprogramming efficiency. Previously, we reported that clonally-expanded mesenchymal stromal/stem cells (MSCs) derived from tooth germs of human third molars efficiently reprogrammed into iPS cells by retroviral transduction of *OCT3/4*, *SOX2*, and *KLF4* without *c-MYC*. Our data indicated that human third molars, which usually discarded as clinical wastes, are a valuable cell source for generation of iPS cells. Here, we describe detailed methods of the MSCs preparation and iPS cells generation from the MSCs.

Keywords Induced pluripotent stem · Mesenchymal stromal/stem cells · Embryonic stem · Tooth germ progenitor cells · Dental pulp stem cells · Stem cells from human exfoliated deciduous teeth

Introduction

Mesenchymal stromal/stem cells (MSCs) can differentiate into osteoblasts, chondrocytes, adipocytes, and various cell lineages. MSCs are widely used in clinical applications (Ohgushi and Caplan, 1999; Ohgushi et al., 2005; Salem and Thiemermann, 2010). However, the abilities of proliferation and differentiation of MSCs are limited; therefore, the use of MSCs for clinical applications has restriction in some cases. In 2006 and 2007, groundbreaking researches were reported that mouse and human somatic cells can reprogram into pluripotent cells by retroviral transduction of four transcription factors (mouse or human *OCT3/4*, *SOX2*, *KLF4*, and *c-MYC*) (Takahashi and Yamanaka, 2006; Takahashi et al., 2007). These reprogrammed cells called induced pluripotent stem (iPS) cells are closely resemble to embryonic stem (ES) cells in many aspects, including unlimited proliferation, genes expression, and differentiation ability into three germ layers in vitro and in vivo. Although *c-Myc* is significant for efficient reprogramming process (Nakagawa et al., 2008), reactivation of *c-Myc* caused carcinogenesis in mice (Okita et al., 2007). Recent studies reported that human iPS cells were generated from various cell origins. One of ideal cell source for induction of iPS cells which can easily obtain from donors. Previously, we and others reported that MSCs derived from third molars or teeth, for example, tooth germ progenitor cells (TGPCs), dental pulp stem cells (DPSCs), and stem cells from human exfoliated deciduous teeth (SHED), showed highly proliferation rather than bone marrow derived MSCs (Gronthos et al., 2000; Ikeda et al., 2006, 2008; Miura et al., 2003; Yagyuu et al., 2010). In this paper, we focus on human third molars which are usually discarded as clinical waste and demonstrate the preparation methods as well as importance of the MSCs from the third molars, which efficiently reprogrammed into iPS cells by retroviral transduction of *OCT3/4*, *SOX2*, and *KLF4* without *c-MYC* (Oda et al., 2010).

H. Ohgushi (✉)
Tissue Engineering Research Group, Health Research Institute, National Institute of Advanced Industrial Science and Technology (AIST), Amagasaki City, Hyogo 661-0974, Japan
e-mail: hajime-ohgushi@aist.go.jp

Materials

Most of our protocols of the iPS cell generation are referred to Center for iPS Cell Research and Application (CiRA) at Kyoto University (http://www.cira.kyoto-u.ac.jp/e/index.html) and are described below with some modifications.

Tissue Preparation

- Partially mineralized and impacted human third molars are removed by raising soft tissue flaps for adequate exposure and removing the alveolar crest bone with high-speed surgical burrs. The procedures can be done under local anesthesia and thus obtained third molars are used for isolation/expansion of MSCs with written informed consent (Ikeda et al., 2008).

Vectors

- pMXs retroviral vectors containing open reading frame (ORF) of *OCT3/4*, *SOX2*, and *KLF4* can be purchased from addgene (http://www.addgene.org/Shinya_Yamanaka) or Cell Biolabs, Inc. (http://www.cellbiolabs.com/retroviral-vectors-ips-cell-generation). More information about pMXs retroviral vectors are shown in the reference (Kitamura et al., 2003).

Cells for Generation of iPS Cell

- Platinum-A (Plat-A) retroviral packaging cells can be purchased from Cell Biolabs, Inc. (http://www.cellbiolabs.com/retroviral-packaging-cells-ips-cell-generation). More information about Plat-A retroviral packaging cells is shown in the reference (Morita et al., 2000).
- SNL feeder cells can be purchased from European Collection of Cell Cultures (ECACC). ECACC is one of the four collections which constitute the Health Protection Agency Culture Collections (http://www.hpacultures.org.uk). You can also purchase from Cell Applications, Inc. (http://www.cellapplications.com).
- Human dermal fibroblasts (HDF) can be purchased from Cell Applications, Inc. (http://www.cellapplications.com).

Reagents

- Phosphate-buffered salines (PBS; 10010-049, Invitrogen)
- Minimum essential medium (MEM) alpha medium (α-MEM; 12571-071, Invitrogen)
- Dulbecco's modified eagle medium (DMEM; 11965-118, Invitrogen)
- D-MEM / F-12 (which supplemented with GlutaMAX-I, 10565-018, Invitrogen)
- Fetal bovine serum (FBS; 171012, Nichirei, Japan)
- KnockOut™ serum replacement (KSR; 10828-028, Invitrogen)
- MEM non-essential amino acids solution (11140-050, Invitrogen)
- Penicillin-Streptomycin (15140-122, Invitrogen)
- 2-Mercaptoethanol (21985-023, Invitrogen)
- Basic fibroblast growth factor (bFGF; 060-04543, Wako, Japan)
- Puromycin (P7255-25MG, Sigma)
- Blasticidin S HCl (R210-01, Invitrogen)
- 0.05% trypsin/0.53 mM EDTA (25300-054, Invitrogen)
- 0.25% trypsin/1 mM EDTA (25200-056, Invitrogen)
- 2.5% trypsin (10×) (15090-046, Invitrogen)
- Collagenase Type IV (17104-019, Invitrogen)
- Gelatin (G1890, Sigma)
- Mitomycin C (134-07911, Wako, Japan)
- FuGENE® HD transfection reagent (E2311, Promega)
- Opti-MEM® I reduced-serum medium (31985-062, Invitrogen)
- Hexadimethrine bromide (Polybrene; H9268-5G, Sigma)
- CELLBANKER®-1 (cell freezing solution; BLC-1, Juji Field, Japan)
- DMSO (D2650, Sigma)
- Acetamide (015-00115, Wako, Japan)
- propylene glycol (164-04996, Wako, Japan)
- 4% Paraformaldehyde Phosphate Buffer Solution (4% PFA solution; 163-20145, Wako, Japan)
- Leukocyte Alkaline Phosphatase Kit (86C-1KT, Sigma)

Reagents Set Up

- **MSC medium (containing 15% FBS)**
  To prepare MSC medium, add 90 ml of FBS and 5 ml of Penicillin-Streptomycin into a 500 ml of α-MEM. Mix gently and stored at 4°C.
- **SNL medium (containing 10% FBS)**
  To prepare SNL medium, add 56 ml of FBS and 5 ml of Penicillin-Streptomycin into a 500 ml of D-MEM. Mix gently and store at 4°C.
- **10 x gelatin stock solution (1% w/v)**
  Dissolve 5 g of gelatin powder in 500 ml of distilled water. Autocrave and store at 4°C.
- **1 x gelatin solution (0.1% w/v)**
  Thaw the 10 x gelatin stock solution in the water bath at 37°C and add 50 ml of the thawed 10 x gelatin stock solution into 450 ml of distilled water, then pass the solution through filter using a 0.22 μm bottle top filter and store at 4°C.
- **1 mg/ml mitomycin C stock solution**
  Dissolve 10 mg of mitomycin in 10 ml of PBS, filter through a 0.22-mm filter. Store at −80°C.
- **10 mg/ml puromycin solution**
  Dissolve 25 mg of puromycin powder in 2.5 ml of distilled water, filter through a 0.22 μm filter. Store at −20°C.
- **10 mg/ml blasticidin-S solution**
  Dissolve 50 mg of Blasticidin S HCl powder in 5 ml of distilled water, and filter through a 0.22 μm filter. Store at −20°C.
- **8 mg/ml polyblene (hexadimethrine bromide) solution**
  For 10 x stock (80 mg/ml polyblene) solution, dissolve 0.8 g of hexadimethrine bromide powder in 10 ml of distilled water. Dilute the 1 ml of 10 x stock solution in 9 ml of distilled water, and filter through a 0.22 μm filter. Store at −20°C.
- **10 μg/ml bFGF stock solution**
  Dissolve 100 μg of bFGF powder in 10 ml of iPS medium (see below). Stock aliquots of 320 μl of the bFGF stock solution in each 1.5 ml tube and store at −20°C.
- **iPS medium**
  To prepare iPS medium, add 125 ml of KSR (final conc. 20%), 6.4 ml of MEM Non-Essential Amino Acids Solution (final conc. 0.1 mM), 6.4 ml of Penicillin-Streptomycin (final conc. 100 U/ml – 100 mg/ml), 1.16 ml of 2-Mercaptoethanol (final conc. 0.1 mM), and 320 μl of 10 μg/ml bFGF (final conc. 5 ng/ml) into a 500 ml of D-MEM/F-12 (which supplemented with GlutaMAX-I) bottle. Mix gently and store at 4°C.
- **1 mg/ml collagenase solution**
  Dissolve 10 mg of collagenase Type IV powder in 10 ml of distilled water and filter through a 0.22 μm filter. Store at −20°C.
- **0.1 M CaCl$_2$**
  Dissolve 0.11 g of CaCl$_2$ in 10 ml of distilled water and filter through a 0.22 μm filter. Store at 4°C.
- **CTK solution**
  Add 10 ml of 1 mg/ml collagenase solution, 1 ml of 0.1 M CaCl$_2$, 10 ml of 2.5% trypsin, and 20 ml of KSR into 60 ml of distilled water. Store at −20°C.
- **10 M acetamide**
  Dissolve 5.9 g of acetamide in 10 ml of distilled water. Store at room temperature.
- **DAP213 solution**
  Mix 1.43 ml of DMSO, 1 ml of 10 M acetamide, and 2.2 ml of propylene glycol in 5.37 ml of iPS medium. Store at −80°C.

Equipment

- PIPETMAN® P-10 (F144802, Gilson)
- PIPETMAN® P-200 (F123601, Gilson)
- 2 ml aspirating pipets (357558, BD Biosciences)
- 5 ml serological pipets (356543, BD Biosciences)
- 10 ml serological pipets (356551, BD Biosciences)
- 25 ml serological pipets (356535, BD Biosciences)
- 50 ml serological pipets (356550, BD Biosciences)
- T-75 tissue culture flasks with vented cap (T75-flask; 353136, BD Biosciences)
- T-225 tissue culture flasks with vented cap (T225-flask; 353138, BD Biosciences)
- 100-mm tissue culture dishes (100-mm dish; 353003, BD Biosciences)
- 96-well tissue culture plate (353072, BD Biosciences)
- 24-well tissue culture plate (353047, BD Biosciences)
- 6-well tissue culture plate (353046, BD Biosciences)
- 60-mm easy-grip cell culture dishes (60-mm dish; 353004, BD Biosciences)
- 15 ml polypropylene conical tube (352096, BD Biosciences)
- 50 ml polypropylene conical tube (352070, BD Biosciences)

- 1.5 ml microtube (MCT-150-C, Axygen)
- 2 ml cryogenic vial (MS-4603, Sumitomo Bakelite, Japan)
- CellBIND® Surface HYPERFlask® M Cell Culture Vessel (10020, corning)
- Costar® 1 L storage bottles (8396, corning)
- 0.22 μm pore size cellulose acetate filter (17597 K, Sartorius)
- 0.45 μm pore size cellulose acetate filter (16555 K, Sartorius)
- 10 ml disposable syringe (SS-10SZ, Termo, Japan)
- Feather disposable scalpel (No.10, Feather)
- FACS Vantage SE (Becton Dickinson)
- Cell Scrapter (9000-220, Iwaki, Japan)

Procedure

Most of our protocols of the iPS cell generation are referred to Center for iPS Cell Research and Application (CiRA) at Kyoto University (http://www.cira.kyoto-u.ac.jp/e/index.html) and are described below with some modifications.

Preparation of Human Third Molars for MSCs Isolation/Clonally-Expansion

Harvest and Primary Culture of Tooth Germs from Human Third Molar

1. Tooth germs of human third molar at the late bell stage with no eruption into oral cavity are extracted during orthodontic treatments (see reference Ikeda et al., 2008).
2. Separate the tooth germ of dental papilla from dental follicle in the extracted third molar using forceps.
3. Finely mince the tooth germ (approximately 0.4 g) using disposable scalpel. Transfer the germ into 10 ml of collagenase solution (4 mg/ml collagenase in PBS supplemented with 1 mM $CaCl_2$) in 15 ml of conical tube.
4. Incubate and gently shake the tube for 30 min at 37°C in the water bath.
5. Centrifuge the tube at $400g$ for 10 min at 4°C.
6. Aspirate the supernatant, resuspend the germ with 10 ml of MSC medium, and seed into the 100-mm dish.
7. Culture the germ at 37°C in a CO_2 incubator. Change the medium every other day. During the culture, the cell debris and floating cells can be removed, thereby majority of the cells show adherent fibroblast-like cell morphology.
8. When cells reach 80–90% confluency (approximately 1 week after cultivation), it's time to passage the cells into larger dish or flask.

Isolation and Expansion of Clonally-Expanded MSCs Derived from Tooth Germs

9. Aspirate the medium, and wash the 100-mm dish with 10 ml of PBS.
10. Add 1 ml of 0.05% Trypsin / 0.53 mM EDTA, and incubate the dish in a CO_2 incubator at 37°C for 5 min.
11. Add 9 ml of MSC medium, and transfer the cell suspension into a 15 ml conical tube.
12. Centrifuge the tube at $180g$ for 5 min at 4°C.
13. Resuspend cell pellet with appropriate amount of MSC medium, and seed directly into 96-well plates at single cell / well using the Clonecyte system of flow cytometry (FACS) Vantage SE. We defined passage-1 at this stage.
14. Select the wells which containing single cell (colony forming efficiency of the single cells was approximately 70%). Change the medium every other day until cells become 80–90% confluency.
15. When clonally-expanded cells (henceforth; clonally-expanded MSCs) reach confluent, trypsinize and divide the cells into three wells of 6-well plates (passage-2). For further expansion, seed the cells at 1×10^5 cells/T-75 flask (passage-3). We usually used passage-7 cells for the iPS cell generation. Typical morphologies of clonally-expanded MSCs are seen in Fig. 9.1.

Cryopreservation of Clonally-Expanded MSCs Derived from Tooth Germs

16. Aspirate the medium, and wash the T-75 flask with 10 ml of PBS.
17. Add 1 ml of 0.05% Trypsin / 0.53 mM EDTA, and incubate at 37°C for 5 min.
18. Add 9 ml of MSC medium, and transfer the cell suspension into a 15 ml conical tube.

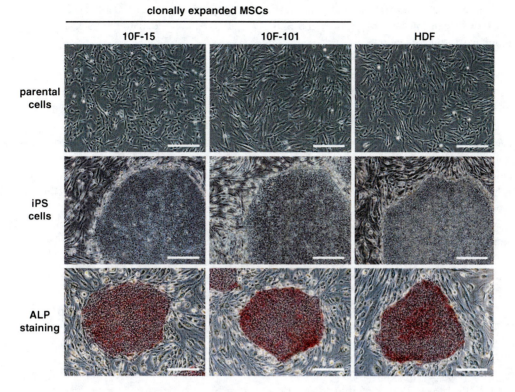

Fig. 9.1 Morphologies of clonally-expanded MSCs, human dermal fibroblasts (HDF), and iPS cells. Parental cells of clonally-expanded MSCs and HDF (*upper panel*), iPS cells from the parental cells (*middle panel*), and ALP staining of each iPS cell (*lower panel*). Scale bars = 100 μm. Reproduced from Oda et al. (2010) with permission of the American Society for Biochemistry and Molecular Biology

19. Count the cell number, and centrifuge the tube at 180g for 5 min at 4°C.
20. Resuspend cell pellet with appropriate amount of CELLBANKER-1 to adjust cell density at 5×10^5 cells/ml.
21. Add 1 ml of the cell suspension into each cryovial.
22. Store these tubes at −80°C in a freezer (up to 3 months) or in liquid nitrogen for more long term of storage.

Thawing of Clonally-Expanded MSCs Derived from Tooth Germs

23. Prepare 9 ml of MSC medium into a 15 ml of conical tube. Pre-warm the medium in water bath at 37°C.
24. Transfer the cryovial containing the frozen stocked cells (Section "Cryopreservation of Clonally-Expanded MSCs Derived from Tooth Germs") into water bath until most of cells are thawed.
25. Wipe the cryovial with 70% ethanol, and transfer the cell suspension into the pre-warmed MSC medium in a 15 ml conical tube.
26. Centrifuge the tube at 180g for 5 min at 4°C.
27. Aspirate the supernatant, resuspend the cells with 10 ml of MSC medium, and seed into 100-mm dish (5×10^5 cells/100-mm dish).
28. Culture the cells at 37°C in a CO_2 incubator. Change the medium every other day until cells become 80–90% confluency.

Preparation of SNL Feeder Cells

Thawing of SNL Feeder Cells

29. Prepare 9 ml of SNL medium into a 15 ml of conical tube. Pre-warm the medium in water bath at 37°C.
30. Transfer the cryovial containing SNL feeder cells into water bath until most of cells are thawed.

31. Wipe the cryovial with 70% ethanol, and transfer the cell suspension into the pre-warmed SNL medium in a 15 ml conical tube.
32. Centrifuge the tube at 180g for 5 min at 4°C.
33. Aspirate the supernatant, resuspend the cells with 60 ml of SNL medium, and seed into 1 x gelatin-coated T-225 flasks (30 ml/flask). We recommend the density of SNL feeder cells at 1–2 × 10^4 cells/cm^2.
34. Culture the cells at 37°C in a CO_2 incubator. Change the SNL medium every other day until cells become 80–90% confluency.

Passaging SNL Feeder Cells

35. Aspirate SNL medium, add 30 ml of PBS into the T-225 flask.
36. Aspirate PBS, add 3 ml of 0.05% Trypsin/0.53 mM EDTA, and incubate the flask in a CO_2 incubator at 37°C for 2–5 min.
37. Add 27 ml of SNL medium, and transfer the cell suspension into a 50 ml conical tube.
38. Centrifuge the tube at 180g for 5 min at 4°C.
39. Aspirate the supernatant, resuspend with 560 ml of SNL medium, and seed all of them in a 1 x gelatin-coated HYPERFlask.
40. Culture the cells at 37°C in a CO_2 incubator. Change the SNL medium every other day. The cells become confluent after 3–4 days.

Treatment of Mitomycin C and Cryopreservation of SNL Feeder Cells

41. Transfer the SNL medium from a HYPER Flask (approximately 560 ml) which culturing SNL feeder cells into a 1 L storage bottle.
42. Add 5.6 ml of 1 mg/ml mitomycin C stock solution into the 1 L storage bottle.
43. Transfer the SNL medium containing mitomycin C (approximately 566 ml) into the SNL feeder cells culturing HYPER Flask. Final concentration of mitomycin C is 10 μg/ml.
44. Incubate the HYPER Flask at 37°C in a CO_2 incubator for 2.5–3 h. Avoid long time incubation (more than 4 h) which reduces the cell viability.
45. Wash the HYPER Flask with 250 ml of PBS. Repeat this step once more.
46. Aspirate PBS, add 100 ml of 0.25% Trypsin/1 mM EDTA, and incubate the flask in a CO_2 incubator at 37°C for 5 min.
47. Add 100 ml of SNL medium, and transfer the cell suspension into several 50 ml conical tubes.
48. Centrifuge the tube at 180g for 5 min at 4°C.
49. Aspirate the supernatant, resuspend the cells with 50 ml of SNL medium.
50. Count the cell number, and centrifuge the tube at 180g for 5 min at 4°C.
51. Resuspend the cells with an appropriate amount of CELLBANKER-1 to adjust concentration to 1 × 10^7 cells/ml.
52. Add the 1 ml of cell suspension into each cryovial.
53. Store these tubes in a −80°C freezer or liquid nitrogen.

Expansion, and Cryopreservation of Plat-A Packaging Cells

Thawing of Plat-A Packaging Cells

54. Thaw Plat-A cells in the cryovial as same as described in steps 23–26 using with SNL medium.
55. Aspirate the supernatant, resuspend the cells with 30 ml of SNL medium, and seed into T-225 flask. Culture the cells in a CO_2 incubator at 37°C.
56. Next day, aspirate the medium and add the 30 ml of fresh SNL medium supplemented with 3 μl of 10 mg/ml of puromycin, and 30 μl of 10 mg/ml of blasticidin-S (Plat-A medium).
57. Change the Plat-A medium every other day until cells become 80–90% confluency.

Passaging Plat-A Packaging Cells

58. Passage the Plat-A cells as same as described in steps 35–38 using with Plat-A medium. We routinely seed Plat-A cells at 1:10 split ratio.
59. Culture the cells in a CO_2 incubator at 37°C.

Cryopreservation of Plat-A Packaging Cells

60. Trypsinize the Plat-A cells as same as steps 35–38.
61. Resuspend appropriate amount of CELLBANKER-1 to adjust concentration to 1 × 10^7 cells/ml.

62. Add 1 ml of cell suspension into each cryovial. Store these tubes in a −80°C freezer or liquid nitrogen.

Generation of iPS Cells from Clonally-Expanded MSCs

Day 1

Thawing of Plat-A Packaging Cells

63. Thaw the Plat-A cells in the cryovial (Section "Cryopreservation of Plat-A Packaging Cells") as same as described in step 54.
64. Aspirate the supernatant, resuspend the cells with 30 ml of SNL medium, and seed into T225 flask (1×10^7 cells / T225 flask). Do not add puromycin and blasticdin-S. Culture the cells in a CO_2 incubator at 37°C.
65. Change the Plat-A medium every other day until cells become 80–90% confluency. It takes around 3 days after thawing of the cells.

Day 2

66. Check the attachment of Plat-A cells in the T-225 flask under a microscope.

Day 3

Thawing of Clonally-Expanded MSCs

67. Thaw the clonnaly-expanded MSCs (Section "Thawing of Clonally-Expanded MSCs Derived from Tooth Germs") as same as described in steps 23–26.
68. Aspirate the supernatant, resuspend the cells with 10 ml of MSC medium, and seed into 100-mm dish (5×10^5 cells / 100-mm dish).
69. Culture the cells in a CO_2 incubator at 37°C. Change the medium every other day until cells become 80–90% confluency. It takes around 3–4 days after plating.

Day 4

Passaging of Plat-A Packaging Cells

70. Trypsinization of the confluent Plat-A cells described in step 58.
71. Aspirate the supernatant, resuspend appropriate amount of SNL medium, and seed them at 8×10^6 cells / 100-mm dish. At least, you need three dishes for next step (pMXs retroviral vectors transfection). Culture the cells overnight in a CO_2 incubator at 37°C.

Day 5

Tansfection of pMXs Retroviral Vectors to Plat-A Packaging Cells

72. Next day, prepare 300 μl of OPTI-MEM I in a 1.5 ml tube. At least, you need three tubes for pMXs retroviral vectors transfection.
73. Add 27 μl of FuGENE HD reagent into each tube containing the OPTI-MEM. Mix gently and incubate 5 min at room temperature.
74. Add 9 μg of each of three pMXs retroviral vectors encoding *OCT3/4*, *SOX2*, and *KLF4* into the three tubes, respectively. Mix gently and incubate 15 min at room temperature.
75. Add the pMXs vectors / FuGENE HD mixture into each dish culturing Plat-A cells, and gently shake the dishes back and forth. Incubate the cells overnight in a CO_2 incubator at 37°C.

Day 6

76. Next day, aspirate the supernatant (containing pMXs vectors and FuGENE HD reagent), and add 10 ml of fresh SNL medium. Incubate the cells overnight in a CO_2 incubator at 37°C.

Preparation of Clonally-Expanded MSCs

77. About 80–90% confluent cells from Section "Thawing of Clonally-Expanded MSCs" are trypsinized, counted and seeded at 5×10^5 cells / 100-mm dish. Culture the cells overnight in a CO_2

incubator at 37°C. Trypsinization and cell counts are described in steps 16–19.

Day 7

Retroviral Transduction to Clonally-Expanded MSCs (First Retroviral Transduction)

78. Collect the viral supernatant (Section "Tansfection of pMXs Retroviral Vectors to Plat-A Packaging Cells") from each dish culturing Plat-A cells using 10 ml of disposable syringe, filter through 0.45 μm pore size cellulose acetate filter, and transfer them into a 50 ml conical tube (i.e. 30 ml of viral mixture containing 10 ml of OCT3/4, 10 ml of SOX2, and 10 ml of KLF4 viral supernatant). Add 10 ml of fresh SNL medium into the dishes culturing Plat-A cells.
79. Add 15 μl of 8 mg / ml polyblene solution in a viral containing 50 ml tube, mix gently by pipetting. The final concentration of polyblene is 4 μg / ml.
80. Aspirate the MSC medium from the dishes (prepared Section "Preparation of Clonally-Expanded MSCs"), and add 10 ml of viral mixture / 100-mm dish. Culture the cells overnight in a CO_2 incubator at 37°C.

Day 8

Retroviral Transduction to Clonally-Expanded MSCs (Second Retroviral Transduction)

81. Collect the viral supernatant (Section "Retroviral Transduction to Clonally-Expanded MSCs (First Retroviral Transduction)") from each Plat-A cultured dish.
82. Repeat the steps 78–80 for second retroviral transduction.

Thawing of Mitomycin C Treated SNL Feeder Cells for Replating of Transduced Cells

83. Thaw the mitomycin C treated SNL feeder cells (prepared in Section "Treatment of Mitomycin C and Cryopreservation of SNL Feeder Cells") described in steps 29–32.

84. Aspirate the supernatant, resuspend the cells with 50 ml of SNL medium (1×10^7 cells / 50 ml), and seed them into 1 x gelatin-coated 100-mm dishes. We recommend the density of mitomycin C treated SNL feeder cells at $1.5–2 \times 10^6$ cells / 100-mm dish. Culture the cells in a CO_2 incubator at 37°C.

Day 9

Culture of Transduced Clonally-Expanded MSCs

85. Aspirate the medium containing viral supernatant from the dishes (from Section "Retroviral Transduction to Clonally-Expanded MSCs (Second Retroviral Transduction)"), and add 10 ml of fresh MSC medium.

Day 10

86. Repeat step 85.

Day 11

Replating of Transduced Clonally-Expanded MSCs onto Mitomycin C-Treated SNL Feeder Cells

87. Trypsinize the transduced MSCs (step 86), and adjust the cells at 5×10^4 or 2×10^5 cells / 10 ml of MSC medium. Trypsinization and cell counts are described in steps 16–19.
88. Seed either 5×10^4 or 2×10^5 cells onto mitomycin C-treated SNL feeder cells (prepared in Section "Thawing of Mitomycin C Treated SNL Feeder Cells for Replating of Transduced Cells"). Culture the cells overnight in a CO_2 incubator at 37°C.

Day 12~

89. Aspirate the culture medium from the dishes, and add 10 ml of fresh iPS medium. Change medium every other day until the iPS cell colonies become large enough to pick up (see Fig. 9.1). It takes about 3–4 weeks after retroviral transduction but the term is different from each lot of clonally-expanded MSCs.

Picking up the iPS Colonies

90. Add 150 μl of iPS medium per well of 96-well plate.
91. Set the adjusting knob of PIPETMAN P-10 at 5 μl, pick up the iPS colonies from the dishes under a microscope, and transfer them into the wells of 96-well plate.
92. Set the adjusting knob of PIPETMAN P-200 at 140 μl, and break these iPS cell colonies to small clumps (20–50 cells/clump) by pipetting. Extensive pipetting causes dispersion of the clumps at single cell level which should be avoided by careful monitoring using microscope. Transfer these iPS cell clumps into 24-well plate which is already seeded with mitomycin C treated SNL feeder cells. Add 400 μl of iPS medium into each well.
93. Culture the cells overnight in a CO_2 incubator at 37°C. Change iPS medium every day until the iPS colonies become large enough to passage. It takes about 4–7 days after colony plating.

Passaging and Expansion of iPS Cells

94. Aspirate iPS medium, and wash each well with 500 μl of PBS.
95. Aspirate PBS, add 100 μl per well of CTK solution, and incubate at room temperature for 1–2 min. When SNL feeder cells begin to dissociate from the plates while iPS colonies still adhere to plate, aspirate the CTK solution and add 500 μl of PBS in each well. If SNL feeder cells still attach to the plate, incubate at room temperature another several minutes.
96. Aspirate PBS, and wash each well with 500 μl of PBS.
97. Aspirate PBS, and add 500 μl of iPS medium into the each well. Scrape the adherent iPS colonies using cell scraper, and break these iPS cell colonies to small clumps (20–50 cells/clump) by pipetting. The clumps are cultured on SNL feeder cells as described in Section "Picking up the iPS Colonies".
98. Further expansions are carried out by repeating the Sections "Picking up the iPS Colonies" and "Passaging and Expansion of iPS Cells". We usually expand iPS cells from 6-well scale to 60-mm dish and 100-mm dish to obtain enough numbers of iPS cells. Figure 9.1 shows typical morphologies of iPS cells derived from clonally-expanded MSCs.

Cryopreservation of iPS Cells

99. Aspirate iPS medium, and wash with 10 ml / 100-mm dish of PBS.
100. Aspirate PBS, add 1 ml / 100-mm dish of CTK solution, and incubate at room temperature for 1–2 min.
101. Aspirate CTK solution, and wash twice with 10 ml of PBS.
102. Aspirate PBS, and add 12 ml of iPS medium. Scrape the adherent iPS colonies using cell scraper. Do not break these iPS cell colonies by pipetting.
103. Transfer 4 ml of scraped iPS cells into three 15 ml conical tubes.
104. Centrifuge the tubes at 180g for 5 min at 4°C.
105. Aspirate the supernatant, add 200 μl of cooled DAP213 solution into each 15 ml conical tube, and gently pipette for 2–3 times.
106. Transfer the iPS cell suspension into each cryovial. Immediately (within 15 s), put these tubes into liquid nitrogen.

Thawing of iPS Cells

107. Prepare 9.8 ml of iPS medium into a 15 ml of conical tube. Pre-warm the tube in the water bath at 37°C.
108. Transfer the cryovial containing iPS cell colonies (Section "Cryopreservation of iPS Cells") into safety cabinet, add 900 μl of pre-warmed iPS medium into each cryovial, and thaw the colonies as soon as possible by pipetting for several times.
109. Transfer the iPS cell colonies suspension into the 15 ml conical tube described in step 107.
110. Centrifuge the tube at 180g for 5 min at 4°C.
111. Aspirate supernatant, resuspend the iPS cell colonies with 10 ml of iPS medium, and transfer into 100-mm dish which is already seeded with mitomycin C treated SNL feeder cells.
112. Culture the cells in a CO_2 incubator at 37°C. Change iPS medium every day.

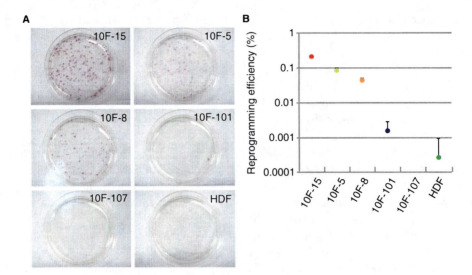

Fig. 9.2 Reprogramming efficiencies of clonally expanded MSCs and HDF. (**a**) ALP staining of clonally expanded MSCs and HDF derived iPS cells. Cells were stained after 30 days of first retroviral transduction. (**b**) Reprogramming efficiencies of clonally-expanded MSCs and HDF. The efficiencies were determined as the number of total iPS-like ALP positive colonies per the total number of transduced cells. The *closed circles* represent average of two independent experiments and *bars* indicate standard derivation ($n = 8$). As seen in this figure, reprogramming efficiencies from each parental cell are different. Some clonally-expanded MSCs from human third molar show excellent reprogramming efficiency. Reproduced from Oda et al. (2010) with permission of the American Society for Biochemistry and Molecular Biology

Alkaline Phosphatase (ALP) Staining for Count ALP-Positive iPS Colonies

113. Pre-warm 4% PFA solution and Leukocyte Alkaline Phosphatase Kit at room temperature.
114. Aspirate iPS medium from the 100-mm dish, wash twice with 10 ml of PBS.
115. Aspirate PBS, add 5 ml of 4% PFA solution into the dish, and incubate for 10 min at room temperature.
116. While waiting for cell fixation, prepare 5.6 ml of distilled water into the 15 ml conical tube.
117. Add 125 μl of Sodium Nitrite Solution and 125 μl of FRV-Alkaline Solution into the 1.5 ml tube, and incubate 2 min at room temperature (these solutions supplied in the kit).
118. Transfer these mixed solution into the 15 ml conical tube containing 5.6 ml water, and add 125 μl of Naphthol AS-BI Alkaline Solution (supplied in the kit). Mix gently.
119. Add all mixed solution into the fixed iPS cell dish.
120. Incubate for 30 min at 37°C. Protect from light.
121. Wash three times with 10 ml of PBS or distilled water, and then count ALP positive iPS colonies (Typical ALP positive colonies are seen in Figs. 9.1 and 9.2). The number of ALP positive iPS cell colonies can be used for measuring the reprogramming efficiency as seen in Fig. 9.2b.

References

Gronthos S, Mankani M, Brahim J, Robey PG, Shi S (2000) Postnatal human dental pulp stem cells (DPSCs) in vitro and in vivo. Proc Natl Acad Sci USA 97:13625–13630

Ikeda E, Hirose M, Kotobuki N, Shimaoka H, Tadokoro M, Maeda M, Hayashi Y, Kirita T, Ohgushi H (2006) Osteogenic differentiation of human dental papilla mesenchymal cells. Biochem Biophys Res Commun 342:1257–1262

Ikeda E, Yagi K, Kojima M, Yagyuu T, Ohshima A, Sobajima S, Tadokoro M, Katsube Y, Isoda K, Kondoh M, Kawase M, Go MJ, Adachi H, Yokota Y, Kirita T, Ohgushi H (2008) Multipotent cells from the human third molar: feasibility of cell-based therapy for liver disease. Differentiation 76:495–505

Kitamura T, Koshino Y, Shibata F, Oki T, Nakajima H, Nosaka T, Kumagai H (2003) Retrovirus-mediated gene transfer and expression cloning: powerful tools in functional genomics. Exp Hematol 31:1007–1014

Miura M, Gronthos S, Zhao M, Lu B, Fisher LW, Robey PG, Shi S (2003) SHED: stem cells from human exfoliated deciduous teeth. Proc Natl Acad Sci USA 100:5807–5812

Morita S, Kojima T, Kitamura T (2000) Plat-E: an efficient and stable system for transient packaging of retroviruses. Gene Ther 7:1063–1066

Nakagawa M, Koyanagi M, Tanabe K, Takahashi K, Ichisaka T, Aoi T, Okita K, Mochiduki Y, Takizawa N, Yamanaka S (2008) Generation of induced pluripotent stem cells without Myc from mouse and human fibroblasts. Nat Biotechnol 26:101–106

Oda Y, Yoshimura Y, Ohnishi H, Tadokoro M, Katsube Y, Sasao M, Kubo Y, Hattori K, Saito S, Horimoto K, Yuba S, Ohgushi H (2010) Induction of pluripotent stem cells from human third molar mesenchymal stromal cells. J Biol Chem 285:29270–29278

Ohgushi H, Caplan AI (1999) Stem cell technology and bioceramics: from cell to gene engineering. J Biomed Mater Res 48:913–927

Ohgushi H, Kotobuki N, Funaoka H, Machida H, Hirose M, Tanaka Y, Takakura Y (2005) Tissue engineered ceramic artificial joint—ex vivo osteogenic differentiation of patient mesenchymal cells on total ankle joints for treatment of osteoarthritis. Biomaterials 26:4654–4661

Okita K, Ichisaka T, Yamanaka S (2007) Generation of germline-competent induced pluripotent stem cells. Nature 448: 313–317

Salem HK, Thiemermann C (2010) Mesenchymal stromal cells: current understanding and clinical status. Stem Cells 28: 585–596

Takahashi K, Yamanaka S (2006) Induction of pluripotent stem cells from mouse embryonic and adult fibroblast cultures by defined factors. Cell 126:663–676

Takahashi K, Tanabe K, Ohnuki M, Narita M, Ichisaka T, Tomoda K, Yamanaka S (2007) Induction of pluripotent stem cells from adult human fibroblasts by defined factors. Cell 131:861–872

Yagyuu T, Ikeda E, Ohgushi H, Tadokoro M, Hirose M, Maeda M, Inagake K, Kirita T (2010) Hard tissue-forming potential of stem/progenitor cells in human dental follicle and dental papilla. Arch Oral Biol 55:68–76

Chapter 10

Self-renewal and Differentiation of Intestinal Stem Cells: Role of Hedgehog Pathway

Nikè V.J.A. Büller, Sanne L. Rosekrans, and Gijs R. van den Brink

Abstract The epithelium of the intestine is a rapidly renewing system in which the rate of proliferation of stem cells is in a perfect balance with the number of differentiating cells. In an effort to understand the mechanisms that maintain homeostasis in such dynamic yet stable systems, research has shown that morphogenetic pathways are not only involved in body patterning during embryogenesis but also in orchestrating tissue patterning in adult tissues. In the intestine, fate and proliferation of stem cells is determined by the Wnt signaling pathway. In this review we will discuss recent data that show that the balance between differentiated cells and stem cell proliferation is determined by a negative feedback loop from the differentiated cells to the stem cell compartment that depends on epithelial-mesenchymal interactions. We will elaborate on the evidence that this negative feedback loop depends on Indian hedgehog secreted by differentiated enterocytes which acts to maintain the expression of bone morphogenetic proteins and activins in the mesenchyme which subsequently negatively regulate stem cell fate in the epithelial layer. Furthermore, we will discuss the potential role of this negative feedback loop in wound healing and show how it is inactivated during the development of colorectal cancer.

Keywords Homeostasis · Epithelium · Epithelial-mesenchymal interaction · Activins · Feedback loop · Villi

Introduction

Multicellular organisms consist of a large variety of specialized cells that form organs with complex architecture and tasks. In order to shape or maintain an organ, cells must be tightly instructed to determine their number, position and function. To maintain such complexity cell fate needs to be regulated at the population level by extrinsic signals. How this cell fate is determined and by what signals, remains one of the greatest questions in biology.

The epithelium on the villi of the small intestine is entirely renewed once every 3–5 days from a pool of continuously replicating stem cells which reside in the bottom of small mucosal invaginations called crypts (Potten and Loeffler, 1990). Stem cells can either self renew or generate daughter cells that migrate upwards to become transit amplifying cells which can rapidly proliferate but have lost the capacity to self renew. When they reach the top of the crypt, transit amplifying cells withdraw from the cell cycle and differentiate into one of the four cell types of the small intestine (enterocyte, goblet cell, enteroendocrine cell or Paneth cell). These cells migrate further to their positions on the villus or in the crypt until they are shed off or undergo apoptosis (Potten, 2004) (Fig. 10.1). The morphology of the colon is similar to that of the small intestine, but it lacks villi and Paneth cells.

Thus the intestinal epithelium is a system in which a perfect balance is maintained between different compartments of cells despite a very high flux of cells between these compartments. Such dynamic equilibria depend on the presence of negative feedback loops between compartments. The presence of such feedback loops not only allows the fine tuning of the number of

G.R. van den Brink (✉)
Department of Gastroenterology & Hepathology, Tytgat Institute for Liver and Intestinal Research, Academic Medical Center, Amsterdam, The Netherlands
e-mail: g.r.vandenbrink@amc.nl

the expression of a distinct set of target genes which determine different outcomes in terms of cellular fate. Therefore, dependent on the position of a cell in such concentration gradients it can acquire different characteristics in response to the same signaling molecule. Four families of morphogenetic pathways can roughly be distinguished, the Wnt, Hedgehog (Hh), Tgf-β families and a large group of receptor tyrosine kinases such as fibroblast growth factor, platelet-derived growth factor, epidermal growth factor etcetera, which share similar intracellular signaling pathways. Several of these morphogenetic pathways have now been identified as key regulators of cell fate in the intestinal epithelium. In this chapter we will first briefly review how stem cell fate is maintained by Wnt signaling and then discuss data that show how an epithelial mesenchymal negative feedback loop which involves the Hh and different TGF-β family members acts to maintain homeostasis between differentiated cells and the rate of proliferation in the crypt.

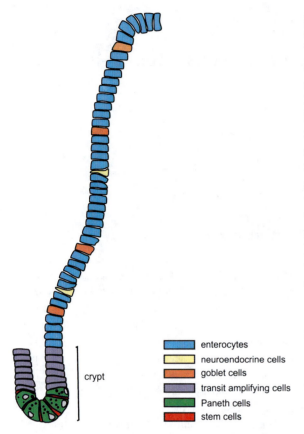

Fig. 10.1 Crypt-villus compartment. In the adult intestine transit amplifying cells are derived from stem cells and either move downwards to form Paneth cells (only in the small intestine), or upwards to form the other intestinal cell lineages

Wnt Signaling and the Intestinal Stem Cell

The Wnt pathway is one of the best studied signaling pathways due to its relevance in biology and carcinogenesis. The knowledge on Wnt signaling was boosted when it was discovered that the *APC* gene, an important regulator of Wnt signalling, was mutated in patients with familial adenomatous polyposis (FAP) (Nishisho et al., 1991). Although FAP is a rare disease, mutations in *APC* have been found in the majority of sporadic colorectal cancers (Bienz and Clevers, 2000).

The pathway turns on cell type specific gene expression programs due to the stabilization and nuclear localization of β-catenin. Wnt ligand binds to its cell surface receptor of the Frizzled family and prevents degradation of β-catenin by a complex of proteins including Axin 1/2 and adenomatous polyposis coli (APC). β-catenin can translocate to the nucleus and interact with TCF/LEF family transcription factors.

In recent years, it has become clear that Wnt signaling is important for the specification of stem cell fate and for stem cell self renewal. Several Wnt targets such as LGR5 and ASCL2 are specifically expressed in the intestinal epithelial stem cells and can now be used as stem cell markers. The discussion of the role of Wnt

differentiated epithelial cells on the villus to the rate of proliferation at the base of the crypt under homeostatic conditions but will also allow a rapid increase in proliferation in case of massive loss of differentiated cells such as in wounding of the mucosal surface. Identifying such loops is crucial to our understanding of biological systems and it can contribute to our knowledge of both tissue homeostasis and disease.

The fate of a cell in an organ is dependent on its position along different spatial axes both during development and in rapidly regenerating tissues in the adult, such as the hematopoietic system, skin and the intestinal epithelium (Van Den Brink and Offerhaus, 2007). Morphogens are the key regulators of such position dependent cell fate regulation. Morphogens are soluble proteins that form a concentration gradient through a tissue. A morphogen receiving cell has one or more concentration thresholds that are coupled to signaling in intestinal stem cell biology is outside the context of this chapter however (for review see Barker et al., 2008).

Hedgehog Signaling During Development

The Hh-pathway was first discovered by Nüsslein-Volhard and Wieschaus (1980) in a genetic screen in Drosophila that identified regulators of body segmentation during embryogenesis. Vertebrates have three Hedgehog genes: Sonic hedgehog (Shh), Desert hedgehog (Dhh) and Indian hedgehog (Ihh). Hh ligand can bind to its transmembrane receptor Patched (Ptch1). In the absence of Hh ligand, Ptch1 suppresses another transmembrane receptor Smoothened (Smo). By binding Hh this suppression is alleviated and allows Smo to transmit the Hh signal, resulting in the transcription of target genes. The Gli transcription factor family is the main downstream activator of Hh signaling. Ptch1 and Hedgehog-interacting protein (Hhip) are transcriptional targets that act as a negative regulator of Hedgehog signaling (Fig. 10.2).

The important function of Hh signaling in the development of the small intestine and colon has been shown in studies with Shh and Ihh deficient mice which both die before or shortly after birth. $Shh^{-/-}$ mice display major abnormalities in foregut development but also show multiple anomalies in the intestine such as intestinal malrotation, duodenal stenosis, reduction of smooth muscle development and abnormal innervation (Litingtung et al., 1998). In $Ihh^{-/-}$ mice the intestinal epithelium fails to organize in a monolayer and there is a lack of good crypt organization (Van Den Brink et al., 2004). In addition, the Ihh mutant mouse show lack of neurons and dilated colon, both features of Hirschsprung's disease (Ramalho-Santos et al., 2000). These results show that Hh signals are essential for organogenesis of the gastrointestinal tract.

Hedgehog Signaling in Adult Intestine

Both Shh and Ihh are expressed in various parts of the gastrointestinal epithelium (Bitgood and McMahon, 1995). In adult small intestine and colon Ihh is the major Hh that is expressed (Van Den Brink et al.,

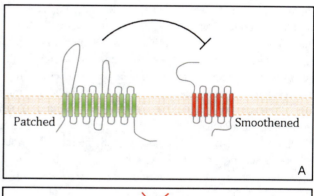

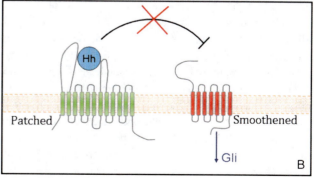

Fig. 10.2 The Hedgehog receptor complex. A model of Ptch-Smo interaction. (**a**) In the absence of Hedgehog Ptch functions as a transmembrane pump that inhibits receptor Smo. (**b**) Binding of Hedgehog to Ptch alleviates this suppression of Smo and results in activation of the pathway

2004; Van Dop et al., 2010). In the small intestine *Ihh* messenger RNA (mRNA) is highly expressed at the crypt-villus junction with gradually diminishing expression towards the tip of the villus and the protein is expressed by the enterocytes on the villi. In colon in situ hybridization showed that *Ihh* mRNA is expressed by the differentiating epithelial cells in the midcrypt region, whereas Ihh protein is expressed by the differentiated enterocytes. The pattern of partially overlapping mRNA and protein is often seen in enterocyte genes and explained by the cells moving up the villus, while still expressing the protein but no longer transcribing mRNA of the gene. A population of rare epithelial cells at the base of the crypt may express Shh as we observed these cells in the human small intestine and colon (Van Den Brink et al., 2002) and similar cells were detected in the mouse intestine using a Shh^{gfp} reporter mouse (Varnat et al., 2009, 2010). However the expression is likely very low as we were unable to detect this *Shh* expression by in situ hybridization in the mouse (Van Dop et al., 2009) and the role of this low Shh expression in normal homeostasis remains obscure.

Using $Ptch1^{LacZ/+}$, $Gli1^{LacZ/+}$ and $Gli2^{LacZ/+}$ reporter mice Kolterud et al. (2009) reported that Hh receptor Ptch1 and its direct targets Gli1 and Gli2 are exclusively expressed in the underlying mesenchyme. Therefore, it can be concluded that Hh signaling is strictly paracrine from epithelium to mesenchyme. Functional evidence for exclusive paracrine signaling was provided in *Villin-Cre;Smo$^{flox/flox}$* mice in which the Hh signaling receptor Smo was specifically deleted in intestinal epithelial cells. These mice exhibited a normal intestinal and colonic architecture, normal cell lineages and unaffected Wnt signaling (Kosinski et al., 2010). Hh-responsive cells in the mesenchyme include smooth muscle precursor cells, smooth muscle cells of the villus cores and muscularis mucosae, myofibroblasts and pericytes (Kolterud et al., 2009). It has also been described that myeloid cells, including dendritic cells are Hh responsive (Lees et al., 2008; Zacharias et al., 2010).

Intestinal myofibroblasts are located below the epithelium in close proximity to the smooth muscle cells. These cells at the base of the crypt are thought to be a part of the stem cell niche and have the ability to modulate epithelial proliferation and differentiation via membrane molecules as well as paracrine acting factors (Kedinger et al., 1998). Several studies have demonstrated that increased Hh signaling in the adult intestine leads to accumulation of myofibroblasts and smooth muscle cells. Van Dop et al. (2009) showed that induced $Ptch^{flox/flox}CreERT2^{+/-}$ mice exhibited a strong increase in the mesenchyme of α-smooth muscle actin (α-SMA) positive cells, which is a marker for myofibroblasts. However, no staining for desmin was performed leaving the possibility that these Hh responsive cells could also be smooth muscle precursor cells. Kolterud et al. (2009) described an accumulation of α-SMA and desmin double positive smooth muscle cells and α-SMA positive and desmin negative smooth muscle precursor cells in the villus cores of adult *Villin-Hhip* mice. Studies in mice with disrupted Hh signaling resulted in depletion of smooth muscle cells from the villus core (Zacharias et al., 2010; van Dop et al., 2010), as was also shown in the developing intestine by Madison et al. (2005). Taken together, these data indicate that Hh signaling controls the size of the smooth muscle cell and possibly the myofibroblast population in the villus core and the colonic lamina propria. However, it is unclear exactly what factors are expressed by these Hh-responsive cells and how they are involved in orchestrating homeostasis.

Negative Regulator of Wnt Signaling

Similar to the Hh pathway, the Wnt pathway was initially identified in genetic screens for patterning genes in fruit flies. Wnt signaling is the most important driving force for maintenance of ISC proliferation and cell fate of intestinal precursor cells (Korinek et al., 1998). The pathway turns on cell type specific gene expression programs due to the stabilization and nuclear localization of β-catenin. Wang et al. (2002) were the first to show that Hh signaling was involved in regulating ISC proliferation during postnatal development of the intestine. Hh signaling was disrupted with a Hh neutralizing antibody which resulted in hyperproliferation of crypt epithelial cells and the appearance of ectopic crypts in the villus compartment. In studies in which Hh was chemically inhibited by Smo antagonist cyclopamine (van den Brink et al., 2004) or genetically altered (Madison et al., 2005; Kosinski et al., 2010; van Dop et al., 2010), it was shown that Hh acts as an antagonist of Wnt signaling. Rats treated with cyclopamine showed disturbed enterocyte maturation in the colon, with loss of enterocyte differentiation markers such as brush-border staining for villin and carbonic anhydrase IV. Furthermore target genes of Wnt signaling were upregulated in the treated rats.

Madison et al. (2005) studied the developing intestine using an intestine specific overexpression of Hh inhibiting protein (Hhip). The *Villin-Hhip* transgenic mouse showed features similar to mice treated with a Hh neutralizing antibody with epithelial hyperplasia, ectopic crypt-like structures, poorly differentiated brush border and increased Wnt signaling. Similar results were obtained by Kosinski et al. (2010) using the same Villin promoter but specifically deleting Ihh using *VillinCre-Ihh$^{-/-}$* mice which clearly established that Ihh is the major Hh to regulate the development of the intestinal epithelium both before birth and during postnatal development. We conditionally deleted Ihh in the adult small intestine epithelium using the *Cyp1a1-Cre* promoter and observed a proliferative response of the intestinal epithelium with crypt fissioning and lengthening. This was accompanied by increased Wnt signaling as evidenced by nuclear accumulation of β-catenin, increased expression of Wnt targets and accumulation of stem cells. Interestingly, we found that these epithelial hallmarks of a wound healing response which we observed upon deletion of Ihh from the adult intestinal epithelium were accompanied by a mesenchymal wound healing response i.e. the recruitment of macrophages and fibroblasts. Thus, loss of a single signaling molecule derived from the differentiated epithelial cells is sufficient to induce multiple aspects of a wound healing response. This indicates that Ihh may act as a significant molecular indicator of epithelial integrity in the intestine. Loss of differentiated epithelial cells will result in a reduction of the concentration of Ihh which subsequently results in recruitment of mesenchymal cells critical to the wound healing response and loss of inhibition of proliferation of stem cells at the base of the crypt.

After prolonged disrupted Ihh signaling we and others observed loss of smooth muscle cells from the villus core with subsequent loss of villi and development of villus atrophy. Following this loss of villi we found that mice developed an enteritis characterized by a mixed inflammatory infiltrate (Van Dop et al., 2010). Our interpretation of these results is that this inflammation was due to the loss of villi and resulting mucosal damage rather than a direct result of the loss of Ihh signaling but this will not be further discussed in the context of this chapter (further reading: Lees et al., 2008; Zacharias et al., 2010; Kosinski et al., 2010).

We were able to obtain further evidence for a major role of the Hh signaling pathway as a negative regulator of Wnt signaling and stem cell fate in mice in which we conditionally deleted the Hh binding receptor Ptch1 in *Rosa26CreERT2-Ptch1$^{fl/fl}$* mice resulting in conditional activation of the pathway. In these mice we observed inhibition of Wnt signaling with premature maturation of stem cells to a precursor of the enterocyte lineage and colonic crypt hypoplasia (Van Dop et al., 2009). In conclusion, these data indicate that Hh signaling is involved in regulating proliferation of epithelial precursor cells and differentiation of enterocytes through negative regulation of Wnt signaling.

The Bmp/Activin Signaling Pathways Are Mesenchymal Targets of Hh Signaling

Since intestinal Hh signaling is exclusively epithelial to mesenchymal, effects on Wnt signaling in the stem cells at the base of the crypt have to depend on mesenchymal targets of Hh signaling. Bitgood and McMahon (1995) were the first to suggest a close link between Hh signaling and the expression of members of the Bmp pathway based on the adjacent gene expression of Hhs and Bmp2 and Bmp4 in many organs of the developing embryo. Later, Roberts et al. (1995, 1998) found that Bmp4 is indeed a mesenchymal target of Hh signaling in chick intestine and Madison et al. (2005) and Van Dop et al. (2009, 2010) showed that both Bmp4 and Bmp7 are mesenchymal targets of Hh signaling in adult mice. Intestinal specific expression of Bmp antagonist Noggin in Villin-Noggin transgenic mice allowed normal development of the intestinal epithelium but several weeks after birth these mice developed lesions that are similar to hamartomas, a rare type of polyp that is sometimes observed in humans. Similar lesions were observed in *Mx1-Cre-Bmpr1a$^{fl/fl}$* mice in which the Bmp receptor Bmpr1a was conditionally deleted from the adult intestinal epithelium and mesenchyme. It is important to realize however that such hamartomas are mainly characterized by an abnormally expanded mesenchymal component and show a relatively normal epithelial layer (Hardwick et al., 2008). Indeed, Auclair et al. (2007) deleted Bmpr1a specifically from the intestinal epithelium and observed a modest effect on epithelial proliferation and no polyp development indicating that hamartoma development depends on loss of mesenchymal Bmp signaling. This makes sense as we (Hardwick et al., 2004) and others (Haramis et al., 2004) have previously found that Bmp signaling occurs mainly in the differentiated epithelial in the colon and small intestine and not in the proliferating cells as judged by the phosphorylation status of Smad1,5,8. In Ihh mutant mice we observed loss of Bmp4 expression and loss of phosphorylated Smad1,5,8 from the villi. However, since loss of Ihh expression leads to a profound proliferative response in the crypts, the fact that Bmp signaling occurs mainly in the differentiated cells suggests that factors other than loss of Bmp signaling may be responsible for this. We therefore examined the localization of the active (phosphorylated) form of Smad2 and 3 which mediate signaling by the Tgfβ and activin receptors. Interestingly, the active forms of Smad1,5,8 and Smad2,3 were present in non-overlapping patterns in wild type mice with Smad1,5,8 being active in the differentiated cells as described and Smad2,3 active in the proliferating cells in the crypt. In *Ihh* mutant mice Smad2,3 phosphorylation was lost from the crypts. When we examined the expression of Tgfβ1-3 and all activin subunits we observed a generalized loss of Activin expression and loss of expression of the activin target Goosecoid.

These data strongly suggest that negative regulation of proliferation downstream of Hh signaling is mediated primarily via activin and not Bmp signaling.

Together these data suggest that Ihh produced by the differentiated cells on the villus induces both Bmps and activin expression which subsequently signal back to the epithelium. Bmps signal mainly to the differentiated cells whereas activins signal mainly towards the proliferating cells in the crypts (Fig. 10.3). Further experiments are now needed to test this concept.

Hedgehog Signaling and Carcinogenesis

Wnt pathway activating mutations in *APC* have been found in the majority of sporadic colorectal cancers (Bienz and Clevers, 2000). Since the Ihh-Bmp/activin signaling loop is a feedback loop that negatively regulates Wnt signaling, this loop may act as a tumor supressor mechanism. Indeed, both the BMP and Activin pathways are frequently inactivated in colorectal cancer. Loss of BMP signaling occurs either through loss of SMAD4 expression or loss of expression of BMPR2 which are mutually exclusive events. Loss of BMPR2 occurred mainly in microsattelite instable colon cancer and we found that the microsattelite mutations were present in the 3'-UTR of the *BMPR2* gene and resulted in instability of the *BMPR2* mRNA (Kodach et al., 2008). Mutations in the TGFβ type II receptor as well as in Activin type II receptor are similarly associated with microsatellite instability in colon cancer (Markowitz et al., 1995; Jung et al., 2004). We found that loss of BMP activity was present in 70% of colorectal cancers and occurred mainly at the transition from late adenoma to early carcinoma (Kodach et al., 2008). Thus it is clear that the cancer cells become unresponsive to the BMPs and Activins that are induced in the mesenchyme by Hh signaling.

What is less clear however is the role of Hh signaling itself in colorectal carcinomas. There are several reports on the role of Hh signaling in CRC but data are often conflicting. This is partly due to problems with antibody specificity of most commercially available antibodies for components of the Hh pathway and the fact that many results depend on the use of the Smo inhibitor cyclopamine which has important off-target effects when used at higher doses as done in most studies (Yauch et al., 2008).

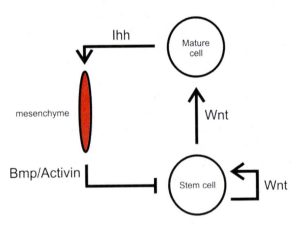

Fig. 10.3 Interaction between Hh and Wnt signaling. Proposed model of negative feedback signaling in the intestinal epithelial crypt. Ihh secreted by the differentiated cells acts on the mesenchymal cells, which secrete factors that subsequently negatively regulate precursor cells at the base of the crypt, possibly through Bmp and Activin

It has been shown that, in contrast to normal epithelium, mRNA levels of *Ptch1*, *Smo* and *Gli1* are detectable at least by PCR in colorectal cancer cell lines and xenografts derived from patients with colon carcinoma (Qualtrough et al., 2004). However, in the case of the xenografts the expression of Hh pathway components as detected by RT-PCR may well be derived from small contaminations of mesenchymal cells. Although it was found that the Smo antagonist cyclopamine resulted in apoptosis of colon cancer cell lines (Qualtrough et al., 2004), this occurred at doses that were later found to be 100 fold higher than the dose required for maximal inhibition of Hh signaling (Yauch et al., 2008) and may be the result of significant off-target effects of cyclopamine (Yauch et al., 2008). On the other hand, Varnat et al. found corroborating evidence for expression of Hh pathway components in colorectal cancers (Varnat et al., 2009). Since Hh signaling normally occurs in the mesenchyme, it may be that Hh responsiveness is related to features of epithelial-to-mesenchymal transition (EMT) in colon cancer. Varnat et al. (2009) went on to show that proliferation of a variety of colon cancer cell lines may depend on Hh signaling as their growth was impeded by expression of shRNA for Gli transcription factors or Smo and overexpression of a Gli3 repressor form. Furthermore overexpression of Gli1 and an shRNA against the inhibitory Hh receptor Ptch1 stimulated growth of colon cancer cell lines. It was not shown if these interventions altered the activity of the Hh pathway in terms of the expression of established targets of the pathway or a Gli-luciferase reporter assay. Also in some of the experiments using CD133 as a single marker to identify colon cancer stem cells it is unsure that there is no contamination of CD133+ cells from the mesenchyme. When colon cancer cell lines were transfected with Gli1, features of EMT were seen such as loss of epithelial morphology and increased expression of EMT markers *FOXC2*, *VIMENTN*, *SNAIL1* and *ZFHX1B* (Varnat et al., 2009). In a subsequent study Varnat et al. (2010) showed that CD133+ fraction of colon cancers lose the expression of Wnt targets such as *LGR5*, *AXIN2* and *c-MYC* at more advanced TNM stages. Instead the CD133+ cells acquired expression of Hh targets such as *GLI1* and *HHIP*. Again the caveat of this experiment is that CD133 was used as a single marker of colon cancer stem cells which risks contamination of mesenchymal cells. In an intriguing follow-up experiment however the authors show that activation of Hh signaling can overcome the dependence on Wnt signaling in Ls147T colon cancer cells. Based on their data the authors hypothesize that there is a switch from Wnt dependence to Hh dependence as colon cancer cells acquire metastatic potential. Further experiments are needed to confirm these intriguing results.

In conclusion, it is clear that Hh mediated negative feedback signaling by BMPs and activins is inactivated via mutational loss of either SMAD4 or the TGF-β family of receptors. Data from Varnat et al. suggest that colon cancer cells may acquire Hh responsiveness at higher TNM stages and that growth and metastatic potential depends on Hh signaling. Conflicting data have been published however and this concept awaits further confirmation.

References

Auclair BA, Benoit YD, Rivard N, Mishina Y, Perreault N (2007) Bone morphogenetic protein signaling is essential for terminal differentiation of the intestinal secretory cell lineage. Gastroenterology 133(3):887–896

Barker N, van de Wetering M, Clevers H (2008) The intestinal stem cell. Genes Dev 22(14):1856–1864

Bienz M, Clevers H (2000) Linking colorectal cancer to Wnt signaling. Cell 103:311–320

Bitgood MJ, McMahon AP (1995) Hedgehog and Bmp genes are co-expressed at many diverse sites of cell-cell interaction in the mouse embryo. Dev Biol 172:126–138

Haramis AP, Begthel H, van den Born M, van Es J, Jonkheer S, Offerhaus GJ, Clevers H (2004) De novo crypt formation and juvenile polyposis on BMP inhibition in mouse intestine. Science 303:1684–1686

Hardwick JC, Van Den Brink GR, Bleuming SA, Ballester I, Van Den Brande JM, Keller JJ, Offerhaus GJ, Van Deventer SJ, Peppelenbosch MP (2004) Bone morphogenetic protein 2 is expressed by, and acts upon, mature epithelial cells in the colon. Gastroenterology 126(1):111–121

Hardwick JC, Kodach LL, Offerhaus GJ, van den Brink GR (2008) Bone morphogenetic protein signalling in colorectal cancer. Nat Rev Cancer 8(10):806–812

Jung B, Doctolero RT, Tajima A, Nguyen AK, Keku T, Sandler RS, Carethers JM (2004) Loss of activin receptor type 2 protein expression in microsatellite unstable colon cancers. Gastroenterology 126(3):654–659

Kedinger M, Duluc I, Fritsch C, Lorentz O, Plateroti M, Freund JN (1998) Intestinal epithelial–mesenchymal cell interactions. Ann NY Acad Sci 859:1–17

Kodach LL, Bleuming SA, Musler AR, Peppelenbosch MP, Hommes DW, van den Brink GR, van Noesel CJ, Offerhaus GJ, Hardwick JC (2008) The bone morphogenetic protein pathway is active in human colon adenomas and inactivated in colorectal cancer. Cancer 112(2):300–306

Kodach LL, Wiercinska A, de Miranda NF, Bleuming SA, Musler AR, Peppelenbosch MP, Dekker E, Van Den Brink GR, van Noesel CJ, Morreau H, Hommes DW, Ten Dijke P, Offerhaus GJ, Hardwick JC (2008) The bonemorphogenetic protein pathway is inactivated in the majority of sporadic colorectal cancers. Gastroenterology 134(5):1332–1341

Kolterud A, Grosse AS, Zacharias WJ, Walton KD, Kretovich KE, Madison BB, Waghray M, Ferris JE, Hu C, Merchant JL, Dlugosz AA, Kottmann AH, Gumucio DL (2009) Paracrine Hedgehog signaling in stomach and intestine: new roles for hedgehog in gastrointestinal patterning. Gastroenterology 137(2):618–628

Korinek V, Barker N, Moerer P, van Donselaar E, Huls G, Peters PJ, Clevers H (1998) Depletion of epithelial stem-cell compartments in the small intestine of mice lacking Tcf-4. Nat Genet 19(4):379–383

Kosinski C, Stange DE, Xu C, Chan AS, Ho C, Yuen ST, Mifflin RC, Powell DW, Clevers H, Leung SY, Chen X (2010) Indian Hedgehog regulates intestinal stem cell fate through epithelial–mesenchymal interactions during development. Gastroenterology 139(3):893–903

Lees CW, Zacharias WJ, Tremelling M, Noble CL, Nimmo ER, Tenesa A, Cornelius J, Torkvist L, Kao J, Farrington S, Drummond HE, Ho GT, Arnott ID, Appelman HD, Diehl L, Campbell H, Dunlop MG, Parkes M, Howie SE, Gumucio DL, Satsangi J (2008) Analysis of germline GLI1 variation implicates hedgehog signalling in the regulation of intestinal inflammatory pathways. PLoS Med 5:e239

Litingtung Y, Lei L, Westphal H, Chiang C (1998) Sonic hedgehog is essential to foregut development. Nat Genet 20:58–61

Madison BB, Braunstein K, Kuizon E, Portman K, Qiao XT, Gumucio DL (2005) Epithelial hedgehog signals pattern the intestinal crypt-villus axis. Development 132(2):279–289

Markowitz S, Wang J, Myeroff L, Parsons R, Sun L, Lutterbaugh J, Fan RS, Zborowska E, Kinzler KW, Vogelstein B, Brattain M, Willson JKV (1995) Inactivation of the type II TGF-beta receptor in colon cancer cells with microsatellite instability. Science 268(5215):1336–1338

Nishisho I, Nakamura Y, Miyoshi Y, Miki Y, Ando H, Horii A, Koyama K, Utsunomiya J, Baba S, Hedge P (1991) Mutations of chromosome 5q21 genes in FAP and colorectal cancer patients. Science 253(5020):665–669

Nüsslein-Volhard C, Wieschaus E (1980) Mutations affecting segment number and polarity in Drosophila. Nature 287(5785):795–801

Potten CS (2004) Radiation, the ideal cytotoxic agent for studying the cell biology of tissues such as the small intestine. Radiat Res 161:123–136

Potten CS, Loeffler M (1990) Stem cells: attributes, cycles, spirals, pitfalls and uncertainties. Lessons for and from the crypt. Development 110:1001

Qualtrough D, Buda A, Gaffield W, Williams AC, Paraskeva C (2004) Hedgehog signalling in colorectal tumour cells: induction of apoptosis with cyclopamine treatment. Int J Cancer 110(6):831–837

Ramalho-Santos M, Melton DA, McMahon AP (2000) Hedgehog signals regulate multiple aspects of gastrointestinal development. Development 127:2763–2772

Roberts DJ, Johnson RL, Burke AC, Nelson CE, Morgan BA, Tabin C (1995) Sonic hedgehog is an endodermal signal inducing Bmp-4 and Hox genes during induction and regionalization of the chick hindgut. Development 121(10):3163

Roberts DJ, Smith DM, Goff DJ, Tabin CJ (1998) Epithelial–mesenchymal signaling during the regionalization of the chick gut. Development 125(15):2791–2801

van den Brink GR, Offerhaus GJ (2007) The morphogenetic code and colon cancer development. Cancer Cell 11(2):109–117

van den Brink GR, Hardwick JC, Nielsen C, Xu C, ten Kate FJ, Glickman J, van Deventer SJ, Roberts DJ, Peppelenbosch MP (2002) Sonic hedgehog expression correlates with fundic gland differentiation in the adult gastrointestinal tract. Gut 51(5):628–633

van den Brink GR, Bleuming SA, Hardwick JC, Schepman BL, Offerhaus GJ, Keller JJ, Nielsen C, Gaffield W, van Deventer SJ, Roberts DJ, Peppelenbosch MP (2004) Indian Hedgehog is an antagonist of Wnt signaling in colonic epithelial cell differentiation. Nat Genet 36(3):277–282

Van Dop WA, Uhmann A, Wijgerde M, Sleddens-Linkels E, Heijmans J, Offerhaus GJ, van den Bergh Weerman MA, Boeckxstaens GE, Hommes DW, Hardwick JC, Hahn H, van den Brink GR (2009) Depletion of the colonic epithelial precursor cell compartment upon conditional activation of the hedgehog pathway. Gastroenterology 136(7):2195–2203

Van Dop WA, Heijmans J, Büller NVJA, Snoek SA, Rosekrans SL, Wassenberg EA, van den Bergh Weerman MA, Lanske B, Clark AR, Winton DJ, Wijgerde M, Offerhaus GJ, Hommes DW, Hardwick JC, de Jonge WJ, Biemond I, Van Den Brink GR (2010) Loss of Indian hedgehog activates multiple aspects of a wound healing response in the mouse intestine. Gastroenterology 139(5):1665–1676

Varnat F, Duquet A, Malerba M, Zbinden M, Mas C, Gervaz P, Altaba A (2009) Human colon cancer epithelial cells harbour active HEDGEHOG-GLI signalling that is essential for tumour growth, recurrence, metastasis and stem cell survival and expansion. EMBO Mol Med 1:338–351

Varnat F, Siegl-Cachedenier I, Malerba M, Gervaz P, Ruiz i Altaba A (2010) Loss of WNT-TCF addiction and enhancement of HH-GLI1 signalling define the metastatic transition of human colon carcinomas. EMBO Mol Med 2(11):440–457

Wang LC, Nassir F, Liu ZY, Ling L, Kuo F, Crowell T, Olson D, Davidson NO, Burkly LC (2002) Disruption of hedgehog signaling reveals a novel role in intestinal morphogenesis and intestinal-specific lipid metabolism in mice. Gastroenterology 122(2):469–482

Yauch RL, Gould SE, Scales SJ, Tang T, Tian H, Ahn CP, Marshall D, Fu L, Januario T, Kallop D, Nannini-Pepe M, Kotkow K, Marsters JC, Rubin LL, de Sauvage FJ (2008) A paracrine requirement for hedgehog signalling in cancer. Nature 455:406–410

Zacharias WJ, Li X, Madison BB, Kretovich K, Kao JY, Merchant JL, Gumucio DL (2010) Hedgehog is an anti-inflammatory epithelial signal for the intestinal lamina propria. Gastroenterology 138:2368–2377

Chapter 11

Hematopoietic Stem Cell Repopulation After Transplantation: Role of Vinculin

Tsukasa Ohmori and Yoichi Sakata

Abstract Hematopoietic stem cells (HSCs) are the most thoroughly characterized type of stem cells, and reconstitution of the hematopoietic system after HSC transplantation has demonstrated the self-renewal and differentiation capabilities of stem cells in vivo. HSCs must undergo several steps to achieve reconstitution after transplantation, e.g., homing to the bone marrow, lodging in the bone marrow niche, and proliferation and multilineage differentiation (repopulation). Identification of the factors required for HSCs to perform these reconstitution functions might improve our understanding of stem cell biology, as well as leading to more efficient HSC transplantation protocols. The gold standard for analyzing the function of target genes in HSCs is the creation of gene-deficient, knockout mice by gene targeting, while silencing of target gene expression by RNA interference is an attractive alternative strategy. In this chapter, we will explain the RNA interference methods available for silencing genes in HSCs using lentiviral vectors, and discuss the role of vinculin in HSC repopulation after transplantation.

Keywords Hematopoietic stem cells · Vinculin · Lentiviral vector · Short hairpin RNA · Repopulation · Stem cells

T. Ohmori (✉)
Research Division of Cell and Molecular Medicine, Center for Molecular Medicine, Jichi Medical University, Shimotsuke, Tochigi 329-0498, Japan
e-mail: tohmori@jichi.ac.jp

Introduction

Hematopoietic stem cells (HSCs) are multipotent adult stem cells that are characterized by their abilities to self-renew and differentiate into all hematopoietic cell lineages. HSCs are historically the most thoroughly characterized type of adult stem cell, and reconstitution of the hematopoietic system by HSC transplantation has provided the main means of confirming the multipotent abilities of HSCs. Transplantation of HSC populations has been shown to be sufficient for long-term multilineage reconstitution of blood cells in clinical patients with hematologic malignancies and bone marrow failure, as well as in experimental animal models. Identification of the factors required for HSC function would improve our understanding of stem cell biology, and also lead to the development of more efficient procedures for HSC transplantation in clinical settings.

The ideal method for investigating the role of a specific molecule in HSC function is to create gene-deficient, knockout mice. A number of studies using HSCs from knockout mice have demonstrated the critical roles of cell surface receptors and cell cycle modulators in HSC functions, including homing, niche interaction, hibernation, repopulation, and differentiation. Although the creation of such knockout mice and the transplantation of HSCs from these mice are valuable techniques for studying the roles of specific genes in HSC function, the production of knockout mice is an expensive and time-consuming process. In addition, we sometimes have to further establish the conditional gene-deficient mouse to avoid the neonatal lethality. To solve these limitations, lentiviral vector (LV)-mediated expression of short hairpin RNA (shRNA) sequences in HSCs can be used to inhibit the expression of specific genes, as a promising alternative strategy for HSC research. In this chapter, we review the methods available for HSC research using LVs, and focus on the novel roles of the cytoskeletal protein vinculin in HSC repopulation.

Fate of Hematopoietic Stem Cells After Transplantation

The characterization and/or isolation of HSCs using specific cell surface markers has been an important advance in HSC research. CD34 has been used as a marker for human HSCs. CD34$^+$ cells in the bone marrow and umbilical cord blood possess colony-forming potential and can differentiate into blood cells in vitro, and are used as a source of cells for HSC transplantation in clinical protocols. However, some studies have also demonstrated the existence of HSCs in the CD34$^-$ cell fraction. In mice, the HSC fraction positive for c-kit and Sca-1 antigen, but not for lineage-specific markers (KSL cells), was found to contain a primitive stem cell fraction (Nakauchi et al., 2001). KSL cells were further subdivided according to their surface expression of CD34. CD34$^{low/-}$ c-kit$^+$ Sca-1$^+$ Lin$^-$ (CD34^{low}KSL) cells were highly enriched for HSCs with long-term marrow-repopulating ability, whereas CD34$^+$ c-kit$^+$ Sca-1$^+$ Lin$^-$ (CD34$^+$KSL) cells represented progenitors with short-term reconstitution capacity. These results suggest that CD34^{low}KSL cells have a higher rank in the hematopoietic hierarchy in mice than CD34$^+$KSL cells (Nakauchi et al., 2001). Furthermore, a subpopulation of bone marrow cells ("side population") able to efflux fluorescent dyes, including Hoechst 33342, has been identified as a HSC fraction (Golebiewska et al., 2011). This side population of cells can efflux Hoechst dye through ABC family transporter activity.

Following transplantation into a recipient, HSCs home to and then lodge in specialized niches in the bone marrow microenvironment (Wilson and Trumpp, 2006). Homing of HSCs after transplantation is the first critical stage in the reconstitution of blood cells (Srour et al., 2001). The mechanisms whereby the transplanted HSCs recognize their home (bone marrow and spleen in mice) has not yet been elucidated, although the importance of stromal cell-derived factor-1α (SDF-1α) and its counter receptor CXCR4 expressed on HSCs have been implicated in the selective direction of HSC homing. In addition, adhesion molecules on HSCs, such as integrins and selectins, also appear to be involved in the process of homing into the bone marrow environment (see below).

HSCs lodge in the bone marrow environment "niche" (Wilson and Trumpp, 2006), which can be characterized as a region in which the stem cells are maintained through self-renewal in the absence of differentiation (Wilson and Trumpp, 2006). Transplanted HSCs need to undergo clonal expansion without differentiation (self-renewal) in order to reconstitute the hematopoietic system. Some daughters of dividing stem cells separate from the niche environment and produce differentiating progenitors (differentiation) (Wilson and Trumpp, 2006). This proliferation within the bone marrow is essential for the reconstitution of transplanted HSC, and is generally termed "repopulation". However, the niche microenvironment also provides signals that repress cell division (Li, 2011). The niche retains some HSCs in a quiescent state in G$_0$ phase of the cell cycle, in so-called hibernation. It is still unclear if these opposing stem cell-niche functions can be provided by a single molecular interaction or involve different anatomical zones, and the way in which the niche controls the balance between self-renewal and differentiation required to reconstitute the hematopoietic system after transplantation remains unknown.

The existence of two types of niche within the bone marrow has been proposed, the endosteal niche and the vascular niche (Wilson and Trumpp, 2006). The endosteum is the inner surface of the bone that directly interacts with the bone marrow. It is covered with osteoblasts and osteoclasts able to produce large amounts of cytokines to regulate HSC functions. Manipulation of osteoblast numbers directly affects the maintenance of HSCs in vivo. Although little is known about the signals that are exchanged between HSCs and osteoblasts, several receptors, membrane proteins, and secreted factors have been proposed to support niche functions, e.g., Notch signaling, osteopontin, membrane-bound stem cell factor, N-cadherin, and Tie-2 signaling (Wilson and Trumpp, 2006; Yin and Li, 2006). These interactions are believed to be involved in maintaining HSCs in a quiescent state. In the other specialized niche, the vascular niche, bone marrow sinusoidal endothelial cells constitutively express cytokines, including SDF-1α and adhesion molecules, that are important for the function of HSCs (Yin and Li, 2006).

Lentiviral Vectors: Effective Viral Vector System for Hematopoietic Stem Cells

LVs have become some of the most widely-used vectors, not only for fundamental biological research, but also for human gene therapy. LVs are a subclass of gamma retroviral vectors (γRVs) able to integrate into the target cell genome, resulting in the stable expression of the gene of interest over a prolonged period. γRVs produce DNA from the RNA virus genome by reverse transcription, and this is then incorporated into the host genome by an integrase enzyme. These vectors are replication-defective, and lack the coding regions of the genes required for additional rounds of virion replication and packaging.

Compared with γRV, LVs can transduce non-dividing cells and thus allow more efficient gene transfer into HSCs than γRVs (Frecha et al., 2008). Furthermore, LVs are less sensitive to silencing than γRVs, leading to more stable expression of the target protein. Targeting of HSCs with LVs is an increasingly important therapeutic approach for human immunodeficiencies and thalassemia because of its improved safety, compared with the use of γRVs (Kohn, 2008). Previous human clinical trials demonstrated promising therapeutic effects of γRVs for the treatment of some immunodeficiency syndromes (Kohn, 2008). However, the risk of insertional mutagenesis resulting from proviral integration is the main limiting factor in applying these viral vectors to clinical treatments (Kohn, 2008). Current efforts have focused on reducing the oncogenic potential of integrated gene vectors by modifying the vector design. Compared with γRVs, LVs show a stronger preference for integration within active transcriptional units, with no obvious bias towards proliferation-associated genes or transcriptional start sites, suggesting a lower potential for triggering adverse oncogenic events. Self-inactivating (SIN) vector systems, in which the promoter activity in the U3 region of the viral long-terminal repeat (LTR) is deleted, have been used in a variety of studies, because the promoter activity of the viral LTR has long been associated with transcriptional activation of oncogenes in γRVs (Montini et al., 2009). It is possible that the use of a cell-lineage-specific targeting promoter as the internal promoter in a SIN vector may be safer than using a viral or ubiquitous viral promoter.

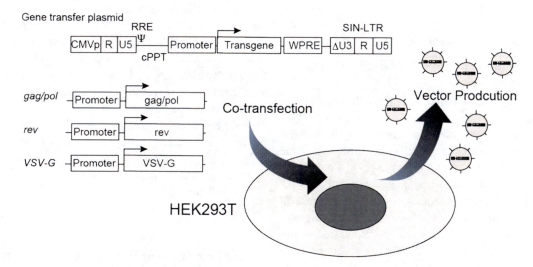

Fig. 11.1 Production of third-generation LVs. A minimal LV plasmid consisting of the CMV/LTR chimera promoter followed by the packaging signal (ψ), rev-responsive element (RRE) for cytoplasmic export of the RNA, the transgene expression package consisting of the internal promoter and transgene, and the 3' self-inactivating LTR. All genes coding for enzymatic or structural proteins have been removed. Together with the vector plasmid, a packaging plasmid encoding *gal-pol*, *rev*, and an envelope-expressing plasmid (*VSV-G*) are co-transfected into HEK293T cells. The LV is produced in the supernatant from the HEK293T cells (Ohmori et al.)

Most LVs used in recent studies and clinical trials have been so-called third-generation LVs, in which all the accessory genes (*vif, vpr, vpu, nef*) have been deleted. In addition, the two key regulatory genes, *tat* and *rev*, have been either deleted or separated from the packaging construct; these modifications are critically important for ensuring that the corresponding LV becomes replication-defective after transduction. The most common method of generating LVs is by cotransfection of HEK293T cells with the gene transfer vector together with the *gag-pol, rev*, and *env* packaging constructs (Fig. 11.1). Several types of third-generation LVs with SIN-LTRs, including human immunodeficiency virus (HIV), simian immunodeficiency virus (SIV), and feline immunodeficiency virus vectors (FIV), are now commercially available.

The native lentivirus envelope in LVs is generally replaced by a helper plasmid expressing a heterologous envelope glycoprotein (*env*). This process is termed pseudotyping, and can greatly affect the host-cell tropism of LVs. Pseudotyping with the vesicular stomatitis virus glycoprotein (*VSV-G*) has been extensively used to transduce many types of cells, including HSCs. Other viral envelopes have been used to successfully pseudotype LV particles, including those from lyssaviruses, arenaviruses, flaviviridae, baculovirus, and alphaviruses.

Application of Lentiviral Vectors for Inhibiting Target Gene Expression

RNA interference (RNAi) was originally described in the nematode worm *Caenorhabditis elegans* by Fire and colleagues in 1998, and is now recognized as an evolutionarily-conserved mechanism that permits the selective post-transcriptional down-regulation of target genes. RNAi is an essential and powerful tool for inhibiting specific protein expression in mammalian cells. A number of vector systems have been proposed to mediate shRNA sequence expression within the cells. Expressed shRNA sequences derived from the vector were converted into small interfering RNAs by Dicer, to form an RNA-induced silencing complex (RISC) that cleaves target mRNA by its slicer activity (Cullen, 2006). RNAi represents a powerful and promising technology for both basic research and therapeutic interventions.

Recent strategies aimed at expressing shRNA sequences in cells are mediated by RNA polymerase III promoters (pol III), such as U6 and H1 promoters (as in the case of LentiLox) or RNA polymerase II promoters (pol II). While artificial shRNAs are directly transcribed by pol III, the generalized RNA polymerase II promoter mediates the transcription of microRNAs (miRNA). RNA pol II can transcribe primary miRNAs (pri-miRNAs) that are processed into pre-miRNAs by the action of the RNase Drosha. The design of shRNA transcripts as miRNA mimics driven by tissue- or cell type-specific RNA pol II promoters significantly expands the possibilities for conditional RNAi in mammalian cells (Cullen, 2006).

LVs can now be used to regulate the expression of specific proteins to mediate shRNA sequences within the cells. We have used an LV system called LentiLox (pLL3.7 plasmid commercially available from American Type Culture Collection (ATCC)) (Rubinson et al., 2003). The main characteristic of this vector is the ability to identify transduced cells by their expression of enhanced green fluorescent protein (EGFP). Peripheral blood cells derived from transduced HSCs can be easily identified as EGFP-positive cells by flow cytometry (Fig. 11.2). It is also possible to visualize the cell fate in an in vivo imaging system by replacing the EGFP gene with the luciferase gene (Fig. 11.2) (Ohmori et al., 2010a). Previous studies by ourselves and others have identified important factors in HSC function by transplanting HSCs transduced with LVs expressing shRNA sequences (Rawls et al., 2007; Ogaeri et al., 2009; Ohmori et al., 2010a). We demonstrated that transduction of HSCs with LentiLox resulted in the inhibition of specific protein expression in terminally-differentiated anucleate blood platelets, suggesting that shRNA expression could be maintained during megakaryopoiesis from HSCs (Ohmori et al., 2007). The existence of miRNAs and their processing proteins in anucleate platelets has also been reported by other researchers (Landry et al., 2009).

Role of Integrin in Hematopoietic Stem Cell Function

Adhesive interactions between cells and the extracellular matrix (ECM) play important roles in a number of biological processes, including cell survival and

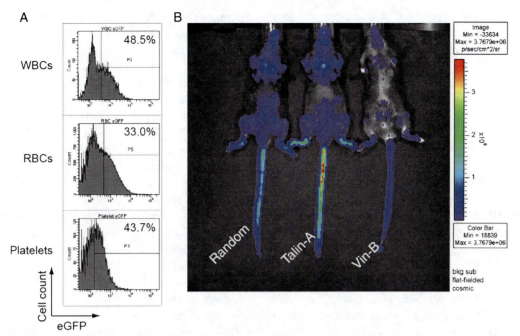

Fig. 11.2 Reconstitution capacities of KSL HSCs transduced with LentiLox vectors. (**a**) KSL HSCs transduced by LentiLox expressing EGFP, together with non-transduced bone marrow cells, were transplanted into lethally-irradiated recipient mice. EGFP expression in peripheral blood cells was assessed at 1 month after transplantation. (**b**) The *EGFP* gene of the LentiLox vector was replaced with a *luciferase* gene. KSL HSCs were transduced with a LentiLox vector expressing a control shRNA sequence (Random) or shRNA sequences against talin (Talin-A) or vinculin (Vin-B). Transduced KSL cells, together with competitor cells, were transplanted into lethally-irradiated recipient mice. Photons transmitted through the body were collected after transplantation using an IVIS Imaging System (Ohmori et al.)

growth, differentiation, migration, platelet aggregation, inflammation, and tumor invasion (Takada et al., 2007). These interactions are mediated by the cell surface receptors known as integrins. Integrins are heterodimeric cell surface receptors, composed of α and β subunits. There are at least 24 different combinations of subunits, each of which can bind to a specific ligand, including ECM and soluble ligands (Takada et al., 2007). The conformation of integrins can change from a low- to a high-affinity state for ligand interactions, through so-called "inside-out signaling" pathways (Coller and Shattil, 2008). Ligand interaction triggers further signaling that promotes cytoskeletal changes, leading to stabilization of the binding through "outside-in signaling" (Coller and Shattil, 2008). Proteins able to directly bind β-integrin cytoplasmic tails are important factors in these signaling pathways. Recent studies using knockout mice revealed that talin and kindlins act as key proteins in the regulation of integrin affinity status, by binding to β-integrin cytoplasmic tails (Moser et al., 2009).

Previous reports suggested that HSCs mainly express integrins α4, α5 and α6, which can associate with integrin β1(reviewed in Chan and Watt, 2001; Imai et al., 2010). Integrin β1-null HSCs fail to engraft in irradiated recipient mice, because of sequestration of the HSCs into the circulation (i.e., failure of HSCs to home into the bone marrow). Although fundamental roles for integrin α4 in the development of the hematopoietic system have previously been proposed, it appears to have a trivial influence in the construction of the hematopoietic system. However, conditional ablation of integrin α4 in hematopoietic cells results in sustained and significant increases in circulating progenitors. Administration of a function-blocking antibody or blocking peptide against integrin α4 or integrin β1 also reduces HSC homing and leads to HSC release into the blood. Similar phenotypes perturbing homing or sequestration of HSCs or progenitors have been reported in integrin α6- or integrin β7-knockout mice. These data suggest that the main function of integrin in HSCs is in regulating their homing and anchoring within the marrow. Integrin α4β1-mediated adhesion of HSCs to fibronectin has also been shown to promote their proliferation and survival potential (Yokota et al., 1998).

Vinculin is Indispensable for Hematopoietic Stem Cell Repopulation

The cytoplasmic domain of integrin can form focal adhesions that transmit cellular signals via binding with the ECM. The signaling complex at the focal adhesion directly modulates integrin functions, and consists of several proteins, including talin, vinculin, α-actinin, paxillin, and integrin-associated kinase. Among these proteins, talin directly binds to the cytoplasmic tail of integrins, and this binding represents the final step in increasing the affinity of integrin for the ECM. Indeed, the ablation of talin using the conditional Cre-loxP system in platelets confirmed the importance of talin for integrin function; talin-deficient platelets were unable to aggregate with each other because of the functional loss of integrin αIIbβ3 activation (Nieswandt et al., 2007; Petrich et al., 2007). Although previous reports have suggested a critical role for integrin in HSC function, as described above, the role of the signaling complex in directly affecting HSC function has not yet been elucidated. We have previously focused on the well-known focal adhesion proteins, talin and vinculin, and identified an important role for vinculin in the repopulation of transplanted HSCs, possibly acting independently of integrin function (Ohmori et al., 2010a).

In contrast to the case of talin, the role of vinculin in integrin function is controversial. Vinculin is a highly-conserved actin-binding protein that is frequently used as a general marker for focal adhesion complexes in many types of cells. Vinculin contains a globular head domain, a flexible hinge, and a tail domain (Ziegler et al., 2006). These authors indicate that conformational changes lead to dissociation of the head-to-tail association of vinculin, resulting in interaction with other cytoskeletal proteins. The activation status of vinculin has been reported to be mediated by talin and actin. Although vinculin does not interact directly with the integrin cytoplasmic tail, the activation status of vinculin (conformational change) is believed to be involved in integrin function (Ziegler et al., 2006).

Overexpression of the active form of vinculin induced integrin activation (Ohmori et al., 2010b), and fibroblasts from knockout embryos showed strong inhibition of cell adhesion and invasion on ECM (Marg et al., 2010). In contrast, the conditional loss of vinculin in platelets did not affect integrin αIIbβ3 activation induced by agonist stimulation (Mitsios et al., 2010), and the inhibition of vinculin by RNAi did not affect cell adhesion to the ECM (Ohmori et al., 2010b; Peng et al., 2010). Vinculin deficiency leads to embryonal lethality in mice as a result of heart and brain defects. In addition, heart-specific deletion of the vinculin gene causes cardiomyopathy and ventricular tachycardia, leading to sudden death. These abnormalities in knockout mice are believed to result from defects in integrin-dependent cell functions, although the involvement of a specific function of vinculin that is independent of integrins could not be ruled out.

To investigate the role of focal adhesion proteins in HSC function, we created LVs (LentiLox) with shRNA sequences for talin and vinculin (Ohmori et al., 2010a). LentiLox allows blood cells derived from transduced HSCs to be identified after transplantation (Fig. 11.2). The transplantation of HSCs transduced with LentiLox with a shRNA sequence for vinculin unexpectedly resulted in a marked reduction in the numbers of peripheral blood cells derived from transduced HSCs after transplantation. Bone marrow cells in the various differentiated stages were also reduced, while granulocyte- and granulocyte-macrophage-colony-forming units in vitro, and homing to the bone marrow were unaffected by the loss of vinculin. The reconstitution failure was correlated with the frequencies of long-term culture-initiating cells (LTC-IC) and cell cycle modulation in vitro. HSCs transduced with LentiLox with a shRNA sequence for talin also showed reduced reconstitution activity, but the inhibitory effects were much weaker than those associated with vinculin inhibition. Interestingly, adhesion to the ECM was significantly inhibited by the loss of talin, but not vinculin, suggesting that vinculin is an indispensable factor for stem cell functioning in the bone marrow, independent of any perturbation of integrin function. These data support the existence of integrin-independent roles for vinculin in cellular function.

Questions regarding which HSC signaling pathway(s) are modified by vinculin to enable efficient repopulation in the bone marrow remain to be answered. Vinculin reportedly exists not only at integrin-mediated focal adhesions, but also at cadherin-mediated cell-cell contacts, and directly regulates cadherin expression and cell-cell interactions (Peng et al., 2010). Because N-cadherin expressed on HSCs is thought to be an important regulator of bone marrow niche function, vinculin might regulate HSC maintenance in the niche via cadherin. Vinculin might also directly regulate the intrinsic molecular machinery to control the fate choices of individual HSCs. Several transcription factors are implicated in the regulation of HSC function, including in self-renewal and quiescence (Kiel and Morrison, 2006; Wilson and Trumpp, 2006). Although no data are available regarding the involvement of vinculin in HSC quiescence, vinculin silencing significantly abolished the frequency of LTC-IC and cell cycle modulation of HSC in vitro. These data suggest that vinculin is directly involved in the spatial and temporal control processes responsible for maintaining the intrinsic balance of HSC self-renewal. Further studies are required to address these issues.

Future Directions

This chapter summarizes the method of LV-mediated RNAi for examining the functions of transplanted HSCs, and also the rationale for identifying vinculin as an important regulator of HSC repopulation. However, the LV transduction process involves ex vivo culture, with the use of a combination of cytokines, and the possibility that the primary characteristics of stem cells may decline with increasing time in culture cannot be ruled out. An efficient and simple transduction procedure for HSCs is required that will allow the direct transduction of HSCs in vivo. Despite these disadvantages, however, the use of LVs to inhibit target gene expression is a time- and cost-effective strategy, and is thus a useful method for performing preliminary studies, prior to the more time-consuming and costly creation of knockout mice. Further studies are currently underway to investigate the precise mechanism whereby vinculin modulates HSC repopulation, and to examine its integrin-independent cellular functions.

References

Chan JY, Watt SM (2001) Adhesion receptors on haematopoietic progenitor cells. Br J Haematol 112:541–557

Coller BS, Shattil SJ (2008) The GPIIb/IIIa (integrin alphaIIb-beta3) odyssey: a technology-driven saga of a receptor with twists, turns, and even a bend. Blood 112:3011–3025

Cullen BR (2006) Induction of stable RNA interference in mammalian cells. Gene Ther 13:503–508

Frecha C, Szecsi J, Cosset FL, Verhoeyen E (2008) Strategies for targeting lentiviral vectors. Curr Gene Ther 8: 449–460

Golebiewska A, Brons NH, Bjerkvig R, Niclou SP (2011) Critical appraisal of the side population assay in stem cell and cancer stem cell research. Cell Stem Cell 8:136–147

Imai Y, Shimaoka M, Kurokawa M (2010) Essential roles of VLA-4 in the hematopoietic system. Int J Hematol 91: 569–575

Kiel MJ, Morrison SJ (2006) Maintaining hematopoietic stem cells in the vascular niche. Immunity 25:862–864

Kohn DB (2008) Gene therapy for childhood immunological diseases. Bone Marrow Transplant 41:199–205

Landry P, Plante I, Ouellet DL, Perron MP, Rousseau G, Provost P (2009) Existence of a microRNA pathway in anucleate platelets. Nat Struct Mol Biol 16:961–966

Li J (2011) Quiescence regulators for hematopoietic stem cell. Exp Hematol 39:511–520

Marg S, Winkler U, Sestu M, Himmel M, Schonherr M, Bar J, Mann A, Moser M, Mierke CT, Rottner K, Blessing M, Hirrlinger J, Ziegler WH (2010) The vinculin-DeltaIn20/21 mouse: characteristics of a constitutive, actin-binding deficient splice variant of vinculin. PLoS One 5:e11530

Mitsios JV, Prevost N, Kasirer-Friede A, Gutierrez E, Groisman A, Abrams CS, Wang Y, Litvinov RI, Zemljic-Harpf A, Ross RS, Shattil SJ (2010) What is vinculin needed for in platelets? J Thromb Haemost 8:2294–2304

Montini E, Cesana D, Schmidt M, Sanvito F, Bartholomae CC, Ranzani M, Benedicenti F, Sergi LS, Ambrosi A, Ponzoni M, Doglioni C, Di Serio C, von Kalle C, Naldini L (2009) The genotoxic potential of retroviral vectors is strongly modulated by vector design and integration site selection in a mouse model of HSC gene therapy. J Clin Invest 119: 964–975

Moser M, Legate KR, Zent R, Fassler R (2009) The tail of integrins, talin, and kindlins. Science 324:895–899

Nakauchi H, Sudo K, Ema H (2001) Quantitative assessment of the stem cell self-renewal capacity. Ann NY Acad Sci 938:18–24, discussion 24-15

Nieswandt B, Moser M, Pleines I, Varga-Szabo D, Monkley S, Critchley D, Fassler R (2007) Loss of talin1 in platelets abrogates integrin activation, platelet aggregation, and thrombus formation in vitro and in vivo. J Exp Med 204: 3113–3118

Ogaeri T, Eto K, Otsu M, Ema H, Nakauchi H (2009) The actin polymerization regulator WAVE2 is required for early bone marrow repopulation by hematopoietic stem cells. Stem Cells 27:1120–1129

Ohmori T, Kashiwakura Y, Ishiwata A, Madoiwa S, Mimuro J, Sakata Y (2007) Silencing of a targeted protein in in vivo platelets using a lentiviral vector delivering short hairpin RNA sequence. Arterioscler Thromb Vasc Biol 27: 2266–2272

Ohmori T, Kashiwakura Y, Ishiwata A, Madoiwa S, Mimuro J, Furukawa Y, Sakata Y (2010a) Vinculin is indispensable for repopulation by hematopoietic stem cells, independent of integrin function. J Biol Chem 285:31763–31773

Ohmori T, Kashiwakura Y, Ishiwata A, Madoiwa S, Mimuro J, Honda S, Miyata T, Sakata Y (2010b) Vinculin activates inside-out signaling of integrin alphaIIbbeta3 in Chinese hamster ovary cells. Biochem Biophys Res Commun 400:323–328

Peng X, Cuff LE, Lawton CD, DeMali KA (2010) Vinculin regulates cell-surface E-cadherin expression by binding to beta-catenin. J Cell Sci 123:567–577

Petrich BG, Marchese P, Ruggeri ZM, Spiess S, Weichert RA, Ye F, Tiedt R, Skoda RC, Monkley SJ, Critchley DR, Ginsberg MH (2007) Talin is required for integrin-mediated platelet function in hemostasis and thrombosis. J Exp Med 204:3103–3111

Rawls AS, Gregory AD, Woloszynek JR, Liu F, Link DC (2007) Lentiviral-mediated RNAi inhibition of Sbds in murine hematopoietic progenitors impairs their hematopoietic potential. Blood 110:2414–2422

Rubinson DA, Dillon CP, Kwiatkowski AV, Sievers C, Yang L, Kopinja J, Rooney DL, Ihrig MM, McManus MT, Gertler FB, Scott ML, Van Parijs L (2003) A lentivirus-based system to functionally silence genes in primary mammalian cells, stem cells and transgenic mice by RNA interference. Nat Genet 33:401–406

Srour EF, Jetmore A, Wolber FM, Plett PA, Abonour R, Yoder MC, Orschell-Traycoff CM (2001) Homing, cell cycle kinetics and fate of transplanted hematopoietic stem cells. Leukemia 15:1681–1684

Takada Y, Ye X, Simon S (2007) The integrins. Genome Biol 8:215

Wilson A, Trumpp A (2006) Bone-marrow haematopoietic-stem-cell niches. Nat Rev Immunol 6:93–106

Yin T, Li L (2006) The stem cell niches in bone. J Clin Invest 116:1195–1201

Yokota T, Oritani K, Mitsui H, Aoyama K, Ishikawa J, Sugahara H, Matsumura I, Tsai S, Tomiyama Y, Kanakura Y, Matsuzawa Y (1998) Growth-supporting activities of fibronectin on hematopoietic stem/progenitor cells in vitro and in vivo: structural requirement for fibronectin activities of CS1 and cell-binding domains. Blood 91:3263–3272

Ziegler WH, Liddington RC, Critchley DR (2006) The structure and regulation of vinculin. Trends Cell Biol 16:453–460

Chapter 12

Static and Suspension Culture of Human Embryonic Stem Cells

Guoliang Meng and Derrick Rancourt

Abstract Since the first generation of human embryonic stem cells (hESCs) in 1998, they have excited great interest among scientists and doctors, and become a powerful tool in both basic and applied research, as their capacity for unlimited self-renewal and differentiation into any cell type in the body. In this review, we summarize the current state of derivation, propagation and expansion of hESCs in static and suspension cultures and focus on recent advances in generation and expansion of these cells in xeno-free, chemically defined conditions. We also give an overview of the application of ROCK inhibitor, Y-27632 in both static and suspension culture by single cell enzymatic dissociation. Based on the previous studies, we speculate the methodologies for derivation and expansion of hESC lines in xeno-free, chemically defined conditions under current good manufacturing process (cGMP) standards that will enable the generation of clinical-grade hESC lines for the clinical purposes.

Keywords Human embryonic stem cells · Current good manufacturing process · Mouse embryonic fibroblasts · Fetal bovine serum · Knockout serum replacement · Cell-conditioned medium

D. Rancourt (✉)
Department of Biochemistry and Molecular Biology, Faculty of Medicine, University of Calgary, Calgary, AB, Canada
T2N 4N1
e-mail: rancourt@ucalgary.ca

Introduction

Since the first derivation of human embryonic stem cells (hESCs) in 1998 (Thomson et al., 1998), more and more researchers have been attracted to this area. The unique properties of hESCs to self-renew indefinitely or to differentiate to any cell type in the body have great potential for transplantation therapy, regenerative medicine, drug screening, and basic research (Gearhart, 1998). Originally, hESCs were isolated and cultured on inactivated mouse embryonic fibroblasts (MEFs) in fetal bovine serum (FBS) containing medium. Then researchers developed a variety of culture methods for growing and expanding hESCs for different specific purposes.

At present, two main culture systems are being widely used to maintain hESCs in an undifferentiated state. One is feeder dependent culture system consisting of Knockout Serum Replacement (KSR) medium and feeder layer cells, which containing mouse fibroblasts and human cells. Another is feeder-free culture system consisting of mTeSR1 medium or feeder cell-conditioned medium (CM) and Matrigel coating matrix. Both culture systems are not suitable for clinical trials or future clinical applications, as they are not xeno-free, chemically defined culture systems. Such as, KSR and mTeSR1 media contain large amount of xenogeneic BSA; Matrigel is a kind of xenogeneic product derived from murine tumors; MEFs are prepared directly from mouse embryos. Although human feeder cells are strictly detested for virus and pathogens, probably they still carry unknown pathogenic species. For the purpose of clinical applications, some progress in the design of xeno-free culturing practices and components have been made in recent years (Villa-Diaz et al., 2010; Melkoumian et al., 2010; Rajala et al., 2010).

Xeno-free culture media and recombinant human protein matrices are commercially available from several companies. As hESCs undergo massive cell death after single cell dissociation in culture, they are routinely passaged and cryopreserved in cell clumps, produced by mechanical cutting or mild enzymatic treatment. To address this problem, the researchers found a high efficiency and safe reagent, ROCK inhibitor, Y27632, which can greatly enhance the cell survival rate after single dissociation and significantly improve the recovery of freeze-thawed hESCs in singles or in clumps (Watanabe et al., 2007; Li et al., 2008). However, a major limitation of adherent culture is low cell yield, which is insufficient to meet the requirements of the future clinical purposes. The need for large-scale expansion in clinical therapies could be overcome by propagation in suspension. Recently, researchers tried to expand hESCs in suspension for prolonged culture and have made some interesting progress on this (Krawetz et al., 2010; Steiner et al., 2010).

Derivation of hESC Lines

Human embryonic stem cell (hESC) lines are mainly derived from the inner cell masses (ICMs) of preimplantation blastocysts. They can also be derived from 4-cell embryos or morulae. The unique properties of hESCs, indefinite propagation and the capacity to produce all cell types in the body, make them have the potential to provide an unlimited source of cells for transplantation therapy, regenerative medicine, drug screening, and basic research. Recently, hESCs have been moved into clinical trials within North America and with the recent shift in the United States Policy on stem cell research, we can only assume that more trials will begin in the coming years. While it is true that hESCs hold great promise for human cell replacement therapy, the major challenge is that the overwhelming majority of hESC lines have been directly or indirectly exposed to materials containing animal-derived components during their derivation, propagation and cryopreservation.

For hESC derivation, immunosurgery has been routinely adopted to isolate ICMs by selectively killing surrounding trophoblasts within blastocysts. This method, which requires animal-sourced antibodies and complement, runs the risk of contaminating resulting hESC lines with animal pathogens and foreign molecules. In addition, this technique wastes human embryos by testing suitable concentrations of each batch of antibody and complement used for immunosurgery. Two alternative approaches eliminate the need for animal-derived products. First, the ICMs can be isolated mechanically by microdissection with sharpened metal needles (Ström et al., 2007) or syringe needles (Meng et al., 2011). This mechanical method proved to be an effective way to derive hESC lines; however, this technique requires specialized metal needles and complicated operation. Meng et al. have also explored the blastocyst microsurgery as an option for removing trophoblast cells prior to seeding ICM on feeder cells. Here, a 30G1/2 needle attached to a 1 mL syringe was substituted for the sharpened steel needles and used to remove the majority of trophoblast cells prior to transferring ICM to feeder cells. Moreover, this syringe needle approach is also convenient for cutting hESC colonies for subsequent nonenzymatic passaging in the early derivation stage.

Several groups developed laser-assisted systems for the isolation of the inner cell masses (ICMs) that can give rise to hESC lines, thereby avoiding immunosurgery that utilizes animal-derived products. One group (Chen et al., 2009) reported that the derivation efficiency of hESC lines can reach as high as 52% by using laser-assisted system when isolating ICMs from day 6 blastocysts.

Derivation of hESC lines from ICMs has raised political and ethical issues. In order to address this issue, much work has been devoted to isolating hESC cells from earlier stage embryos without embryo destruction. Klimanskaya et al. (2006) found a way to generate hESC lines from single blastomeres removed from 8-cell embryos. However, the method required co-culture of blastomeres with existed hESCs derived in xenogeneic conditions previously. The same group (Chung et al., 2008) reported the derivation of five hESC lines without embryo destruction, by using a modified approach using culture media supplemented with laminin, was suggested to be simulation of the natural ICM niche, which prevented polarization of the blastomeres into ICM and trophectoderm. In addition, by using the optimal culture conditions, one blastomere-derived hESC cell line was established without hESC co-culture in feeder-free conditions. This strategy substantially improved the efficiency of the hESC derivation to rates comparable to whole embryo derivations. Based on this study, probably new hESC lines can be generated without hESC co-culture in xeno-free, chemically defined conditions.

Feeder Dependent Culture of hESCs

Traditionally, hESCs were grown on inactivated mouse embryonic fibroblasts (MEFs) derived from day 12.5 to 13.5 postcoitum fetuses. However, MEFs have a limited lifespan in culture and have great variation from batch to batch, animal products can contain toxic proteins or immunogens, which may evoke an immune response that can lead to rejection upon transplantation, and the use of animal products, increase the risk of hESC contamination from animal pathogens, such as viruses or prions. To overcome this problem, several kinds of human tissue-derived cells, such human embryonic fibroblasts (Richards et al., 2002), newborn foreskin fibroblasts (Hovatta et al., 2003), autologous hESC-derived fibroblasts (Stojkovic et al., 2005), and human placental fibroblasts (Genbacev et al., 2005), etc. were successfully used as feeder cells to maintain existing hES cell lines as well as derive new hESC lines.

Compared to primary MEFs, human feeders enhance the maintenance of hESCs because of the extended lifespan, and lower the risk of animal pathogen contamination. However, most of the previously reported human feeder cells were derived and cultured in medium containing fetal bovine serum (FBS), using culture vessels coated with gelatin and trypsin for dissociation. Recently, few groups reported the xeno-free derivation of human fibroblasts supporting hESC growth (Meng et al., 2008; Kibschull et al., 2011). Although human feeder cells derived and expanded under xeno-free conditions can still carry unknown human pathogens, this is an important step forward to clinical purposes. However, although these culture systems are xeno-free, are still not chemically defined. In accordance, hESCs culture medium has changed substantially since the first derivation of hESCs.

FBS containing medium, which was first used for culturing hESCs was soon replaced by KSR or human serum. While SR is able to promote undifferentiated growth, it unfortunately contains high amounts of animal protein, BSA. In contrast, human serum can cause extensive differentiation of hESCs, presumably due to human serum batch variations and human serum containing unknown factors that promote the differentiation of hESCs. In addition, culture media containing animal-derived components still have above mentioned drawbacks and are suboptimal for clinical purposes. Even if animal components can be completely removed from hESC media, we are still limited by the feeder cells for maintaining hESCs in an undifferentiated state. While feeder cells have proven the best at supporting hESC pluripotency and genetic stability, while suppressing spontaneous differentiation (Draper et al., 2004), they still present several complications in hESC culture, the most important being cellular contamination and pathogen contamination; furthermore, establishment of clinical grade feeder cell lines for hESC culture carries with it enormous costs.

Feeder-Free Culture of hESCs

Although human feeder cells were shown to support hESCs for prolonged cultures while maintaining hESC properties, they still have some disadvantages: first, the need of feeder cells will limit the large-scale culture of hESCs; second, the culture system cannot be precisely defined because of unknown factors secreted by feeder cells; and third, there exist large variations from batch to batch of feeder cells. So, the optimal culture method for hESCs should be a combination of a serum-free, animal-free, and feeder-free culture system. Xu et al's work (Xu et al., 2001) is a milestone in feeder-free culture of hESCs. In this paper, they described a successful feeder-free hESC culture system in which undifferentiated hESCs are cultured on Matrigel or laminin in medium conditioned by MEFs. The hESCs cultured in this culture system maintained a normal karyotype, stable proliferation rate, and high telomerase activity; expressed specific hESC markers; and have the capacity to differentiate into three germ layers in vivo and in vitro. In spite of this progress, this culture system doesn't lower the risk of animal pathogen contamination, as the animal products, MEF-conditioned medium and Matrigel, derived from Engelbreth-Holm-Swarm mouse tumor probably carry animal pathogens. In addition, the culture system cannot be accurately defined due to the use of conditioned medium and poor defined Matrigel.

To ensure a feeder layer-free, chemically defined environment for the growth of hESCs, the chemically defined medium mTeSR1 was used quickly to substitute for MEF-conditioned medium by many research groups all over the world. This serum-free, feeder-free culture system including Matrigel matrix and mTeSR1 medium simplified and standardized the procedure of hESC culture in the lab and has been used by many groups. Unfortunately, both Matrigel and mTeSR 1 are not xeno-free and suboptimal for future clinical purposes. To address this issue, human extracellular matrix (ECM) from human tissues has been used as an alternative in conjunction with several chemically defined culture media. The purified extracellular matrix, a combination of fibronectin, laminin, collagen IV, and vitronectin was firstly reported to culture hESCs in a defined culture system (Ludwig and Thomson, 2007). However, the ECM derived from human tissues still cannot rule out the possibility of human pathogen contamination and generally are not xeno free.

Recombinant protein matrices (such as laminin and vitronectin) produced in animal-free conditions have been reported to support long-term growth of hESCs. Recently as an alternative, a novel method using poly-d-lysine and the ROCK inhibitor has also been employed (Harb et al., 2008). This culture method broke new ground in the expansion of hESCs. However, since then there is no further progress reported on culture of hESCs using similar method under xeno-free, chemically defined conditions. In the year 2010, both groups (Villa-Diaz et al., 2010; Melkoumian et al., 2010) reported that they successfully grew hESCs on synthetic polymer and synthetic peptide-acrylate coated surfaces in xeno-free, defined culture media.

Currently, feeder-free culture systems of hESCs can be divided into four types: 1) xenogeneic medium and xenogeneic matrix (Xu et al., 2001; Klimanskaya et al., 2005); 2) xeno-free medium and xenogeneic matrix (Yao et al., 2006); 3) xenogeneic medium and xeno-free matrix (Braam et al., 2008); 4) both xeno-free medium and matrix (Rajala et al., 2010). The development of xeno-free, feeder-free, chemically defined culture systems will promote clinical trials and applications of hESCs in the future. For xeno-free culture of hESCs, all animal components should be eliminated from their derivation, expansion, freezing and thawing. The hESCs grown under xeno-free conditions should have hESC and colony morphology, normal karyotype, express specific hESC markers, and have the capacity to differentiate into three germ layers in vivo and in vitro.

Passaging hESCs

In the process of deriving hESCs and early passages of newly isolated hESC colonies, a mechanical dissociation was used to passage ICM-derived colonies or putative hESC colonies by dissecting them into cell clumps with finely drawn glass pipettes or steel needles. This mechanical method can also be used to eliminate the differentiated areas appeared within colonies in the process of establishment of hESC lines. As the number of cells increase, mechanical dissection is insufficient to meet scale up expansion of hESCs. Therefore, enzymatic dissociation was used as the main method for expansion of hESCs in culture. For enzymatic dissociation, collagenase IV and dispase are most commonly used to detach and dissociate hESC colonies into cell clumps.

A combination of mechanical and enzymatic methods is very useful and practical for hESC propagation. The differentiated colonies and differentiated areas appeared within colonies should be removed with mechanical dissection before enzyme dissociation of hESC colonies, as propagation of hESCs only with enzymatic dissociation can easily accumulate differentiated cells in hESC population. In addition, many of these proteolytic enzymes are derived from animal products and cannot be used to dissociate hESCs grown in xeno-free condition. Two commercially available xeno-free enzymes, Accutase (Innovative Cell Technologies) and TrypLE (Invitrogen) were used to dissociate hESCs to single cells and were reported to provide higher cell survival after passage (Bajpai et al., 2008; Ellerström et al., 2010). These products may prove to be useful in expansion of cell lines under xeno-free conditions.

Maintenance of Undifferentiated hESCs in Adherent Culture

In static culture conditions, hESCs have been cultured in feeder-dependent or feeder-free systems. No matter which culture system is used, spontaneous differentiation of hESCs is unavoidable. According to reports and our experience, suboptimal and nonstandard growth conditions, such as expired growth factors and reagents, inappropriate feeder cell density or poor quality feeder layers, unsuitable culture systems, inappropriate handling, freezing/thawing, derivation of new hESC lines, or selection following gene transfection can cause extreme differentiation in hESC colonies. Routinely, the partially differentiated areas in hESC colonies could be removed using a finely drawn glass pipette or steel needle attached to a syringe (Kim et al., 2005; Baharvand et al., 2010). Although this method works well in removing partially differentiated areas of hESC colonies, this approach is not effective for extremely differentiated (>80%) hESC colonies. If extreme differentiation occurs in hESC colonies, it has been nearly impossible to remove completely differentiated areas.

To address this problem, our group developed a novel method to isolate remaining undifferentiated hESCs from highly differentiated colonies (Meng et al., 2011). The key to this technique is to use a combined method to excise differentiated areas first as much as possible with cutting tool and then separate undifferentiated hESC clusters from differentiated cells with enzymatic dissociation. Using this method, it is quick and easy to derive completely undifferentiated hESC populations from extremely differentiated colonies.

ROCK Inhibitor and hESC Expansion

As hESCs undergo massive cell death in culture after single cell dissociation and are very sensitive to the routine manipulations, such as passaging, cryopreservation and gene transfection. These defects illustrate the need for new reagent and technical improvement for hESC expansion. A major breakthrough for solving this problem was the identification of Y-27632, a selective inhibitor of the p160-Rho-associated coiled kinase (ROCK). Up to now, many reports confirmed that ROCK inhibitor, Y27632 is a high efficiency and safe reagent, which can dramatically enhance the cell survival rate after single dissociation and significantly improve the recovery of freeze-thawed hESCs in singles or in clumps (Watanabe et al., 2007; Li et al., 2008).

However, the molecular mechanism of action of Y-27632 has not been fully understood. Based on previous studies (Xu et al., 2010), we can assume that 1) The Rho-ROCK-Myosin II axis plays an important role in mediating cell-cell adhesion; 2) Rho-ROCK signaling regulates E-cadherin-mediated cell-cell adhesion in ECM-free conditions; 3) E-cadherin is the primary cell-cell adhesion molecule and a highly expressed protein in hESCs; 4) Inhibition of the Rho-ROCK pathway prevents hESCs from death following single cell dissociation; 5) Cell-ECM interaction could also regulates cell-cell interaction by modulating Rho-ROCK pathway; 6) Cell-ECM interaction has been implicated to play an important role for hESC survival and self-renewal; 7) E-Cadherin signaling and integrin signaling regulate each other through modulating Rho activities and both are required for survival and self-renewal of hESCs.

In static culture, the process of colony formation consists of 4 steps: attachment of individual cells, migration, reaggregation, proliferation and formation of colonies. If single hESCs were seeded without addition of Y27632, some of the single cells could physically attach to the substrate, but failed to migrate toward each other and form cell aggregates. Without cell-cell communication or cell-cell contact, adherent cells would detach from culture substrate and die totally in short time. If hESCs grown at low cell density (2000 cells/cm^2) in the medium supplemented with Y27632, only few colonies in each dish were observed under the microscope. This means that it is hard for cells to migrate toward each other and form aggregates, as the distance between them is too far to contact and aggregate each other. So we speculated that cell-cell contact, not anti-apoptosis, predominantly responsible for the hESC growth in static culture system. As Y27632 can greatly promotes hESC attachment and viability but not proliferation, Y27632 containing medium should be replaced with fresh medium without Y27632 the second day after seeding or thawing dissociated cells. As for its role in hESC suspension culture, we will discuss in next section.

Expansion of hESCs in Suspension

One of the serious drawbacks of hESCs cultured in static conditions is low cell yield, which will not meet the actual demand of the clinic in the future. Recent several years, researchers reported different culture methods for the scale-up of hESCs in suspension culture. Suspension culture of hESCs results in the formation of aggregates, a process which can be controlled by several parameters, such as starting cell concentration, passage time, stirring speed, culture medium and addition of growth factors. In recent studies, some investigators focused on adaptation of 2D hESC cultures to 3D suspension by microcarriers. Microcarriers are support matrix allowing for the growth of adherent cells in bioreactors by providing an enlarged attachment surface. For the first time, Phillips et al. (2008) reported their developed method for maintaining hESCs on trimethyl ammonium-coated polystyrene microcarriers for feeder-free, 3-dimensional suspension culture. However, they only achieved initial hESC expansion, cell growth ceased over successive passages.

Oh et al. (2009) described a simple and robust method for maintaining undifferentiated hESCs in suspension cultures on Matrigel-coated microcarriers yielding 2- to 4-fold cells than those in static cultures. They also successfully expanded hESCs on Microcarriers in two serum-free defined media (StemPro and mTeSR1) with high cell yield. In these studies, hESC attachment and proliferation depended on matrix coated microcarriers. Trimethyl ammonium may not be an ideal matrix for supporting hESC growth in this suspension culture system and Matrigel, a poorly defined matrix is also not suitable for expansion of hESCs utilized for the clinical purposes. In addition, the use of microcarriers might increase technical and operational difficulties with respect to hESC generation for clinical purposes.

To establish a system for hESC propagation and expansion in scalable, suspension cultures, independent of additional matrix, Krawetz et al. (2010) developed a novel bioreactor protocol that yields a 25-fold expansion of hESCs over 6 days by using mTeSR1 supplemented with 10 uM ROCK inhibitor, Y-27632 and 0.1 nM Rapamycin. They demonstrated that hESCs cultured in bioreactor retained high levels of pluripotency and a normal karyotype. Singh et al. (2010) reported a method of forming controlled aggregates in suspension from single hESC inoculations in mTeSR1 medium by using Y-27632 in combination with heat shock treatment. In this study, single hESCs were treated with Y27632 and a heat shock, and formed aggregates in 2 ml static cultures and progressively up-scaled to 10 ml, and finally 50 ml stirred suspension cultures. However, mTeSR1 supports long-term expression of pluripotency markers in two hESC lines, but not in one cell line.

Most recently, Steiner et al. (2010) described the derivation and expansion of hESCs in a suspension culture system using Neurobasal medium supplemented with KSR, beta D-xylopyranose, growth factors (Activin A, FGF2), neurotrophic factors, and ECM components (laminin, fibronectin, and gelatin). Although hESCs could be maintained and expanded in this system, the cell harvest was lower relative to monolayer culture on feeder cells due to increased cell loss.

Amit et al. (2010) developed a radically different method for expansion of hESCs in suspension cultures. To initiate suspension cultures, hESCs were removed from culture dishes using type IV collagenase, broken into small clumps and cultured in suspension in Petri dishes. Before transferring to a 125 ml Erlenmeyer, cell clumps were cultured in Petri dishes for at least one passage. In their experiments, the researchers found that even at high doses of 10–40 ng/ml bFGF led to differentiation of hESCs after five passages, and the combination of full-length IL6RIL6 chimera and bFGF, supported hESC and hiPSC expansion in suspension for long-term culture. However, in this report, the researchers didn't give further information that whether their culture system could support single cell expansion. In conclusion, the suspension culture enables the propagation and expansion of hESCs in the absence of feeder cells and matrices, which makes a big step forward in facilitating the clinical application of hESCs.

Prospects for Deriving and Expanding hESC Lines

To date, nearly a thousand of hESC lines have been derived from donated embryos. The cell lines generated and cultured in chemically defined conditions can be used in basic research, such as signaling pathways and regulations in undifferentiated and differentiated hESCs, drug screening, human development, screening toxins, and building differentiated models in vitro and human gene functions, etc., as the defined culture conditions would eliminate interference from both the feeder cells and unknown factors. Almost all cell lines have been directly or indirectly exposed to animal-derived products, which would prevent the use of hESCs for clinical purposes, due to the possibility of xenogeneic bimolecule and pathogen contamination. Therefore, for establishment of clinical-grade hESC lines in xeno-free, defined conditions, mechanical or laser-assisted isolation of the ICMs from the blastocysts avoiding exposure to animal products is the first and key step. To circumvent political and ethical issues, hESC lines can also be generated from earlier stage embryos without embryo destruction, such as from single blastomeres removed from 8-cell embryos under xeno-free, chemically defined conditions.

Up to now, recombinant protein matrices (such as laminin and vitronectin) produced in animal-free conditions and synthetic matrices (synthetic polymer and synthetic peptide-acrylate) have been reported to support long-term growth of hESCs. As for animal-free culture media, HEScGRO (Millipore), TeSR2 (Stemcells Techniligies), XF/FF culture medium (Stemgent) and Knockout xeno-free serum replacement are commercially available. We believe that more and more xeno-free matrices and media will be released. However, a medium or matrix, working well in one culture system probably doesn't work in other culture systems. It is hard to say which medium or matrix is optimal for maintaining hESCs in xeno-free, defined culture conditions. It depends on the synergistic effect of both.

The working together of culture medium, matrix and factors should provide an adequate supply of nourishment and signaling pathways for supporting undifferentiated hESC growth and self-renewal. The hESC lines can be generated and cultured at early passages in adherent conditions under xeno-free, chemically defined culture system and then transferred into small bioreactors, progressively up-scaled to large stirred suspension cultures before clinical trials and applications. As above mentioned, to avoid the ethical problem, the modified method used for generation of xeno-free hESC lines from single blastomeres without destruction of embryos is a good choice. Other procedures and manipulations related to the derivation, expansion of hESCs, such as cell dissociation, freezing and thawing also should be performed under xeno-free, chemically defined conditions. Animal and human-derived products should be eliminated completely from each steps performed on hESCs.

For clinical purposes in the future, the generation, expansion, freezing and thawing of hESC lines should be manipulated under current good manufacturing process (cGMP) standards. Only cGMP hESC lines generated and expanded under xeno-free, defined conditions can be used as candidates for the clinical applications. In addition, these cell lines must meet the defining criteria for pluripotent stem cells after long-term culture, including specific hESC and colony morphology, the expression of pluripotency markers, stable karyotype and three-germ layer differentiation in vivo and in vitro. Here, one of the most important things is to establishing a therapeutic human embryonic stem cell bank using these cGMP hESC lines, as enough numbers of hESC lines can meet the need of different patients.

References

Amit M, Chebath J, Margulets V, Laevsky I, Miropolsky Y, Shariki K, Peri M, Blais I, Slutsky G, Revel M, Itskovitz-Eldor J (2010) Suspension culture of undifferentiated human embryonic and induced pluripotent stem cells. Stem Cell Rev 6:248–259

Baharvand H, Salekdeh GH, Taei A, Mollamohammadi S (2010) An efficient and easy-to-use cryopreservation protocol for human ES and iPS cells. Nat Protoc 5:588–594

Bajpai R, Lesperance J, Kim M, Terskikh AV (2008) Efficient propagation of single cells Accutase-dissociated human embryonic stem cells. Mol Reprod Dev 75:818–827

Braam SR, Zeinstra L, Litjens S, Ward-van Oostwaard, D van den, Brink S, van Laake L, Lebrin F, Kats P, Hochstenbach R, Passier R, Sonnenberg A, Mummery CL (2008) Recombinant vitronectin is a functionally defined substrate that supports human embryonic stem cell self-renewal via alphavbeta5 integrin. Stem Cells 26:2257–2265

Chen AE, Egli D, Niakan K, Deng J, Akutsu H, Yamaki M, Cowan C, Fitz-Gerald C, Zhang K, Melton DA, Eggan K (2009) Optimal timing of inner cell mass isolation increases the efficiency of human embryonic stem cell derivation and allows generation of sibling cell lines. Cell Stem Cell 4:103–106

Chung Y, Klimanskaya I, Becker S, Li T, Maserati M, Lu SJ, Zdravkovic T, Ilic D, Genbacev O, Fisher S, Krtolica A, Lanza R (2008) Human embryonic stem cell lines generated without embryo destruction. Cell Stem Cell 2:113–117

Draper JS, Smith K, Gokhale P, Moore HD, Maltby E, Johnson J, Meisner L, Zwaka TP, Thomson JA, Andrews PW (2004) Recurrent gain of chromosomes 17q and 12 in cultured human embryonic stem cells. Nat Biotechnol 22:53–54

Ellerström C, Hyllner J, Strehl R (2010) Single cell enzymatic dissociation of human embryonic stem cells: a straightforward, robust, and standardized culture method. Methods Mol Biol. 584:121–134

Gearhart J (1998) New potential for human embryonic stem cells. Science 282:1061–1062

Genbacev O, Krtolica A, Zdravkovic T, Brunette E, Powell S, Nath A, Caceres E, McMaster M, McDonagh S, Li Y, Mandalam R, Lebkowski J, Fisher SJ (2005) Serum-free derivation of human embryonic stem cell lines on human placental fibroblast feeders. Fertil Steril 83:1517–1529

Harb N, Archer TK, Sato N (2008) The Rho-ROCK-Myosin signaling axis determines cell–cell integrity of self-renewing pluripotent stem cells. PLoS One 3:e3001

Hovatta O, Mikkola M, Gertow K, Stromberg AM, Inzunza J, Hreinsson J, Rozell B, Blennow E, Andang M, Ahrlund-Richter L (2003) A culture system using human foreskin fibroblasts as feeder cells allows production of human embryonic stem cells. Hum Reprod 18:1404–1409

Kibschull M, Mileikovsky M, Michael IP, Lye SJ, Nagy A (2011) Human embryonic fibroblasts support single cell enzymatic expansion of human embryonic stem cells in xeno-free cultures. Stem Cell Res 6:70–82

Kim HS, Oh SK, Park YB, Ahn HJ, Sung KC, Kang MJ, Lee LA, Suh CS, Kim SH, Kim DW, Moon SY (2005) Methods for derivation of human embryonic stem cells. Stem Cells 23:1228–1233

Klimanskaya I, Chung Y, Meisner L, Johnson J, West MD, Lanza R (2005) Human embryonic stem cells derived without feeder cells. Lancet 365:1636–1641

Klimanskaya I, Chung Y, Becker S, Lu SJ, Lanza, R (2006) Human embryonic stem cell lines derived from single blastomeres. Nature 444:481–485

Krawetz R, Taiani JT, Liu S, Meng G, Li X, Kallos MS, Rancourt DE (2010) Large-scale expansion of pluripotent human embryonic stem cells in stirred-suspension bioreactors. Tissue Eng C Methods 16:573–582

Li X, Meng G, Krawetz R, Liu S, Rancourt DE (2008) The ROCK inhibitor Y-27632 enhances the survival rate of human embryonic stem cells following cryopreservation. Stem Cells Dev 17:1079–1085

Ludwig T, Thomson JA (2007) Defined, feeder-independent medium for human embryonic stem cell culture. Curr Protoc Stem Cell Biol Chapter 1, p. Unit 1C 2

Melkoumian Z, Weber JL, Weber DM, Fadeev AG, Zhou Y, Dolley-Sonneville P, Yang J, Qiu L, Priest CA, Shogbon C, Martin AW, Nelson J, West P, Beltzer JP, Pal S, Brandenberger R (2010) Synthetic peptide-acrylate surfaces for long-term self-renewal and cardiomyocyte differentiation of human embryonic stem cells. Nat Biotechnol 28:606–610

Meng G, Liu S, Krawetz R, Chan M, Chernos J, Rancourt DE (2008) A novel method for generating xeno-free human feeder cells for human embryonic stem cell culture. Stem Cells Dev 17:413–422

Meng G, Liu S, Rancourt DE (2011) Rapid isolation of undifferentiated human pluripotent stem cells from extremely differentiated colonies. Stem Cells Dev. 20:583–591

Oh SK, Chen AK, Mok Y, Chen X, Lim UM, Chin A, Choo AB, Reuveny S (2009) Long-term microcarrier suspension cultures of human embryonic stem cells. Stem Cell Res 2:219–230

Phillips BW, Horne R, Lay TS, Rust WL, Teck TT, Crook JM (2008) Attachment and growth of human embryonic stem cells on microcarriers. J Biotechnol 138:24–32

Rajala K, Lindroos B, Hussein SM, Lappalainen RS, Pekkanen-Mattila M, Inzunza J, Rozell B, Miettinen S, Narkilahti S, Kerkelä E, Aalto-Setälä K, Otonkoski T, Suuronen R, Hovatta O, Skottman H (2010) A defined and xeno-free culture method enabling the establishment of clinical-grade human embryonic, induced pluripotent and adipose stem cells. PLoS One 5:e10246

Richards M, Fong CY, Chan WK, Wong PC, Bongso A (2002) Human feeders support prolonged undifferentiated growth of human inner cell masses and embryonic stem cells. Nat Biotechnol 20:933–936

Singh H, Mok P, Balakrishnan T, Rahmat SN, Zweigerdt R (2010) Up-scaling single cell-inoculated suspension culture of human embryonic stem cells. Stem Cell Res 4:165–179

Steiner D, Khaner H, Cohen M, Even-Ram S, Gil Y, Itsykson P, Turetsky T, Idelson M, Aizenman E, Ram R, Berman-Zaken Y, Reubinoff B (2010) Derivation, propagation and controlled differentiation of human embryonic stem cells in suspension. Nat Biotechnol 28:361–364

Stojkovic P, Lako M, Stewart R, Przyborski S, Armstrong L, Evans J, Murdoch A, Strachan T, Stojkovic M (2005) An autogeneic feeder cell system that efficiently supports growth of undifferentiated human embryonic stem cells. Stem Cells 23:306–314

Ström S, Inzunza J, Grinnemo KH, Holmberg K, Matilainen E, Stromberg AM, Blennow E, Hovatta O (2007) Mechanical isolation of the inner cell mass is effective in derivation of new human embryonic stem cell lines. Hum Reprod 22:3051–3058

Thomson JA, Itskovitz-Eldor J, Shapiro SS, Waknitz MA, Swiergiel JJ, Marshall VS, Jones JM (1998) Embryonic stem cell lines derived from human blastocysts. Science 282:1145–1147

Villa-Diaz LG, Nandivada H, Ding J, Nogueira-de-Souza NC, Krebsbach PH, O'Shea KS, Lahann J, Smith GD (2010) Synthetic polymer coatings for long-term growth of human embryonic stem cells. Nat Biotechnol 28:581–583

Watanabe K, Ueno M, Kamiya D, Nishiyama A, Matsumura M, Wataya T, Takahashi JB, Nishikawa S, Nishikawa S, Muguruma K, Sasai Y (2007) A ROCK inhibitor permits survival of dissociated human embryonic stem cells. Nat Biotechnol 25:681–686

Xu C, Inokuma MS, Denham J, Golds K, Kundu P, Gold JD, Carpenter MK (2001) Feeder-free growth of undifferentiated human embryonic stem cells. Nat Biotechnol. 19: 971–974

Xu Y, Zhu X, Hahm HS, Wei W, Hao E, Hayek A, Ding S (2010) Revealing a core signaling regulatory mechanism for pluripotent stem cell survival and self-renewal by small molecules. Proc Natl Acad Sci USA 107:8129–8134

Yao S, Chen S, Clark J, Hao E, Beattie GM, Hayek A, Ding S (2006) Long-term self-renewal and directed differentiation of human embryonic stem cells in chemically defined conditions. Proc Natl Acad Sci USA 103:6907–6912

Chapter 13

Generation of Marmoset Induced Pluripotent Stem Cells Using Six Transcription Factors (Method)

Ikuo Tomioka and Erika Sasaki

Abstract The four transcription factors Oct-3/4, Sox2, Klf4, and c-Myc induce pluripotency in somatic cells. These embryonic stem (ES) cell-like induced pluripotent stem (iPS) cells have potential for therapeutic applications in humans, and iPS cell technology has shown dramatic advances in recent years. The common marmoset (*Callithrix jacchus*) offers many advantages over other laboratory primates for medical studies, including reproductive biology studies. In this chapter, we introduce a generation of marmoset iPS cells from fetal liver cells by the retrovirus-mediated introduction of six human transcription factors Oct-3/4, Sox2, Klf4, c-Myc, Nanog, and Lin28. The common marmoset and its iPS cells will provide a powerful preclinical model for regenerative medicine studies.

Keywords Embryonic stem cell · Induced pluripotent stem cell · Common marmoset · Liver cell · Lin28

Introduction

Induced pluripotent stem (iPS) cell technology, which was first reported by Takahashi and Yamanaka (2006), has progressed dramatically in recent years and now promises the development of regenerative medicine for humans. Thus, this technology will soon be applied to medical use, and the safety and efficacy of therapies using iPS cells must be evaluated in nonhuman primates closely related to human species through autogenic or allogenic transplantation. One of the deepest concerns is the oncogenicity of iPS-derived cells transplanted into a patient, but the life span of mice is too short to assess the long-term side effects of regenerative medicine using iPS cells. Thus, a long-term follow-up of patients transplanted with autogenic or allogenic iPS cells is required before this technology can be applied in clinical use.

Nonhuman primates have great potential for human disease studies. The common marmoset (*Callithrix jacchus*), a non-endangered New World primate native to Brazil, offers many advantages over other laboratory primates for use in human disease studies because its neurophysiological functions, metabolic pathways, and drug sensitivities are similar to those of humans. In fact, the number of common marmoset-based publications has been increasing and has more than tripled in the last two decades (Torres et al., 2010). This increase in the use of the common marmoset is also attributable to its moderate body size, reproductive rate, ease of handling, and long life span. Using marmosets enabled us to observe the long-term side effects of iPS cell-derived cell transplantation. Moreover, we recently reported creating the first transgenic marmosets with germline transmission through lentiviral vector-mediated gene transfer (Sasaki et al., 2009), followed by the establishment of marmoset iPS cells in 2010 (Tomioka et al., 2010). Hence, we can produce many kinds of model marmosets for human disease using this gene transfer technology. Combined with the model marmosets, establishing iPS cells in this species will dramatically accelerate the development of preclinical regenerative medicine studies. In this

E. Sasaki (✉)
Central Institute for Experimental Animals, Kawasaki, Kanagawa 216-0001, Japan; School of Medicine, Keio University, Tokyo, Japan; PRESTO Japan Science and Technology Agency, Tokyo, Japan
e-mail: esasaki@ciea.or.jpm

chapter, we introduce the methodology for establishing marmoset iPS cells.

Virus Production

Retroviral pMX vectors for human Oct-3/4, Sox2, Klf4, c-Myc, Nanog, and Lin28 were kindly provided by Dr. Yamanaka (Takahashi et al., 2007). Retroviruses of these transcription factors were produced using the Retroviral Gene Transfer and Expression System (Clontech, Tokyo, Japan) according to the manufacturer's instructions. Briefly, GP-2 cells were plated at 3×10^6 cells per 100-mm poly-L-lysine-coated dish (Sigma, St. Louis, MO, USA) and reached 80–90% confluence the following day. The cells were transfected with 6 μg of pMX vector and 6 μg of pVSV-G vector using the FuGENE 6 Transfection Reagent (Roche, Basel, Switzerland), and the medium was replaced the next day. The medium was collected 48 and 72 h after transfection, as a virus-containing supernatant, and filtered through a 0.45-μm-pore cellulose acetate filter (Sartorius, Göttingen, Germany). Virus stocks were stored at −80°C until use. We were able to generate marmoset iPS cells using frozen virus stocks stored for up to 1 month.

Virus Infection of Marmoset Cells

Common marmoset fetal liver cells, which were isolated from a miscarried female fetus, were seeded at 1×10^6 cells per 10-cm dish 1 day before transduction, and the cells reached 70–80% confluence the following day. Equal volumes of the virus-containing supernatant with Oct-3/4, Sox2, Klf4, c-Myc, Nanog, Lin28, and GFP were mixed. The medium was replaced with the virus-containing mixture supplemented with 4 μg/ml polybrene (Nacalai Tesque, Kyoto, Japan), and the cells were incubated for 12 h. Infection rates assessed by green fluorescent protein (GFP) fluorescence should be more than 30% (Fig. 13.1a). Seven days after the introduction, the cells were harvested by trypsinization and plated onto irradiated mouse embryonic fibroblasts (MEFs) at $1–2 \times 10^5$ cells per 10-cm gelatin-coated dish. At the same time, Dulbecco's modified Eagle's medium (DMEM) containing 10% fetal bovine serum (FBS) and 1% antibiotic–antimycotic solution was replaced with Knockout™ DMEM (ES cell culture medium), supplemented with 10% Knockout™ Serum Replacement (KSR; Invitrogen, Carlsbad, CA, USA), 1 mM L-glutamine, 0.1 mM MEM nonessential amino acids, 0.1 m β-mercaptoethanol (2-ME; Sigma), 1% antibiotic–antimycotic solution, and 10 ng/ml leukemia inhibitory factor (Millipore, Billerica, MA, USA). The medium was changed every other day.

Picking Colonies

Three to five weeks after we introduced the six transcription factors, several colonies morphologically resembling ES cells emerged (Fig. 13.1c), consistent with a report on rhesus monkey iPS cells (Liu et al., 2008). Each colony was picked up in 0.2 ml of ES cell culture medium and dissociated mechanically into small clumps by pipetting up and down. The cell suspension was transferred onto MEFs in gelatin-coated 12-well plates and cultured in ES cell culture medium. For cell splitting, undifferentiated iPS cell colonies were detached from feeder cells using 0.25% trypsin supplemented with 1 mM $CaCl_2$ and 20% KSR (Sasaki et al., 2005). The removed colonies were dissociated mechanically into 10–50 cells and re-plated on a new MEF feeder layer. All iPS cell colonies had a flat, packed, and tight colony morphology and a high nucleus-to-cytoplasm ratio (Fig. 13.1d). Continuous cultures of iPS cells have been sustained for more than 1 year.

The reason why we used six human transcription factors is that no iPS cells were established after we introduced Yamanaka's four transcription factors: Oct-3/4, Sox2, Klf4, and c-Myc. In contrast, when six transcription factors were introduced into fetal liver cells, colonies resembling marmoset ES cells emerged 4–5 weeks later. Especially, we realized that Lin28 in addition to Yamanaka's four transcription factors improved the efficiency of iPS cells established after several experiments using Nanog plus those four factors (Nanog 5-factors) or Lin28 plus those four factors (Lin28 5-factors). We only obtained iPS cells from the Lin28 5-factor combination.

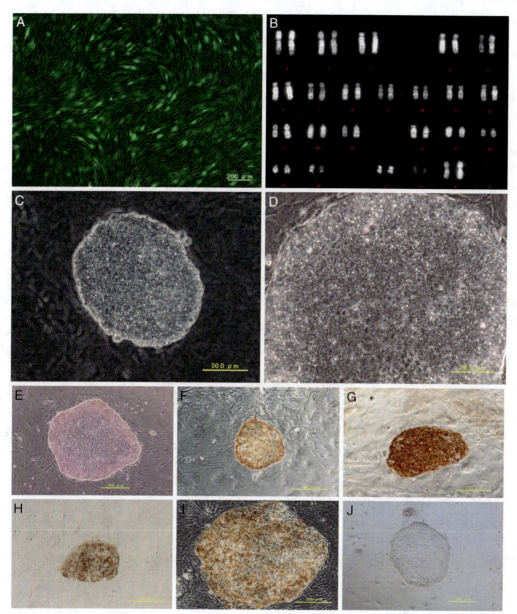

Fig. 13.1 (a) Green fluorescent protein (GFP) fluorescence 2 days after virus infection. About 33% of the cells fluoresced in this figure. (b) The induced pluripotent stem (iPS) cells retained the normal 46, XX karyotype after a 2-month culture. (c, d) All iPS cells had a flat, packed, tight colony morphology and a high nucleus-to-cytoplasm ratio. The iPS cells showed alkaline phosphatase activity (e) and expressed SSEA-3 (f), SSEA-4 (g), TRA-1-60 (h), and TRA-1-81 (i), but not SSEA-1 (j). Parts of these figures are from Tomioka et al. (2010)

Characterization of Established iPS Cells

Immunocytochemical Staining

To confirm the undifferentiated status of the iPS cells, we examined cell surface marker expression on cultured marmoset iPS cells and detected alkaline phosphatase using the Alkaline Phosphatase Detection Kit (Millipore) according to the manufacturer's instructions. Immunocytochemical staining followed a previous report (Sasaki et al., 2005). Briefly, iPS cells were fixed with 4% paraformaldehyde in phosphate-buffered saline (PBS) for 10 min at room temperature. The primary antibodies against stage-specific embryonic antigen (SSEA)-1, SSEA-3, SSEA-4 (Developmental Studies Hybridoma Bank, Iowa City, IA, USA), TRA-1-60, and TRA-1-81 (Millipore) were diluted with Antibody Diluent (Dako ChemMate; Dako, Glostrup, Denmark), and the cells were incubated for 1 h at room temperature in a solution containing each antibody. The following are the dilutions for each primary antibody: anti-SSEA-1 (1:100), anti-SSEA-3 (1:100), anti-SSEA-4 (1:200), anti-TRA-1-60 (10 μg/ml), and anti-TRA-1-81 (10 μg/ml). After three washes with PBS, the cells were incubated for 30 min at room temperature in a solution containing the biotinylated secondary antibody using the Simple Stain MAX-PO Multi system (Nichirei Corporation, Tokyo, Japan). The samples were washed three times with PBS, and the bound monoclonal antibodies were located using the 3,3′-diaminobenzidine tetrahydrochloride-horseradish peroxidase complex.

As a result, iPS cells showed alkaline phosphatase activity (Fig. 13.1e) and expressed SSEA-3 (Fig. 13.1f), SSEA-4 (Fig. 13.1g), TRA-1-60 (Fig. 13.1h), and TRA-1-81 (Fig. 13.1i), but not SSEA-1 (Fig. 13.1j). These results are consistent with a previous report on common marmoset ES cells (Sasaki et al., 2005). The cells had many similarities to human and other nonhuman primate ES cells in terms of morphology, surface antigens, and cellular characteristics (Thomson et al., 1995, 1998; Reubinoff et al., 2000; Suemori et al., 2001).

Karyotypic Analysis

Numerous abnormalities develop while establishing iPS cells because iPS cells are artificial products. One of the abnormalities is a karyotype abnormality that occurs with high frequency. Hence, all iPS cell lines were subjected to karyotype analysis using a modification of the Q-banding technique (Sugawara et al., 2006). Briefly, iPS cells were incubated with medium containing 100 ng/ml colcemid (Invitrogen) for 90 min. Then, they were washed in PBS, dissociated using trypsin–EDTA solution, and centrifuged. The slides were stained with 0.01 μg/ml Hoechst 33258 for 5 min and with 5.0 g/ml quinacrine mustard for 20 min. The stained slides were mounted in a mount solution for observation through a DMRXA2 fluorescent microscope (Leica, Wetzlar, Germany) and analyzed using Leica CW4000. As a result, five (83.3%) of six iPS cell lines retained a normal 46, XX karyotype (Fig. 13.1b) after a 2-month culture.

Reverse Transcription-PCR

RNA was isolated using the RNeasy Mini Kit (Qiagen, Valencia, CA, USA) according to the manufacturer's instructions. First-strand cDNA was synthesized from RNA using the QuantiTect Reverse Transcription kit (Qiagen). As a negative control, RNA was allowed to react with the cDNA synthesis reaction mixture in the absence of reverse transcriptase. After cDNA synthesis, the cDNA synthesis reaction mixture was used as the PCR template. The primers used were described in our previous report (Tomioka et al., 2010). The PCR reaction mixture (20 μl) contained 1× PCR buffer (10 mM Tris-HCl [pH 9.0], 1.5 mM $MgCl_2$, 50 mM KCl), 0.2 mM dNTP, 0.5 μM of each primer, and 2.5 U *Taq* polymerase. The amplification was performed for 35 cycles at 98°C for 20 s, 60°C for 25 s, and 72°C for 25 s. The reverse transcription-PCR revealed that all iPS cells also expressed endogenous Oct4, Sox2, Klf4, c-Myc, Nanog, and Lin28 genes, whereas all of the transgenes were silenced, showing that they maintained undifferentiated states of their own.

In Vitro Differentiation

Embryoid Body Formation In Vitro

Embryoid body (EB) formation is an assessment of the spontaneous differentiation potency of ES cells and iPS cells in vitro. To form the EB, iPS cell colonies were detached from feeder cells using 0.25% trypsin supplemented with 1 mM $CaCl_2$ and 20% KSR, and dissociated mechanically into 10–50 cells. The cells were subjected to a floating culture in DMEM supplemented with 10% FBS for 7–28 days. Half of the medium was changed every 2 days. Then, we examined the formation of EBs and the expression of several genes for the three germ layers.

As a result, simple EBs formed several days after the start of the suspension cultures, and cystic EBs formed within 2 weeks (Fig. 13.2a). EBs from iPS

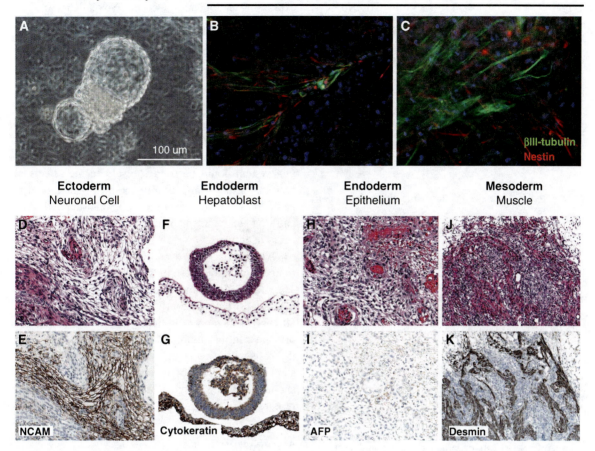

Fig. 13.2 (a) Embryoid body formation. (b, c) After a 24-day culture on PA6 cells, cells positive for the neural progenitor marker nestin (*red*) and neuronal marker βIII-tubulin (*green*) were observed. (d–k) NCAM-positive cells were observed as neuronal cells, showing evidence of induced pluripotent stem (iPS) cell differentiation into ectodermal cells (d, e). The presence of a columnar epithelium (f, g) consisting of cytokeratin-positive cells and hepatoblasts (h, i), which were AFP-positive, suggested endodermal differentiation. The muscle-like structures expressed desmin (m, n). Parts of these figures are from Tomioka et al. (2010)

cells expressed several genes for all three germ layers, showing that all of the iPS cells had the developmental potential to give rise to differentiated derivatives of all three primary germ layers. Moreover, spontaneously beating cells were found in the cultures, showing their capacity to differentiate into functional cardiomyocytes.

Neural Differentiation of Marmoset iPS Cells In Vitro

We cultured marmoset iPS cells using the modified SDIA method to induce neural differentiation (Kawasaki et al., 2000). Several colonies of marmoset iPS cells were picked up, partially dissociated, and cocultured with semi-confluent PA6 cells. The cells were plated onto gelatin-coated coverslips at a density of 9×10^3 cells/cm^2 and cultured in a differentiation medium consisting of Glasgow's modified Eagle's medium (GMEM) supplemented with 10% KSR, 2 mM glutamine, 1 mM sodium pyruvate, 0.1 mM nonessential amino acids, and 0.1 mM 2-ME. The medium was changed every 2 days. On day 17, the differentiation medium was switched to GMEM supplemented with N2, 100 μM tetrahydrobiopterin, 200 μM ascorbic acid, 2 mM glutamine, 1 mM sodium pyruvate, 0.1 mM nonessential amino acids, and 0.1 mM 2-ME. On day 24, the cells were fixed with 4% paraformaldehyde and processed for immunocytochemical analysis with anti-nestin (rabbit IgG, 1:4000; GenBank Accession No. X65964) and anti-βIII-tubulin (mouse IgG, 1:1000; Sigma) antibodies.

After a 24-day culture on PA6 cells, cells positive for the neural progenitor marker nestin and the neuronal marker βIII-tubulin were observed in all of the iPS cell lines tested (Fig. 13.2b, c).

Teratoma Formation

We injected $1–5 \times 10^6$ iPS cells into the kidneys capsules of 5-week-old immunodeficient NOG mice to examine teratoma formation (Ito et al., 2002). Four to eight weeks after the injection, the tumors were removed from the mice. The resected tumors were fixed in neutral buffered formalin, embedded in paraffin blocks, sectioned, and subjected to immunohistochemical staining. The specimens were incubated with primary antibodies against cytokeratin, desmin, NCAM, and AFP (Dako) followed by incubation with the biotinylated secondary antibody Simple Stain MAX-PO Multi system. Localization of the bound monoclonal antibodies was detected using the Envision System (Dako), and several sections were stained with Alcian blue.

The NCAM-positive cells were neuronal cells, as evidence of iPS cell differentiation into ectodermal cells (Fig. 13.2d, e). The presence of columnar epithelium (Fig. 13.2f, g), which consisted of cytokeratin-positive cells, and hepatoblasts (Fig. 13.2h, i), which consisted of AFP-positive cells, suggested endodermal differentiation. The teratomas frequently differentiated into mesodermal tissues, such as muscle, blood vessels, and cartilage. The muscle-like structures expressed desmin (Fig. 13.2j, k). These results showed that all of the iPS cells had the developmental potential to produce differentiated derivatives of all three primary germ layers.

Summary

In this study, we established common marmoset iPS cells from fetal liver cells through the retrovirus-mediated introduction of six human transcription factors: Oct-3/4, Sox2, Klf4, c-Myc, Nanog, and Lin28. The cells maintained an undifferentiated state expressing endogenous Oct-3/4, Sox2, Klf4, c-Myc, Nanog, and Lin28 and revealed a normal ability to differentiate into the three germ cell layers both in vitro and in vivo. Moreover, we successfully induced neural cells in vitro, which produced a very precise system to assess safety and efficacy for regenerative medicine. Using this system, both human and marmoset iPS cell-derived cells could be transplanted into marmosets of a human disease model such as spinal cord injury (Iwanami et al., 2005). Furthermore, this system could be used to evaluate the effects of both major histocompatibility complex-matching allogenic transplantation (marmoset iPS cell-derived cells) and xenogenic transplantation (human iPS cell-derived cells) in animals.

Over the past few decades, numerous medical and reproductive biology studies have involved marmosets. The availability of marmosets and their ease of breeding suggest that these primates represent a promising alternative to more traditional Old World nonhuman primates. In the future, common marmosets and their iPS cells will provide a powerful preclinical model for studies in the field of regenerative medicine, which should lead to a surge in interest among biological researchers.

Acknowledgements This study was supported by the Strategic Research Program for Brain Sciences, the Global COE program for Education and Research Centre for Metabolomic Systems Biology, the Precursory Research for Embryonic Science and Technology (PRESTO), Funding Program for World-Leading Innovatve R&D on Science and Technology (FIRST), the Ministry of Education, Culture, Sports, Science and Technology (MEXT), and the Japan Science and Technology Agency (JST).

References

Ito M, Hiramatsu H, Kobayashi K, Suzue K, Kawahata M, Hioki K, Ueyama Y, Koyanagi Y, Sugamura K, Tsuji K, Heike T, Nakahata T (2002) NOD/SCID/gamma(c)(null) mouse: an excellent recipient mouse model for engraftment of human cells. Blood 100:3175–3182

Iwanami A, Yamane J, Katoh H, Nakamura M, Momoshima S, Ishii H, Tanioka Y, Tamaoki N, Nomura T, Toyama Y and Okano, H (2005) Establishment of graded spinal cord injury model in a nonhuman primate: the common marmoset. J Neurosci Res 80:172–181

Kawasaki H, Mizuseki K, Nishikawa S, Kaneko S, Kuwana Y, Nakanishi S, Nishikawa SI, Sasai Y (2000) Induction of midbrain dopaminergic neurons from ES cells by stromal cell-derived inducing activity. Neuron 28:31–40

Liu H, Zhu F, Yong J, Zhang P, Hou P, Li H, Wei Jiang W, Cai J, Liu M, Cui K, Qu X, Xiang T, Lu D, Chi X, Gao G, Ji W, Ding M, Deng H (2008) Generation of induced pluripotent stem cells from adult rhesus monkey fibroblasts. Cell Stem Cell 3:587–590

Reubinoff BE, Pera MF, Fong CY, Trounson A, Bongso A (2000) Embryonic stem cell lines from human blastocysts: somatic differentiation *in vitro*. Nat Biotechnol 18:399–404

Sasaki E, Hanazawa K, Kurita R, Akatsuka A, Yoshizaki T, Ishii H, Tanioka Y, Ohnishi Y, Suemizu H, Sugawara A, Tamaoki N, Izawa K, Nakazaki Y, Hamada H, Suemori H, Asano S, Nakatsuji N, Okano H, Tani K (2005) Establishment of novel embryonic stem cell lines derived from the common marmoset (*Callithrix jacchus*). Stem Cells 23:1304–1313

Sasaki E, Suemizu H, Shimada A, Hanazawa K, Oiwa R, Kamioka M, Tomioka I, Sotomaru Y, Hirakawa R, Eto T, Shiozawa S, Maeda T, Ito M, Ito R, Kito C, Yagihashi C, Kawai K, Miyoshi H, Tanioka Y, Tamaoki N, Habu S, Okano H, Nomura T (2009) Generation of transgenic non-human primates with germline transmission. Nature 459:523–527

Suemori H, Tada T, Torii R, Hosoi Y, Kobayashi K, Imahie H, Kondo Y, Iritani A, Nakatsuji N (2001) Establishment of embryonic stem cell lines from cynomolgus monkey blastocysts produced by IVF or ICSI. Dev Dyn 222:273–279

Sugawara A, Goto K, Sotomaru Y, Sofuni T, Ito T (2006) Current status of chromosomal abnormalities in mouse embryonic stem cell lines used in Japan. Comp Med 56:31–34

Takahashi K, Yamanaka S (2006) Induction of pluripotent stem cells from mouse embryonic and adult fibroblast cultures by defined factors. Cell 126:663–676

Takahashi K, Tanabe K, Ohnuki M, Narita M, Ichisaka T, Tomoda K, Yamanaka S (2007) Induction of pluripotent stem cells from adult human fibroblasts by defined factors. Cell 131:861–872

Thomson JA, Kalishman J, Golos TG, Durning M, Harris CP, Becker RA, Hearn JP (1995) Isolation of a primate embryonic stem cell line. Proc Natl Acad Sci USA 92:7844–7848

Thomson JA, Itskovitz-Eldor J, Shapiro SS, Waknitz MA, Swiergiel JJ, Marshall VS, Jones JM (1998) Embryonic stem cell lines derived from human blastocysts. Science 282:1145–1147

Tomioka I, Maeda T, Shimada H, Kawai K, Okada Y, Igarashi H, Oiwa R, Iwasaki T, Aoki M, Kimura T, Shiozawa S, Shinohara H, Suemizu H, Sasaki E, Okano H (2010) Generating induced pluripotent stem cells from common marmoset (*Callithrix jacchus*) fetal liver cells using defined factors, including Lin28. Genes Cells 15:959–969

Torres LB, Silva Araujo BH, Gomes de Castro PH, Romero Cabral F, Sarges Marruaz K, Silva Araujo M, Gomes da Silva S, Muniz JA, Cavalheiro EA (2010) The use of new world primates for biomedical research: an overview of the last four decades. Am J Primatol 72:1055–1061

Chapter 14
MYC as a Multifaceted Regulator of Pluripotency and Reprogramming

Keriayn N. Smith and Stephen Dalton

Abstract Pluripotent stem cells have the ability to generate cellular descendants of the three primary germ layers. For this reason, they are a viable resource in the generation of specialized cells for tissue regeneration and drug development. In the embryo and in vitro culture, pluripotent cells express specific factors that maintain the pluripotent state. Such factors promote the expression of other pluripotency genes to maintain self-renewal and impede differentiation. The proto-oncogene Myc is a central regulator that holds multiple roles in the control of pluripotency. Key functions include maintenance of the pluripotent cell cycle, metabolic regulation and suppression of differentiation pathways. Myc target genes number in the thousands, so it is likely that novel aspects of Myc function in pluripotent stem cell biology remain to be fully elucidated. This chapter deals with our current understanding of Myc's contribution to pluripotency, its involvement in reprogramming and its contribution to cancer stem cell biology.

Keywords Pluripotent stem cells · Murine embryonic development · Inner cell mass · Embryonic stem cells · Epiblast stem cells · Embryonic germ cells

Pluripotent Stem Cells

Several well-defined pluripotent cell populations transiently exist throughout early murine embryonic development. The earliest of these is the inner cell mass (ICM) that is specified at around E3.5. Cells of the early epiblast develop at approximately E5 and primordial germ cells are specified at around E7. Under the appropriate conditions, these embryo-derived pluripotent cells can be cultured in vitro and retain the characteristics of the embryonic cells from which they were derived.

The best studied of these cell populations, embryonic stem cells (ESCs) are derived from the inner cell mass of blastocysts. When cultured in vitro, ESCs retain the ability to undergo self-renewal whilst retaining the capacity to form any cellular derivative of the embryonic germ layers. Upon reintroduction into a blastocyst, murine ESCs (mESCs) reintegrate into the embryo and contribute to differentiating tissues, including the germ line.

Epiblast stem cells (EpiSCs) have been more recently characterized and represent pluripotent cells equivalent to the primitive ectoderm stage of development. EpiSCs differ from ESCs in their gene expression signature and in cellular morphology and therefore represent a distinct pluripotent cell population (Tesar et al., 2007). Similar to human ESCs (hESCs), EpiSCs grow as a single layered, epithelial-like sheet. This contrasts with mESCs that grow as a domed-shaped colony. Unlike mESCs, EpiSCs express early differentiation markers including T-Brachyury and Fgf5 in addition to classic pluripotency markers such as Oct4 and Nanog. While EpiSCs represent a distinctly different pluripotent state when compared to

S. Dalton (✉)
Department of Biochemistry and Molecular Biology, Paul D. Coverdell Center for Biomedical and Health Sciences, University of Georgia, Athens, GA 30602, USA
e-mail: sdalton@uga.edu

ESCs, they can be converted into an ESC-like state by prolonged culture in media containing LIF (Bao et al., 2009). EpiSCs can also be reprogrammed to an ESC-like state through the expression of pluripotency regulators or via the introduction of small molecules (Hanna et al., 2009; Zhou et al., 2010). Although EpiSCs can differentiate into germ layer derivatives in vitro and are able to form teratomas when introduced into immunocompromised animals, they are unable to incorporate into a blastocyst and generate chimeras. Initially, this was not surprising considering that EpiSCs have a different spatiotemporal origin than ESCs. However, more recent studies have demonstrated that EpiSCs can also be derived from pre-implantation blastocysts (Najm et al., 2011). It remains to be determined whether blastocyst-derived EpiSCs will reincorporate into blastocyst-stage embryos and contribute to chimeras.

Embryonic germ cells (EGCs) and germ cell stem cells (GSCs) are derived from primordial germ cells and spermatogonial stem cells in the male neonatal gonads, respectively. The derivation of EGCs from primordial germ cells requires the addition of LIF, bFGF and SCF that stimulates the expression of pluripotency factors such as Myc and Klf-4. Similar to ESCs, EGCs and GSCs hold the ability to differentiate into specialized cell types in vitro and in vivo (Guan et al., 2006; Labosky et al., 1994).

Of the abovementioned pluripotent cell types, ESCs presently hold the most therapeutic potential mainly because they are easy to isolate and because of their proven wide-ranging differentiation potential. Still, using human embryos to generate pluripotent stem cells for therapies is hindered by ethical issues and remains a major barrier to their therapeutic application. This issue may be overcome however, by the use of induced pluripotent stem cells (iPSCs). iPSCs in principle, are generated by the reprogramming of differentiated somatic cells back to a pluripotent state (Takahashi and Yamanaka, 2006). These ESC-like pluripotent cells offer the advantage of being a potential source of patient-specific stem cells.

MYC Family of Proteins

The major Myc family members, c-myc, N-myc and L-myc and the lesser studied B-myc and S-myc are members of the basic helix-loop-helix leucine zipper family of proteins (Dang, 1999). The association of dysregulated c-, N-, and L-myc with many cancers including lymphoma, neuroblastoma, breast and ovarian carcinomas and cancers of the lung, liver, bladder and prostate is well established. Oncogenic activation of Myc can involve a range of genetic changes including gene amplification, chromosomal translocation and point mutations. These genomic alterations often result in mitogen-independence, genomic instability and immortalization (Meyer and Penn, 2008).

While Myc family members are often key oncogenes in human tumor development, they also play important roles in regulation of normal cellular processes during development and cellular homeostasis. Numerous studies have implicated Myc in regulation of cellular growth, senescence escape, differentiation, maintenance of cellular structure, cellular motility and apoptosis (Meyer and Penn, 2008).

General Modes of MYC Function

The Myc proteins have been traditionally thought of as transcriptional activators, but they are also able to repress transcription in certain contexts. Transcriptional activation is primarily mediated by binding DNA in a sequence-specific manner at canonical and non-canonical E-boxes with their binding partner, the leucine zipper protein, Max. Myc proteins can also regulate transcription in a sequence-independent manner, but this is less well understood than regulation through E-boxes. Even though they are relatively weak trans-activators, Myc has widespread effects on transcriptional activity. For example, genome-wide studies show that Myc potentially regulates the expression of 10–15% of all cellular genes (Fernandez et al., 2003).

The mechanism behind Myc-dependent repression of target genes is not well understood and is likely to involve multiple mechanisms. The best example of Myc-dependent repression involves the sequestration of Miz-1 away from its transcriptional targets. Alternatively, by forming a complex with co-repressor Dnmt3a and Miz-1 on the p21Cip1 promoter, Myc is able to actively repress transcription (Brenner et al., 2005; Wu et al., 2003). The end result of these mechanisms is to reduce the expression of Miz-1 targets, some of which include cell cycle inhibitors.

In addition to regulation of protein coding target genes, Myc also regulates non-coding RNAs, including miRNAs (Smith and Dalton, 2010). As miRNAs regulate their target genes post-transcriptionally by impeding translation or causing degradation of mRNAs, Myc indirectly controls post-transcriptional regulation of some transcripts through stimulation or repression of miRNA targets.

Myc also influences gene expression by regulating the cellular epigenetic state through extensive binding to broad chromatin domains where it functions to maintain euchromatin (Cotterman et al., 2008). This ability is based on interactions between Myc and a wide array of epigenetic regulators including histone modifying enzymes and chromatin remodeling complex factors (Smith et al., 2011). Through interactions with these proteins, Myc impacts chromatin accessibility.

Regulation of Pluripotent Stem Cells by MYC

Myc is a well-established regulator of pluripotent cells in vivo and in vitro. In mESCs that require exogenous LIF to maintain self-renewal, Myc is a downstream target of the LIF signaling pathway (Cartwright et al., 2005). LIF binding to the gp130 receptor activates Stat3 expression that in turn, stimulates Myc transcription. LIF signaling thus maintains high levels of Myc protein, which declines upon LIF withdrawal and cellular differentiation. Differentiation also ensues when a dominant negative Myc, presumably affecting both c- and N-myc activity is expressed in mESCs. Additionally, expression of a constitutively active c-myc mutant promotes self-renewal and reduces the need for LIF signaling (Cartwright et al., 2005). These data highlight the importance of Myc in the maintenance of pluripotent cells.

c- and N-myc have at least partially redundant functions, consistent with the ability of mESCs to self-renew when c-myc is inactivated (Baudino et al., 2002; Malynn et al., 2000). c-myc$^{-/-}$ N-myc$^{-/-}$ knockout cells however, are unable to maintain self-renew and lose pluripotency, spontaneously differentiating into primitive endoderm (Smith et al., 2010). In this context, Myc functions as a transcriptional repressor blocking differentiation through repression of the primitive endoderm master regulator, Gata6 (Smith et al., 2010). L-myc is not able to rescue pluripotency in this experimental model (Smith et al., 2010). This highlights differential properties of c- and N-myc compared to L-myc in functionally regulating pluripotency.

The role of Myc in hESCs is not fully understood and all three major family members are expressed in hESCs (Kelly and Rizzino, 2000). Unlike mESCs, LIF/Stat3 signaling is not a requirement for hESC maintenance raising the possibility that Myc may not be involved (Humphrey et al., 2004). However, since Myc promotes the establishment of pluripotency in human somatic cells (Takahashi et al., 2007) (discussed later), it remains likely that Myc is involved in hESCs maintenance but this awaits further experimentation.

Although Myc is clearly implicated as a regulator of pluripotency, multiple studies have failed to find a key link that defines how Myc contributes to pluripotency, outside of cell cycle regulation and metabolic control (Smith et al., 2011). Relative to the common targets shared by key pluripotency regulators Oct4, Sox2 and Nanog (OSN), Myc target gene lists are surprisingly distinct. The OSN factors are central pluripotency regulators that stimulate the expression of key target genes to maintain self-renewal. They also simultaneously occupy the promoters of specification factors to block differentiation (Boyer et al., 2006). Therefore Myc and OSN primarily operate in separate regulatory networks and importantly, the lack of overlap between OSN and Myc targets highlight the combinatorial approach utilized to maintain the pluripotent state.

Only a small number of factors that regulate differentiation seem to be directly controlled by Myc. Notable targets however, include the PRC2 regulatory component, Suz12 (Kim et al., 2008; Lin et al., 2009b; Smith et al., 2010). Regulation of PRC2 by Myc may therefore promote repression of lineage specification targets.

The majority of Myc target genes identified in pluripotent cells perform roles in cell proliferation, nucleic acid metabolism and protein metabolism (Smith et al., 2011). Considering Myc's historic role in the regulation of growth and the cell cycle in normal and tumor cells, this finding was not unexpected.

Pluripotent cells divide rapidly and have a characteristic cell cycle structure where ~60% of the cell cycle is devoted to S-phase with a minority of the population residing in G1. This is in contrast to differentiated populations that spend the majority of time in G1 (Singh and Dalton, 2009). The rapid cycling of mouse pluripotent cells may be related to the need for rapid expansion of pluripotent cells during early development but, it may also be related to maintenance of the pluripotent state.

From studies in other cell types, Myc is known to regulate multiple cell cycle regulators at the transcriptional and post-transcriptional level. Since Myc levels are elevated in pluripotent cells, persistent stimulation of these cell cycle targets are believed to promote constitutive Cdk activity, unlike that normally observed in differentiated cells.

Myc also negatively regulates cell cycle inhibitors including members of the INK4/Arf family in pluripotent stem cells (Smith et al., 2011). Moreover, Myc also indirectly represses the activity of cell cycle inhibitors through regulation of miRNAs (Smith and Dalton, 2010). Suppression of these inhibitors allows cyclin-dependent kinases to operate in an unrestricted manner, analogous to that seen in tumor cells.

As pluripotent cells differentiate, their cell cycle structure is remodeled so that cell division times increase and the length of G1 elongates. This is due in part to a reduction in transcriptional stimulation of cyclins A, B, E and D in addition to the derepression of cell cycle inhibitors (Singh and Dalton, 2009). An important consequence of G1 elongating is that cells acquire a restriction (R-) point and become regulated by external mitogenic signals for the first time. Prior to this, pluripotent cells divide in a cell autonomous manner reminiscent of mitogen-independent, transformed cells.

Of the miRNAs regulated by Myc in ESCs, the miR-17-92 cluster is of special interest with regards to cell cycle control. Cell cycle regulators such as the proliferation inhibitors Cip1^{p21} and Rb2 are negatively regulated by members of the miR17-92 cluster, allowing for rapid cell division. The miR-290 family members are also stimulated by Myc. Interestingly, members of this miRNA family are able to act as a Myc substitute to improve the efficiency of cellular reprogramming (Judson et al., 2009).

Myc also occupies the presumed promoter regions of miR-141, miR-200, miR-338 and miR-429 in pluripotent cells (Lin et al., 2009a). Interestingly, these miRNAs are functional components of a pluripotency network that inhibits differentiation by targeting specification factors.

Besides activation, Myc represses a variety of miRNAs in pluripotent cells such as Let-7, a miRNA that promotes differentiation. Let-7 levels increase during differentiation, coinciding with loss of Myc (Chang et al., 2009).

Pluripotent cells are highly euchromatic and display widespread acetylation of histones H3, H4 and trimethylated H3K4 (H3K4me3), properties indicative of an open chromatin configuration. Heterochromatic regions bearing marks of repressed chromatin that include trimethylated H3K9 and H3K27 (H3K27me3) constitute a more minor fraction (Meshorer and Misteli, 2006). This open chromatin state is thought to support the developmental plasticity of pluripotent cells and facilitates rapid activation of lineage specification programs upon receipt of the appropriate signals. During differentiation, there is remodeling of chromatin as illustrated by a marked reduction in euchromatin accompanied by increases in heterochromatic foci. This is thought to be due to a global decrease in active histone modifications concurrent with increases in repressive modifications (Meshorer and Misteli, 2006).

Genes encoding enzymes that modify histone residues or regulate chromatin accessibility are regulated by Myc in pluripotent cells. These include the histone modifying enzymes and chromatin remodeling complex components Ash2l, Setd8 and Smarcc1 (Lin et al., 2009b; Smith et al., 2010). In addition to direct transcriptional regulation, Myc influences chromatin activity through interaction with epigenetic modifiers. These include lysine-specific demethylase 1 (LSD1), members of the NuA4/Tip60 histone acetyltransferase complex and the repressive NURD complex (Smith et al., 2011). LSD1 demethylates di- or mono-methylated histone H3K4 or H3K9 and can therefore positively or negatively influence transcription (Shi et al., 2005). The acetyltransferase activity of NuA4/Tip60 serves to promote transcription while NURD functions as a repressor. These interactions suggest that by interacting in different complexes, Myc can activate and repress target genes in a context-dependent manner in pluripotent cells. It is unclear whether Myc establishes epigenetic marks on histones, is involved in the maintenance of these marks or, if it is simply recruited by these marks to a wide range of promoters.

Another unique aspect of pluripotent stem cell biology that speaks to their developmental plasticity is the presence of bivalent marks that is, genes that have both active and inhibitory histone modifications (Mikkelsen et al., 2008). Bivalent marks are typically found at genes involved in lineage specification. Upon loss of pluripotency, bivalency is resolved so that only activating (H3K4me3) or repressive marks (H3K27me3) are retained (Mikkelsen et al., 2008). Only a low percentage of such bivalently marked genes are Myc targets in pluripotent cells (Kim et al., 2008).

Overall, these transcriptional, post-transcriptional and epigenetic regulatory functions help to account for Myc's importance in maintenance of pluripotency (see Fig. 14.1). They also explain why Myc is able to promote the establishment of pluripotent cell lines from genetic backgrounds that are traditionally non-permissive (Hanna et al., 2009).

Cellular Reprogramming by MYC

The exogenous expression of Oct4, Sox2, Klf4 and Myc, as well as other factor combinations, was used to generate a pluripotent stem cell type (iPSCs) from

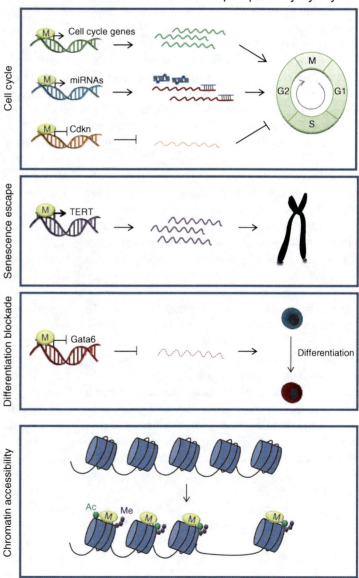

Fig. 14.1 Myc controls multiple cellular processes to maintain pluripotent stem cells

somatic cells (Takahashi and Yamanaka, 2006). iPSCs hold similar developmental potential to ESCs, and early studies revealed that their gene expression profiles are fairly similar (Mikkelsen et al., 2008). For this reason, and since they can be derived from the somatic cells of an individual, they can be used in the development of personalized therapies for diseases such as Parkinson's, Alzheimer's and heart disease. Studies have begun in which researchers have generated iPSCs using somatic cells from individuals with diseases such as Parkinson's, Down syndrome, Hungtinton's, type 1 diabetes, SMA and ALS as a first step towards developing therapies. Other studies have taken this a step further to correct genetic abnormalities to treat diseases including sickle cell anemia and hemophilia in mouse models.

Although these results are encouraging, more recent examinations have revealed more significant variations in gene expression signatures and epigenetic differences between ESCs and iPSCs particularly in terms of methylation marks (Doi et al., 2009). On the other hand, work from another group of researchers has suggested that the differences between ESCs and iPSCs fall within a reasonable variation range (Bock et al., 2011). Some of these differences also seem to be resolved over time with passaging of iPSCs. Even though this cell type holds promise as an alternative to the use of embryonic stem cells derived from human embryos, these anomalies need to be resolved before they can replace hESCs as the preferred starting point in cell therapy.

For successful reprogramming to occur, the expression of differentiated cell specification factors must be silenced and the pluripotency regulatory circuit must be activated. This is no small feat as changes that need to occur center around global chromatin reorganization. For example, heterochromatin needs to be remodeled to euchromatin, DNA methylation needs to be reversed, poised bivalent chromatin needs to be reestablished, the inactive X chromosome needs to be reactivated and reprogramming trangenes need to be silenced. Studies have shown that this dedifferentiation occurs in a stepwise fashion with epigenetic changes driven by Myc leading the way.

Myc has the capacity to regulate the first steps of successful cellular reprogramming through epigenetic remodeling of cellular chromatin and repression of specification. Indeed, extensive gene expression changes occur upon introduction of Myc alone, and the ability of Myc to recruit chromatin regulators could provide accessibility of the reprogramming factors to cellular targets.

Exogenous Myc is not an absolute requirement for cellular reprogramming, perhaps due to endogenous Myc being present in cycling cells (Smith and Dalton, 2010). Increases in Myc levels during reprogramming would facilitate cell cycle entry and subsequent remodeling of the cell cycle along the dedifferentiation pathway.

MYC in Cancer Stem Cells

Many cancer biologists now agree that tumors arise from 'cancer stem cells' that hold the capacity to regenerate the tumor if differentiated derivatives are eliminated without eradicating the stem cell source (Jordan, 2004). Such cancer stem cells have been identified as the driving force behind cancers of the blood and solid tumors. There remain differences in opinion as to how cancer stem cells arise. For example, are cancer stem cells the result of changes in tissue-specific adult stem cells or are non-stem cells reprogrammed back to a stem-like state? Both scenarios may apply.

Regardless of their origin, cancer stem cells are similar to normal stem cell populations. For instance, cancer stem cells are multipotential and they express an overlapping set of stem cell genes (Ben-Porath et al., 2008). Cancer stem cells also hold the ability to self-renew and potentially constitute a replenishing source of rogue cells that define the tumor. Another commonality is the rarity of such cancer stem cells, which are often found to be a very minor component of tumors (Jordan, 2004). Cancer stem cells can also adopt a dormant state. This, together with their rarity makes it challenging to eradicate them by present chemotherapeutic approaches.

As discussed previously, Myc is important in sustaining normal stem cell populations. Given this property and the connection with cellular transformation, it is not surprising that Myc also has ties with cancer stem cells. Similar to observations made in analyses of somatic cell reprogramming, Myc activation can stimulate a stem cell profile in cancer cells and it is therefore able to facilitate the potent generation of cancer initiating cells. For instance, it promotes the growth and survival of glioma cancer stem cells (Wang et al., 2008) and has also been implicated in the development of liver cancer (Shachaf et al., 2004). Thus, Myc and Myc-stimulated transcriptional modules may be the link between normal stem cell populations, cancer stem cells and the progression of cancer.

Therapy Implications

Pluripotent stem cells are a potential source of differentiated cell types that can be used in the treatment of many diseases and debilitating injuries. The use of embryo-derived stem cells however, faces a number of ethical barriers. While iPSCs could potentially generate patient-specific transplantable cells, such therapies are several years from being translated into a clinical context. Recent studies have sparked a debate on significant differences between ESCs and iPSCS at the epigenetic level that may impact on their differentiation capacity. Other reports have highlighted potential issues relating to their genomic instability. Problems associated with the use of integrating viruses can probably be overcome with small molecular compounds, RNA mediated delivery or by excision of trangenes from the genome using recombinase-based approaches. Besides reprogramming back to a pluripotent state, interest has recently shifted to the direct trans-differentiation of cells. Several reports have described the direct conversion of fibroblasts to functional cardiomyocytes and hematopoietic progenitors without the need to first pass through a pluripotent iPSC-like state. Formation of tumors has long been recognized as a potential problem with transplanted cells originating from pluripotent populations. To prevent this, all undifferentiated cells must be removed for any therapeutic purpose and so drug and mechanical selection seem to be a potential way to circumvent this problem. Safety issues represent a major barrier for clinical development in cell therapy. Myc is unlikely to be part of any therapeutic pathway for reprogramming due to its oncogenic potential- small molecules and miRNAs may be used to substitute for Myc. Despite these barriers, the promise of cell-based therapies, particularly those utilizing pluripotent cells as a starting point, represents a major frontier in biomedical research. Research into pluripotent cells has not only given hope for new therapies, it has acted as an engine to drive basic biological research in a wide range of disciplines.

References

Bao S, Tang F, Li X, Hayashi K, Gillich A, Lao K, Surani MA (2009) Epigenetic reversion of post-implantation epiblast to pluripotent embryonic stem cells. Nature 461:1292–1295

Baudino TA, McKay C, Pendeville-Samain H, Nilsson JA, Maclean KH, White EL, Davis AC, Ihle JN, Cleveland JL (2002) c-Myc is essential for vasculogenesis and angiogenesis during development and tumor progression. Genes Dev 16:2530–2543

Ben-Porath I, Thomson MW, Carey VJ, Ge R, Bell GW, Regev A, Weinberg RA (2008) An embryonic stem cell-like gene expression signature in poorly differentiated aggressive human tumors. Nat Genet 40:499–507

Bock C, Kiskinis E, Verstappen G, Gu H, Boulting G, Smith ZD (2011) Reference maps of human ES and iPS cell variation enable high-throughput characterization of pluripotent cell lines. Cell 144:439–452

Boyer LA, Plath K, Zeitlinger J, Brambrink T, Medeiros LA, Lee TI, Levine SS, Wernig M, Tajonar A, Ray MK, Bell GW, Otte AP, Vidal M, Gifford DK, Young RA, Jaenisch R (2006) Polycomb complexes repress developmental regulators in murine embryonic stem cells. Nature 441:349–353

Brenner C, Deplus R, Didelot C, Loriot A, Vire E, De Smet C, Gutierrez A, Danovi D, Bernard D, Boon T, Pelicci PG, Amati B, Kouzarides T, de Launoit Y, Di Croce L, Fuks F (2005) Myc represses transcription through recruitment of DNA methyltransferase corepressor. EMBO J 24:336–346

Cartwright P, McLean C, Sheppard A, Rivett D, Jones K, Dalton S (2005) LIF/STAT3 controls ES cell self-renewal and pluripotency by a Myc-dependent mechanism. Development 132:885–896

Chang TC, Zeitels LR, Hwang HW, Chivukula RR, Wentzel EA, Dews M, Jung J, Gao P, Dang CV, Beer MA (2009) Lin-28B transactivation is necessary for Myc-mediated let-7 repression and proliferation. Proc Natl Acad Sci 106:3384

Cotterman R, Jin VX, Krig SR, Lemen JM, Wey A, Farnham PJ, Knoepfler PS (2008) N-Myc regulates a widespread euchromatic program in the human genome partially independent of its role as a classical transcription factor. Cancer Res 68:9654–9662

Dang CV (1999) c-Myc target genes involved in cell growth, apoptosis, and metabolism. Mol Cell Biol 19:1

Doi A, Park IH, Wen B, Murakami P, Aryee MJ, Irizarry R, Herb B, Ladd-Acosta C, Rho J, Loewer S (2009) Differential methylation of tissue-and cancer-specific CpG island shores distinguishes human induced pluripotent stem cells, embryonic stem cells and fibroblasts. Nat Genet 41:1350–1353

Fernandez PC, Frank SR, Wang L, Schroeder M, Liu S, Greene J, Cocito A, Amati B (2003) Genomic targets of the human c-Myc protein. Genes Dev 17:1115–1129

Guan K, Nayernia K, Maier LS, Wagner S, Dressel R, Lee JH, Nolte J, Wolf F, Li M, Engel W (2006) Pluripotency of spermatogonial stem cells from adult mouse testis. Nature 440:1199–1203

Hanna J, Markoulaki S, Mitalipova M, Cheng AW, Cassady JP, Staerk J, Carey BW, Lengner CJ, Foreman R, Love J (2009) Metastable pluripotent states in NOD-mouse-derived ESCs. Cell Stem Cell 4:513–524

Humphrey RK, Beattie GM, Lopez AD, Bucay N, King CC, Firpo MT, Rose-John S, Hayek A (2004) Maintenance of pluripotency in human embryonic stem cells is STAT3 independent. Stem Cells 22:522–530

Jordan CT (2004) Cancer stem cell biology: from leukemia to solid tumors. Curr Opin Cell Biol 16:708–712

Judson RL, Babiarz JE, Venere M, Blelloch R (2009) Embryonic stem cell-specific microRNAs promote induced pluripotency. Nat Biotechnol 27:459–461

Kelly DL, Rizzino A (2000) DNA microarray analyses of genes regulated during the differentiation of embryonic stem cells. Mol Reprod Dev 56:113–123

Kim J, Chu J, Shen X, Wang J, and Orkin SH (2008) An extended transcriptional network for pluripotency of embryonic stem cells. Cell 132:1049–1061

Labosky PA, Barlow DP, Hogan BL (1994) Embryonic germ cell lines and their derivation from mouse primordial germ cells. Ciba Found Symp 182:157–168; discussion 168-178

Lin CH, Jackson AL, Guo J, Linsley PS, Eisenman RN (2009a) Myc-regulated microRNAs attenuate embryonic stem cell differentiation. EMBO J 28:3157–3170

Lin CH, Lin CW, Tanaka H, Fero ML, Eisenman RN (2009b) Gene regulation and epigenetic remodeling in murine embryonic stem cells by c-Myc 4:e7839

Malynn BA, de Alboran IM, O'Hagan RC, Bronson R, Davidson L, DePinho RA, Alt FW (2000) N-myc can functionally replace c-myc in murine development, cellular growth, and differentiation. Genes Dev 14:1390–1399

Meshorer E, Misteli T (2006) Chromatin in pluripotent embryonic stem cells and differentiation. Nat Rev Mol Cell Biol 7:540–546

Meyer N, Penn LZ (2008) Reflecting on 25 years with MYC. Nat Rev Cancer 8:976–990

Mikkelsen TS, Hanna J, Zhang X, Ku M, Wernig M, Schorderet P, Bernstein BE, Jaenisch R, Lander ES, Meissner A (2008) Dissecting direct reprogramming through integrative genomic analysis. Nature 454:49–55

Najm FJ, Chenoweth JG, Anderson PD, Nadeau JH, Redline RW, McKay RDG, Tesar PJ (2011) Isolation of epiblast stem cells from preimplantation mouse embryos. Cell Stem Cell 8:318–325

Shachaf CM, Kopelman AM, Arvanitis C, Karlsson Å, Beer S, Mandl S, Bachmann MH, Borowsky AD, Ruebner B, Cardiff RD (2004) MYC inactivation uncovers pluripotent differentiation and tumour dormancy in hepatocellular cancer. Nature 431:1112–1117

Shi YJ, Matson C, Lan F, Iwase S, Baba T, Shi Y (2005) Regulation of LSD1 histone demethylase activity by its associated factors. Mol Cell 19:857–864

Singh AM, Dalton S (2009) The cell cycle and Myc intersect with mechanisms that regulate pluripotency and reprogramming. Cell Stem Cell 5:141–149

Smith K, Dalton S (2010) Myc transcription factors: key regulators behind establishment and maintenance of pluripotency. Regen Med 5:947–959

Smith KN, Singh AM, Dalton S (2010) Myc represses primitive endoderm differentiation in pluripotent stem cells. Cell Stem Cell 7:343–354

Smith KN, Lim JM, Wells L, Dalton S (2011) Myc orchestrates a regulatory network required for the establishment and maintenance of pluripotency. Cell Cycle 10:592–597

Takahashi K, Yamanaka S (2006) Induction of pluripotent stem cells from mouse embryonic and adult fibroblast cultures by defined factors. Cell 126:663–676

Takahashi K, Tanabe K, Ohnuki M, Narita M, Ichisaka T, Tomoda K, Yamanaka S (2007) Induction of pluripotent stem cells from adult human fibroblasts by defined factors. Cell 131:861–872

Tesar PJ, Chenoweth JG, Brook FA, Davies TJ, Evans EP, Mack DL, Gardner RL, McKay R (2007) New cell lines from mouse epiblast share defining features with human embryonic stem cells. Nature (London) 448:196

Wang ZX, Teh CH, Chan CM, Chu C, Rossbach M, Kunarso G, Allapitchay TB, Wong KY, Stanton LW (2008) The transcription factor Zfp281 controls embryonic stem cell pluripotency by direct activation and repression of target genes. Stem Cells 26:2791–2799

Wu S, Cetinkaya C, Munoz-Alonso MJ, von der Lehr N, Bahram F, Beuger V, Eilers M, Leon J, Larsson LG (2003) Myc represses differentiation-induced p21CIP1 expression via Miz-1-dependent interaction with the p21 core promoter. Oncogene 22:351–360

Zhou H, Li W, Zhu S, Joo JY, Do JT, Xiong W, Kim JB, Zhang K, Schöler HR, Ding S (2010) Conversion of mouse epiblast stem cells to an earlier pluripotency state by small molecules. J Biol Chem 285:29676

Part II
Cancer Stem Cells

Chapter 15

Human Thyroid Cancer Stem Cells

Veronica Catalano, Antonina Benfante, Giorgio Stassi, and Matilde Todaro

Abstract Increasing advances in stem cell research have opened new chances for treatment of many types of cancers. The identification of Cancer Stem Cells (CSCs) will provide a better knowledge of the molecular events governing carcinogenesis and the establishment of more accurate diagnostic methods and effective therapies. Parallel to other tumors, it has been demonstrated the presence of CSCs in thyroid cancers. Here, we will discuss the origin of human thyroid cancer stem cells and what is known about the molecular and the cellular aspects of their biology. We will also explore the potential traits of CSCs in thyroid cancer which give hope for the development of new therapeutic approaches in treatment-resistant thyroid cancer.

Keywords Cancer stem cells · Thyroid cancer stem cells · Papillary carcinoma · Follicular carcinoma · Undifferentiated anaplastic thyroid carcinoma · Medullary thyroid Carcinoma

Introduction

Cancers that arise in the thyroid gland are the most common malignancies of endocrine organs and their incidence rates have steadily increased over recent years. Most thyroid cancers originate from thyroid follicular cells. They encompass the most common well-differentiated papillary carcinoma (∼80% of all thyroid cancers) and follicular carcinoma (∼15%), further subdivided into conventional and oncocytic (Hüthle cell) types, as well as poorly differentiated carcinoma (<1%) and anaplastic carcinoma (∼<2%) (Nikiforova and Nikifrov, 2009).

Both papillary (PTC) and follicular (FTC) carcinomas have a good prognosis and the treatment of election is the surgical resection, followed by chemo and/or radioiodotherapy. On the contrary, rare undifferentiated anaplastic thyroid carcinoma (UTC) has a higher aggressive clinical outcome and unfavourable prognosis due to the high invasiveness and insensitivity to radioactive iodine treatment, because it does not express the iodine symporter. Paclitaxel appears to be the only agent with significant clinical systemic activity against UTC. However, it is not capable of improving the lethality of this malignancy, suggesting the need for additional therapeutic innovations.

In addition to those derived from follicular cell differentiation, there exists another group of thyroid tumors derived by parafollicular C cell differentiation. This minority of tumors (5%), referred to as medullary thyroid carcinoma (MTC), has a much lower cure rate than does the "well differentiated" thyroid cancers showing local or distant metastasis in the liver, lung, bone, brain and tumor recurrence after surgery (Zhu et al., 2010).

Recent studies have provided proofs that tumorigenesis is driven by a rare population of abnormal cells, the so called cancer stem cells (CSCs), necessary and sufficient to initiate and sustain tumor growth. Even though these tumor-initiating cells have been identified in various types of solid tumors, among which breast

---

G. Stassi (✉)
Laboratory of Cellular and Molecular Pathophysiology, Department of Surgical and Oncological Sciences, University of Palermo, 90127 Palermo, Italy
e-mail: gstassi@gmail.com

(Al-Hajj et al., 2003) and colon (O'Brien et al., 2007; Ricci-Vitiani et al., 2007) carcinomas, new data underlie the existence of CSCs in thyroid tumors (Todaro et al., 2010). For these reasons, understanding the complexity of stem cells and their malignant CSCs counterpart represents an essential step for the development of more targeted, selective, and individualized treatment regimes for thyroid cancers.

Thyroid Stem Cells

The thyroid gland has been known for a long time for its self-renewal ability; however, only recently the proven presence of adult stem cells has explained its potentiality.

The existence of thyroid stem cell populations within the mature thyroid was first proven by Dumont et al. (1992), since the injection of a minimum number of cells in mouse models led to the growth of thyroid transplants and also foci formation in cloning assays was very inefficient (Dumont et al., 1992). This finding was reinforced when Thomas et al. (2006) detected a subpopulation of adult stem cells expressing the pluripotent marker Oct-4, the endodermal markers Gata-4 and HNF4a, together with the TTF, Pax8, within human goitrous thyroid (Thomas et al., 2006).

Later, this hypothesis was confirmed by Lan et al. (2007), because thyroid stem cells isolated from primary thyroid cultures demonstrated its ability to differentiate into thyroid cells in vitro and grow either as a monolayer or embedded in collagen (Lan et al., 2007). Several sources of stem cells have been described in literature: the progenitor of follicular cells, which originates from the floor of the foregut (endodermal origin); the progenitor of C cells, which arise from the ultimo-branchial bodies (neural crest origin); and a bipotential progenitor of both follicular cells and C cells. These different types of thyroid stem cells could undergo genetic alterations triggering thyroid tumors (Zhang et al., 2006 Gibelli et al., 2009).

The classical multistep tumorigenesis model proposed that thyroid carcinomas are generated by thyrocytes that accumulate multiple genomic damages to their genome, in oncogenes or tumor suppressors, that could promote neoplastic phenotype. According to this hypothesis, thyrocytes could give rise to PTC by *RAS* and *BRAF* mutations or *RET/ PTC* and *Trk* rearrangements and to FTC by point mutations of the *RAS* gene and *PAX8/ PPARγ* rearrangement. In contrast, UTC are derived from differentiated carcinomas by mutations in *p53* gene (Takano et al. 2005; Nikiforova and Nikiforov, 2009) (Fig. 15.1).

The existence of common genomic changes between differentiated carcinomas and anaplastic carcinomas, direct proof of the multistep carcinogenesis hypothesis, was questioned by Tallini et al. (1998) since they found that rearrangement of the *RET* gene is detected only in papillary carcinomas but not in anaplastic carcinomas (Tallini et al., 1998). Moreover, it has been shown that the *PAX8-PPARγ* rearranged gene is limited to follicular tumors and never observed in anaplastic carcinomas (Kroll et al., 2000). Recent studies also revealed that mutations in the *p53* gene, closely related to the aggressiveness of anaplastic variants, have been observed in other types of tumors, even follicular adenomas (Takano et al., 2005).

The above findings lead to raise a question regarding the succession of genomic changes from differentiated thyroid carcinomas to anaplastic thyroid cancer supported by the multi-step thyroid carcinogenesis. So, several studies have proposed a different view of thyroid tumorigenesis, the fetal-stem cell carcinogenesis hypothesis, according to which cancer cells derive from the remnants of fetal thyroid cells with self-renewal capacity, but not from well-differentiated cells. Follicular, papillary and anaplastic carcinomas are believed to be generated, respectively, from the remnants of prothyrocytes, thyroblasts and thyroid stem cells. Genomic changes, including *RET/ PTC* and *PAX8-PPARγ* rearrangements and mutations in *BRAF* gene, should prevent fetal thyroid cells from differentiating and confer proliferation advantages.

Even though Thyroid Stem Cells (TSCs) represent the origin of anaplastic carcinomas, they have the ability to generate thyroblasts and prothyrocytes. When TSCs themselves proliferate, the resulting tumor acts as an undifferentiated carcinoma; otherwise, when TSCs give rise to thyroblasts and prothyrocytes, the proliferating tumors act as differentiated variants (Fig. 15.2).

From a therapeutic point of view, thyroid tumors composed of cells with limited ability of proliferation can be shrunk after surgical dissection, whereas those derived from remnants of fetal thyroid cells have a fatal course because they are likely to grow back as they

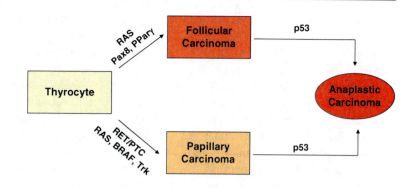

Fig. 15.1 Thyroid cancer multi-step hypothesis. According to the classical multistep carcinogenesis, thyroid carcinomas could generated from normal thyroid follicular cells (thyrocytes) by multiple genomic damages

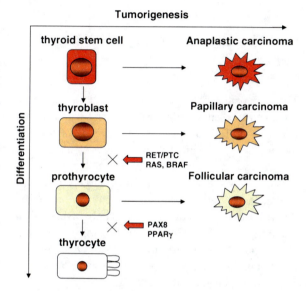

Fig. 15.2 Fetal cell carcinogenesis of thyroid carcinoma. In the novel hypothesis of thyroid carcinogenesis, the cellular target for malignant transformation is the remnants of three types of fetal thyroid cells with self-renewal ability

are characterized by illimited proliferative potential (Takano and Amino, 2005).

Emerging Concepts in Thyroid Carcinogenesis: Thyroid Cancer Stem Cells

The hypothesis that thyroid cancer might be initiated by CSCs with acquired proliferation advantages has been proposed by several authors (Takano and Amino, 2005; Zhang et al., 2006); however, only recently thyroid CSCs (TCSCs) have been identified (Todaro et al., 2010).

The exciting discoveries in thyroid cancer research are focused on stem cell characterization thanks to the identification of suitable markers for TCSCs. Even though CD133 has been suggested as a marker to identify the stem cell-like population within UTC cell lines (Klonisch et al., 2009), Todaro's data pointed that CD133 is not present in the putative stem cell population of epithelial thyroid cancer specimens (Todaro et al., 2010). On the contrary, increased aldehyde dehydrogenase 1 (ALDH1) activity has been associated with primitive cells from breast (Ginestier et al., 2007), pancreatic (Jelski et al., 2007), multiple myeloma (Matsui et al., 2004), acute myeloid leukemia (Pearce et al., 2005), and lung (Ucar et al., 2009) carcinomas.

The presence and the amount of the population with ALDH enzymatic activity in the thyroid gland has been detected following the digestion, by ALDEFLUOR assay that provides an easy and accurate analysis during the cell sorting procedure. The three histological thyroid cancer variants show cells with high ALDH expression with the highest percentage in UTC spheres, maybe correlated with higher malignancy.

A prerequisite of putative CSCs is the ability to grow indefinitely in vitro as tumor spheres and retain the tumorigenic potential upon injection in immunocompromised mice.

Accordingly, the ALDH^{high} population, seeded under nondifferentiating conditions, demonstrates a higher number of clonogenic cells within UTC populations in comparison with normal counterparts, that reveals the self-renewal capability. In order to evaluate whether these cells retain tumor-initiating capacity and recapitulate the clinical and pathological behaviour of parental tumors, including the aggressive features of undifferentiated thyroid carcinomas, ALDH^{high} spheres were isolated from PTC, FTC and

UTC and injected into the thyroid gland of immunocompromised mice.

Animals inoculated with ALDH[high] PTC spheres revealed local tumor growth, whereas those injected with FTC spheres exhibited thyroid gland infiltration and compression of adjacent structures, such as larynx and trachea. Moreover, whole-body in vivo imaging analysis of thyroid tumors generated by ALDH[high] UTC indicated orthotopic tumor growth and a high rate of lung metastasis. In comparison with the corresponding parental tumors, the pattern of ALDH1, CK19, and thyroglobulin expression and the percentage of tumorigenic cells did not change significantly in primary thyroid cancer xenografts, thus suggesting that xenografts derived from thyroid sphere maintain the same hierarchy of thyroid cancer.

The characterization of tumorigenic clones from thyroid cancer has considerable implications: the identification of the specific genetic alterations contributing to tumor growth and invasion but also the creation of orthotopic models of thyroid cancer exploited for development and preclinical validation of novel targeted therapies.

Study of the transcriptional program awarding tumorigenic and metastatic potential of TCSCs population indicated the important relationships between Met/Akt pathway and the invasive behaviour of TCSCs. In particular, Todaro's group demonstrated that the activation of Akt, Met, and β-catenin, together with down-regulation of E-cadherin, confers an aggressive phenotype and a major migratory ability to UTC stem cells. Interestingly, Akt or Met silencing represses Twist and Snail expression, two key transcription factors that characterize epithelial-mesenchymal transition (EMT), abolishing migration and metastatic activity of UTC stem cells.

These promising effects of Akt and Met for the treatment of invasive malignant thyroid cancers have been confirmed with in vivo results. UTC sphere cells transduced with ShMet or ShAkt were allowed to orthotopically grow into mouse thyroid gland. The bioluminescence analysis detected by Photon imaging system revealed that both ShMet and ShAkt determined the complete abrogation of the metastatic potential of TCSCs (Todaro et al., 2010).

Many other research groups are committed to understand how the aberrant activation of PI3K/Akt signaling pathways could contribute to the onset and/or progression of thyroid cancer and investigate the therapeutic potential of inhibiting their oncogenic activity. Liu et al. (2009) show that the Akt-specific inhibitor (perifosine) blocks proliferation and induces apoptosis in thyroid cancer cells characterized by PI3K/Akt-activating genetic alterations sparing those harbouring no mutations. Temsirolimus, the inhibitor of mTOR, a serine-threonine protein kinase involved in the regulation of thyrocyte proliferation, determines the same effects providing access to Akt and mTOR inhibitors as effective therapeutic strategies (Liu et al., 2009).

New Therapeutic Strategies for Thyroid Cancers

The therapeutic procedures for thyroid cancers have remained the same in the last 20 years: patients with papillary or follicular carcinomas receive a dose of radioactive iodine after their surgery in an attempt to destroy any remaining thyroid cells except the advanced thyroid variants in which surgery resection is unable to eradicate tumor. In contrast, anaplastic thyroid carcinoma has a higher aggressive clinical outcome and unfavorable prognosis, as it is characterized by rapid growth, local invasion and resistance to radioiodine or chemotherapeutic treatment lacking of radioiodine uptake (Todaro et al., 2010).

The increasing knowledge of the pathogenesis of thyroid tumors may contribute to an improved management of the treatment-resistant thyroid variants. It has been previously reported that in thyroid cancer resistance to death ligand- and chemotherapy-induced cell death correlates with autocrine production of interleukin (IL)-4 and IL-10, through the up-regulation of anti-apoptotic molecules such as cFLIP, Bcl-xL and PED (Stassi et al., 2003; Todaro et al., 2006). Next, it has been demonstrated that in UTC, the propagation of the survival signalling and the related refractoriness to death is likely to depend on impaired expression of suppressors cytokine signalling (SOCS) molecules that control the expression levels of Bcl-2 family members through Akt down-modulation. Exogenous expression of SOCS-3 and SOCS-5 genes reduces tumor growth and potently enhances the efficacy of chemotherapy both in vitro and in vivo by altering the balance of pro-apoptotic and anti-apoptotic molecules. These results indicated that SOCS regulation of cytokine-prosurvival programs might be a new strategy to overcome the resistance to chemotherapy in the most aggressive variant of thyroid cancer (Francipane et al., 2009).

TCSCs represents an exciting area of research bringing with it important implications both for the diagnosis and for the treatment of thyroid cancer. Given that CSCs have unlimited proliferative potential (attributed to unlimited self-renewal capacity and multi linage differentiation), the challenge will be to render them the primary target for chemotherapy. Current anti-thyroid therapies, such as surgery, chemotherapy, and radiation, rapidly kill growing differentiated thyroid tumor cells but spare quiescent cancer initiating cells. An ideal treatment regime should kill differentiated cancer cells, and at the same time, TCSCs opposing their mutagenic potential (Fig. 15.3).

Although the idea of drugs targeting CSCs may look exciting, it is not easy. CSCs have been widely described to evade death signals induced by therapeutic drugs through the evolvement of multiple mechanisms including up-regulation of ATP-binding cassette (ABC) transporters, active DNA-repair capacity and over-expression of anti-apoptotic molecules. In this context, the identification of thyroid cancer-initiating cells provide powerful tools for a better understanding of specific gene and signaling transduction pathways involved in stem cell renewal and chemoresistance of CSCs, such as the Wnt/β-catenin pathway. In anaplastic thyroid cancers deregulation of this pathway appears to be associated with antineoplastic effects of the selective tyrosine kinase inhibitor imatinib mesylate (gleevec) which it is not effective as monotherapy, despite it is able to target β-catenin and reduce invasiveness and proliferation of thyroid cancer cells (Klonisch et al., 2009).

Several agents have been studied and have been promising at least in the experimental systems.

They include specific tyrosinkinase inhibitors, e.g. the pyrozolopyrimided PP2 for RET/PTC or RET signalling (Carlomagno et al., 2003) and imatinib for Wnt/β-catenin signalling (Rao et al., 2005) as well as thiazolididione for stimulation of PPARγ signalling (Park et al., 2005; Martelli et al., 2002). In the next future, the challenge will be to develop novel specific inhibitors able to antagonize signal activation through the most recently identified thyroid oncogenes *BRAF* in papillary thyroid cancers and PI3K in anaplastic thyroid cancers (Fagin, 2004; Garcia-Rostan et al., 2005). In the management of aggressive MTCs, recent data demonstrate the therapeutic efficacy of specific agents against RET and FGF receptors to inhibit tumor growth in vitro and in vivo, suggesting the combined genetic and pharmacologic approaches as effective forms of therapy (Zhu et al., 2010).

Future Directions

The studies reviewed here highlight recent novel findings on TCSCs which emphasize future challenges in thyroid cancer therapy. An extensive characterization of tumor-initiating cells may allow to study their potential role in tumorigenesis and how they are involved in the resistance to current anticancer therapies. Moreover, these cells can be used for the creation

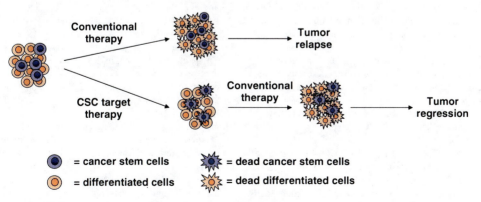

Fig. 15.3 Clinical implications of CSCs. The CSC hypothesis suggests that a small population of tumorigenic CSCs have escaped the normal limits of self-renewal giving rise to abnormally differentiated cancer cells that contribute to tumor growth and progression. Since CSCs are more resistant to conventional chemotherapy, it is important to use targeted therapies in order to cure cancer

of animal model systems useful to elucidate in vivo molecular occurrences that mediate thyroid carcinogenesis and fully understand the strengths and limitations of new individualized treatment regiments, especially against the invasive malignant thyroid cancers.

References

Al-Hajj M, Wicha MS, Benito-Hernandez A, Morrison SJ, Clarke MF (2003) Prospective identification of tumorigenic breast cancer cells. Proc Natl Acad Sci USA 100: 3983–3988

Carlomagno F, Vitagliano D, Guida T, Basolo F, Castellone MD, Melillo RM, Fusco A, Santoro M (2003) Efficient inhibition of RET/papillary thyroid carcinoma oncogenic kinases by 4-amino-5-(4-chloro-phenyl)-7-(t-butyl)pyrazolo[3,4-d]pyrimidine (PP2). J Clin Endocrinol Metab 88:1897–1902

Dumont JE, Lamy F, Roger P, Maenhaut C (1992) Physiological and pathological regulation of thyroid cell proliferation and differentiation by thyrotropin and other factors. Physiol Rev 72:667–697

Fagin JA (2004) Challenging dogma in thyroid cancer molecular geneticsole of RET/PTC and BRAF in tumor initiation. J Clin Endocrinol Metab 89:4264–4266

Francipane MG, Eterno V, Spina V, Bini M, Scerrino G, Buscemi G, Gulotta G, Todaro M, Dieli F, De Maria R, Stassi G (2009) Suppressor of cytokine signaling 3 sensitizes anaplastic thyroid cancer to standard chemotherapy. Cancer Res 69:6141–6148

Garcia-Rostan G, Costa AM, Pereira-Castro I, Salvatore G, Hernandez R, Hermsem MJ, Herrero A, Fusco A, Cameselle-Teijeiro J, Santoro M (2005) Mutation of the PIK3CA gene in anaplastic thyroid cancer. Cancer Res 65:10199–10207

Gibelli B, El-Fattahi AMA, Giugliano G, Proh M, Grosso E (2009) Thyroid stem cells – anger or resource? Acta Otorhinolaryngol Ital 29:290–295

Ginestier C, Hur MH, Charafe-Jauffret E, Monville F, Dutcher J, Brown M, Jacquemier J, Viens P, Kleer CG, Liu S, Schott A, Hayes D, Birnbaum D, Wicha MS, Dontu G (2007) ALDH1 is a marker of normal and malignant human mammary stem cells and a predictor of poor clinical outcome. Cell Stem Cell 1:555–567

Jelski W, Chrostek L, Szmitkowski M (2007) The activity of class I, II, III, IV of alcohol dehydrogenase isoenzymes and aldehyde dehydrogenase in pancreatic cancer. Pancreas 35:142–146

Klonisch T, Hoang-Vu C Hombach-Klonisch S (2009) Thyroid tem ells and ancer. Thyroid 19:1303–1315

Kroll TG, Sarraf P, Pecciarini L, Chen CJ, Mueller E, Spiegelman BM, Fletcher JA (2000) PAX8–PPARgamma1 fusion oncogene in human thyroid carcinoma. Science 289:1357–1360

Lan L, Cui D, Nowka K Derwahl M (2007) Stem cells derived from goiters in adults form spheres in response to intense growth stimulation and require TSH for differentiation into thyrocytes. J Clin Endocrinol Metab 92: 3681–3688

Liu D, Hou P, Liu Z, Wu G, Xing M (2009) Genetic alterations in the phosphoinositide 3-kinase/Akt signaling pathway confer sensitivity of thyroid cancer cells to therapeutic targeting of Akt and mammalian target of rapamycin. Cancer Res 69:7311–7319

Martelli ML, Iuliano R, Le Pera I, Sama I, Monaco C, Cammarota S, Kroll T, Chiariotti L, Santoro M, Fusco A (2002) Inhibitory effects of peroxisome poliferator-activated receptor gamma on thyroid carcinoma cell growth. J Clin Endocrinol Metab 7:4728–4735

Matsui W, Huff CA, Wang Q, Malehorn MT, Barber J, Tanhehco Y, Smith BD, Civin CI, Jones RJ (2004) Characterization of clonogenic multiple myeloma cells. Blood 103:2332–2336

Nikiforova M Nikiforov YE (2009) Molecular iagnostics and redictors in hyroid ancer. Thyroid 19:1351–1361

O'Brien CA, Pollet A, Gallinger S, Dick JE. 2007. A human colon cancer capable of initiating tumour growth in immunodeficient mice. Nature 445:106–110

Park JW, Zarnegar R, Kanauchi H, Wong MG, Hyun WC, Ginzinger DG, Lobo M, Cotter P, Duh QY, Clark OH (2005) Troglitazone, the peroxisome proliferator-activated receptor gamma agonist, induces antiproliferation and redifferentiation in human thyroid cancer cell lines. Thyroid 15: 222–231

Pearce DJ, Taussig D, Simpson C, Allen K, Rohatiner AZ, Lister TA, Bonnet D (2005) Characterization of cells with a high aldehyde dehydrogenase activity from cord blood and acute myeloid leukemia samples. Stem Cells 23:752–760

Rao AS, Kremenevskaja N, von Wasielewski R, Jakubcakova V, Kant S, Resch J, Brabant G (2005) Wnt/{beta}-catenin signalling mediates anti-neoplastic effects of Imatinib mesylate (Glivec) in anaplastic thyroid cancer. J Clin Endocrinol Metab 91:159–168

Ricci-Vitiani L, Lombardi DG, Pilozzi E, Biffoni M, Todaro M, Peschle C, De Maria R. 2007. Identification and expansion of human colon-cancer-initiating cells. Nature 445:111–115

Stassi G, Todaro M, Zerilli M, Ricci-Vitiani L, Di Liberto D, Patti M, Florena A, Di Liberto D, Patti M, Florena A, Di Gaudio F, Di Gesù G, De Maria R (2003) Thyroid cancer resistance to chemotherapeutic drugs via autocrine production of interleukin-4 and interleukin-10. Cancer Res 63:6784–6790

Takano T Amino N (2005) Fetal Cell Carcinogenesis. A New Hypothesis for Better Understanding of Thyroid Carcinoma. Thyroid 15:432–438

Tallini G, Santoro M, Helie M, Carlomagno F, Salvatore G, Chiappetta G, Carcangiu ML, Fusco A (1998) RET/PTC oncogene activation defines a subset of papillary thyroid carcinomas lacking evidence of progression to poorly differentiated or undifferentiated tumor phenotypes. Clin Cancer Res 4:287–294

Thomas T, Nowka K, Lan L, Derwahl M (2006) Expression of endoderm stem cell markers: evidence for the presence of adult stem cells in human thyroid glands. Thyroid 16: 537–544

Todaro M, Zerilli M, Ricci-Vitiani L, Bini M, Perez Alea M, Maria Florena A, Miceli L, Condorelli G, Bonventre S, Di Gesù G, De Maria R, Stassi G (2006) Autocrine production of interleukin-4 and interleukin-10 is required for survival and growth of thyroid cancer cells. Cancer Res 66:1491–1499

Todaro M, Iovino F, Eterno V, Cammareri P, Gambara G, Espina V, Gulotta G, Dieli F, Giordano S, De Maria R Stassi G (2010) Tumorigenic and etastatic ctivity of uman hyroid ancer tem ells. Cancer Res 70:8874–8885

Ucar D, Cogle CR, Zucali JR, Ostmark B, Scott EW, Zori R, Gray BA, Moreb JS (2009) Aldehyde dehydrogenase activity as a functional marker for lung cancer. Chem Biol Interact 178:48–55

Zhang P, Zuo H, Ozaki T, Nakagomi N, Kakudo K (2006) Cancer stem cell hypothesis in thyroid cancer. Pathol Int 56:485–489

Zhu W, Hai T, Ye L, Cote GJ (2010) Medullary thyroid carcinoma cell lines contain a self-renewing CD133+ population that is dependent on ret proto-oncogene activity. J Clin Endocrinol Metab 95:439–444

Chapter 16
Tumor Stem Cells: CD133 Gene Regulation and Tumor Stemness

Kouichi Tabu, Tetsuya Taga, and Shinya Tanaka

Abstract Tumors are composed of diverse types of cells that exhibit distinct morphologies and biological phenotypes; these characteristics are significantly relevant to therapeutic effects of tumors. Although tumor heterogeneity has been classically explained by the stochastic clonal evolution model, recent evidence has revived an alternative tumor stem cell (TSC) hierarchy model, which hypothesizes that tumors contain a rare subset of stem-like cells that can differentiate into multiple lineages for the architecture of tumors. TSCs are highly tumorigenic, metastatic, chemo/radiation-resistant, and are characterized by elevated expression of cell surface antigen CD133 in many, if not all, human neoplasms. CD133 expression is regulated by several extrinsic factors, including TGF-β or environmental conditions (e.g., hypoxia), and possibly via Ras/ERK-dependent signaling pathways through alternative promoters, which suggests multi-directional regulation of TSC features and tumor stemness. A comprehensive understanding of molecular and cellular networks that govern CD133-expressing tumor cells could help to elucidate TSC stemness and contribute to the development of more effective cancer therapies.

Keywords Tumor stem cell · Tumor hierarchy · Promoter · DNA methylation · Transcription · Signal transduction

Introduction

Over the past several decades, it has been suggested that tumor tissues are heterogeneous and are composed of multiple subpopulations of cells that differ in morphology, proliferation rate, metastatic potential, marker expression, and sensitivity to chemo/radiation therapies. Tumor heterogeneity has been classically explained by the "stochastic (or clonal evolution) model," which suggests that tumor cells asynchronously acquire genetic mutations that allow for subsequent selection of more aggressive clones. However, the alternative "tumor stem cell (TSC) (or hierarchy) model" was recently revived, which suggests that, similar to normal tissues, rare stem cell populations can proliferate and differentiate into various lineages, which contribute to architectural organization of tumors (Jordan et al., 2006).

Since the 1970s, a large number of studies, which focused on direct introduction of viral oncogenes and mutated genes isolated from patient tumors, demonstrated that normal cells are susceptible to genetic mutations, thereby leading to neoplastic transformation for tumor initiation and expansion. In addition, many tumors retain features of surrounding differentiated epithelium, suggesting that oncogenic gene mutations occur in terminally differentiated cells. However, there remains some controversies concerning the origin of tumor cells. For example, malignant tumors histologically contain a certain degree of undifferentiated components. However, cell differentiation has been regarded as a unidirectional process under normal physiological conditions, and nuclear reprogramming was only recently described following successful nuclear transfer, ES cell-fusion, or the establishment

K. Tabu (✉)
Department of Stem Cell Regulation, Medical Research Institute, Tokyo Medical and Dental University, 1-5-45, Yushima, Bunkyo-ku, Tokyo 113-8510, Japan
e-mail: k-tabu.scr@mri.tmd.ac.jp

of induced pluripotent stem (iPS) cells (Yamanaka and Blau, 2010). In addition, terminally differentiated cells do not normally proliferate in vivo, and therefore the possibility that quiescent cells can acquire oncogenic gene mutations remains low, although the cells often undergo spontaneous immortalization in vitro and proliferate infinitely as cell lines.

TSC presence in many, if not all, solid tumors is supported by numerous studies, and the TSC theory helps to explain the controversies surrounding tumor initiation and heterogeneity. This review summarizes the basic TSC concepts and the characteristics of the TSC marker CD133 gene, as well as potential therapeutic approaches within the framework of the CD133 regulatory pathway.

Concepts of Tumor Stem Cells

The TSC model is not a new concept. Indeed, in the 1970s, efforts were made to gain insight into the potential of tumor malignancy through the use of specimens from patients with myeloma and ovarian cancer. Technological advances in flow cytometry, as well as the discovery of stem cell surface antigens, accelerated research in this field, starting with human leukemia and the subsequent identification of breast and brain tumors (Jordan et al., 2006).

The 2006 AACR Workshop on Cancer Stem Cells defined TSCs as "a small subset of malignant cells that constitute a pool of self-sustaining cells with the exclusive ability to maintain the tumor" (Clarke et al., 2006). TSCs share fundamental properties with normal stem cells specific to their original organs; e.g., brain tumor and neural stem cells. Normal stem cells are capable of continuously replenishing normal tissues throughout life in certain organs, and stem cells are characterized by two main hallmarks — multipotential and self-renewal. Multipotential stem cells can produce multiple types of functional progenies, and the differentiation into these cell types is often associated with growth-arrest. Self-renewing stem cells can produce new stem cells, which are identical to the original cells and retain the two main hallmarks, thereby maintaining the stem cell pool. Likewise, tumors are organized into a hierarchy, where rare TSCs are at the top of pyramid and exhibit extensive potential for proliferation and self-renewal, as well as the homeostasis maintenance of the tumor bulk. However, TSCs proliferate and self-renew in a disorderly fashion, which results in increased cell numbers.

The current gold standard assay for testing whether a cell population fulfills the definition of a TSC (self-renewal and tumor propagation) is the orthotopic xenograft experiment; cells are transplanted at limiting dilutions into NOD/Shi-scid/IL2Rγ-null (NOG) mice, and the frequency of cancer stem cells is determined. In particular, serial transplantation into NOG mice is regarded as the best functional assay for testing long-term, self-renewal capacity.

The TSC model has important implications for clinical treatment of tumors, because some features of TSCs make them particularly difficult to eliminate. TSCs reside in a relatively quiescent cell cycle state referred to as a state of "dormancy," which allows them to evade typical chemotherapeutic agents that actively target proliferating cells. Many studies have attempted to kill tumor cells independently of the cell cycle, or to selectively induce the tumor cells enter the cell cycle. In addition, TSCs express high levels of multi-drug resistant proteins and transporters associated with detoxification, which consequently confers multidrug resistance by expelling chemotherapeutic reagents. Moreover, TSCs are frequently resistant to standard radiotherapy regimens, because of elevated expression of reactive oxygen species (ROS) scavenging (Haraguchi et al., 2010) and DNA damage response genes (Bao et al., 2006). Interestingly, conventional chemo/radiotherapy results in an increased proportion of TSCs and a rapid relapse of the original tumor. It is imperative that future studies establish an effective therapeutic approach for enhancing sensitivity to chemotherapeutic drugs and radiation in TSCs.

Detection of Tumor Stem Cells

TSCs have been isolated from tumor tissues and cell lines through the use of diverse experimental techniques. Based on the functional properties of stem cells, two methods using fluorescence-activated cell sorting (FACS) have contributed to TSC selection; the Hoechst 33342 dye effluxing side population (SP) technique and ALDEFLUOR to measure aldehyde dehydrogenase (ALDH) activity. Hoechst 33342 is a fluorescent dye that binds to AT-rich regions of DNA and accumulates in most cells. However, stem cells express high levels of ABC transporter family genes, which result in dye efflux. For example, human fetal neural stem/progenitor cells express high levels of multidrug resistance 1 (MDR1, also known as ABCB1, P-gp) and ATP-binding cassette sub-family G member 2 (ABCG2, also known as Bcrp), which are downregulated during differentiation (Islam et al., 2005). These transporters exhibit important roles in active efflux of xenobiotics from normal cell bodies, thereby protecting cells from cytotoxic agents. Cells with the ability to efflux dye were initially identified in mouse bone marrow (Goodell et al., 1996). Following staining with Hoechst 33342 dye and exposure to a UV laser during FACS, a population of cells that displays decreased red and blue fluorescence is sorted from the other cells. This population is referred to as side population (SP) cells, because it appears as a "side" relative to the positively stained "main" population in the FACS plots. Since this discovery (Goodell et al., 1996), the SP technique has been utilized to enrich putative stem cells and progenitors from a number of normal tissues and malignant tumors. SP cells preferentially express high levels of stemness genes and are capable of differentiating into multiple lineages. Therefore, these cells are considered to function as stem cells in original tissues and tumors.

ALDH activity measurements have been more recently utilized for isolation of putative TSCs. The ALDH enzyme oxidizes intracellular aldehydes, and several isoforms of the ALDH family have been identified in humans, although ALDH1 is the primary isoform isolated from human hematopoietic progenitors. Recent studies have shown that human and murine hematopoietic progenitors can be isolated using BODIPY-aminoacetaldehyde (BAAA, commercially available as ALDEFLUOR), which is a fluorescent-labeled substrate specific for ALDH activity (Ginestier et al., 2007). ALDH1 has a role in early differentiation of hematopoietic stem cells (HSCs) by converting retinol to retinoic acid. Increased ALDH activity has also been detected in normal neural stem cells and TSCs in several malignant tumors.

Alternatively, potential TSCs can be identified by a variety of cell surface markers or the combination of these markers; e.g., CD34+/CD38 for AML, CD44+/CD24(−/low) for breast tumor, and CD133+ for brain tumor (Jordan et al., 2006). However, these methods, which are based on surface molecules, have increased some contradictions. For instance, different stem cell markers identify distinct subpopulations of cells in one tumor, and in melanoma, at least four subpopulations (CD20+, CD133+, label-retaining slow-cycling cells, and SP cells) have been separately identified, all of which exhibit stem cell features (Zabierowski and Herlyn, 2008). The diversity of TSC markers suggests that a cell population isolated by specific surface molecules could remain heterogeneous, and that complete TSC enrichment is not successfully achieved in some tumor types. In addition, TSC frequency is highly variable, even within the same type of tumors. In colon cancer, the frequency of tumor-initiating cells in NOD/SCID mice represents a broad range from 1.8 to 24.5% (O'Brien et al., 2007), demonstrating the need for more refined markers (or combinations), as well as assay systems. Nevertheless, it is evident that surface markers and the involved mechanisms are important keys for a better understanding of the regulatory pathways that maintain tumor stemness.

The significance of CD133 as a TSC marker, as well as a predictor of patient prognosis, has become important in various human neoplasms, and CD133 expression is still utilized as a marker of high-efficiency enrichment of TSCs. Indeed, in many studies of human brain tumors, TSCs have been isolated by elevated expression of CD133 and the CD133+ subpopulation exhibits a greater ability to regenerate original tumors in immunodeficient mice compared with other cell populations. CD133 could, therefore, provide important clues for the establishment of therapeutic targets against TSCs in certain types of human neoplasms.

CD133 Gene Structure

CD133 (also called AC133, PROM1, or PROML1) is one of the two members of the pentaspan transmembrane glycoprotein prominin family. In 1997, mouse Prominin-1 was isolated as a protein selectively localized at the apical surface of murine neuroepithelial stem cells and was named for its "prominent" location on cell membrane protrusions. CD133 was detected the same year by a monoclonal antibody (AC133) and was identified as an antigen expressed at the cell surface of HSCs from human fetal liver, bone marrow, and cord blood. CD133 is the human homologue of mouse prominin-1, which was confirmed by cloning of cDNA encoding AC133 antigen.

The CD133 gene is located on chromosome 4p15.32 in the human (Entrez Gene ID: 8842) and 5B3 in the mouse (Entrez Gene ID: 19126); the gene spans approximately 160 kb. CD133 genes have similar genomic structures (e.g., exon/intron boundaries) between species and are composed of at least 37 exons in the human and 34 exons in the mouse. The human CD133 protein contains five transmembrane regions and two extracellular loops with eight glycosylated sites, and has a total molecular weight of 97–120 kDa. A human AC133 isoform of 856-amino acid (aa), which lacks exon 3 of 27 nucleotides, is referred to as ACC133-2 (CD133s1), while the 865-aa longer isoform is named AC133-1 (CD133s2). Although the function of CD133 remains unclear, CD133s1 expression is predominant in a variety of human fetal tissue, adult tissues, and several tumors. In contrast, CD133s2 mRNA is more prominent in fetal brain and adult skeletal muscle, but not in fetal liver and kidney, adult pancreas, kidney, and placenta, suggesting different roles for the two isoforms in fetal development and adult tissue homeostasis.

The transcript size of CD133 is approximately 4.4 kb. In 2004, at least 10 exons from exon 1 (Exon 1A, B, C, D1, D2, D3, E1, E2, E3, and E4) were found to be transcribed within the 5′-untranslated region (UTR) of the human CD133 gene (Shmelkov et al., 2004). Analysis using different tissues and cell lines revealed that at least seven CD133 transcripts with alternative exon 1s are driven by five alternative promoters (P1, P2, P3, P4, and P5). In addition, all CD133 promoters are TATA-less, and three of them (P1, P2, and P3) are located within a cytosine-guanine rich DNA region (CpG island). Expression of 5′-UTR CD133 isoforms exhibits tissue-dependent patterns; liver, kidney, pancreas, placenta, lung, spleen, and colon express exon 1A- and exon 1B-containing transcripts; brain, ovary, and fetal liver express only the exon 1A-containing transcript; and prostate and small intestine express only the exon 1B-containing transcript. Exon 1D is detected only in the testis, and Exon 1A, 1B, or 1D isoforms have not been detected in heart, skeletal muscle, thymus, or bone marrow. In addition, exon 1C and exon 1E isoforms were not detected in any examined tissues of the Schmelkov et al. study. Our group recently showed that CD133 expression levels correlate with glioma WHO grading and that malignant gliomas predominantly express exon 1A, 1B, and 1C isoforms (Tabu et al., 2008). In addition, at least three novel exon 1s, designated as exon 1C2, 1D4, and 1E5, and at least five elongated forms of known exon 1s, were discovered, all of which conform to the GT-AG exon-intron consensus rule. All splicing patterns of CD133 transcripts are summarized in Fig. 16.1.

DNA Methylation

To date, DNA methylation, RTKs/Ras/ERK signaling, and hypoxic environments are considered the major regulators of the human CD133 gene, as shown in Fig. 16.2. Human CD133 promoters P1, P2, and P3 have 54 CpG sites at the high percentage (50%, 68%, and 69%, respectively). Abnormal DNA hypomethylation status of the CpG islands in the P1-P3 promoter positively correlates with increased CD133 expression in multiple types of TSCs, including colorectal, ovarian, gastric, neuroblastoma, and glial tumors. DNA methylation is an important component of gene expression in numerous cellular processes, including embryonic development, genomic imprinting, X-chromosome inactivation, and preservation of chromosome stability, and is directly regulated by DNA methyltransferases (DNMTs) possessing de novo DNA methylation activity. Genomic hypomethylation contributes to tumorigenesis by inducing oncogene activation and/or genomic instability. For instance, DNMT1 hypomorphic mice exhibiting genomic hypomethylation develop aggressive T-cell lymphoma, and the tumors typically display increased chromosome instability (Gaudet et al., 2003). Similarly, global hypomethylation, via induction of a hypomorphic DNMT1 allele, accelerates onset of sarcoma formation in Nf1$^{+/-}$p53$^{+/-}$mice (Eden et al., 2003). These studies demonstrated that DNA hypomethylation could initiate tumorigenesis. Therefore, genomic hypomethylation might be associated with the development and/or maintenance of TSCs, as well as CD133 gene expression.

Interestingly, via inhibition of DNMT1 and DNMT3b expression, TGF-β/Smad2/3/4 signaling induces DNA demethylation of the CD133 P1 promoter and its expression (You et al., 2010). TGF-β has recently been identified as a candidate extracellular signal in the regulation of HSC hibernation in bone marrow (Yamazaki et al., 2009), and bone morphogenetic proteins (BMPs), which belong to a subset of the TGF-β superfamily, maintain self-renewal and

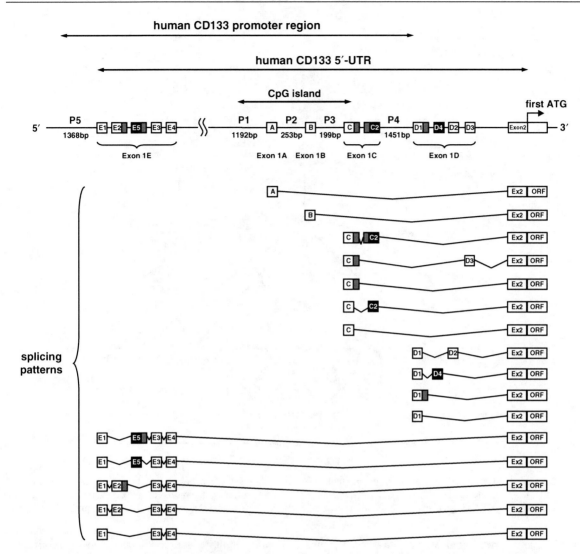

Fig. 16.1 Structure of the human CD133 gene and its various splicing patterns of 5′-UTR. Closed boxes and gray boxes represent novel exon 1s and elongation of known exon 1s, respectively, which were discovered in a human glioma species (Tabu et al., 2008). The CD133 gene possesses five promoters (P5, P1 through P4, in this order), yielding different spliced transcripts with five alternated first exons (Exon 1A to 1E). A CpG island resides in the P1 through P3 promoter region

multi-lineage differentiation potential of neural stem cells within the subventricular zone (SVZ) of the adult brain. TGF-β has been proposed to play important roles in TSC maintenance; TGF-β confers stem cell-like properties and tumorigenic activity through induction of epithelial-mesenchymal transition (EMT) in human mammary epithelial cells (HMECs) (Mani et al., 2008). Moreover, a recent study provided evidence that TGF-β signals are crucial for maintenance of self-renewal and tumorigenicity in glioma cells. In addition, the TGF-β receptor I inhibitor SB431542 significantly decreases CD133+/Nestin+ population sizes and decreases sphere-forming activity, self-renewal, and in vivo tumorigenic potential via Sox4 down-regulation (Ikushima et al., 2009). The efficacy and safety of trabedersen (AP 12009), a TGFβ2-specific antisense oligonucleotide, have been successfully evaluated in high-grade glioma patients in clinical Phase I/II/IIb studies, as well as ongoing Phase I/II studies for patients with pancreatic carcinoma and malignant melanoma (Schlingensiepen et al., 2008). The combination of TGF-β inhibitors with

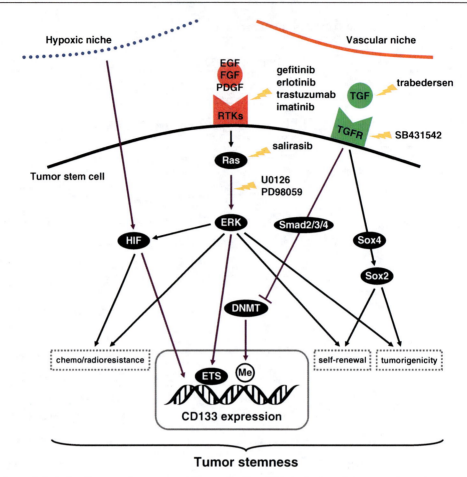

Fig. 16.2 Intracellular signaling regulates tumor stemness. TGF and RTKs/Ras/ERK signals and hypoxic environment are major regulators of CD133 gene expression (purple arrows). In addition, these pathways regulate other stem cell features, such as self-renewal, tumorigenicity, and chemo/radioresistance. Possible inhibitors for disruption of tumor stemness are denoted

conventional pharmacological and radiation therapies could be a promising approach for eliminating a specific stem cell population. Further studies focused on the regulatory mechanisms underlying CD133 hypomethylation could promote the development of chemotherapeutic agents.

Previous studies have utilized demethylating drugs, such as decitabine (also known as 5-aza-2′deoxycytidine) and 5-azacytidine (5-AC), as anti-cancer agents. Actually, differentiated cells are predisposed to malignant transformation by silencing of tumor suppressor genes through promoter hypermethylation. However, treatment with 5-AC restores CD133 gene transcription (Tabu et al., 2008). Interestingly, ESCs from Dnmt1-deficient mice or Dnmt3a/Dnmt3b double-knockout mice proliferate as undifferentiated stem cells, which suggests that self-renewal is preserved in ESCs with hypomethylated genomes (Tsumura et al., 2006). In addition, the mutant ESCs fail to undergo differentiation in vitro, possibly due to a failure to repress pluripotent-related genes, such as Oct4 and Nanog. DNA methylation might result in the opposite effect on the differentiation and self-renewal of stem cells. Therefore, it is possible that demethylating drugs might be effective in a major population of differentiated tumor cells, but not in a rare population of TSCs. The treatment of tumor cells with conventional therapy, followed by selective DNA methylation of stemness genes, could suppress growth of the remaining TSCs.

RTKs/Ras/ERK Signaling Pathway

Although transcriptional machinery of the human CD133 gene remains poorly understood, our group recently characterized a CD133 promoter region to determine the molecular basis of human tumor stemness. Our results revealed the Ras/ERK/ETS pathway as a regulator of CD133 transcription via two E26 transformation-specific (ETS) binding sites (Tabu et al., 2010). The ETS family of transcriptional factors comprises over 35 members, and some are nuclear targets of the receptor tyrosine kinases (RTKs)/Ras/Raf/MEK/ERK signaling pathway, which is involved in various biological processes, including cell proliferation, apoptosis, differentiation, hematopoiesis, tissue remodeling, angiogenesis, metastasis, and oncogenic transformation. Ras mutations have been observed in 45% of colon carcinomas and 90% of pancreatic cancers, and Raf mutations has been found in two-third of melanomas. Inhibition of the ERK pathway through the use of U0126 (a potent and specific inhibitor of MEK1/2) results in downregulated CD133 expression and decreased SP size (Tabu et al., 2010). In addition, studies have shown that the Ras/ERK pathway is directly relevant to stem cell regulation. Undifferentiated human embryonic stem cells (hESCs) require basic fibroblast growth factor (FGF-2), which transmits signals via the Ras/ERK pathway. ERK is activated in undifferentiated hESCs, and U0126 treatment results in extensive cell death and differentiation (Armstrong et al., 2006). In addition, sophisticated mouse tumor models, triggered by oncogenic Ras, have demonstrated the contribution of the Ras/ERK pathway in the acquisition of tumor stem cell properties in primary HMECs (Morel et al., 2008). H-RasV12 also induces p53-knockout mouse-derived astrocyte transformation into brain tumor stem cells, and the MEK/ERK pathway is responsible for neurosphere formation (Lee et al., 2008). Our study also confirmed that transduction of the oncogenic Ras gene (RasV12) into immortalized normal human astrocytes induces CD133 gene expression, as well as sphere-forming activity, self-renewal, and in vivo tumor formation (Tabu et al., 2010). Importantly, expression of MDR1 and ABCG2 genes is regulated by the same ERK signaling, both of which are cell surface transporters causing multiple drug resistance in tumor cells. MDR1 and ABCG2 genes also exhibit high-affinity with various anti-neoplastic agents, such as doxorubicin, etoposide, vincristine, paclitaxel, imatinib, and mitoxantrone, and subsequently extrude them from the cell body. In addition, Ras can also control radioresistance in some normal and malignant cells, and its inhibition results in radiosensitization of tumor cells that expressed activated Ras. Moreover, Ras plays a central role in multiple downstream stem cell features, including CD133 expression and chemo/radioresistance. Salirasib (S-trans, trans-farnesylthiosalicylic acid) has been shown to disrupt Ras membrane anchoring and is currently in Phase I/II clinical trials; the combination with the standard drug gemcitabine results in longer survival expectancy for patients with pancreatic cancer (Bustinza-Linares et al., 2010). In addition, gefitinib (Iressa) and erlotinib (Tarceva), which are selective inhibitors of Ras-activating epidermal growth factor (EGF) receptor, have been widely utilized in patients with advanced non-small cell lung cancer, resulting in inhibition of RTKs/Ras/ERK signaling.

Hypoxia

Cells that surround stem cells provide extrinsic cues, including TGF-β and growth factors, and this specialized microenvironment is referred to as the "stem cell niche". Cellular communication with this niche is essential for the maintenance of proper stem cell numbers and functions. An initial report on the TSC niche proposed a perivascular niche, where glioma stem cells closely interact with vascular endothelium (Calabrese et al., 2007), which was verified by subsequent studies showing that glioma cells express high levels of laminin receptor integrinα6β1 in the perivascular niche and CD133+/integrinα6 (high) enriches tumor cells with stem cell properties (Lathia et al., 2010). In addition, secreted nitric oxide (NO) from the vascular endothelium regulates adjacent Nestin+ glioma cells (Charles et al., 2010). Although the perivascular niche is well accepted, low oxygen areas away from tumor vessels are also recognized as secondary niches that play a role in TSC regulation. CD133 expression increases by approximately two-fold when primary glioma spheres are incubated in physiological concentrations of oxygen (7%) (McCord et al., 2009). In addition, additional stem cell genes, such as Sox2, Oct4, and Nestin, are also simultaneously up-regulated.

The HIF-1 transcription factor adapts to changes in oxygen concentrations and has more than 60 putative downstream genes that are involved in angiogenesis, glucose transport, glycolysis, cell survival, and metastasis. Interestingly, Ras increases nuclear HIF-1α phosphorylation via ERK activation and superoxide production; superoxide scavenging by superoxide dismutase (SOD), as well as inhibition of ERK activity by PD98059, has been shown to decrease HIF-1α activation (Wang et al., 2004). Some chemotherapeutic agents target RTKs, such as gefitinib (Iressa, an inhibitor of EGFR/ERBB1), trastuzumab (Herceptin, an inhibitor of ERBB2/HER2), and imatinib (Glivec, an inhibitor of Bcr-Abl and PDGFRβ), have been shown to inhibit HIF-1 activity, and further evidence has shown that hypoxia mediates resistance to chemotherapy and radiation. Therefore, RTK inhibition is expected to result in dual effects against Ras-mediated tumor stemness and hypoxia-mediated aspects of tumor progression.

Conclusion

TGF-mediated DNA demethylation, RTKs/Ras/ERK signaling, and hypoxic environments are major regulators of CD133 gene expression and tumor stemness in some human malignant tumors; these intracellular signals interact closely with each other. Further studies focused on regulatory mechanisms of important stemness genes, including CD133, MDR1, and ABCG2, could help to identify promising molecular and cellular targets against TSCs.

References

Armstrong L, Hughes O, Yung S, Hyslop L, Stewart R, Wappler I, Peters H, Walter T, Stojkovic P, Evans J, Stojkovic M, Lako M (2006) The role of PI3K/AKT, MAPK/ERK and NFkappabeta signaling in the maintenance of human embryonic stem cell pluripotency and viability highlighted by transcriptional profiling and functional analysis. Hum Mol Genet 15:1894–1913

Bao S, Wu Q, McLendon RE, Hao Y, Shi Q, Hjelmeland AB, Dewhirst MW, Bigner DD, Rich JN (2006) Glioma stem cells promote radioresistance by preferential activation of the DNA damage response. Nature 444:756–760

Bustinza-Linares E, Kurzrock R, Tsimberidou AM (2010) Salirasib in the treatment of pancreatic cancer. Future Oncol 6:885–891

Calabrese C, Poppleton H, Kocak M, Hogg TL, Fuller C, Hamner B, Oh EY, Gaber MW, Finklestein D, Allen M, Frank A, Bayazitov IT, Zakharenko SS, Gajjar A, Davidoff A, Gilbertson RJ (2007) A perivascular niche for brain tumor stem cells. Cancer Cell 11:69–82

Charles N, Ozawa T, Squatrito M, Bleau AM, Brennan CW, Hambardzumyan D, Holland EC (2010) Perivascular nitric oxide activates notch signaling and promotes stem-like character in PDGF-induced glioma cells. Cell Stem Cell 6:141–152

Clarke MF, Dick JE, Dirks PB, Eaves CJ, Jamieson CH, Jones DL, Visvader J, Weissman IL, Wahl GM (2006) Cancer stem cells—perspectives on current status and future directions: AACR workshop on cancer stem cells. Cancer Res 66:9339–9344

Eden A, Gaudet F, Waghmare A, Jaenisch R (2003) Chromosomal instability and tumors promoted by DNA hypomethylation. Science 300:455

Gaudet F, Hodgson JG, Eden A, Jackson-Grusby L, Dausman J, Gray JW, Leonhardt H, Jaenisch R (2003) Induction of tumors in mice by genomic hypomethylation. Science 300:489–492

Ginestier C, Hur MH, Charafe-Jauffret E, Monville F, Dutcher J, Brown M, Jacquemier J, Viens P, Kleer CG, Liu S, Schott A, Hayes D, Birnbaum D, Wicha MS, Dontu G (2007) ALDH1 is a marker of normal and malignant human mammary stem cells and a predictor of poor clinical outcome. Cell Stem Cell 1:555–567

Goodell MA, Brose K, Paradis G, Conner AS, Mulligan RC (1996) Isolation and functional properties of murine hematopoietic stem cells that are replicating in vivo. J Exp Med 183:1797–1806

Haraguchi N, Ishii H, Mimori K, Tanaka F, Ohkuma M, Kim HM, Akita H, Takiuchi D, Hatano H, Nagano H, Barnard GF, Doki Y, Mori M (2010) CD13 is a therapeutic target in human liver cancer stem cells. J Clin Invest 120:3326–3339

Ikushima H, Todo T, Ino Y, Takahashi M, Miyazawa K, Miyazono K (2009) Autocrine TGF-beta signaling maintains tumorigenicity of glioma-initiating cells through Sry-related HMG-box factors. Cell Stem Cell 5:504–514

Islam MO, Kanemura Y, Tajria J, Mori H, Kobayashi S, Shofuda T, Miyake J, Hara M, Yamasaki M, Okano H (2005) Characterization of ABC transporter ABCB1 expressed in human neural stem/progenitor cells. FEBS Lett 579:3473–3480

Jordan CT, Guzman ML, Noble M (2006) Cancer stem cells. N Engl J Med 355:1253–1261

Lathia JD, Gallagher J, Heddleston JM, Wang J, Eyler CE, Macswords J, Wu Q, Vasanji A, McLendon RE, Hjelmeland AB, Rich JN (2010) Integrin alpha 6 regulates glioblastoma stem cells. Cell Stem Cell 6:421–432

Lee JS, Gil JE, Kim JH, Kim TK, Jin X, Oh SY, Sohn YW, Jeon HM, Park HJ, Park JW, Shin YJ, Chung YG, Lee JB, You S, Kim H (2008) Brain cancer stem-like cell genesis from p53-deficient mouse astrocytes by oncogenic Ras. Biochem Biophys Res Commun 365:496–502

Mani SA, Guo W, Liao MJ, Eaton EN, Ayyanan A, Zhou AY, Brooks M, Reinhard F, Zhang CC, Shipitsin M, Campbell

LL, Polyak K, Brisken C, Yang J, Weinberg RA (2008) The epithelial–mesenchymal transition generates cells with properties of stem cells. Cell 133:704–715

McCord AM, Jamal M, Shankavaram UT, Lang FF, Camphausen K, Tofilon PJ (2009) Physiologic oxygen concentration enhances the stem-like properties of CD133+ human glioblastoma cells in vitro. Mol Cancer Res 7:489–497

Morel AP, Lievre M, Thomas C, Hinkal G, Ansieau S, Puisieux A (2008) Generation of breast cancer stem cells through epithelial–mesenchymal transition. PLoS One 3:e2888

O'Brien CA, Pollett A, Gallinger S, Dick JE (2007) A human colon cancer cell capable of initiating tumor growth in immunodeficient mice. Nature 445:106–110

Schlingensiepen KH, Fischer-Blass B, Schmaus S, Ludwig S (2008) Antisense therapeutics for tumor treatment: the TGF-beta2 inhibitor AP 12009 in clinical development against malignant tumors. Recent Results Cancer Res 177:137–150

Shmelkov SV, Jun L, St Clair R, McGarrigle D, Derderian CA, Usenko JK, Costa C, Zhang F, Guo X, Rafii S (2004) Alternative promoters regulate transcription of the gene that encodes stem cell surface protein AC133. Blood 103:2055–2061

Tabu K, Sasai K, Kimura T, Wang L, Aoyanagi E, Kohsaka S, Tanino M, Nishihara H, Tanaka S (2008) Promoter hypomethylation regulates CD133 expression in human gliomas. Cell Res 18:1037–1046

Tabu K, Kimura T, Sasai K, Wang L, Bizen N, Nishihara H, Taga T, Tanaka S (2010) Analysis of an alternative human CD133 promoter reveals the implication of Ras/ERK pathway in tumor stem-like hallmarks. Mol Cancer 9:39

Tsumura A, Hayakawa T, Kumaki Y, Takebayashi S, Sakaue M, Matsuoka C, Shimotohno K, Ishikawa F, Li E, Ueda HR, Nakayama J, Okano M (2006) Maintenance of self-renewal ability of mouse embryonic stem cells in the absence of DNA methyltransferases Dnmt1, Dnmt3a and Dnmt3b. Genes Cells 11:805–814

Wang FS, Wang CJ, Chen YJ, Chang PR, Huang YT, Sun YC, Huang HC, Yang YJ, Yang KD (2004) Ras induction of superoxide activates ERK-dependent angiogenic transcription factor HIF-1alpha and VEGF-A expression in shock wave-stimulated osteoblasts. J Biol Chem 279:10331–10337

Yamanaka S, Blau HM (2010) Nuclear reprogramming to a pluripotent state by three approaches. Nature 465:704–712

Yamazaki S, Iwama A, Takayanagi S, Eto K, Ema H, Nakauchi H (2009) TGF-beta as a candidate bone marrow niche signal to induce hematopoietic stem cell hibernation. Blood 113:1250–1256

You H, Ding W, Rountree CB (2010) Epigenetic regulation of cancer stem cell marker CD133 by transforming growth factor-beta. Hepatology 51:1635–1644

Zabierowski SE, Herlyn M (2008) Melanoma stem cells: the dark seed of melanoma. J Clin Oncol 26:2890–2894

Chapter 17

Cripto-1: A Common Embryonic Stem Cell and Cancer Cell Marker

Maria Cristina Rangel, Nadia P. Castro, Hideaki Karasawa, Tadahiro Nagaoka, David S. Salomon, and Caterina Bianco

Abstract Human Cripto-1 has been implicated in embryogenesis and tumorigenesis. During early embryonic development, Cripto-1 functions as a co-receptor for transforming growth factor-β family members, including Nodal/growth differentiation factors 1 and 3, and is essential for mesoderm and endoderm formation and anterior/posterior and left-right axis establishment. In normal adult tissues Cripto-1 is expressed at very low levels, while its expression significantly increases in approximately 50–80% of different types of human carcinomas. Overexpression of Cripto-1 in mouse mammary epithelial cells leads to their transformation in vitro and enhances migration, invasion, branching morphogenesis and epithelial to mesenchymal transition. Transgenic mouse studies have shown that overexpression of Cripto-1 in the mammary gland results in mammary hyperplasias and papillary adenocarcinomas. Furthermore, Cripto-1 is expressed at high levels in different types of human tumors. In conclusion, while during embryogenesis Cripto-1 performs specific and regulatory functions related to cell and tissue patterning, inappropriate expression of Cripto-1 in adult tissues leads to cell transformation and tumor progression.

Keywords Cripto-1 · Epidermal growth factor · Embryonic development · Mammary hyperplasias · Papillary adenocarcinomas · Embryonic stem cells

C. Bianco (✉)
Mammary Biology and Tumorigenesis Laboratory, Center for Cancer Research, National Cancer Institute, National Institutes of Health, Bethesda, MD, USA
e-mail: biancoc@mail.nih.gov

Human Cripto-1, a Member of the EGF-CFC Family

Human Cripto-1, also known as teratocarcinoma-derived growth factor-1 (TDGF-1), is a member of the Epidermal Growth Factor (EGF)-Cripto-1-FRL-1-Cryptic (CFC) protein family and plays important roles in embryonic development and tumor progression (de Castro et al., 2010). The EGF-CFC family includes also monkey Cripto-1, mouse Cripto-1 (Cr-1/cfc2), chicken Cripto-1, zebrafish one-eyed pinhead (*oep*), *Xenopus* XCR1/FRL-1, XCR2, XCR3, mouse cryptic (Cfc1) and human Cryptic (CFC1) (Bianco et al., 2010; de Castro et al., 2010). Structurally, these proteins are composed of a NH2-terminal signal peptide, a modified EGF-like domain, a CFC cysteine-rich domain and a short hydrophobic COOH-terminus containing a sequence for glycosylphosphatidylinositol (GPI) cleavage and attachment (Fig. 17.1). GPI anchoring determines membrane localization of Cripto-1 in lipid rafts microdomains and within caveolae (Bianco et al., 2010; de Castro et al., 2010; Watanabe et al., 2007). Cripto-1 protein can be released from the cell membrane upon treatment with phosphatidylinositolphospholipase C (PI-PLC), and by the activity of the endogenous enzyme GPI-phospholipase D (GPI-PLD) (Fig. 17.1) (Bianco et al., 2010; de Castro et al., 2010). Therefore, this controlled release mechanism regulates the ability of Cripto-1 to function as a membrane-associated co-receptor or as soluble ligand. In fact, soluble forms of Cripto-1 have been reported to be active in a number of different in vitro and in vivo assays, while the GPI-anchor is required by Cripto-1 to function as a co-receptor for transforming growth factor (TGF)-β-related protein

M.A. Hayat (ed.), *Stem Cells and Cancer Stem Cells, Volume 2*,
DOI 10.1007/978-94-007-2016-9_17, © Springer Science+Business Media B.V. 2012

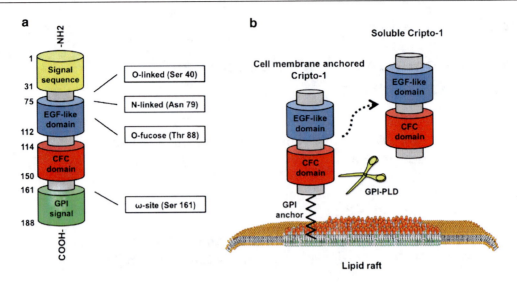

Fig. 17.1 (a) Structure of human Cripto-1 protein (amino acid 1-188) with post-translational modifications. (b) Cripto-1 is a GPI-anchored membrane protein that can be cleaved by glycosylphosphatidylinositol phospholipase D (GPI-PLD) and released into the supernatant of the cells as a soluble protein

Nodal (Bianco et al., 2010; de Castro et al., 2010). Furthermore, Cripto-1 protein has several glycosylation sites, including O-linked glycosylation at Ser40 and Ser161 (which is the ω-site for GPI-attachment), N-linked glycosylation at Asn79 and O-linked fucosylation at Thr88 (Fig. 17.1a) (Bianco et al., 2010; de Castro et al., 2010). Among them, O-linked fucosylation of EGF-CFC proteins is necessary for their ability to function as co-receptors for Nodal (de Castro et al., 2010). However, Cripto-1 O-fucosylation mutants are fully functional with regard to activation of Nodal-independent signaling pathways, including MAPK and AKT signaling pathways (Bianco et al., 2008a). In addition, another study has demonstrated that it is the Thr88 residue within the EGF-like domain of Cripto-1 and not O-fucosylation of this residue that is required for Cripto-1 to function as a Nodal co-receptor (Shi et al., 2007).

Cripto-1 and Embryonic Development

During embryonic development EGF-CFC proteins function as co-receptors for the TGF-β ligands Nodal and growth and differentiation factors 1 and 3 (GDF-1/GDF-3) (Bianco et al., 2010; de Castro et al., 2010). Genetic studies in zebrafish and mice have defined an essential role for Nodal that functions through oep/Cripto-1 in the formation of the primitive streak, patterning of the anterior-posterior (A/P) axis, and specification of mesoderm and endoderm (mesoendoderm) (Bianco et al., 2010; de Castro et al., 2010). In later stages of embryonic development the EGF-CFC family member, Cryptic, regulates the establishment of left/right (L/R) axis, allowing asymmetric development of visceral organs. Biochemical studies have demonstrated that EGF-CFC proteins bind directly to both Nodal/GDF-1/GDF-3 and the Activin type I receptor ALK4 (ActRIB), recruiting the Activin type II receptor and inducing activation and phosphorylation of Smad-2/Smad-3 intracellular signaling pathway (Fig. 17.2a) (Bianco et al., 2002). However, Cripto-1 can also regulate A/P axis specification independently of Nodal signaling (D'Andrea et al., 2008). In fact, Cripto-1$^{F78A/F78A}$ mouse embryos carrying the amino acid substitution F78A are unable to activate the Nodal signaling pathway, but clearly form an A/P axis and initiate germ layer formation and gastrulation movements (D'Andrea et al., 2008). During early mouse embryogenesis, Cripto-1 can first be detected prior to the gastrulation stage in the inner cell mass and in extra-embryonic trophoblast cells at day 4 of development. Cripto-1 expression increases on day 6.5 of embryonic development, and is found in the primitive streak in epiblast cells undergoing epithelial to mesenchymal transition (EMT), which eventually give rise to the mesoderm and endoderm (Bianco et al., 2010; de Castro et al., 2010). Cripto-1 is also detected in

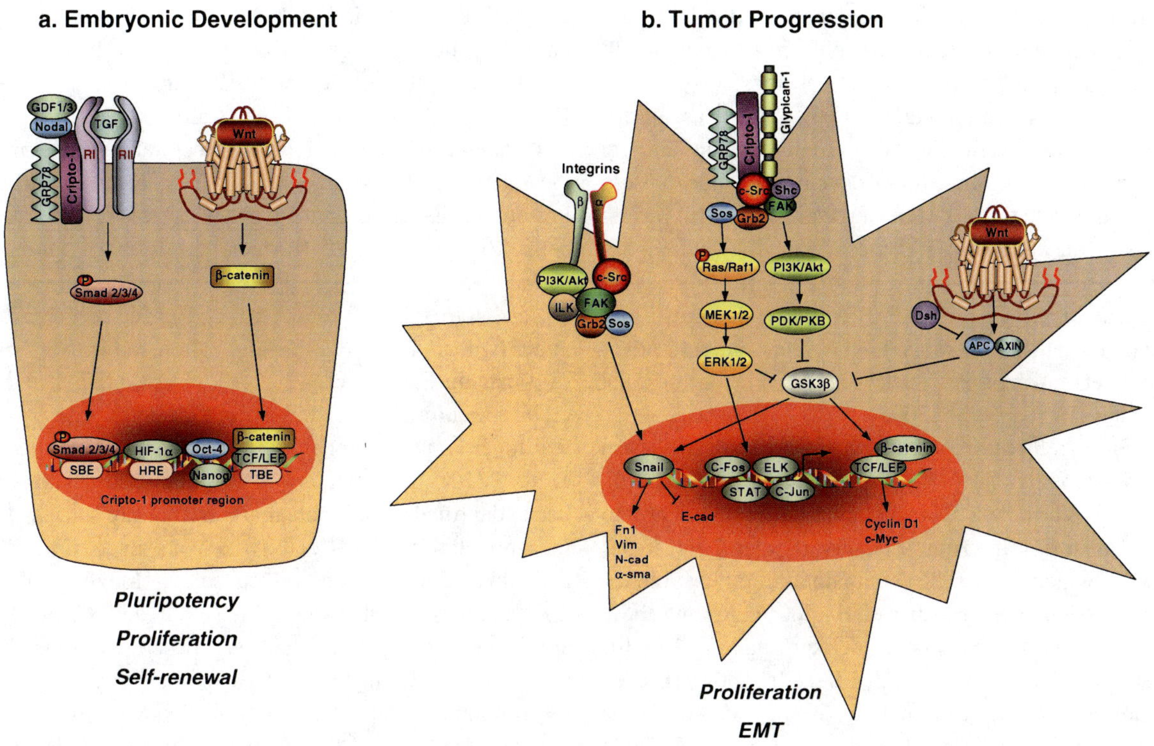

Fig. 17.2 Schematic diagram of Cripto-1 signaling pathway during embryonic development and tumor progression. (**a**) Cross-talk of Cripto-1/Nodal, *Wnt*/β-catenin and HIF-1α signaling pathways during embryonic development. Activated Smad-2/3/4 complex binds to SBE within the Cripto-1 promoter and positively regulates its expression. HIF-1α binds to HRE within the Cripto-1 promoter and directly enhances Cripto-1 expression in hypoxic conditions. Oct-4 and Nanog can also directly interact with the Cripto-1 promoter. Canonical *Wnt*/β-catenin signaling pathway cross-talks with Cripto-1/Nodal signaling during embryonic development. (**b**) During tumor progression, Cripto-1 upon binding to Glypican-1 activates MAPK and AKT signaling pathways, which inhibit GSK3β that consecutively induces nuclear localization and protein stabilization of Snail and β-catenin. Epithelial cells lose the expression of epithelial-specific genes, such as E-cadherin and acquire the expression of mesenchymal genes. Cripto-1 increases expression of α and β integrins during EMT. GRP78 can enhance Cripto-1/Nodal-dependent and Nodal-independent signaling pathways and potentially might modulate Cripto-1 signaling during embryogenesis and tumorigenesis. HIF-1α: hypoxia inducible factor-1 α; SBE: Smad binding elements; HRE: hypoxia responsive elements; TCF/LEF: T-cell factor/lymphoid enhancer factor; TBE: TCF/LEF binding elements; EMT: epithelial to mesenchymal transition, MAPK: mitogen activated protein kinase; GDF: growth and differentiation factor; GSK3β: glycogen synthase kinase 3β

the ectoplacental cone at this stage. Expression then decreases on day 7 when Cripto-1 is detected mostly in the truncus arterious of the developing heart. With the exception of the developing heart, little if any expression of Cripto-1 can be detected in the embryo after day 8 (Bianco et al., 2010; de Castro et al., 2010). Disruption of Cripto-1 in Cripto-1$^{-/-}$ embryos is embryonically lethal and results in the formation of embryos that possess a head without a trunk, demonstrating that there is a severe deficiency in embryonic mesoderm and endoderm without a loss of anterior neuroectoderm formation (de Castro et al., 2010). Initiation of the primitive heart tube in Cripto-1$^{-/-}$ null mice is severely inhibited due to failure in the development of functional beating cardiomyocytes, as demonstrated by the absence of expression of terminal myocardial differentiation genes (de Castro et al., 2010).

Cripto-1 and Embryonic Stem Cells

Stem cells are characterized by two unique properties that differentiate them from other cell types: the ability for self-renewal through symmetric (embryonic stem cells) or asymmetric (adult or somatic stem cells) cell division and the capability to generate mature cells of a particular tissue through differentiation (Bendall et al., 2008). Embryonic stem (ES) cells are pluripotent and may be isolated from the inner cell mass or from the epiblast of an early-stage embryo, known as blastocyst, whereas adult stem cells are multipotent and are found in adult tissues. In the developing embryo, stem cells give rise to cells of the three primary germ layers: ectoderm, endoderm and mesoderm. In adult organisms, stem cells and progenitor cells function as an internal tissue repair system, dividing to replenish specialized cells and also maintaining the normal turnover of regenerative organs, such as blood, skin, or intestinal tissues (Bendall et al., 2008).

Stem cell research has made several progresses in understanding the molecular mechanisms regulating ES cell pluripotency. Such studies have shed light into a number of transcription factors, such as Oct4, Rex1, Sox2, which are essential in maintaining pluripotency of ES cells (Koestenbauer et al., 2006). Among these genes, Cripto-1 is also considered a marker of undifferentiated and pluripotent ES cells and has been referred as stem cell marker (Bianco et al., 2010; de Castro et al., 2010; Hough et al., 2009). In 2007 the International Stem Cell Initiative characterized 59 human ES cell lines and all of them exhibited similar expression profile for strongly developmentally regulated genes including Nanog, Oct4 (POU5F1), Cripto-1, DNMT3B, GABRB3 and GDF3 (Bianco et al., 2010; de Castro et al., 2010). Interestingly, chromatin immunoprecipitation analysis of the mouse ES cell genome has identified Oct-4 and Nanog binding loci within the Cripto-1 promoter, suggesting that Cripto-1 is downstream of key modulators of ES cell undifferentiated and pluripotential state (Bianco et al., 2010; de Castro et al., 2010). Comparison of the transcriptional profile across species has demonstrated conserved pathways regulating self-renewal between mouse and human ES cells, and genes such as Oct-4, Lefty, Nodal, Sox-2, Utf-1 (undifferentiated embryonic cell transcription factor-1), tert (telomerase reverse transcriptase), and Cripto-1 are highly enriched in both mouse and human ES cells (Wei et al., 2005).

Additionally, Cripto-1 has been shown to cross-talk with other genes that are critical for early embryonic development and essential for stem cell proliferation, maintenance and differentiation, including the *Wnt* signaling pathway, TGF-β family members, the Notch pathway and hypoxia inducible factor-1 α (HIF-1α) (Fig. 17.2a) (Bianco et al.; de Castro et al., 2010). Activation of the canonical *Wnt*/β-catenin pathway can trigger transcription of genes that regulate ES cell pluripotency and differentiation, such as Oct-4, Nanog and Sox-2 (Cole et al., 2008). Cripto-1 has also been identified as a direct target gene in the canonical *Wnt*/β-catenin signaling pathway during embryonic development and in colon carcinoma cells (Bianco et al., 2010). In addition, the Cripto-1 ortholog XCR1/FRL-1 in *Xenopus* can function as a co-receptor for *Wnt*11 together with frizzled receptor 7 and Glypican-4, leading to stabilization and activation of β-catenin (Bianco et al., 2010). Nodal, GDF-1 and GDF-3 require Cripto-1 for signaling and they are critical for ES cell maintenance and self-renewal (Bianco et al., 2010). In particular, GDF-3 and Cripto-1 have been identified as ES cell markers that are enriched in a population of ES cells which are uncommitted and have high self-renewal capacity (Hough et al., 2009). Cross-talk between the Notch and Cripto-1 signaling pathways has also been described (Bianco et al., 2010). Using a yeast two-hybrid system and by coimmunoprecipitation analysis, Watanabe and colleagues (2009) have demonstrated that Cripto-1 can directly bind to all four mammalian Notch receptors and facilitates the intracellular posttranslational maturation of Notch receptors, enhancing ligand-induced activation of Notch signaling (Watanabe et al., 2009). Finally, hypoxia and the transcription factor HIF-1α can increase Cripto-1 expression by binding of HIF-1α to hypoxia-responsive elements (HREs) within the mouse and human Cripto-1 promoters in mouse ES cells and in human embryonal carcinoma cells, respectively (Fig. 17.2a) (Bianco et al., 2009). Additionally, hypoxia stimulation can significantly enhance cardiomyocyte differentiation of mES cells in comparison with mES cells grown under normoxic conditions.

Cripto-1 and Cancer Stem Cells

Recent studies have suggested that tumor growth and survival is dependent upon the existence of a subpopulation of chemo- and radio-resistant cells within the tumor, also known as cancer stem cells or tumor initiating cells (Bianco et al., 2010; de Castro et al., 2010). Cancer stem cells were first identified in the hematopoietic system and after they have also been identified in solid cancers, including cancers of the breast, lung, prostate, colon, brain, head and neck, and pancreas (Bianco et al., 2010; de Castro et al., 2010). A cancer cell can be defined as a cancer stem cell based upon its ability to self-renew and regenerate the original phenotype of the tumor when implanted into immunodeficient mice (Visvader and Lindeman, 2008).

Several studies have demonstrated that cell fate regulation during embryonic development and cell transformation during oncogenesis share common signaling pathways, suggesting that uncontrolled reactivation of embryonic signaling pathways might drive cell transformation and tumor progression in adult tissues (Bianco et al., 2010).

Recent evidence clearly suggests that tumors can grow and metastasize from tumor-initiating cells, and our laboratory has reported that Cripto-1 might represent a novel cell surface marker for cancer cells with stem-like cell characteristics (Watanabe et al., 2010). Embryonal carcinoma (EC) cells are pluripotent stem cells derived from germ cell teratocarcinomas and are considered to represent the malignant counterparts of human ES cells. A heterogeneous expression of Cripto-1 in EC cells allowed us to identify two distinct subpopulations of high and low expressing Cripto-1 EC cells. Interestingly, these two subpopulations showed different in vitro and in vivo tumorigenic abilities. The Cripto-1 high subpopulation of EC cells formed tumor spheres in a serum-free suspension culture with an efficiency significantly higher than the Cripto-1 low expressing EC cells. Furthermore, Cripto-1 high expressing cells, when injected subcutaneously into nude mice, gave rise to tumors larger in size and displaying a shorter tumor latency period compared with tumors derived from Cripto-1 low expressing cells. Finally, key regulators of pluripotent ES cells, such as Activin/Nodal and the transcription factors Nanog and Oct-4, modulated Cripto-1 expression in this subpopulation of Cripto-1 high expressing EC cells (Watanabe et al., 2010). Furthermore, Cripto-1 has been proposed as a novel marker for the identification of cancer stem cells in melanoma (Strizzi et al., 2008) and in prostate cancer (Cocciadiferro et al., 2009). Altogether, these findings suggest that Cripto-1 might represent a promising candidate for the identification and potential therapeutic targeting of cancer stem cells within aggressive tumors.

Cripto-1 and EMT

EMT is a fundamental process that occurs during embryogenesis, tumor progression and metastasis. During EMT epithelial cells undergo dramatic morphological changes that allow them to acquire migratory and invasive properties of mesenchymal cells, ultimately leading to tumor progression and metastasis (Thiery et al., 2009). EMT is a property which has also been shown to be associated with cancer stem cells (Hollier et al., 2009). Cripto-1 is involved in embryonic development during gastrulation, when epiblastic cells undergo EMT, and Cripto-1 increased expression has been shown to promote EMT in vitro in mouse mammary epithelial cells and in vivo in mouse mammary tumors (Strizzi et al., 2004). Moreover, Cripto-1 can enhance migration, invasion and branching morphogenesis of several mouse mammary epithelial cell lines (Wechselberger et al., 2001). NMuMG mouse mammary epithelial cells overexpressing the transcription factor Msx2 undergo morphological changes suggestive of EMT. Interestingly, Cripto-1 was found overexpressed in NMuMG Msx2 cells suggesting that Cripto-1 might promote EMT in mouse mammary epithelial cells (di Bari et al., 2009). Furthermore, Cripto-1 has been reported to be a key EMT regulator together with Snail/Slug/Twist, and Six1 (Micalizzi et al., 2010). During EMT, activation of TGF-β and *Wnt* signaling pathways at the leading edge of the tumor together with expression of EMT regulators is critical for tumor cells to acquire a mesenchymal phenotype that allow them to locally invade and escape from the primary tumor site, setting the stage for metastatic dissemination (Micalizzi et al., 2010).

These studies clearly suggest that Cripto-1 is involved in epithelial plasticity and EMT during embryonic development and cancer, leading to induction of a comprehensive program of proprieties necessary for tumor progression.

Cripto-1 and Cancer

Since its original discovery in 1989, Cripto-1 has been clearly involved in tumor progression, inducing transformation, migration and invasion of normal mammary epithelial cells, as well as stimulating tumor angiogenesis in vitro and in vivo (Bianco et al., 2010;

de Castro et al., 2010). Additionally, transgenic mouse models have demonstrated that Cripto-1 overexpression promotes hyperplasias and adenocarcinomas of the mammary gland and leiomyosarcoma of the uterus. Finally, Cripto-1 is overexpressed at the mRNA and protein level in a wide variety of human carcinomas (de Castro et al., 2010).

Cripto-1 Oncogenic Activities In Vitro

The first in vitro studies suggesting the involvement of Cripto-1 in tumorigenesis showed that murine fibroblasts and mammary epithelial cells transfected with a Cripto-1 expression vector acquired a transformed phenotype in vitro, as observed by their ability to grow in an anchorage-independent manner in soft agar (Bianco et al., 2010; de Castro et al., 2010). Cripto-1 overexpression has also been shown to enhance migration and invasion in mouse mammary EpH4, NOG-8, TAC-2 or NMuMG cells, MCF-7 human breast cancer cells and Caski human cervical carcinoma cells, as assessed by Boyden chamber migration and invasion assays (Bianco et al., 2010; de Castro et al., 2010). These results suggest that Cripto-1 overexpression might be associated with progression towards a more aggressive phenotype. More recently, Lawrence and colleagues (2011) have demonstrated that Cripto-1 is expressed in 6 human prostate cancer cell lines (Lawrence et al., 2011). Interestingly, Nodal, in a Cripto-1 dependent manner, could enhance the growth of LNCaP prostate cancer cells in anchorage-independent conditions. Cripto-1 is also expressed at high levels in nasopharyngeal carcinoma (NPC) cell lines as compared to immortalized nasopharyngeal epithelial cells, and inhibition of endogenous Cripto-1 using lentivirus-mediated RNAi silencing technique strongly suppressed NPC cell growth and invasion in vitro (Wu et al., 2009). Cripto-1 may also be involved in glioma tumorigenesis. In fact, in vitro studies using U87MG and GBM glioma cell lines have shown that Nodal together with Cripto-1 induces Smad-2 activation and promotes glioma cell proliferation (Lee et al., 2010). Cripto-1 expression is also significantly induced in cells transformed by different oncogenes, such as rat embryo fibroblasts (CREF) or Fischer rat thyroid cells (FRTL) transformed by c-Ha-*ras* or c-Ki-*ras* (de Castro et al., 2010).

In addition to promoting cellular transformation, Cripto-1 can also function as a potent angiogenic protein both in vitro and in vivo. Cripto-1 is able to enhance proliferation, migration and invasion of human umbilical endothelial cells (HUVECs), stimulating their differentiation into vascular-like structures in matrigel. Furthermore, Cripto-1 promotes neovascularization in vivo as assessed by a directed in vivo angiogenic assay (DIVAA) and by a breast cancer xenograft mouse model (Bianco et al., 2005). More recently, HIF-1α has been shown to enhance Cripto-1 expression in murine embryonic stem cells and in human embryonal carcinoma cells through the direct binding of HIF-1α to the Cripto-1 promoter under hypoxic conditions (Bianco et al., 2009). Since low oxygen conditions are often responsible for the induction of several angiogenic molecules in growing tumors, such as vascular endothelial growth factor (VEGF) and basic-fibroblast growth factor (b-FGF), it is possible that low oxygen conditions within a growing tumor might trigger Cripto-1 expression, which in turn induces new vessel formation to sustain tumor growth.

Signaling Pathways Activated by Cripto-1 During Oncogenic Transformation

In addition to functioning as a Nodal co-receptor, Cripto-1 can function independently of Nodal modulating a variety of intracellular signaling pathways (de Castro et al., 2010). Cripto-1 upon binding to Glypican-1, a GPI-linked heparan sulphate proteoglycan (HSPG), activates the cytoplasmic tyrosine kinase c-Src, which in turn triggers activation of the ras/raf/MAPK and PI3K/AKT signaling pathways (Fig. 17.2b) (Bianco et al., 2003). Interaction of Cripto-1 and Glypican-1 might occur within lipid raft microdomain regions of the cell membrane that are enriched in GPI-linked proteins (Bianco et al. 2003). Within lipid rafts, Cripto-1 directly interacts with another membrane protein, Caveolin-1 (Cav-1), a protein that acts as a tumor suppressor in the mammary gland (Bianco et al., 2008b). Cav-1 inhibits activation of c-Src and MAPK/AKT signaling pathways induced by Cripto-1 in mouse mammary epithelial cells, reducing the ability of Cripto-1 to enhance migration, invasion and formation of branching structures of mouse mammary epithelial cells. In addition, mammary tumors derived from transgenic mice overexpressing the human Cripto-1 transgene under the control of the mouse mammary tumor virus promoter (MMTV-Cripto-1 mice) show a dramatic reduction in Cav-1 expression, suggesting that loss of Cav-1 is an essential step in the cellular transformation induced by Cripto-1 in the mouse mammary gland (Bianco et al., 2008b). In addition to Glypican-1, Cripto-1 mitogenic signaling is also dependent upon binding to glucose-regulated protein 78 (GRP78), an endoplasmic reticulum (ER) heat shock chaperone protein that can be also expressed on tumor cells membranes (Fig. 17.2b) (de Castro et al., 2010). Indeed, disruption of the Cripto-1/GRP78 complex at the cell membrane interferes with Cripto-1 oncogenic activity in vitro, preventing Cripto-1 activation of MAPK/AKT signaling pathway. Interestingly, unlike Glypican-1, GRP78 is also important for Nodal-dependent Cripto-1 signaling, enhancing activation of the Smad-2/Smad-3 signaling pathway (Fig. 17.2a) (de Castro et al., 2010).

Cripto-1 Oncogenic Activities In Vivo

Beside performing an important role in cellular transformation in vitro, Cripto-1 can function as an oncogene in vivo. Kenney and colleagues (1996) reported that mammary tumors derived from transgenic mice overexpressing a variety of different oncogenes, including neu (erbB-2), TGF-α, int-3, polyoma middle T (PyMT), or simian virus 40 large T antigens, showed a significant increase in Cripto-1 expression, suggesting the involvement of Cripto-1 in the promotion or progression of mammary tumors induced by these oncogenes (Kenney et al., 1996). Subsequently, overexpression of a human Cripto-1 transgene in the mouse mammary gland under the control of the MMTV or whey acidic protein (WAP) promoter, has directly implicated Cripto-1 in mammary transformation (Sun et al., 2005; Wechselberger et al., 2005). Wechselberger and colleagues (2005) demonstrated that the majority of nulliparous MMTV-Cripto-1 transgenic mice exhibited enhanced ductal branching, intraductal hyperplasias and hyperplastic alveolar nodules, and about 30–40% of aged multiparous female mice developed multifocal hyperplasias and papillary adenocarcinomas. The relatively long latency period of mammary tumor formation implies that additional genetic or regulatory alterations in combination with Cripto-1 overexpression are necessary to facilitate tumorigenesis (Wechselberger et al., 2005). Moreover, it has been shown that mammary gland hyperplasias and tumors derived from MMTV-Cripto-1 transgenic mice express molecular markers and signaling molecules characteristics of EMT (Strizzi et al., 2004). N-cadherin, vimentin, cyclin-D1, Snail, α-smooth muscle actin, fibronectin and β-catenin protein expression was significantly increased in MMTV-Cripto-1 tumors as compared to mammary tissue from control FVB/N multiparous mice. In contrast, E-cadherin was decreased in MMTV-Cripto-1 mammary tumors as compared to normal mammary tissues. Additionally, expression of phosphorylated (P)-c-Src, P-focal adhesion kinase (FAK), P-AKT, P-glycogen synthase kinase 3β (GSK3β), dephosphorylated (DP)-β-catenin, and integrins, such as, α3, αv, β1, β3, and β4 was also increased in MMTV-Cripto-1 tumors, suggesting that Cripto-1 might play an important role in facilitating migration and invasion of tumor cells (Fig. 17.2b) (Strizzi et al., 2004). Surprisingly, 20% of the MMTV-Cripto-1 female nulliparous or multiparous transgenic mice developed uterine leiomyosarcomas as compared to control mice over a 24-month observation period. Cripto-1 transgene was expressed at high levels in uterine tumors collected from the MMTV-Cripto-1 mice (Strizzi et al., 2007). Furthermore, western blot analysis showed higher levels of phosphorylated forms of c-Src, AKT, GSK3β and DP-β-catenin in uterine leiomyosarcomas derived from MMTV-Cripto-1 mice as compared to uteri from control mice (Strizzi et al., 2007). Immunostaining also showed increased nuclear localization of β-catenin in the MMTV-Cripto-1 uterine leiomyosarcomas. This study suggests a role for Cripto-1 during uterine tumorigenesis either by activating c-Src and AKT and/or via cross-talk with the canonical Wnt/β-catenin signaling pathway, as suggested by the increased expression of P-GSK3β, DP-β-catenin, and increased nuclear localization of β-catenin in MMTV-Cripto-1 mice leiomyosarcomas. Unlike the MMTV promoter that can drive expression of the Cripto-1 transgene in the virgin mouse, the WAP promoter is maximally active during mid-pregnancy and lactation. Approximately 50% of old nulliparous WAP-Cripto-1 mice developed multifocal intraductal hyperplasias, while more than half of multiparous WAP-Cripto-1 female mice developed multifocal mammary tumors of mixed histological subtypes (Sun et al., 2005). Histological analysis of the WAP-Cripto-1 mammary tumors revealed the presence of tumors of mixed histology, containing glandular, papillary and undifferentiated carcinoma, as well as myoepithelioma and adeno-squamous carcinoma. Mammary tumors of mixed histology have been described in transgenic mice that have alterations in the canonical Wnt/β-catenin pathway. Interestingly, hyperactivation of a canonical Wnt/β-catenin pathway was detected in WAP-Cripto-1 mammary tumors, suggesting that the canonical Wnt/β-catenin pathway together with Cripto-1 promotes mammary tumorigenesis (Sun et al., 2005). This may be significant since activation of the Wnt/β-catenin pathway during early mouse embryogenesis and in human colon carcinoma cells can enhance Cripto-1 expression (Hamada et al., 2007; Morkel et al., 2003).

Cripto-1 Expression in Human Tumors

Cripto-1 is expressed at very low levels in normal tissues with the exception of stem cells and embryonic tissues (de Castro et al., 2010). During oncogenic transformation, Cripto-1 is re-expressed in several types of human cancers, including those of the reproductive and gastrointestinal systems (de Castro et al., 2010). High levels of Cripto-1 expression in a wide variety of human tumors with little expression in normal tissue strongly support Cripto-1 as a promising molecular target in cancer therapy (Bianco and Salomon, 2010). For an extensive review on Cripto-1 expression in human tumors see de Castro et al. (2010).

Tumors of the Reproductive System

Breast Cancer

Cripto-1 expression has been detected in 47% of ductal carcinomas in situ and 73–82% of infiltrating breast ductal carcinomas, while very little expression (13–20%) has been found in normal non-involved breast tissues (de Castro et al., 2010). Interestingly, Cripto-1 can be co-expressed with other EGF-related peptides, such as TGFα, amphiregulin (AREG) and heregulin (HRG) and a positive correlation between nuclear *erb*B-4 and Cripto-1 expression in primary human breast carcinomas has also been described. Statistically significant association between overexpression of Cripto-1 and the Nottingham Prognostic Index, histological grade, pathological tumor type, progesterone receptor status as well as the status of Ki-67 proliferation marker was reported in a study where Cripto-1 was found to be overexpressed in 47.5% of breast cancer patients (de Castro et al., 2010). Cripto-1 overexpression has been also associated with high-grade breast tumors, poor prognosis and decreased survival (de Castro et al., 2010). Breast cancer patients showed high levels of circulating plasma Cripto-1 as compared with a control group (Bianco et al., 2006). High Cripto-1 plasma levels were detected also in breast cancer patients at an early stage, suggesting that Cripto-1 might be useful in the early diagnosis of this disease. Within the benign breast lesions, Cripto-1 plasma levels were higher in those lesions characterized by the presence of sclerosis and in fibroadenomas (Bianco et al., 2006).

Ovarian Cancer

Cripto-1 expression has been detected in 52% of ovarian adenocarcinomas, 33% of mucinous tumors with low malignant potential and 35% of cystadenomas (de Castro et al., 2010). In addition, a significant correlation was observed with advanced tumor stage when Cripto-1 was co-expressed with TGFα and AREG, or with the EGF-receptor, suggesting that co-expression of these EGF-related growth factors and their membrane associated receptors together with Cripto-1 may represent a growth advantage for ovarian cancer cells.

Endometrial Cancer

High levels of Cripto-1 have been detected in both normal human endometrium and endometrial carcinomas, but strong Cripto-1 immunoreactivity is detected in 71% of endometrial carcinomas as well as in the majority of endometrial atypical hyperplasias, an early event in endometrial carcinogenesis (de Castro et al., 2010).

In addition, it has been shown that Nodal and Cripto-1 are co-expressed in normal endometrium during the menstrual cycle and their expression is dramatically up-regulated in endometrial carcinomas. Indeed, Nodal and Cripto-1 expression increases dramatically during transition of endometrial carcinomas from histologic Grade 1 to Grades 2 and 3, suggesting that both Nodal and Cripto-1 are suitable diagnostic markers of endometrial cancer progression (de Castro et al., 2010).

Cervical Cancer

Cripto-1 expression has been detected in the stromal compartment of the normal cervix and in cervical cancers, being overexpressed in 26% of early clinical stage cervical carcinomas when compared with non-neoplastic cervical epithelium (de Castro et al., 2010). Interestingly, Cripto-1 overexpression was significantly correlated with tumor size, involvement of lymphatic vascular space, endometrial and parametrial spread, as well as its expression levels were increased in metastatic lymph nodes compared to corresponding primary tumors.

Leiomyosarcoma of the Uterus

Increased expression of Cripto-1 has been detected in 69.2% of human leiomyosarcomas as compared to 20% of human leiomyoma sections (Strizzi et al., 2007). Augmented expression of P-c-Src, P-AKT, P-GSK3β and increased nuclear localization of β-catenin was also detected by immunostaining in human leiomyosarcomas in comparison with leiomyomas.

Testicular Cancer

Cripto-1 has been detected in 100% of non-seminomatous tumors, such as embryonal carcinomas and malignant undifferentiated teratocarcinomas, as compared to only 31% of seminomas (de Castro et al., 2010). A positive association between Cripto-1 expression and non-seminomatous tumors has been described, suggesting that Cripto-1 expression is associated with a more malignant phenotype in germ cell tumors.

Tumors of the Digestive System

Gastric Cancer

Cripto-1 expression has been detected in patients with long-term *Helicobacter pylori* infection and atrophic gastritis, two important risk factors for gastric carcinogenesis (de Castro et al., 2010). About 35–55% of gastric tumor tissues showed high levels of Cripto-1 expression as compared to normal gastric mucosa. In addition, Cripto-1 expression has been found to correlate with the degree of dysplasia in intestinal metaplasia, as well as with tumor stage and patient prognosis in gastric cancer. In fact, the occurrence of Cripto-1 positive cases is more frequent in late-stage locally invasive tumors (62% of cases) than in early-stage non-invasive cancers (25%). Recently, Cripto-1 has been found to be expressed at high levels in gastric carcinoma (71.3%), chronic atrophic gastritis (65%), intestinal metaplasia (83.3%) and dysplasia (80%) as compared to normal gastric mucosa (43.2%) (de Castro et al., 2010). More importantly, Cripto-1 expression was significantly higher in gastric carcinomas with lymph node metastasis (78.3%) than in those without metastasis (53.1%). Moreover, it has been described a positive correlation between Cripto-1 and P-STAT3 expression in gastric carcinomas, suggesting that up-regulation of Cripto-1 and P-STAT3 might play an important role in gastric carcinogenesis and lymph node metastasis. Finally, up-regulation of Cripto-1 expression and down-regulation of E-cadherin expression were found to be positively associated with tumor progression and poor prognosis in gastric cancer (de Castro et al., 2010). A positive correlation between high levels of Cripto-1 expression and tumor size, depth of invasion, positive lymph node metastasis, liver metastasis and TNM stage was also found. Combined analysis of Cripto-1 and E-cadherin had a significant value in predicting the metastatic potential of gastric cancer and patient prognosis.

Colon Cancer

Cripto-1 has been detected at high levels in 62–79% of primary and metastatic colon carcinomas in comparison to 3–16% of noninvolved adjacent mucosa, whereas Cripto-1 was not detected in normal colon samples (de Castro et al., 2010). The level of Cripto-1 expression in adenomas is directly related to the degree of dysplasia with higher levels of Cripto-1 expression in tubulovillous adenomas than tubular adenomas. Furthermore, Cripto-1 expression has been detected in 84% of colon carcinomas, 55% of colon adenomas and 62% of high-risk colon mucosa samples, while only 20% of non-high risk colon specimens were positive for Cripto-1. More recently, Cripto-1 expression was evaluated in a set of paired primary colon tumors and adjacent non-cancerous mucosa, revealing higher levels of Cripto-1 expression in 31% of colorectal tumors when compared with paired normal tissues (de Castro et al., 2010). In addition, high levels of Cripto-1 expression were found to be associated with venous and lymphatic invasion and metastasis. Furthermore, disease-free survival rate was significantly lower in patients with high Cripto-1 expression than in patients with low Cripto-1 expression, identifying Cripto-1 as a predictor for metachronous metastasis and selection of patients with poor prognosis. Moreover, a truncated form of Cripto-1, lacking the first two exons of the Cripto-1 gene, was isolated from a colon carcinoma cell line (de Castro et al., 2010). This short form of Cripto-1 has also been detected in primary human colon carcinomas and in liver metastasis from colon cancer. Interestingly, Cripto-1 short form can be directly regulated by the canonical *Wnt*/β-catenin signaling and since β-catenin activation is present in more than 70% of colon cancers, Cripto-1 up-regulation by β-catenin might contribute to the oncogenic activity of the canonical *Wnt*/β-catenin pathway during colon epithelial cell transformation (Hamada et al., 2007).

Pancreatic Cancer

Cripto-1 is overexpressed in approximately 44% of pancreatic ductal adenocarcinomas and in chronic pancreatitis, and has been shown to have positive association with advanced tumor stage (de Castro et al., 2010). Cripto-1 overexpression may also be involved in the tumorigenesis of gastric-type and pancreatobiliary-type intraductal papillary mucinous neoplasms (IPMNs) of the pancreas, since Cripto-1 was found to be up-regulated in 59.5% of pancreatic carcinomas and significantly increased in pancreatobiliary (80%) and gastric-type (68.4%) IPMNs. In fact, Cripto-1 expression might be associated with a growth advantage of pancreatic tumor cells, as well as with differentiation to form duct-like structures.

Non-small-cell Lung Cancer

Cripto-1 is expressed at high levels in 91% of stage I-IIIA adenocarcinomas of non-small-cell lung (NSCL) (de Castro et al., 2010). Moreover, a statistically significant association between overexpression of Cripto-1 and TGFα and AREG expression has been described. Consequently, evaluation of these growth factors might be useful, in addition to conventional pathological staging, to identify high-risk NSCLC patients who might benefit from post-surgical systemic therapies.

Other Tumors

Gall Bladder Cancer

Cripto-1 has been detected in hyperplasias (67%), adenomas (58%) or adenocarcinomas (68%) of the gall bladder (de Castro et al., 2010). Nevertheless, the incidence of cases with Cripto-1 expression was significantly higher in papillary and well-differentiated adenocarcinomas, as compared to moderately and poorly differentiated adenocarcinomas, suggesting that Cripto-1 expression might be associated with tumor differentiation.

Uveal Melanoma

Cripto-1 is expressed in uveal melanomas in comparison to non-neoplastic ocular tissues (de Castro et al., 2010). Cripto-1 was expressed in 94% of uveal melanomas with no intrascleral or extrascleral extension, whereas 77.7% of uveal melanomas with intrascleral/extrascleral extension and liver metastasis expressed Cripto-1.

Bladder Cancer

Bladder tumors, including areas of carcinoma in situ, express Cripto-1, whereas no detection of Cripto-1 has been reported in benign control tissue specimens (de Castro et al., 2010). Approximately 60% of bladder tumors had areas of papillary tumor with high levels of Cripto-1 expression as compared to 29% of normal urothelium adjacent to the tumors.

Skin Carcinomas

Cripto-1 overexpression has been detected in 80% of basal cell carcinomas samples as compared to normal skin samples (de Castro et al., 2010).

Nasopharyngeal Cancer

Cripto-1 has been recently associated with tumorigenesis and progression of nasopharyngeal carcinomas (NPC). High expression levels of Cripto-1 were detected in 54–76% NPC tissue samples and its overexpression was significantly associated with lymph node and distant metastasis, providing strong evidences that Cripto-1 might be involved in NPC malignant progression (de Castro et al., 2010).

Conclusions

Cripto-1 is an example of an embryonic gene that is re-expressed in an aberrant spatial and temporal manner in a variety of human tumors. Recent evidence has clearly demonstrated that Cripto-1 is expressed by a subset of cancer cells with stem-like characteristics (Watanabe et al., 2010). Cancer stem cells are considered to be a major obstacle in the complete eradication of tumors due their innate resistance to conventional therapy and therefore identification of surface markers that might differentiate cancer stem cells from the bulk population of tumor cells is under active investigation. Therefore, Cripto-1 targeting in human tumors might have a major breakthrough in cancer therapy. Several approaches have been used to target Cripto-1 in cancer cells in vitro and in vivo, from antisense oligonucleotides to blocking monoclonal antibodies (Bianco and Salomon, 2010). Finally, translation of Cripto-1 research to a clinical setting has been recently achieved. In fact, a humanized anti-Cripto-1 antibody conjugated with a potent cytotoxin is currently being evaluated in a Phase I clinical study in cancer patients.

References

Bendall SC, Stewart MH, Bhatia M (2008) Human embryonic stem cells: lessons from stem cell niches in vivo. Regen Med 3:365–376

Bianco C, Salomon DS (2010) Targeting the embryonic gene Cripto-1 in cancer and beyond. Expert Opin Ther Pat 20:1739–1749

Bianco C, Rangel MC, Castro NP, Nagaoka T, Rollman K, Gonzales M, Salomon DS (2010) Role of Cripto-1 in stem cell maintenance and malignant progression. Am J Pathol 177:532–540

Bianco C, Adkins HB, Wechselberger C, Seno M, Normanno N, De Luca A, Sun Y, Khan N, Kenney N, Ebert A, Williams KP, Sanicola M, Salomon DS (2002) Cripto-1 activates nodal- and ALK4-dependent and -independent signaling pathways in mammary epithelial cells. Mol Cell Biol 22: 2586–2597

Bianco C, Strizzi L, Rehman A, Normanno N, Wechselberger C, Sun Y, Khan N, Hirota M, Adkins H, Williams K, Margolis RU, Sanicola M, Salomon DS (2003) A Nodal- and ALK4-independent signaling pathway activated by Cripto-1 through Glypican-1 and c-Src. Cancer Res 63:1192–1197

Bianco C, Strizzi L, Ebert A, Chang C, Rehman A, Normanno N, Guedez L, Salloum R, Ginsburg E, Sun Y, Khan N, Hirota M, Wallace-Jones B, Wechselberger C, Vonderhaar BK, Tosato G, Stetler-Stevenson WG, Sanicola M, Salomon DS (2005) Role of human cripto-1 in tumor angiogenesis. J Natl Cancer Inst 97:132–141

Bianco C, Strizzi L, Mancino M, Rehman A, Hamada S, Watanabe K, De Luca A, Jones B, Balogh G, Russo J, Mailo D, Palaia R, D'Aiuto G, Botti G, Perrone F, Salomon DS, Normanno N (2006) Identification of cripto-1 as a novel serologic marker for breast and colon cancer. Clin Cancer Res 12:5158–5164

Bianco C, Mysliwiec M, Watanabe K, Mancino M, Nagaoka T, Gonzales M, Salomon DS (2008a) Activation of a Nodal-independent signaling pathway by Cripto-1 mutants with impaired activation of a Nodal-dependent signaling pathway. FEBS Lett 582:3997–4002

Bianco C, Strizzi L, Mancino M, Watanabe K, Gonzales M, Hamada S, Raafat A, Sahlah L, Chang C, Sotgia F, Normanno N, Lisanti M, Salomon DS (2008b) Regulation of Cripto-1 signaling and biological activity by caveolin-1 in mammary epithelial cells. Am J Pathol 172:345–357

Bianco C, Cotten C, Lonardo E, Strizzi L, Baraty C, Mancino M, Gonzales M, Watanabe K, Nagaoka T, Berry C, Arai AE, Minchiotti G, and Salomon DS (2009) Cripto-1 is required for hypoxia to induce cardiac differentiation of mouse embryonic stem cells. Am J Pathol 175:2146–2158

Bianco C, Rangel MC, Castro NP, Nagaoka T, Rollman K, Gonzales M, Salomon DS (2010) Role of Cripto-1 in stem cell maintenance and malignant progression. Am J Pathol 177:532–540

Cocciadiferro L, Miceli V, Kang KS, Polito LM, Trosko JE, Carruba G (2009) Profiling cancer stem cells in androgen-responsive and refractory human prostate tumor cell lines. Ann NY Acad Sci 1155:257–262

Cole MF, Johnstone SE, Newman JJ, Kagey MH, Young RA (2008) Tcf3 is an integral component of the core regulatory circuitry of embryonic stem cells. Genes Dev 22:746–755

D'Andrea D, Liguori GL, Le Good JA, Lonardo E, Andersson O, Constam DB, Persico MG, Minchiotti G (2008) Cripto promotes A–P axis specification independently of its stimulatory effect on Nodal autoinduction. J Cell Biol 180:597–605

de Castro NP, Rangel MC, Nagaoka T, Salomon DS, and Bianco C (2010) Cripto-1: an embryonic gene that promotes tumorigenesis. Future Oncol 6:1127–1142

di Bari MG, Ginsburg E, Plant J, Strizzi L, Salomon DS, Vonderhaar BK (2009) Msx2 induces epithelial-mesenchymal transition in mouse mammary epithelial cells through upregulation of Cripto-1. J Cell Physiol 219:659–666

Hamada S, Watanabe K, Hirota M, Bianco C, Strizzi L, Mancino M, Gonzales M, Salomon DS (2007) beta-Catenin/TCF/LEF regulate expression of the short form human Cripto-1. Biochem Biophys Res Commun 355:240–244

Hollier BG, Evans K, Mani SA (2009) The epithelial-to-mesenchymal transition and cancer stem cells: a coalition against cancer therapies. J Mammary Gland Biol Neoplasia 14:29–43

Hough SR, Laslett AL, Grimmond SB, Kolle G, Pera MF (2009) A continuum of cell states spans pluripotency and lineage commitment in human embryonic stem cells. PLoS One 4:e7708

Kenney NJ, Smith GH, Maroulakou IG, Green JH, Muller WJ, Callahan R, Salomon DS, Dickson RB (1996) Detection of amphiregulin and Cripto-1 in mammary tumors from transgenic mice. Mol Carcinog 15:44–56

Koestenbauer S, Zech NH, Juch H, Vanderzwalmen P, Schoonjans L, Dohr G (2006) Embryonic stem cells: similarities and differences between human and murine embryonic stem cells. Am J Reprod Immunol 55:169–180

Lawrence MG, Margaryan NV, Loessner D, Collins A, Kerr KM, Turner M, Seftor EA, Stephens CR, Lai J, Postovit LM, Clements JA, Hendrix MJ (2011) Reactivation of embryonic nodal signaling is associated with tumor progression and promotes the growth of prostate cancer cells. Prostate. 71:1198–1209

Lee CC, Jan HJ, Lai JH, Ma HI, Hueng DY, Lee YC, Cheng YY, Liu LW, Wei HW, Lee HM (2010) Nodal promotes growth and invasion in human gliomas. Oncogene 29:3110–3123

Micalizzi DS, Wang CA, Farabaugh SM, Schiemann WP, Ford HL (2010) Homeoprotein Six1 increases TGF-beta type I receptor and converts TGF-beta signaling from suppressive to supportive for tumor growth. Cancer Res 70:10371–10380

Morkel M, Huelsken J, Wakamiya M, Ding J, van de Wetering M, Clevers H, Taketo MM, Behringer RR, Shen MM, Birchmeier W (2003) Beta-catenin regulates Cripto- and Wnt3-dependent gene expression programs in mouse axis and mesoderm formation. Development 130:6283–6294

Shi S, Ge C, Luo Y, Hou X, Haltiwanger RS, Stanley P (2007) The threonine that carries fucose, but not fucose, is required for Cripto to facilitate Nodal signaling. J Biol Chem 282:20133–20141

Strizzi L, Bianco C, Normanno N, Seno M, Wechselberger C, Wallace-Jones B, Khan NI, Hirota M, Sun Y, Sanicola M, Salomon DS (2004) Epithelial mesenchymal transition is a characteristic of hyperplasias and tumors in mammary gland from MMTV-Cripto-1 transgenic mice. J Cell Physiol 201:266–276

Strizzi L, Bianco C, Hirota M, Watanabe K, Mancino M, Hamada S, Raafat A, Lawson S, Ebert A, D'Antonio A, Losito S, Normanno N, Salomon D (2007) Development of leiomyosarcoma of the uterus in MMTV-CR-1 transgenic mice. J Pathol 211:36–44

Strizzi L, Abbott DE, Salomon DS, Hendrix MJ (2008) Potential for cripto-1 in defining stem cell-like characteristics in human malignant melanoma. Cell Cycle 7:1931–1935

Sun Y, Strizzi L, Raafat A, Hirota M, Bianco C, Feigenbaum L, Kenney N, Wechselberger C, Callahan R, Salomon DS (2005) Overexpression of human Cripto-1 in transgenic mice delays mammary gland development and differentiation and induces mammary tumorigenesis. Am J Pathol 167:585–597

Thiery JP, Acloque H, Huang RY, Nieto MA (2009) Epithelial-mesenchymal transitions in development and disease. Cell 139:871–890

Visvader JE, Lindeman GJ (2008) Cancer stem cells in solid tumours: accumulating evidence and unresolved questions. Nat Rev Cancer 8:755–768

Watanabe K, Bianco C, Strizzi L, Hamada S, Mancino M, Bailly V, Mo W, Wen D, Miatkowski K, Gonzales M, Sanicola M, Seno M, Salomon DS (2007) Growth factor induction of cripto-1 shedding by GPI-phospholipase D and enhancement of endothelial cell migration. J Biol Chem 282:31643–31655

Watanabe K, Nagaoka T, Lee JM, Bianco C, Gonzales M, Castro NP, Rangel MC, Sakamoto K, Sun Y, Callahan R, Salomon DS (2009) Enhancement of Notch receptor maturation and signaling sensitivity by Cripto-1. J Cell Biol 187:343–353

Watanabe K, Meyer MJ, Strizzi L, Lee JM, Gonzales M, Bianco C, Nagaoka T, Farid SS, Margaryan N, Hendrix MJ, Vonderhaar BK, Salomon DS (2010) Cripto-1 is a cell surface marker for a tumorigenic, undifferentiated subpopulation in human embryonal carcinoma cells. Stem Cells 28:1303–1314

Wechselberger C, Ebert AD, Bianco C, Khan NI, Sun Y, Wallace-Jones B, Montesano R, Salomon DS (2001) Cripto-1 enhances migration and branching morphogenesis of mouse mammary epithelial cells. Exp Cell Res 266:95–105

Wechselberger C, Strizzi L, Kenney N, Hirota M, Sun Y, Ebert A, Orozco O, Bianco C, Khan NI, Wallace-Jones B, Normanno N, Adkins H, Sanicola M, Salomon DS (2005) Human Cripto-1 overexpression in the mouse mammary gland results in the development of hyperplasia and adenocarcinoma. Oncogene 24:4094–4105

Wei CL, Miura T, Robson P, Lim SK, Xu XQ, Lee MY, Gupta S, Stanton L, Luo Y, Schmitt J, Thies S, Wang W, Khrebtukova I, Zhou D, Liu ET, Ruan YJ, Rao M, Lim B (2005) Transcriptome profiling of human and murine ESCs identifies divergent paths required to maintain the stem cell state. Stem Cells 23:166–185

Wu Z, Li G, Wu L, Weng D, Li X, Yao K (2009) Cripto-1 overexpression is involved in the tumorigenesis of nasopharyngeal carcinoma. BMC Cancer 9:315

Part III
Diseases

Chapter 18

Treatment of Heart Disease: Use of Transdifferentiation Methodology for Reprogramming Adult Stem Cells

Milán Bustamante, Macarena Perán, Juan Antonio Marchal,
Fernando Rodríguez-Serrano, Pablo Álvarez, and Antonia Aránega

Abstract Despite significant progress in medical research, cardiovascular diseases (CVDs) continue to be the largest contributors to morbidity and mortality in both developed and developing countries. The discovery of multipotent cell populations in adult tissues has opened up new therapeutic possibilities for diseases that cannot be successfully treated by conventional medical therapies. The scientific community is developing new methods to improve clinical outcomes, including the transplantation of stem cells in a pre-differentiated state. In vivo studies have demonstrated the capacity of these cells to differentiate into another cell type through the triggering of a genetic switch by pathological or inductive conditions. This process, whereby one cell type committed to and progressing along a specific developmental lineage switches into another cell type of a different lineage, is designated transdifferentiation and takes place in tissues generated from neighbouring regions during normal embryonic development. In this chapter, we review the current methods of transdifferentiation including guided cardiopoiesis, cellular extracts, co-culture techniques, viral vectors, hyperpolarization, among others.

Keywords Cardiovascular diseases · Myocardial infarction · Stem cells · Cardiomyocytes · Troponin · Sarcomere

Introduction

Major advances in medical science have reduced infant mortality and increased life expectancy in the developed world through the control of numerous diseases. However, the aging of populations has brought about an increase in chronic and degenerative diseases and a high incidence of cancer and cardiovascular diseases (CVDs). CVDs are characterized as multifactorial in origin and pose a complex and important public health challenge worldwide. In this regard, biomedical research efforts and investment have focused on the search for heart transplantation options. This approach is indicated in patients who have suffered end-stage heart failure and are unresponsive to conventional therapy. However, there are a number of preoperative and postoperative risks, besides the major challenge of finding an optimal donor heart and the elevated healthcare costs involved (currently ranging from € 27,839 to 51,575 per case), given the uncertain long-term outcomes of the procedure (Pérez Romero et al., 2010).

A large proportion of CVDs are attributable to ischemic heart disease, and approximately two-thirds of patients surviving acute myocardial infarction (AMI) are left with debilitating congestive heart failure. AMI causes apoptosis and necrosis and produces the ventricular remodeling of non-ischemic myocardium with scar formation, increasing the likelihood of a new crisis, progressive ventricular dilatation, and heart failure, ending in death (Torella et al., 2007). Regenerative medicine has emerged as a promising tool for the treatment of AMI through cardiac regeneration. Scientific evidence in the fields of cell therapy

A. Aránega (✉)
Biopathology and Medicine Regenerative Institute (IBIMER),
Granada, Spain
e-mail: aranega@ugr.es

and regenerative medicine has demonstrated the possibilities of obtaining therapeutic solutions to pathological situations without current treatment or enhancing existing therapies with the utilization of stem cells from the patients themselves or from compatible individuals. Valuable scientific data are expected to become available in the near future on the mechanisms that regulate the viability, proliferation, and differentiation of cells in normal and pathological conditions.

Many different cell types have been considered for myocardial repair, but the ideal candidate has yet to be identified. Adult cardiomyocytes are unable to survive even when transplanted into the normal myocardium, and resident populations of cardiac progenitors are inadequate in AMI cases. Because fetal or neonatal cardiomyocytes are not a feasible source of cells, due to ethical issues and donor availability, research has focused on pluripotent stem cells as a source for myocardial repair and regeneration, and various stem cell types have been proposed. Researchers remain engaged in the search for the optimal cell type for myocardial repair, and a greater understanding of the development of the heart has led to novel therapeutic strategies that emulate the cardiogenic program, currently undergoing pre-clinical trials. Knowledge of the cellular components of the heart and their response to injury is crucial for the design of experiments and therapies in myocardial repair and regeneration.

Characterization of Cardiac Cells

Embryo-Molecular Features

The vascular system of the human embryo appears halfway through the third week, when embryos are no longer able to meet their nutritional requirements solely by diffusion. Cardiac progenitor cells are found in the epiblast and migrate to form the ventricles and the sinus, reaching the splanchnic plate of the lateral mesoderm. Endocardial cells (angioblasts) also appear in the mesoderm, where they proliferate and coalesce forming angiocysts, small clumps that eventually grow and join together, forming a horseshoe-shaped tube lined with endothelium (surrounded by myoblasts), known as the cardiogenic field, which then connects with the dorsal aorta to form the heart tube (Moore and Persaud, 2000).

Figure 18.1 represents the heart development pathways and the factors involved in each one. Early cardiac tube myocytes derive from at least two cardiac progenitor cell populations. Stem cells derived from the First Heart Field (FHF) of the Primary Heart Tube are responsible for initiating differentiation in the growing stage. The Second Heart Field (SHF) corresponds to a population of cardiac multipotent progenitor cells from the pharyngeal epithelium and the splanchnic mesoderm, which proliferate and contribute dynamically to the heart tube growth at both poles, providing the majority of right ventricular myocytes (RV), the outflow tract, left ventricular (LV), and atrium (Buckingham et al., 2005).

Recent studies identified a group of epicardial progenitor cells, a cell population that contributes to the atrium, ventricular myocardium, coronary smooth muscle, and cardiac fibroblasts, but which could not be tracked due to the lack of specific molecular markers. However, it has been shown that stem cells derived from SHF, myocardial, smooth muscle, and endothelial cells may express a characteristic cardiac stem cell transcription factor, the LIM-homeodomain factor ISLT-1. There have also been reports of a third group of epicardial progenitors that express the transcription factors Tbx18 or Wt1 (Zhou et al., 2008).

A number of factors have been involved in the development of SHF progenitor cells, including transcription factors Tbx1, Foxh1, MEF2C, and Hand2, which, along with ISLT-1 and Fgf8 and FGF10 growth factors, are responsible for the negative regulation of SHF progenitor cell differentiation (Buckingham et al., 2005). These growth factors are positively regulated by Tbx1 transcription factor (part of the T-box family). ISLT-1, Gata4, and Foxh1, control the expression of MEF2C, a transcription factor essential to cardiomyocyte and endothelial cell lineages (Xu et al., 2004). The development of SHF also critically depends on bone morphogenetic protein (BMP) signaling. BMP 2.4, 6, and 7 have expression patterns of ISLT-1 accumulation; therefore, deletions of these regions result in multiple defects in SHF-derived structures.

Morphofunctional Features

Cardiomyocytes, responsible for muscle contraction, are cylindrical cells 80–90 μm in length and 15 μm in width. One or two oval nuclei are arranged in

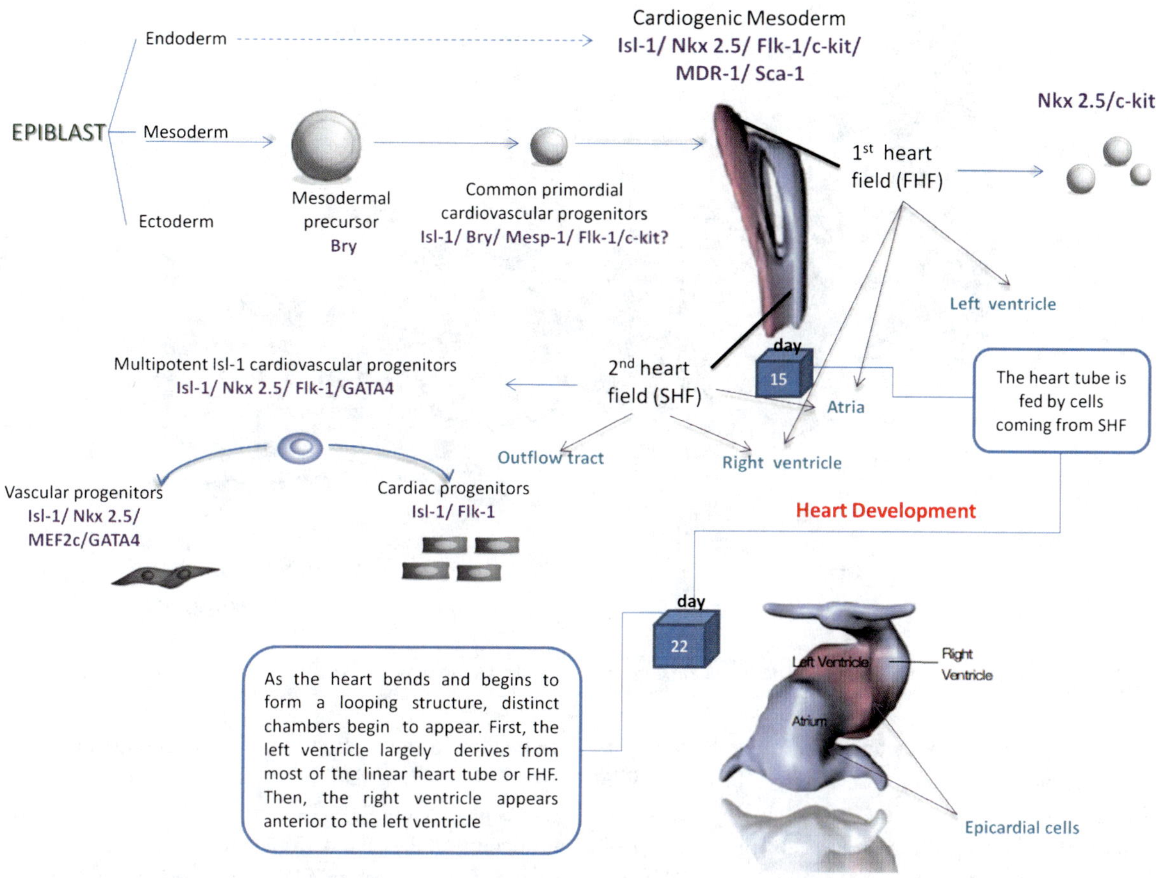

Fig. 18.1 Cell markers involved in heart development

the middle of the cell, whose ends are joined by intercalated discs, with most of its volume occupied by myofibrils, structures responsible for cell contractility. Intercalated discs include desmosomes, which connect cells (gap junctions) and establish communication between the two neighboring sarcoplasmic spaces, facilitating the transmission of depolarizing waves between cells and regulating the timing of their contractions. They also play a structural role in fixing thin myofilaments (which is why they correspond to sarcomeric Z-discs) to those that guide transverse or T tubules, corresponding to long and wide invaginations of the sarcolemma (cell membrane) (Pasek et al., 2008).

The sarcoplasmic reticulum is formed by a set of tubules and saccules arranged along the longitudinal axis of the cell, and it serves the important function of storing calcium ion, which is necessary for contraction of the myofibril. Contraction is therefore the result of the release of intracellular calcium from the sarcoplasmic reticulum or from outside the cell, while relaxation corresponds to its absence in the sarcoplasm.

The myocardiocyte cytoskeleton comprises a complex network of protein filaments in the cytoplasm, which are responsible for stabilizing the situation and relationships of intracellular components and for controlling cell size, shape, and movements, including the muscle contraction process. The cytoskeleton contains three different types of protein filaments: actin filaments, microtubules, and intermediate filaments (Fig. 18.2), a common organization to all eukaryotic cells, but especially well-developed in muscle cells. The myofibril, the element that endows heart cells with the ability to contract, is made up of sarcomeres, structural units 2.5 μm in length that are visible under light microscopy. They are aligned, giving the characteristic striated cell appearance, and show a pattern of alternating light and dark bands under electron microscopy,

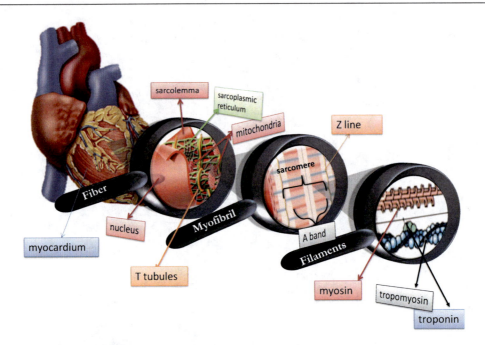

Fig. 18.2 Heart structures showing in detail the protein composition of the cardiomyocyte cytoskeleton

with the dark band (A or anisotropic band) having a central location and length of 1.5 μm. In the middle of this band is a clear region called the H zone, which is divided in two by the M line. The light band (I or isotropic band), located on both sides of the A band, has a variable length.

In the centre of the M line is the Z disk or line, which separates one sarcomere from the next. The sarcomere contains two groups of partially overlapping protein filaments, thin filaments and thick ones. The thin filaments have a length of 1.0 μm and diameter of 8 nm and extend from the Z line of the I band, which they penetrate without reaching the H zone. They are composed of actin, a contractile protein whose subunit, the polypeptide globular actin or G (43,000 Da), is related to one Ca^{+2} ion (which stabilizes the globular configuration), one molecule of ATP and F-actin double-stranded coiled helix (resulting from the polymerization of actin G), which is closely connected with myosin and tropomyosin, responsible for regulating contraction through Ca^{+2}. Troponin (Tn) is a complex of proteins: troponin C (TnC), troponin I (TnI) and troponin T (TnT). Calcium binds to TnC (18,459 Da) and carries the signal to TnT (38,000 Da) and TnI (23,550 Da). The interactions between the three troponin subunits are of primary interest, because their binding to Ca^{+2} and phosphorylation triggers a cascade of changes in the interaction of other members of the myofibril proteins, leading to contraction. The thick filaments have a length of 1.6 μm and diameter of 15 nm and occupy the A band from one end to the other. In summary, both types of filaments overlap the A band, only thin filaments are found in the I band, and only thick filaments in the H band (Pasek et al., 2008).

Cell Replacement in Normal Myocardium and Pathogenesis of Acute Myocardial Infarction (AMI)

We now know that cardiomyocytes represent ∼20–30% of the total cell population of the human heart. The number of cells entering the mitotic cycle every day is the same as that, entering apoptosis, i.e., ∼0.06% of the total population of cardiomyocytes, implying a total renewal of heart tissue over 4–5 years under normal conditions and over a longer period in patients with cardiac hypertrophy or aortic stenosis (Rubart and Field, 2006).

Cardiac stem cells (CSCs) have been shown to re-enter the cell cycle and differentiate into cardiomyocytes in cases of cardiac stress, with increased frequency in cases of acute cardiac stress. This acute injury results in an increase in myocardial mass due to the combination of cardiomyocyte hypertrophy and hyperplasia. The functions of these cells have been reported to include the regulation of cardiac homeostasis in healthy individuals, with the cells being responsible for maintaining the balance between loss and cell division, which is lost when the number of cardiomyocytes undergoing apoptosis and necrosis exceeds the capacity of the progenitors to divide (Torella et al., 2007).

Molecular cardiologists have studied the cascade of intracellular mechanisms that leads to AMI, which can be understood as the dysregulation of signal cascade beta-adrenergic proteins, specifically beta adrenergic receptor βAR, responsible for regulating heart rate and contractility in response to catecholamines (agonists). The binding of an agonist activates the heterotrimeric G-protein second messenger system, which results in stimulatory G-protein alpha-subunit (G S) dissociation. This stimulates adenylyl cyclase (AC) to increase cyclic adenosine monophosphate (cAMP) production, which then activates protein kinase A (PKA). The PKA-dependent phosphorylation of several downstream targets such as troponin-1, phospholamban (PLB), and L-type calcium channels mediates the physiological effects of βAR stimulation. A defect in this pathway leads to an increased sympathetic response resulting in βAR overstimulation, which is initially compensatory but results in chronic heart failure over the long term (Hung et al., 2007).

In cardiomyocytes, membrane excitation results in the entry of calcium via the L-type calcium channel, triggering the release of intracellular stores of calcium from the sarcoplasmic reticulum (SR) via the ryanodine receptor, a calcium release channel. The resulting rise in intracellular calcium causes sarcomeric shortening and muscle contraction. Conversely, muscle relaxation is initiated by a fall in intracellular calcium, a process that is largely driven by sarcoplasmic endoreticulum Ca-ATPase (SERCA)-mediated reuptake of calcium into the SR. The activity of SERCA is modulated by phospholamban (PLN), a SR transmembrane protein. Increased SERCA activity due to PLN phosphorylation results in increased SR calcium reuptake and subsequent release. A second mechanism involved in the intracellular homeostasis of cardiomyocytes is the dysregulation of calcium handling proteins SERCA2a (endoreticulum sarcoplasmic Ca-ATPase), responsible for transporting 75% of calcium from the sarcoplasmic reticulum, allowing the process of muscular contraction and relaxation. Dysregulation of SERCA2a leads to an inability of the cell to recapture calcium from sarcoplasmic reticulum, which affects muscular contraction and relaxation and produces long-term heart failure, as reported in transplant patients (Rengo et al., 2009).

Estimates of cardiac replacement after AMI range from 0.0005 to 3%. However, although cardiomyocytes in the infarcted area die in the first few hours, inducing ischemic damage of vascular and avascular components of the interstitium, Ki-67-measured mitotic activity is still observed. The proliferation of cardiomyocytes at the edge of the infarcted area is two-fold normal rates, and tissue oxygenation is maintained. At molecular level, the extent of AMI is determined by the presence of microRNA associated with myocardial death. Mir-1 is muscle-specific, being expressed abundantly in heart and skeletal muscles with little expression in other tissues, and it is known that the increase in circulating Mir-1 in AMI patients is related to its release by necrotic cardiomyocytes. The aberrant expression of Mir-1 has been associated with arrhythmogenesis in various heart diseases. One of the known mechanisms of arrhythmia is the action of Mir-1 on genes that encode proteins connexin 43 and Kir2.1, which play a crucial role in maintaining cardiac conduction (Ai et al., 2010). Greater understanding of the embryological mechanisms and molecular factors involved in the development of the vascular system and increased knowledge of the growth factors that regulate the proliferation of stem cell populations have considerably advanced the therapeutic possibilities of regenerative medicine in heart disease.

Fundamentals of Cardiac Regeneration

Regenerative Biomedicine efforts have focused on attempts to reverse the failure of the heart muscle by increasing the amount of human functional heart muscle through the transplantation of various adult stem cell types, notably cardiac stem cells, skeletal myoblasts, endothelial stem cells, and mesenchymal stem cells. Drawbacks of embryonic stem cells, besides ethical and legal issues, include problems of allograft rejection and their tendency, due to their totipotency, to form teratomata. In contrast, adult stem

Table 18.1 Sources for adult stem cell heart regeneration

Cell type	Identification	Cell marker expression	Sources
Hematopoietic stem cells	HSCs	Lineage-, c-kit +, SCA-1+, CD34, CD38, CD 31, CD 133	Peripheral blood (PB), bone marrow (BM), umbilical cord blood (UCB)
Endothelial progenitor cells	EPCs	CD133, CD34, KDR+	PB; BM; UCB
Mesenchymal stem cells	MSCs	CD105, CD73, CD90	BM; adipose tissue, umbilical cord (UC), UCB
Muscle-derived stem cells	Myoblasts, satellite cells	Pax 7+, Wht ++, Vim+, Desm+	Basal membrane of muscle fibers
Cardiac stem cells	CSCs	SCA-1, ISL-1, C-kit +	Myocardium

cells are considered a potential therapeutic tool due to their ability to proliferate and self-renew in vitro and their capacity to differentiate into specialized cell types. Table 18.1 shows the different sources of cells that have been tested for cardiac regeneration, indicating the specific cellular markers used for their isolation.

Cardiac Stem Cells

Cardiac Stem Cells are scattered in specific niches in the heart wall thickness, with a larger population in the atrium. These clusters are intimately connected by gap junctions and zonula adherens to myocytes and fibroblasts, with both types of cells fulfilling a support function in these niches. There have also been observations of symmetric and asymmetric division due to the uniform and dispersed location, respectively, of the proteins Numb and α-adaptin in these niches during mitosis and of the co-expression of stem cell marker c-kit (receptor growth factor or SCF stem cells, Stem Cell Factor), myocyte transcription factors, and sarcomere proteins. CSCs have also been shown to be negative for hematopoietic markers. The expression of other stem cell markers has also been reported, including stem cell antigen 1 (Sca-1), P-glycoprotein (involved in the Multi-Drug Resistance phenomenon), and ISLT-1. CSCs are multipotent cells that can generate cardiac progenitors (PgCs) committed to any of the heart lineages (cardiomyocytes, smooth muscle cells, and endothelial cells). PgCs have the capacity to proliferate, becoming precursors (PrC) and, finally, differentiated cells. It has also been found that HGF and IGF-1 growth factors are responsible for promoting the migration, proliferation, and survival of CSCs in cases of an acute injury (Chien et al., 2008).

High expectations have been raised by resident CSCs for the treatment of ischemic cardiovascular disease. Novel strategies are under development, including new drugs, with the aim of mobilizing and encouraging CSCs to generate cardiomyocytes in situ. There is greater knowledge of the localization, isolation, and characterization of CSC populations and on isolation methods and their cloning in the adult heart. However, the difficulty with their therapeutic use, in terms of feasibility and patient safety, is the variability in this cell population as a function of age, sex, and pathophysiological state of the heart.

Evaluation of the Use of Adult Stem Cells from Other Tissues

Adult stem cells, e.g., mesenchymal stem cells, and hematopoietic stem cells, are found in almost every tissue in the body, can differentiate into more than one cell type, and can be isolated and grown in vitro. Clinical trials have been conducted using bone marrow derived cells (BM-SCs). Initial results were interpreted in terms of the transdifferentiation of BM-SCs into cardiomyocytes but it now appears that the beneficial effects of this treatment are more realistically linked to an increased angiogenesis or to the secretion of paracrine factors by the transplanted cells. Thus, endothelial cell precursors might produce capillaries that could help preserve more cardiomyocytes around the infarction area, and the infused cells might produce trophic factors that would prevent cell death and/or stimulate the proliferation of resident stem cells, as shown in Fig. 18.3. However, the interpretation of the clinical trials is complicated by the heterogeneity of results, probably derived from differences in

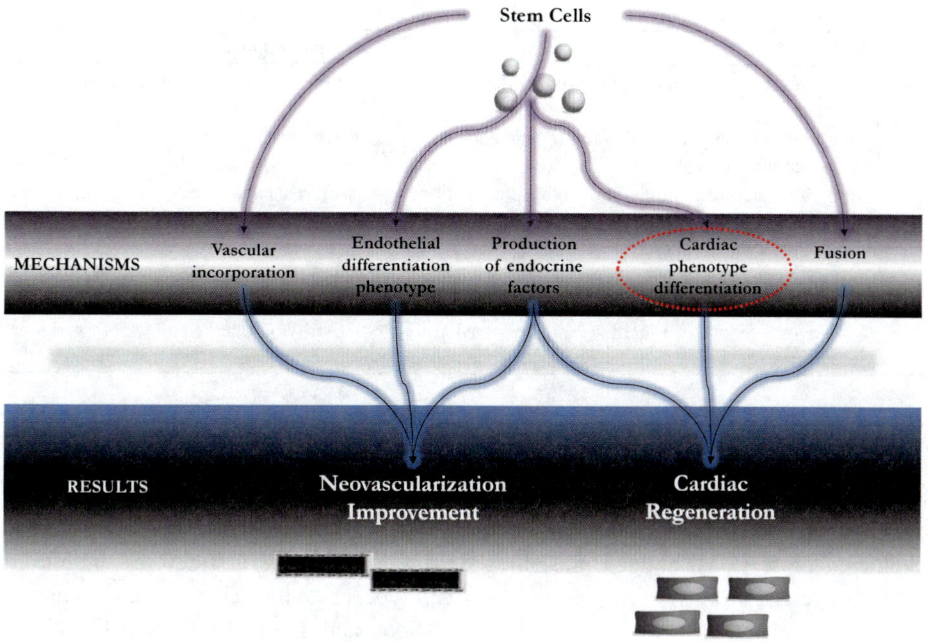

Fig. 18.3 Possible mechanisms of action of stem cells in myocardial infarction

design, selection, cell source, dose, route, and timing, hampering comparisons.

Limitations of pre-clinical studies in the field of cardiovascular disease include the production of arrhythmogenesis with the use of skeletal myoblast precursors and controversy over the real scope of BM-SCs transdifferentiation. There is a need for researchers to follow strict criteria in the selection of an appropriate source of stem cells, taking account of patient safety, methods for their production, and ethical and legal norms. Human mesenchymal stem cells (hMCSs) appear to be promising candidates given their multipotency and ready availability, e.g., via liposuction. It is necessary to establish an in vitro differentiation strategy to transform these cells into functional cardiomyocytes that can integrate in a damaged heart and exert therapeutic action. Table 18.2 summarizes the advantages and disadvantages of using stem cells for myocardial regeneration in vivo.

Mesenchymal Stem Cells (MSCs) Features: Paracrine and Immunology Activity

There have been clinical trials on the use of cultured MSCs in the regeneration of cartilage and bone regeneration, finding that they participated in the formation of new tissue via paracrine signal-induced differentiation into endogenous cells. Investigation of the paracrine effect of MSCs in rat AMI models, using intramyocardial injection of culture medium with MSC-secreted growth factors and cytokines (conditioned medium), demonstrated their role in stromal network creation, neovascularization enhancement, angiogenesis promotion, and cardiac function improvement (Parekkadan and Milwid, 2010). Paracrine effects of MSCs may include the activation of different mechanisms against cell damage. Ex vivo therapeutic models have shown that MSCs are recruited to infarction areas by the hepatocyte growth factor (HGF), which is released during necrosis and apoptosis and acts as a "homing signal"; this migration of MSCs depends on interaction with c-Met, an HGF receptor (Kauser et al., 2007).

MSC-derived conditioned medium was found to promote the proliferation of CSCs and inhibit the apoptosis of CSCs induced by hypoxia and serum starvation. It also upregulated expression of cardiomyocyte-related genes in CSCs, including b-myosin heavy chain (b-MHC) and atrial natriuretic peptide (ANP), demonstrating the protective effects of this medium on CSCs and its enhancement of their migration and

Table 18.2 Advantages and disadvantages of using stem cells for myocardial regeneration in vivo

Cell type	Advantages	Disadvantages
HSCs	Autologous, easy isolation and high proliferation rate	Questionable role in cardiomyogenesis and angiogenesis
EPCs	Autologous, readily available, angiogenic and vasculogenic potential	Uncertain functional activity
MSCs	Autologous, reduced antigenicity, multiple locations for extraction, easy isolation and cryopreservation, paracrine potential	Fibrosis and calcification, and the dependence of their expansion and differentiation on cell age
CSCs	Essential role in myocardial regeneration	Population kinetics, differentiation and apoptosis unknown. Low rate of isolation
Myoblasts	Autologous, reduced antigenicity, high expansion rate	Arrhythmogenic and lack of gap junction

differentiation (Nakanishi et al., 2008). With regard to their immunomodulatory properties, MSCs inhibit T cell proliferation and influence the maturation and expression profile of professional antigen presenting cells such as dendritic cells.

Transdifferentiation and Mesenchymal Stem Cells

Mesenchymal Stem Cells, are self-renewing, multipotent cells present in numerous adult tissues, including bone marrow, trabecular bone, adipose, and muscle. In response to specific culture conditions, MSCs can give rise to multiple mesenchyme-derived cell types, such as osteoblasts, chondrocytes, adipocytes, and myoblasts. Furthermore, in vivo transplantation studies have shown that MSCs can replenish the whole bone marrow system in irradiated rodents and generate not only mesodermal cells but also cells characteristic of neural progenitors and neurons. This type of cross-lineage differentiation, also known as transdifferentiation, is a process whereby one cell type committed to and progressing along a specific developmental lineage switches into another cell type of a different lineage through genetic reprogramming, and it implies that adult stem cells maintain their multidifferentiation potential even after exposure to specific inductive factors (Song and Tuan, 2004).

Transdifferentiation takes place in pathological conditions, such as Barret's Metaplasia, in which the stratified squamous epithelium that normally lines the lower part of the esophagus transdifferentiates into an intestinal-like tissue with an increased risk of tumorigenesis (Tosh and Slack, 2002). Questions remain to be answered. How do cells transdifferentiate? Do differentiated cells dedifferentiate into a primitive cell type first before committing to another cell type, or do they change their phenotype directly?

Song and Tuan (2004) used hMSCs with defined culture medium and observed an extensive proliferation of differentiated cells in the transdifferentiation process, suggesting that pre-committed cells change their phenotype via proliferation by dedifferentiating into a primitive stem cell stage, perhaps through genome reprogramming. Regulation of cell dedifferentiation and transdifferentiation play important roles in the development, maintenance, and regeneration of mammalian tissues. The conversion from adult differentiated cells must involve both the suppression and regulation of different genes in the cells, implying that genes from both cell types are co-expressed at some point. Cell transdifferentiation occurs when the pre-and post-differentiation states are clearly defined, showing the morphological and functional characteristics of both cell types (Tosh and Slack, 2002). Studies on transdifferentiation support the notion that cell fate is controlled by master switch genes, and that one or two factors can be sufficient to direct cells from one lineage to another (Burke and Tosh, 2005).

This technique is beginning to emerge as a recommended strategy for the generation of cardiac cells, supported by the normal occurrence of transdifferentiation in tissues generated from neighboring regions during embryonic development (Tosh and Slack, 2002). Developmental biology studies have identified molecular regulators, such as cell cycle proteins, transcription factors, or other signaling molecules, which control cross-lineage commitment among different cell types. Examples include the well-documented influence of signals released from the cardiac mesoderm on ventral pancreas development, and the blocking of FGF or BMP growth factor signals when the cardiac mesoderm is removed, with the consequent inhibition of liver development (Calmont et al., 2006).

Molecular Mechanisms Involved in Transdifferentiation: Cardiopoiesis

Cardiopoiesis is defined as the definitive engagement of pluripotent or multipotent stem cells in the cardiac differentiation program. Cardiopoietic specification is based on the emulation of natural cardiac development within the embryo, which occurs in the mesoderm under the cardioinductive influence of the neighboring endoderm. This potential influence was found to be enhanced by the cytokine tumor necrosis factor (TNF), allowing the recognition of a combination of factors that can drive naive stem cells towards the cardiac program. With high throughput screening, cardiogenic instructive signals were deciphered and found to be efficacious in inducing expression and nuclear translocation of cardiac master genes, indicating definitive cardiac commitment and lineage specification. There is also evidence that cardiac master genes GATA4, Nkx2.5, and MEF2C are involved in the acquisition of the cardiac phenotype by stem cells (Behfar et al., 2008).

Cardiopoietic guidance emulates natural cardiac differentiation and can be achieved by stimulating stem cells with TGF-β1, BMP-2/4, FGF-2/4, IL-6, IGF-1/2, VEGF-A, EGF, and activin-A. These factors, used as a recombinant cocktail regimen in 5% platelet human lysate, allowed the nuclear translocation of Nkx2.5 by day 2 of differentiation and of later cardiac transcription factors MEF-2C and GATA4 by day 4, which is a critical step in the differentiation of stem cells into the cardiac phenotype. Nuclear transport plays a vital role in tissue specificity. At molecular level, the cardiac phenotype is associated with an increased density of pores, whose constant remodeling depends on active nuclear transport. The energy requirements to support this process derive from a change in metabolic mechanism from anaerobic glycolytic to mitochondrial oxidative type (Behfar et al., 2008).

Methods to Direct Transdifferentiation of Stem Cells to Cardiomyocytes

MSCs have shown promising results in cardiomyoplasty techniques. Knowledge of the molecular machinery and paracrine signals of both mesenchymal populations (MSCs and adult cardiomyocytes) has permitted the generation of cardiomyocytes through transdifferentiation. The strategies adopted are described below.

Guided Cardiopoiesis: Generation of Cardiopoietic Stem Cells, An Enriched Population of MSCs

Currently over a thousand patients worldwide have participated in clinical trials exploring the therapeutic value of MSCs obtained from bone marrow, using strategies that emulate the embryogenic program to recruit cardiac progenitors of these adult cells. The first approach was to use induction with BMP or TGF- β, two prototypic cardiotrophins, which resulted in upregulation of cytosolic expression of cardiac transcription factors Nkx2.5 and MEF2C but not in promotion of the nuclear translocation necessary for definitive cardiac specification. The upregulation of these factors in the cytosol after cardiogenic stimulation evidences the cardiogenic aptitude of human MSCs (Fig. 18.4), but induction with individual cardiotrophic factors is suboptimal because it does not secure definitive engagement in the cardiac program, which requires the importation of cardiac transcription factors into the nucleus of the differentiating stem cell (Behfar and Terzic, 2007). Consequently, researchers have designed a cocktail of cardiogenic induction proteins similar to those produced by the endoderm in order to change the mesenchymal progenitor phenotype into a cardiac phenotype of potential clinical value.

Behfar et al. (2010) studied the timeline of cardiac differentiation by systematic dissection of the stem cell differentiation process, mapping the molecular underpinnings of stem cell-based cardiogenesis. They identified a novel cell phenotype, the cardiopoietic stem cell, an enriched BM-MSC population with the definitive capacity to generate de novo heart muscle for repair when plated at a density of 25,000 cells

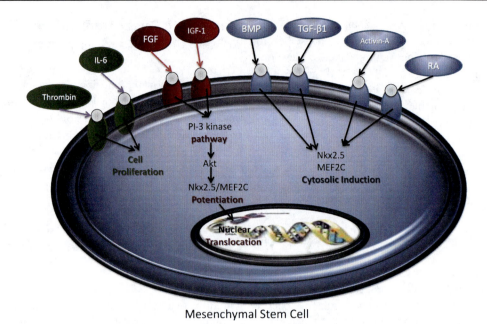

Fig. 18.4 Cardiogenic cocktail, applied in a combined regimen, induced and potentiated nuclear translocation of Nkx-2.5 and MEF2C while maintaining cell cycle activity

per 25-cm² flask. Then, a cardiopoietic cell population was generated by treating hMSCs with recombinant cardiotrophic agents applied alone or in combination, following a schedule, for up to 21 days.

On the way to achieving sarcomerogenesis, cardiopoietic stem cells are an "intermediate" progenitor phenotype distinguished by the nuclear translocation of cardiac transcription factors. The recruited cardiopoietic population can be enriched by using a dual interface Percoll gradient to separate sarcomere-rich high density cardiomyocytes from a lower density sarcomere-poor cardiopoietic phenotype. Specifically, when day 4 cardiopoietic stem cells at 10,000 cells/ml are continuously cultured in monolayer in the presence of a cardiogenic cocktail, sarcomeric differentiation can be achieved by day 7 in ~10% of cells and by day 12 in ~65% of cells. Electron microscopy revealed the intermediate morphology between the stem cell and cardiopoietic state, with a change from a high nucleus-to-cytosol ratio to a progressively mature cardiac structure (Behfar et al., 2008).

Preclinical studies were conducted on the guided cardiopoiesis method using MSCs. The results shows that a complete cardiac phenotype was achieved by using the endoderm-like cocktail protein with hMSCs harvested from patients with coronary artery disease.

The hMSCs were injected into the myocardium of nude infarcted mice and followed up for 1 year to assess functional and structural end points. The recombinant cardiogenic cocktail guidance secured the cardiopoietic phenotype across the patient cohort, achieving a superior functional and structural benefit in comparison to unguided counterparts, with no adverse side effects (Behfar et al., 2010).

Coculture

It is known that intercellular junctions and cellular plasticity are key factors in organogenesis and that the microenvironment plays a critical role in directing stem cells to a differentiated cell phenotype. However, it has not yet been fully elucidated whether cardiomyocyte differentiation is driven by chemical (soluble) or physical (mechanical) factors or by a combination of both. In experimental models of co-culture with rat cardiomyocytes, MSCs were transformed into cells expressing phenotypic markers of cardiomyocytes. It was observed that the transdifferentiation required not only the presence of soluble factors (e.g., cytokines, ion gradients, and/or growth factors) in the culture microenvironment but also

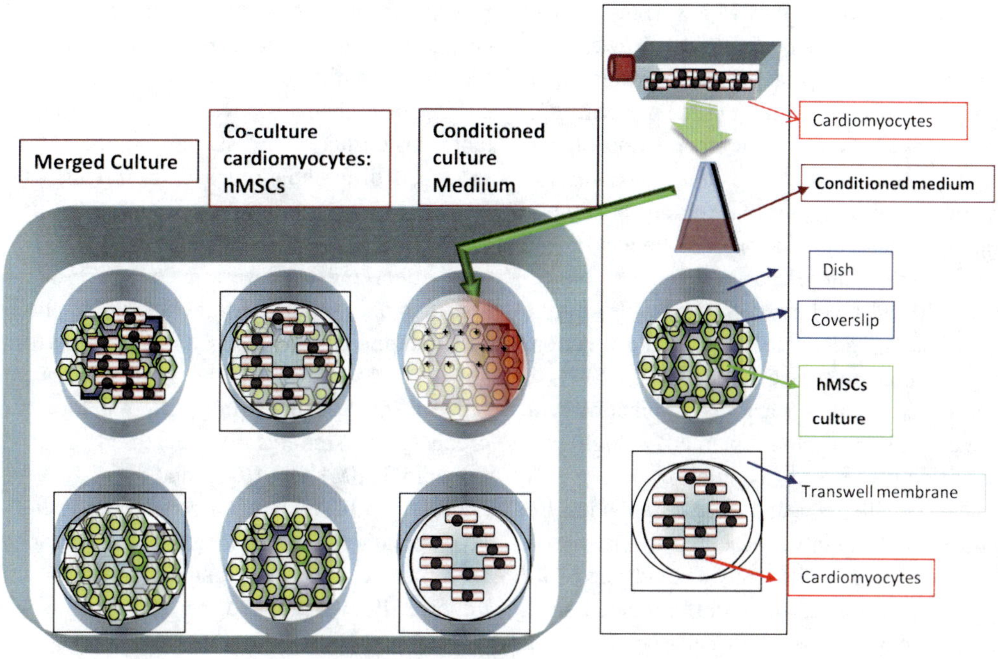

Fig. 18.5 Coculture method

physical intercellular contact between MSCs and cardiomyocytes (Rangappa et al., 2003b). Physical contact allows communication between the cell types for the exchange of membrane fractions and organelles, such as mitochondria and/or other cytoplasmic components, apparently via nano-tubules, and mitochondrial migration from MSCs into cardiomyocytes has even been reported (Plotnikov et al., 2008).

The coculture method (Fig. 18.5) consists of a culture system in which two different types of cells are allowed to grow together. There are some variations in the number of chambers and in the separation between the different cells types. In double-chamber systems, the two cell types are separated by a membrane with a 0.4–0.3 μm pore size to avoid direct cell-to-cell interaction. This system is used to determine whether soluble chemical factors released from one cell type (which can diffuse though the membranes) are sufficient to induce transdifferentiation of the other cell type. In direct co-culture experiments, the two cell types coexist in the same dish or flask with no physical separation between them; the types are differentiated by labeling with a fluorescent tracer before the co-culture (e.g., DAPY; DiI or a specific antibody).

It has also been reported that the participation of adhesion molecules (e.g., E-cadherin) is essential for intercellular contact between human Endothelial Progenitor Cells (EPC) isolated from peripheral blood and isolated cardiomyocytes of newborn rats in the differentiation of EPCs into cardiomyocytes (Koyanagi et al., 2005). Our group has shown the capacity of circulating EPCs, isolated from healthy subjects and patients with cardiovascular disease, to transform into cardiomyocytes in vitro (in press). Rangappa et al. (2003a) demonstrated, in in vitro experiments, the ability of MSCs to rescue damaged myocardial cells and showed the role of the microenvironment in stem cell differentiation. It is important to further explore the paracrine function of MSCs in vivo.

Pretreatment with 5-Azacytidine and Growth Factors

5- Azacytidine (5-aza), a potent inhibitor of DNA methyltransferase (DNMT1), is known to induce demethylation and reactivation of silenced genes. 5-aza-C5 incorporates into DNA, and forms covalent adducts with cellular DNMT1, thereby depleting the cells of enzyme activity and causing demethylation of genomic DNA as a secondary consequence (Christman, 2002).

The in vitro differentiation of MSCs to the cardiac phenotype was achieved with this agent. However, in in vivo studies, specific proteins were expressed in myocytes near the site of injection in the myocardium, but the cells lacked the complete acquisition of cardiac phenotype and were not capable of symmetric contraction. These results may be attributable to heterotypic gap junction channels of connexins 40 and 43, responsible for electromechanical connections between hMSCs and cardiomyocytes, leading to reduced gap junction conductance rates and functionality of the transplanted cells (Valiunas et al., 2004).

Smits et al. (2009) used 5-aza in combination with TGF-β1 and vitamin C and obtained a high percentage of cardiomyocyte differentiation from CSCs. After stimulation with 5-aza and these compounds, the CSCs demonstrated a highly efficacious differentiation into cardiomyocyte like-cells that was evidenced by a shift in gene expression. In the undifferentiated state, expression was observed of stem cell-specific genes (isl-1, c-kit) and of transcription factors that indicate a cardiomyocyte predisposition (e.g., Nkx-2.5, MEF2C, and GATA-4). Then, after the induction of differentiation, CSCs begin to express the genes required to form the complex sarcomeric structures needed in cardiomyocytes for electrophysiological function (SCN5a and Ryr2). CSC-derived cardiomyocytes reveal organized sarcomeric structures, contract spontaneously, and are responsive to adrenergic stimulation, and they show excitation–contraction coupling and action potentials similar to those of ventricular cells. They couple functionally and metabolically through gap junctions, thereby resembling the in vivo myocardium, which consists of large syncytia. Unfortunately, these stimuli cannot be clinically applied due to the unknown effects of DNA demethylation on the overall gene expression pattern and possible bystander effects of growth factors.

Hyperpolarization

Hyperpolarization is a novel cardiac transdifferentiation method that has only been described in CSCs isolated from human biopsies and Embryonic Stem Cells (ESCs). It is based on the major role known to be played by cell membrane potential during development and tissue regeneration, with effects on cell function, proliferation, and differentiation. Each stem cell type exhibits a unique electrophysiological profile in its undifferentiated state. Interestingly, ionic currents and channels have been found to play important roles during myoblast, cardiomyocyte, and neural stem cell differentiation, and the effects of changes in changing membrane potential are highly specific to each cell type (Sundelacruz et al., 2008). Hence, these effects must be investigated in each stem cell type considered a candidate for therapeutic application.

Hyperpolarization of CSCs was performed by reducing extra-cellular potassium concentrations. Subsequent culture in differentiation medium produced a significantly increased expression of troponin T, βMHC, αHCA, and ryanodine receptor 2 (RyR2) by the hyperpolarized CSCs after 5 weeks. Hyperpolarization enhanced intracellular calcium levels and calcineurin signaling in CSCs and, more importantly, upregulated cardiac-specific gene and protein expression, leading to the formation of spontaneously beating cardiomyocytes (Van Vliet et al., 2010). Hyperpolarization studies on MSCs (Sundelacruz et al., 2008) found that membrane potential changes in MSCs induced adipogenic (AD) and osteogenic (OS) differentiation, concluding that treatment with hyperpolarizing reagents upregulated osteogenic markers.

Cellular Extract

The cellular extract method is based on the assumption that more than one transcription factor is needed to change a pattern of cell differentiation to a different one. This method was developed in the lab of Professor Collas and consists of the introduction of the intracellular component of one cell type into another (Fig. 18.6). Purified somatic nuclei or reversibly permeabilized somatic cells are incubated in a nuclear and cytoplasmic extract derived from a different somatic ('target') cell type. The extract is believed to provide nuclear regulatory components that mediate alterations in the gene expression profile of the target genome. Following exposure to the extract, the cells are resealed in culture that contains calcium. By this means, human fibroblasts have been successfully reprogrammed into T-like cells, using the cytoplasmic extract of human T cells (Håkelien et al., 2002), and into beta-like

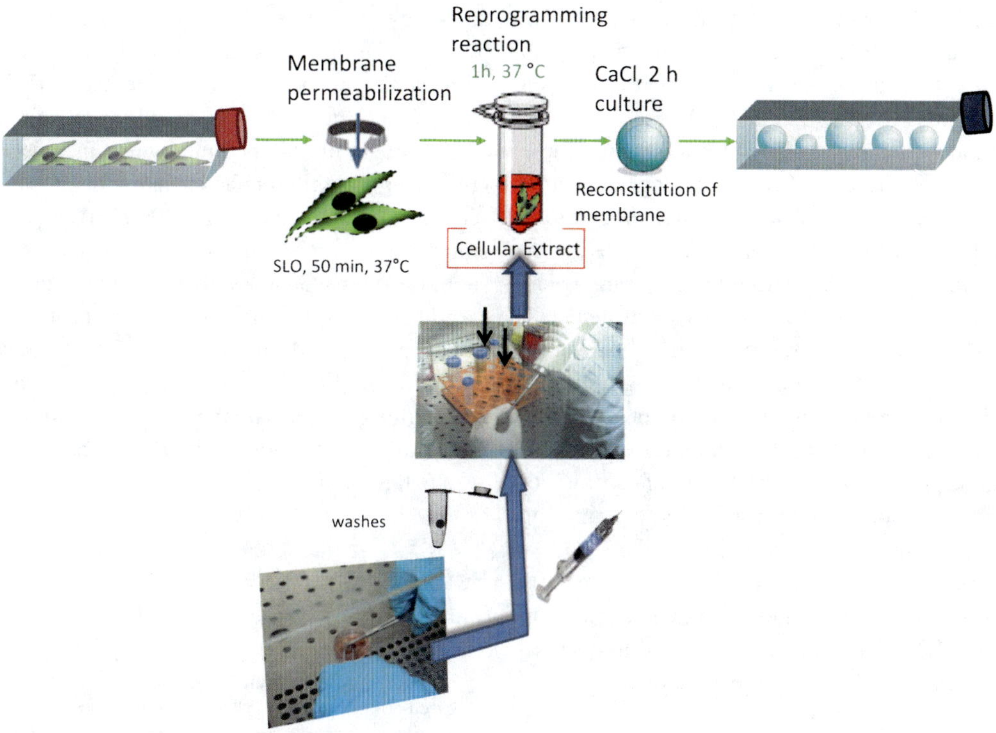

Fig. 18.6 Cellular extract methodology

cells (even able to produce insulin), using the extract of a rat insulin-producing β cell line (Perán et al., 2011). In another experiment, human ADSCs produced cardiomyocyte proteins after incubation with rat cardiomyocyte extracts. The success of these transdifferentiation strategies was demonstrated by phase-contrast microscopy observations of morphological changes, by RT-PCR findings on donor cell-specific genes, and by immunological evidence of alterations in protein expression (Gaustad et al., 2004).

Our group recently reported that adult cardiomyocytes obtained from human donors retain the capacity to induce cardiomyocyte differentiation of mesenchymal stromal cells (Perán et al., 2010). Human Adipose stem cells (hASCs) isolated from lipoaspirates were transiently permeabilized, exposed to human atrial extracts, and allowed to recover in culture. After 21 days, the cells acquired a cardiomyocyte phenotype, as demonstrated by morphologic changes (appearance of binucleate, striated cells, and branching fibers), immunofluorescence detection of cardiac-specific markers (connexin-43, sarcomeric α-actinin, cardiac troponin I and T, and desmin) and the presence of cardiomyocyte-related genes analyzed by reverse transcription – polymerase chain reaction (cardiac myosin light chain 1, α-cardiac actin, cardiac troponin T, and cardiac β-myosin). The relevance of these findings lies in the potential use of autologous extracts to induce stem cell reprogramming. In a therapeutic framework, this is essential to avoid immunologic responses from patients. Other authors have used the cellular extract method to differentiate hASCs into the cardiomyocyte lineage, performing assays with young rodents (Gaustad et al., 2004). In conclusion, the use of autologous extracts for reprogramming adult stem cells may have potential implications for the treatment of heart disease.

Viral Vectors

The genetic modification of MSCs is an interesting option to improve their therapeutic potential. The transfection of master genes or transcription factors that induce differentiation to cardiac phenotype has recently been developed as a transdifferentiation methodology. It has been shown that MSCs of different species can be efficaciously transduced with both adenoviral and retroviral vectors (McMahon et al., 2006). In cardiac research, efforts were made with viral constructions using retroviral vectors that contain the master genes Csx/Nkx2.5 and GATA-4 (extracted hearts of mouse fetus and cloned by RT-PCR). These were transfected in BM-MSCs, showing that three types of cells (cardiac myoblasts, cardiac progenitors, and multipotent stem cells) were differentiated from a single cell, implying that cardiomyocytes are generated stochastically from a single-cell-derived stem cell. Single-cell-derived MSCs overexpressing Csx/Nkx2.5 and GATA4 behaved as cardiac transient amplifying cells and still retained their plasticity in vivo, but 5-azacytidine treatment was needed to achieve a complete cardiac phenotype. The frequency of cardiomyogenic differentiation was increased by co-culturing with fetal cardiomyocytes (Yamada et al., 2007).

For human clinical proposes, Ad- vectors are safer than RV- vectors because they do not integrate into the cellular DNA, and therapy with Ad-transduced MSCs is likely to be less immunogenic than the direct administration of Ad-vectors to affected tissues, due to the anti-inflammatory properties of MSCs. Moreover, transgenic expression in proliferating stem cells is only transient due to the non-integrative properties of Ad-vectors. Nonetheless, short-term therapeutic gene expression may be sufficient or even desirable for the treatment of diseases such as myocardial infarction, in which the transient paracrine effects of MSCs enhance tissue healing and repair responses.

In emulation of the embryological process and in an attempt to determine the true scope of the hypoxia process in the development of heart vascularization and cardiac differentiation, an adenoviral construction was made to evaluate the effects of mutant hypoxia-inducible factor-1α (HIF-1α) adenovirus (Adeno-HIF-1α-Ala402-Ala564) on cardiomyocyte differentiation from MSCs co-cultured with CMCs (Xue et al., 2010). It was concluded that HIF-1α promoted the differentiation of MSCs to cardiomyocytes by upregulating the TGF-β(1)/Smad4 signaling pathway.

Transdifferentiation of Fibroblasts to Cardiomyocytes

Two studies recently reported on the direct reprogramming of murine fibroblast into functional cardiomyocytes. Ding's group obtained cardiomyocytes by virally transducing mouse embryonic fibroblasts with genes encoding for the transcription factors Oct4, Sox2 and Klf4, followed by modified standard reprogramming medium, which included removing leukemia inhibitor factor and adding fetal bovine serum at 1–15% (Efe et al., 2011). Srivastavas' group enforced the expression of developmental cardiac transcription factors Gata4, Mef2c, and Tbx5 and produced cardiomyocytes that matched a normal cardiomyocyte gene expression profile (Ieda et al., 2010). Advances in this field will provide the methodology to obtain a suitable number of cardiomyocyte-like cells for utilization in cardiac disease models, in vitro drug screening, or even cell therapies.

References

Ai, J, Zhang R, Li Y, Pu J, Lu Y, Jiao J, Li K, Yu B, Li Z, Wang R, Wang L, Li Q, Wang N, Shan H, Li Z, Yang B (2010) Circulating microRNA-1 as a potential novel biomarker for acute myocardial infarction. Biochem Biophys Res Commun 391:73–77

Behfar A, Terzic A (2007) Cardioprotective repair through stem cell-based cardiopoiesis. J Appl Physiol 103:1438–1440

Behfar A, Faustino RS, Arrell DK, Dzeja PP, Perez-Terzic C, Terzic A (2008) Guided stem cell cardiopoiesis: discovery and translation. J Mol Cell Cardiol 45(4):523–529

Behfar A, Yamada S, Crespo-Diaz R, Nesbitt JJ, Rowe LA, Perez-Terzic C, Gaussin V, Homsy C, Bartunek J, Terzic A (2010) Guided cardiopoiesis enhances therapeutic benefit of bone marrow human mesenchymal stem cells in chronic myocardial infarction. J Am Coll Cardiol 56(9):721–734

Buckingham M, Meilhac S, Zaffran S (2005) Building the mammalian heart from two sources of myocardial cells. Nat Rev Genet 6:826–835

Burke DZ, Tosh D (2005) Therapeutic Potential of transdifferentiated cells. Science 108:309–321

Calmont A, Wandzioch E, Tremblay KD, Minowada G, Kaestner KH, Martin GR, Zaret KS (2006) An FGF response pathway that mediates hepatic gene induction in embryonic endoderm cells. Dev Cell 11:339–348

Chien KR, Domian IJ, Parker KK (2008) Cardiogenesis and the Complex Biology of Regenerative Cardiovascular Medicine. Science 322(5907):1494–1497

Christman JK (2002) 5-azacytidine and 5-aza-2′-deoxycytidine as inhibitors of DNA methylation: mechanistic studies and their implications for cancer therapy. Oncogene 21:5483–5495

Efe JA, Hilcove S, Kim J, Zhou H, Ouyang K, Wang G, Chen J, Ding S (2011) Conversion of mouse fibroblasts into cardiomyocytes using a direct reprogramming strategy. Nat Cell Biol 13(3):215–222

Gaustad KG, Boquest AC, Anderson BE, Gerdes AM, Collas P (2004) Differentiation of human adipose tissue stem cells using extracts of rat cardiomyocytes. Biochem Biophys Res Commun 314:420–427

Håkelien AM, Landsverk HB, Robl JM, Skålhegg BS, Collas P (2002) Reprogramming fibroblasts to express T-cell functions using cell extracts. Nat Biotechnol. 20:460–466

Hung LY, Kawase Y, Yoneyama R, Hajjar R (2007) Review: gene therapy in the treatment of heart failure. Physiology 22: 81–96

Ieda M, Fu JD, Delgado-Olguin P, Vedantham V, Hayashi Y, Bruneau BG, Srivastava D (2010) Direct reprogramming of fibroblasts into functional cardiomyocytes by defined factors. Cell 142(3):375–386

Kauser K, Zeiher AM, Schuleri KH, Boyle AJ, Hare JM (2007) Mesenchymal stem cells for cardiac regenerative therapy. HEP 180:195–218

Koyanagi M, Urbich C, Chavakis E, Hoffmann J, Rupp S, Badorff C, Zeiher AM, Starzinski-Powitz A, Haendeler J, Dimmeler S (2005) Differentiation of circulating endothelial progenitor cells to a cardiomyogenic phenotype depends on E-cadherin. FEBS Lett 579:6060–6066

McMahon JM, Conroy S, Lyons M, Greiser U, O'Shea C, Strappe P, Howard L, Murphy M, Barry F, O'Brien T (2006) Gene transfer into rat mesenchymal stem cells: a comparative study of viral and nonviral vectors. Stem Cells Dev 15:87–96

Moore KL, Persaud TVN (2000) Embriología Clínica en el desarrollo del ser humano. Ed. Panamericana, Madrid, Spain, pp. 511–521

Nakanishi C, Yamagishi M, Yamahara K, Hagino I, Mori H, Sawa Y, Yagihara T, Kitamura S, Nagaya N (2008) Activation of cardiac progenitor cells through paracrine effects of mesenchymal stem cells. Biochem Biophys Res Commun 374:11–16

Parekkadan B, Milwid JM (2010) Mesenchymal stem cells as therapeutics. Ann Rev Biomed Engineer 12(1):87–117

Pasek M, Brette F, Nelson A, Pearce C, Qaiser A, Christe G, Orchard CH (2008) Quantification of t- tubule area and protein distribution in rat cardiac ventricular myocytes. Prog Biophys Mol Biol 6:244–257

Perán M, Marchal JA, López E, Jiménez-Navarro M, Boulaiz H, Rodríguez- Serrano F, Carrillo E, Sanchez-Espin G, De Teresa E, Tosh D, Aránega A (2010) Human cardiac tissue induces transdifferentiation of adult stem cells towards cardiomyocytes, Cytotherapy 12:332–337

Perán M, Sánchez-Ferrero A, Tosh D, Marchal JA, López E, Alvarez P, Boulaiz H, Rodríguez-Serrano F, Aránega A (2011) Ultrastructural and molecular analyzes of insulin-producing cells induced from human hepatoma cells. Cytotherapy 13(2):193–200

Pérez Romero C, Martín JJ, López del Amo, González MP, Miranda Serrano B, Burgos Rodríguez R, Alonso Gil M (2010) Costes basados en actividades de los programas de trasplantes de riñón, hígado y corazón en siete hospitales españoles. Escuela Andaluza de Salud Pública. <http://www.fundacionsigno.com>. Accessed: 19 de Abril de 2010

Plotnikov EY, Khryapenkova TG, Vasileva AK, Marey MV, Galkina SI, Isaev NK, Sheval EV, Polyakov VY, Sukhikh GT, Zorov, DB. (2008) Cell-to-cell cross-talk between mesenchymal stem cells and cardiomyocytes in co-culture. J Cell Mol Med 12(5A):1622–1631

Rangappa S, Entwistle JW, Wechsler AS, Kresh JY (2003a) Cardiomyocyte-mediated contact programs human mesenchymal stem cells to express cardiogenic phenotype. J Thorac Cardiovasc Surg 126:124–132

Rangappa S, Fen C, Lee EH, Bongso A, Wei ES (2003b) Transformation of adult mesenchymal stem cells isolated from the fatty tissue into cardiomyocytes. Ann Thorac Surg 75:775–779

Rengo G, Lymperopoulos A, Zincarelli C, Donniacuo M, Soltys S, Rabinowitz JE, Koch, WJ. (2009) Myocardial Adeno-Associated Virus Serotype 6-{beta}ARKct Gene Therapy Improves Cardiac Function and Normalizes the Neurohormonal Axis in Chronic Heart Failure. Circulation 119:89–98

Rubart M, Field LJ (2006) Cardiac regeneration: repopulating the heart. Annu Rev Physiol 68:29–49

Smits AM, Van, Vliet P, Metz CH, Korfage T, Sluijter, JPG, Doevendans PA, Goumans MJ (2009) Human Cardiomyocyte progenitor cells differentiate into functional mature cardiomyocytes: an in vitro model for studying human cardiac physiology and pathophysiology. Nat Protoc 4:232–243

Song L, Tuan RS (2004) Transdifferentiation potential of human mesenchymal stem cells derived from bone marrow. FASEB J 18(9):980–982

Sundelacruz S, Levin M, Kaplan DL (2008) Membrane potential controls adipogenic and osteogenic differentiation of mesenchymal stem cells. PLoS One 3(11):e3737

Torella D, Ellison GM, Karakikes I, Nadal-Ginard B (2007) Growth-factor-mediated cardiac stem cell activation in myocardial regeneration. Nat Clin Pract Cardiovasc Med 4:S46–S51

Tosh D, Slack JM (2002) How cells change their phenotype. Nature Rev Mol Cell Biol 3:187–194

Valiunas V, Doronin S, Valiuniene L, Potapova I, Zuckerman J, Walcott B, Robinson RB, Rosen MR, Brink PR, Cohen IS (2004) Human mesenchymal stem cells make cardiac connexins and form functional gap junctions. J Physiol 555:617–626

Van Vliet P, De Boer TP, Van der Heyden MAG, El Tamer MK, Sluijter JPG, Doevendans PA, Goumans MJ (2010) Hyperpolarization induces differentiation in human cardiomyocyte progenitor cells. Stem Cell Rev Rep 6:178–185

Xu H, Morishima M, Wylie JN, Schwartz RJ, Bruneau BG, Lindsay EA, Baldini A (2004) Tbx1 has a dual role in the morphogenesis of the cardiac outflow tract. Development 131:3217–3227

Xue JJ, Wang YS, Ma H, Hu Y, Cheng KL. (2010) Effects of a recombinant adenovirus expressing human hypoxia-inducible factor 1α double-mutant on the in vitro differentiation of bone marrow mesenchymal stem cells to cardiomyocytes. Zhonghua Xin Xue Guan Bing Za Zhi 38(7):638–643

Yamada Y, Sakurada K, Takeda Y, Gojo Z, Umezawa A (2007) Single-cell-derived mesenchymal stem cells overexpressing Csx/Nkx2.5 and GATA4 undergo the stochastic cardiomyogenic fate and behave like transient amplifying cells. Exp Cell Res 313(4):698–706

Zhou B, Ma Q, Rajapoal S, Qing M, Rajagopal S, Wu SM, Domian I, Rivera-Feliciano J, Jiang D, Von Gise A, Ikeda S, Chien K, Pu WT (2008) Epicardial progenitors contribute to the cardiomyocyte lineage in the developing heart. Nature 454:109–113

Chapter 19
Rat Mesenchymal Cell CD44 Surface Markers: Role in Cardiomyogenic Differentiation

Tze-Wen Chung and Ming-Chia Yang

Abstract We reported that hyaluronic acid (HA) containing silk fibroin (SF) patches markedly improved cardiomyogenic differentiation of 5-aza inducing rat mesenchymal stem cells (rMSCs). It is well known that MSCs contain an abundant of CD44 surface markers, and HA is the receptor of those markers. Examining the roles of CD44 markers on cardiomyogenic differentiation of rMSCs might help to design new cardiac patches for cell therapy in infarcted hearts. To study the issue, 5-aza inducing rMSCs with or without a CD44-blockage treatment was cultured in SF/HA cardiac patches; the expressions of cardiac genes and specific cardiac proteins as an index of cardiomyogenic differentiation were examined in the end of the cultivation. It was found that the expressions of cardiac genes such as Gata4 and Nkx2.5 and proteins such as cardiotin and connexion 43, and were significantly decreased for the rMSCs with a CD44-blockage treatment. We conclude that the surface markers of CD44 of rMSCs highly modulate the cardiomyogenic differentiation of the cells when they are cultivated on SF/HA cardiac patches.

Keywords Hyaluronic acid · Osteoblasts · Mesenchymal stem cells · Glycosylation · Hydrogel · Troponin T

T.-W. Chung (✉)
Department of Chemical & Material Engineering, National Yunlin University of Science & Technology, Dou-Liu, Yunlin 640, Taiwan, ROC
e-mail: twchung@yuntech.edu.tw

Introduction

Among various types of cell sources, MSCs have the potential to differentiate into cardiomyocytes, vascular smooth muscle cells and endothelial cells and produce angiogenic factors through paracrine mechanisms (Tan et al., 2009). MSCs can also be differentiated toward the osteoblasts, chondrocytes, or smooth muscle cells lineage pathways under appropriate conditions via interactions with HA (Charbord et al., 2010). It also has been reported that the interactions between CD44 surface markers of rMSCs and extra-cellular hyaluronic acid (HA) would alternate various biological functions such like cell adhesion, matrix assembly, endocytosis, and cell signalling (Herrera et al., 2007; Murphy et al., 2005; Zhou et al., 1999). We reported that rMSCs with a CD44-blockage treatment would significantly decrease the cell proliferations and fibronectin expressions in SF/carbohydrate polymers (e.g., chitosan and HA) cardiac patches (Yang et al., 2009, 2010). It is noticed that rMSCs contain an abundant of CD44 surface markers and HA is one of the major components of the ECM in the myocardium tissues. It is assumable that CD44 of rMSCs might play roles in developing myocardium tissues including the cardiomyogenic differentiation of rMSCs (Hellstrom et al., 2006). However, there is lack report in such issue. In this article, we report the roles of CD44 markers of rMSCs on cardiomyogenic differentiations of rMSCs by determining the expressions of specific cardiac genes such as Gata4 and Nkx2.5 (Fig. 19.1a, b) and specific cardiac proteins such as cardiotin and connexion 43 of the cells after the CD44 markers of rMSCs were blocked, induced by 5-aza and cultured on SF/HA patches.

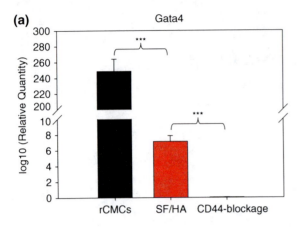

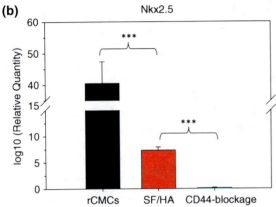

Fig. 19.1 The gene expressions for the specific proteins of cardiac muscles of rMSCs with or without CD44-blockage treatment were shown. After the treatment, rMSCs were further induced by 5-aza and cultured on SF/HA patches for 6 days. Gene expressions of rCMCs group in (**a**) Gata 4 and (**b**) Nkx2.5 were obtained from isolated rat cardiomyocytes, and rMSCs with or without CD44-blockage treatment are presented after they were cultivated on SF/HA patches
(Note: The logarithms values of aforementioned gene expressions for rMSCs without the treatment but cultivated on cell culture wells are assigned as zero; ***$p < 0.001$; Data presented are mean $\pm$ SD, $n = 3$).

CD44 Surface Markers of Mesenchymal Stem Cells

CD44 comprises a large family of transmembrane glycoproteins that exhibit extensive molecular heterogeneity including the standard form of CD44 with a molecular mass of 85–90 kDa, and a multiplicity of iso-form generated by alternative splicing of transcripts and subsequent variable glycosylation (Zhou et al., 1999). The cell adhesion molecule CD44 is involved in a variety of important biological events such as embryogenesis, hematopoiesis, lymphocyte homing and inflammatory reactions (Murphy et al., 2005). Moreover, CD44 is a principal cell surface receptor for extracellular matrix glycosaminoglycan hyaluronan (HA). In our previous report, as positive markers, receptors CD44 in the population of rMSCs were highly expressed (85.7 $\pm$ 2.0%) determined by the flow cytometric spectra (Fig. 19.2).

In previously studies, Herrera et al., derived from their evidences that the expression of CD44 on exogenous cells is important in helping the MSCs to localize to the damaged renal tissue in vivo (Herrera et al., 2007). Wild-type MSCs with CD44 blocked by a neutralizing antibody, as CD44-null cells, were poor at reaching the damaged tissues (Pries et al., 2008). One of the advantages of using an HA-based scaffold is the potential for cell/scaffold interactions via cell surface receptors, which could influence cell behaviours and assist in stem cell differentiation (Zhu et al., 2006). CD44 is a cell surface receptor that binds to HA, providing a means to retain and anchor proteoglycan aggregates to the plasma membrane of a cell (Murphy et al., 2005). In addition, intimate association with the underlying cytoskeleton permits CD44 to initiate intracellular signalling, allowing it to sense changes in the ECM environment and signal a cellular response (Gerecht et al., 2007). Furthermore, CD44 receptor is of particular interest because it is essential for the maintenance of cartilage homeostasis and plays a role in the catabolism of HA via phagocytosis (Knudson and Loeser, 2002). To demonstrate the potential of CD44 of MSCs to interact with HA, the expression of hyaluronidases was observed around MSCs region, indicating the potential to remodel the HA hydrogel. In addition, enzyme of each iso-form plays a specific role in cleaving HA into discrete fragment sizes that regulate different cellular processes (Ostergaard et al., 1997).

Hyaluronic Acid (HA)

Hyaluronic acid (HA), a linear polysaccharide with repeating units of glucuronic acid and N-acetyl glucosamine which is an important component of the extra-cellular matrix (ECM), has widely studied for use in tissue engineering for cartilage, wound healing, implants, and angiogenesis (Tremmel et al., 2009).

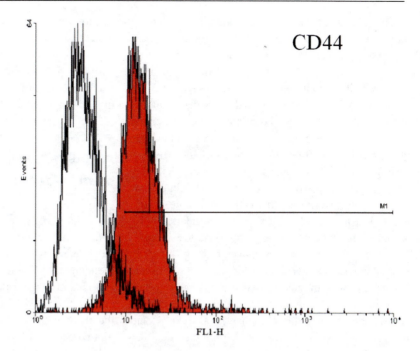

Fig. 19.2 Flow cytometric spectra of isolated rMSCs in this study are immuno-positive to CD44 surface marker

The biological functions of HA have been elucidated including mediating cell proliferation and differentiation during developments (Zhu et al., 2006). HA has diverse biological roles, for instance, being a vital structural component of connective tissues, forming a loose hydrated matrix that allows cells to divide and migrate (Knudson and Loeser, 2002), facilitating cell adhesion and activation (Allison et al., 2007), and playing a role in intracellular signalling (Gerecht et al., 2007). Those functions may be mediated by the interaction of HA with its main receptor CD44 on the surface membrane of various cells (Savani et al., 2001; Ilangumaran et al., 1999). Recent reports in bone regeneration engineering demonstrate that the interaction of HA with CD44 inhibits the induction of MMP-1, MMP-3, and MMP-13 by IL1β or HA in chondrocytes and induces MMP-9 expression in leukocytes (Chung and Burdick, 2009). Hence, HA may able to mediate matrix re-modelling and favouring cell migration to a specific tissue or modulating the engraftment of specific cell types within the bone marrow. Importantly, HA distributes in most parts of heart except the walls of the surrounding large blood vessel and is also one of major components to create the required mechanical properties of a heart (Hellstrom et al., 2006). For example, HA is abundant in a human mitral apparatus that supports mechanical compression of the region such as the posterior leaflet and the free edge of the anterior leaflet (van den Boom et al., 2006). In addition to mechanical support of heart, it is worth of to investigate the roles of HA in cardiomyogenesis in heart regeneration.

CD44: Role in Cardiomyogenic Differentiation

It has been recognized that CD44 can function as a signalling receptor in a variety of cell types. Cell stimulation by monoclonal anti-CD44 antibody or natural CD44 ligands activate signalling pathways that culminate in cell proliferation, cytokine secretion, chemokine gene expression, and cytolytic activator functions (Ilangumaran et al., 1999). Normal endothelial cells (EC) express low levels of CD44, but the expression is up-regulated by activation with cytokines, for example, hyaluronic acid (Savani et al., 2001). Expression of CD44 on EC is associated with homing and migration of leukocytes (i.e., inflammation and migration) (Tremmel et al., 2009). In addition, it has been demonstrated that CD44 plays some roles in new blood vessels formation (or angiogenesis), although its precise role in this process is not clear (Murphy et al., 2005).

The roles of CD44 on the cardiomyogenic differentiations of rMSCs are indexed by examining the gene expressions which are of important committed precursors of cardiac development, and the expressions of contractile proteins of cardiac muscles after 5-aza inducing rMSCs were cultivated in SF/HA patches (Yang et al., 2009, 2010). For the gene expressions of heart development, it is known that Nkx2.5 and Gata4 play essential roles in early heart development by regulating expression of many genes that encode cardiac-specific proteins (Arminan et al., 2009; Ghatpande et al., 2006). Moreover, the Tnnt2 is a gene of troponin T, a protein of adult mammalian hearts, and it regulates muscle contraction in response to variations in intracellular calcium ion concentrations (Arminan et al., 2009; Lemonnier and Buckingham, 2004). Actc1 is a gene present in muscle tissues and is an important constituent of the contractile apparatus (e.g., α-cardiac actin) (Lemonnier and Buckingham, 2004). For examining the expressions of contractile proteins of cardiac muscles, the immunofluorescence stains of troponin T, cardiotin and connexin 43, which is on the actin filament that regulates the force and the velocity of myocardial contraction, contraction-relaxation cycle of the cardiac muscle, and propagation of electrical signals to induce coordinated contraction of the cardiac muscles for blood pumping in the heart (Yoon et al., 2005), respectively, were stained.

Expressions of Various Cardiac Gene Markers as an Index the Roles

It needs to be noticed that, without 5-aza induction, cultivated rMSCs did not express the Gata4, Nkx2.5, Tnnt2 and Actc1 genes. Notably, 5-aza inducing rMSCs expressed the genes of Gata4, Nkx2.5, Tnnt2 and Actc1 in various quantities, indicating that the trends of various cardiomyogenic differentiation of the inducing cells. The expressions of aforementioned specific genes for 5-aza inducing rMSCs cultured on SF/HA patches were significantly higher than those on SF patches (data not shown) although their intensities were less than those of the positive control, rat cardiomyocytes whereas those expressions for the cells with a CD44-blockage treatment were the weakest (Fig. 19.1a, b). Except gene expression of Nkx2.5, the gene expressions of the inducing rMSCs cultured on SF/HA patches were better than those on other patches in our early report (Yang et al., 2009). It is thereby to conclude that 5-aza inducing rMSCs with CD44-blockage treatment would be significantly decreased or nearly no progress in developing the trend in cardiomyogenic differentiation.

Expressions of Various Cardiac Proteins as an Index the Roles of CD44

Regarding to the interactions of CD44 and SF/HA patches, the expressions of cardiac genes and proteins (e.g., troponin T and connexin 43) for 5-aza inducing rMSCs cultivated on SF/HA patches were significantly higher than those cultured on SF patches and culture wells (Yang et al., 2009, 2010). Moreover, the specific cardiac genes and proteins index for cardiomyogenic differentiations of 5-aza inducing rMSCs cultured on SF/HA patches were much better than those cultured on SF/CS patches (Yang et al., 2009, 2010). Therefore, CD44 markers of rMSCs would positively interact with HA of SF/HA patches that promotes the cardiomyogenic differentiations of the cells. For the results of a without CD44-blockage treatment of rMSCs, 5-aza inducing rMSCs markedly expressed troponin T, cardiotin and connexin 43 (Yang et al., 2009, 2010), respectively, after they were cultured on SF/HA patches while those with the treatment, weakly expressed for troponin T, cardiotin and connexin 43 was observed (Fig. 19.3a–c), respectively. Notably, the values of immuno-fluorescent staining for various cardiac proteins for 5-aza inducing rMSCs with or without a CD44-blockage treatment were qualitatively correspondent to those of gene expressions, respectively, cultivated in the same kind of patches (e.g. SF patches). Alternatively, the results suggested that CD44 of rMSCs play an important and unique role in modulating cardiomyogenic differentiations of rMSCs since all of index in examining cardiac genes and proteins of cardiomyogenic differentiations were significantly decreased for the cells with a CD44-blockage treatment in SF/HA cardiac patches tested in this study.

In conclusion, the roles of CD44 on cardiomyogenic differentiation were investigated by culturing 5-aza inducing rMSCs with or without a CD44-blockage treatment in SF/HA cardiac patches. The expressions

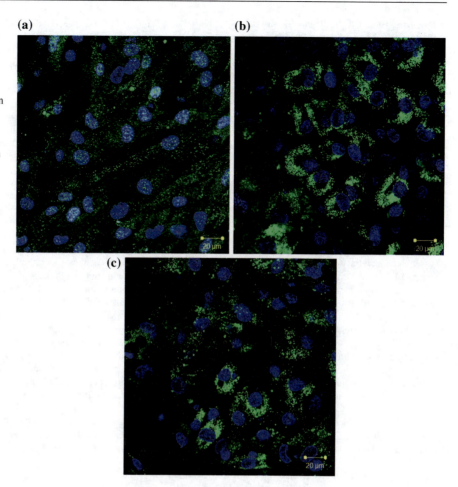

Fig. 19.3 Immuno-fluorescent staining for cardiomyogenic proteins such as troponin T, cardiotin and connexin 43 for rMSCs with a CD44-blockage treatment and then cultured on SF/HA patches for 6 days, respectively. Weak expressions in (**a**) troponin T, (**b**) cardiotin and (**c**) connexin 43 for rMSCs with CD44-blockage treatment were observed, respectively (Note: Colour for troponin T, cardiotin and connexin 43 is *green* and that for nuclei of cells is *blue*; scale bar is 20 μm on each figure).

of cardiac genes and cardiac proteins as an index of cardiomyogenic differentiation were examined in the end of the cultivation. It was found that the expressions of cardiac genes such as Gata4 and Nkx2.5, and cardiac proteins such as cardiotin and connexion 43 were significantly decreased for the rMSCs with a CD44-blockage treatment. It suggests that the surface markers of CD44 of rMSCs highly modulate the cardiomyogenic differentiation of the cells when they are cultivated on SF/HA cardiac patches.

References

Allison DD, Vasco N, Braun KR, Wight TN, Grande-Allen KJ (2007) The effect of endogenous overexpression of hyaluronan synthases on material, morphological, and biochemical properties of uncrosslinked collagen biomaterials. Biomaterials 28:5509–5517

Arminan A, Gandia C, Bartual M, Garcia-Verdugo JM, Lledo E, Mirabet V, Llop M, Barea J, Montero JA, Sepulveda P (2009) Cardiac differentiation is driven by NKX2.5 and GATA4 nuclear translocation in tissue-specific mesenchymal stem cells. Stem Cells Dev 18:907–918

Charbord P, Livne E, Gross G, Haupl T, Neves NM, Marie P, Bianco P, Jorgensen C (2010) Human bone marrow mesenchymal stem cells: a systematic reappraisal via the genostem experience. Stem Cell Rev 7:32–42

Chung C, Burdick JA (2009) Influence of three-dimensional hyaluronic acid microenvironments on mesenchymal stem cell chondrogenesis. Tissue Eng Part A 15, 243–254

Gerecht S, Burdick JA, Ferreira LS, Townsend SA, Langer R, Vunjak-Novakovic G (2007) Hyaluronic acid hydrogel for controlled self-renewal and differentiation of human embryonic stem cells. Proc Natl Acad Sci USA 104:11298–11303

Ghatpande S, Brand T, Zile M, Evans T (2006) Bmp2 and Gata4 function additively to rescue heart tube development in the absence of retinoids. Dev Dyn 235:2030–2039

Hellstrom M, Johansson B, Engstrom-Laurent A (2006) Hyaluronan and its receptor CD44 in the heart of newborn and adult rats. Anat Rec A Discov Mol Cell Evol Biol 288:587–592

Herrera MB, Bussolati B, Bruno S, Morando L, Mauriello-Romanazzi G, Sanavio F, Stamenkovic I, Biancone L, Camussi G (2007) Exogenous mesenchymal stem cells localize to the kidney by means of CD44 following acute tubular injury. Kidney Int 72:430–441

Ilangumaran S, Borisch B, Hoessli DC (1999) Signal transduction via CD44: role of plasma membrane microdomains. Leuk Lymphoma 35:455–469

Knudson W, Loeser RF (2002) CD44 and integrin matrix receptors participate in cartilage homeostasis. Cell Mol Life Sci 59:36–44

Lemonnier M, Buckingham ME (2004) Characterization of a cardiac-specific enhancer, which directs {alpha}-cardiac actin gene transcription in the mouse adult heart. J Biol Chem 279:55651–85565

Murphy JF, Lennon F, Steele C, Kelleher D, Fitzgerald D, Long AC (2005) Engagement of CD44 modulates cyclooxygenase induction, VEGF generation, and proliferation in human vascular endothelial cells. FASEB J 19:446–448

Ostergaard K, Salter DM, Andersen CB, Petersen J, Bendtzen K (1997) CD44 expression is up-regulated in the deep zone of osteoarthritic cartilage from human femoral heads. Histopathology 31:451–459

Pries R, Witrkopf N, Trenkle T, Nitsch SM, Wollenberg B (2008) Potential stem cell marker CD44 is constitutively expressed in permanent cell lines of head and neck cancer. In Vivo 22:89–92

Savani RC, Cao G, Pooler PM, Zaman A, Zhou Z, DeLisser HM (2001) Differential involvement of the hyaluronan (HA) receptors CD44 and receptor for HA-mediated motility in endothelial cell function and angiogenesis. J Biol Chem 276:36770–3678

Tan MY, Zhi W, Wei RQ, Huang YC, Zhou KP, Tan B, Deng L, Luo JC, Li XQ, Xie HQ, Yang ZM (2009) Repair of infarcted myocardium using mesenchymal stem cell seeded small intestinal submucosa in rabbits. Biomaterials 30:3234–3240

Tremmel M, Matzke A, Albrecht I, Laib AM, Olaku V, Ballmer-Hofer K, Christofori G, Heroult M, Augustin HG, Ponta H, Orian-Rousseau V (2009) A CD44v6 peptide reveals a role of CD44 in VEGFR-2 signaling and angiogenesis. Blood 114:5236–5244

van den Boom M, Sarbia M, von Wnuck Lipinski K, Mann P, Meyer-Kirchrath J, Rauch BH, Grabitz K, Levkau B, Schror K, Fischer JW (2006) Differential regulation of hyaluronic acid synthase isoforms in human saphenous vein smooth muscle cells: possible implications for vein graft stenosis. Circ Res 98:36–44

Yang MC, Wang SS, Chou NK, Chi NH, Huang YY, Chang YL, Shieh MJ, Chung TW (2009) The cardiomyogenic differentiation of rat mesenchymal stem cells on silk fibroin-polysaccharide cardiac patches in vitro. Biomaterials 30:3757–3765

Yang MC, Chi NH, Chou NK, Huang YY, Chung TW, Chang YL, Liu HC, Shieh MJ, Wang SS (2010) The influence of rat mesenchymal stem cell CD44 surface markers on cell growth, fibronectin expression, and cardiomyogenic differentiation on silk fibroin – Hyaluronic acid cardiac patches. Biomaterials 31:854–862

Yoon J, Min BG, Kim YH, Shim WJ, Ro YM, Lim DS (2005) Differentiation, engraftment and functional effects of pretreated mesenchymal stem cells in a rat myocardial infarct model. Acta Cardiol 60:277–284

Zhou J, Haggerty JG, Milstone LM (1999) Growth and differentiation regulate CD44 expression on human keratinocytes. In Vitro Cell Dev Biol Anim 35:228–235

Zhu H, Mitsuhashi N, Klein A, Barsky LW, Weinberg K, Barr ML, Demetriou A, Wu GD (2006) The role of the hyaluronan receptor CD44 in mesenchymal stem cell migration in the extracellular matrix. Stem Cells 24:928–935

Chapter 20

Stroke Therapy Using Menstrual Blood Stem-Like Cells: Method

Maria Carolina Oliveira Rodrigues, Svitlana Garbuzova-Davis, Paul R. Sanberg, Júlio C. Voltarelli, Julie G. Allickson, Nicole Kuzmin-Nichols, and Cesario V. Borlongan

Abstract Cerebrovascular diseases are the third leading cause of death and the primary cause of long-term disability in the United States. Most patients, excluded from the available treatment with plasminogen activator (tPA), present permanent neurological impairment and may benefit from restorative treatments with stem cells. Inflammation is a key feature in stroke and it plays a dual role, either increasing injury in early phases or impairing neural survival at later stages. Stem cells can be opportunely used to modulate inflammation, abrogate cell death and, therefore, preserve neural function. To date, there is no consensus about the most adequate cell type, route of delivery or timing for transplantation, as experimental and clinical studies are still inconclusive. Menstrual blood stem cells have been recently studied for their availability, proliferative capacity, pluripotentiality and angiogenic features, which make them a relevant resource for the treatment of stroke.

Keywords Cerebrovascular diseases · Plasminogen activator · Neutrophils · Central nervous system (CNS) · Stem cell · Endometrium

Introduction

Cerebrovascular diseases are the third leading cause of death (Xu et al., 2010) and the primary cause of long-term disability in the United States (CDC, 1999). Although the incidence and mortality have decreased over the years, stroke remains a major concern in the clinical setting largely due to the limited treatment currently available. Fifteen to 30% of first time stroke patients become permanently disabled and 20% still require institutional care three months after stroke (Asplund et al., 1998). Moreover, the disease negatively affects the economic productivity of the society and, therefore, every effort to decrease the incidence of strokes and to, at least, minimize their devastating sequelae is urgently warranted.

To date, the best available therapeutic agent is tissue plasminogen activator (tPA), indicated for ischemic stroke. The drug catalyzes the transformation of plasminogen into plasmin, which acts as a potent thrombolytic agent and is used to restore the blood flow, thus minimizing immediate tissue death. According to the National Institute of Neurological Disorders and Stroke (NINDS, 1995), patients treated with tPA within 3 h of beginning of symptoms present less disability in the following months. The therapeutic window of 3 h, however, is a major barrier to tPA clinical application and excludes most of stroke victims from being treated. Kleindorfer et al. (2008) estimated that only 1.8–2.1% of all patients affected by ischemic strokes in the United States had received the therapy. Such report clearly indicates that the majority of stroke patients have to deal with the long-term consequences of the disease. For these, restorative therapies, aiming to provide at least partial neurological recovery, are desired.

C.V. Borlongan (✉)
Department of Neurosurgery and Brain Repair, College of Medicine, Center of Excellence for Aging and Brain Repair, University of South Florida, Tampa, FL, USA
e-mail: cborlong@health.usf.edu

SGD and CVB are consultants, and PRS is co-founder and board member of Saneron-CCEL Therapeutics, Inc. PRS is also a shareholder in Cryo-Cell International, Inc.

Inflammation in Stroke

The injured site of an ischemic stroke comprises the infarct core and the penumbra area. The first undergoes almost instant cell death following the acute interruption of blood supply. Malfunctioning of the Na^+/K^+-ATPase and Ca^{++}/H^+-ATPase pumps increase intracellular Ca^{++} concentrations, activating Ca^{++}-dependent enzymes, which promote cytotoxicity, oxidative stress and, finally, cell death (Durukan and Tatlisumak, 2007). In parallel, ischemia triggers depolarization of neurons, leading to glutamate excitotoxicity, also contributing to neuronal death.

Surrounding the infarct core, the ischemic penumbra comprises the tissue that retains structural integrity, but lacks function. It may either evolve to death or to recovery after stroke, depending on the complex cascade of events initiated by the ischemic insult, among which inflammation plays a decisive role (Emsley et al., 2008). As a first response to ischemia, the microglia become activated and secrete nitric oxide, reactive oxygen species, and inflammatory cytokines (Amor et al., 2010), which stimulate cell infiltration through the expression of adhesion molecules on the endothelial surface. Attracted by the microglia, neutrophils and monocytes are the first leukocytes to migrate into the CNS, followed by dendritic cells and lymphocytes. Neutrophils are considered the main mediators of brain injury after reperfusion, and their accumulation is correlated with the severity of brain tissue damage and poor neurological outcome (Atochin et al., 2000). Once in the cerebral parenchyma, these cells contribute to the amplification of the inflammatory reaction, releasing cytokines, activating resident cells, attracting more cells from the peripheral circulation and stimulating proteases, all of which also lead to cellular death (Jin et al., 2010).

In the last 15 years, research has targeted inflammatory components of stroke, aiming to recover viability of the penumbra area and, therefore, reduce the extension of injury in the central nervous system (CNS). Anti-inflammatory interventions may attenuate the secondary cell death associated with ischemic stroke and, likely, lessen neurological impairments among other progressive disabilities. Experimental studies have shown that suppression of the inflammatory response after stroke leads to reduction of the infarct size (Connolly et al., 1996; Hurn et al., 2007).

Adding some controversy to this idea, inflammation has also beneficial effects and while it can be deleterious to the integrity of the CNS, it is also necessary for repair. At early stages after stroke, inflammation is associated with removal of debris and other products of cell death and production of neurotrophic factors. It also limits the extension of the injury, through the formation of a constraining glial scar surrounding the infarct area. At late stages, however, inflammation becomes deleterious, releasing toxic agents, such as free radicals and detrimental cytokines, and inhibiting tissue repair and angiogenesis. In summary, inflammation may afford benefits to the brain during the early stages of neural cell death. However, during the chronic period, if inflammation persists and no therapeutic intervention is employed to correct this aberrant response, then such host tissue response to injury will exacerbate the disease progression.

In view of therapeutic opportunities for stem cells, injury following stroke can be divided in three consecutive stages, each one associated with different strategies (Hess and Borlongan, 2008). In the hours that immediately follow stroke, attempts to restore the blood flow are neuroprotective, therefore preventing further early neuronal death and restricting the extent of the penumbra area. Thereafter, once the injury is established, the interventions are mainly restorative and cell-based therapies have their best indications. During the first month after stroke the brain produces inflammatory signals, which can be used to opportunely attract stem cells injected in the systemic circulation to the site of injury (Park et al., 2009). It is also during this period that the interventions may restore the viability of the tissue in the penumbra area. Terminated the first month, inflammation decreases and scars and structural damage persist. Stem cells still have a possible therapeutic role in this last phase, but they should be delivered directly into the nervous tissue, through the aid of scaffolds and surgical procedures.

A key feature of stem cells in the inflammatory context is the ability to modulate the immune response, suppressing deleterious mechanisms without affecting beneficial functions. These unique properties are based on the fact that the suppressive capacity of the stem cells is also regulated by the inflammatory environment. In that way, stem cells are able to control the further generation of pro-inflammatory stimuli and, therefore, limit the progression of the inflammatory response. Neural stem cells, for example, decrease the expression of TNF-α and, in consequence, reduce neutrophil infiltration into the CNS of rat models of hemorrhagic stroke (Lee et al., 2008). Later in the course of inflammation, stem cells also suppress reactive lymphocytes, while enhancing the activity and proliferation of their beneficial, regulatory subsets (Kim et al., 2009). Moreover, trophic factors secreted by the stem cells stimulate angiogenesis and repair (Baraniak and McDevitt, 2010). Stem cells are, therefore, a very powerful therapeutic tool that still requires further studies to be properly applied with healing purposes. Their potential effects on either acute or chronic inflammatory settings make them useful not only as treatment for stroke, but also for other neurodegenerative conditions in which inflammation is present.

Targets for Stem Cells in Stroke

Stem cells opportunely interact with the inflammatory dynamics of stroke, modulating its harmful effects and maximizing its regenerative potential. However, although the knowledge about cell-based therapy for stroke and other neurologic diseases has increased over the years, there is no consensus about how the cells should be administered and even about which types of cells are most effective. Significant numbers of studies investigate the therapeutic effects of mature or differentiated cells, but more immature cell lines also have their advantages. Less differentiated cells maintain stem cell markers, including the stem cell factor receptor (SCF-1), which aid in migration to the sites of injury. These cells survive longer and migrate farther in the host tissue than previously differentiated cells. Moreover, immature cells usually have higher plasticity when compared to the already committed predifferentiated cells. This property may allow the differentiation of the transplanted cells into more than one cell type, in response to the cytokine and chemokine profile determined by the injured tissue and, therefore, provide better repair. Finally, more immature cell types are usually able to secrete a wider range of trophic factors, which are also imperative for tissue regeneration.

Embryonic stem cells stand on one of the ends of the cell maturity spectrum, and combine high differentiation potential, ability to migrate to inflammatory sites, secretion of trophic factors and reduced immunogenicity. However, major difficulties, associated to uncontrolled cell proliferation and the risk of malignancy have hindered research using those cells. Since ethical and safety reasons were associated with embryonic stem cells, the last decade has witnessed the wide use of adult stem cells as graft source for cell therapy. In the United States, the previous government moratorium on the use of embryonic stem cells also arguably influenced the shift of cell based-therapies toward the use of adult stem cells.

The optimal source for stem cells is also another subject of discussion. For decades, the bone marrow has been used as the stem cell reservoir for diverse types of therapy and, in this context, most of the knowledge derives from bone marrow transplantation. In the late years, however, new sources of stem cells have been investigated, as an attempt to avoid the hurdles associated to hematopoietic stem cell harvesting. In addition, some disposable tissues, such as the umbilical cord blood, placenta, amniotic fluid and, more recently, the menstrual blood, have provided less mature cells than the bone marrow, some of which expressing embryonic-like markers (Patel et al., 2008; Patel and Silva, 2008; Antonucci et al., 2010).

Applications of Cell-Based Therapy for Stroke

Cell-based therapy for the treatment of stroke is an important and growing field of research. Experimental studies involve the application of cells in variable stages of maturity, through different routes of administration. Immortalized neural stem cells from culture, neural progenitors from fetal tissue or from embryonic cells, hematopoietic and endothelial progenitors and mesenchymal cells from diverse tissue sources show promising, although variable, results when used for treatment of stroke (Bliss et al., 2010). Pre-differentiated cells tend to be administrated locally, mostly due to their impaired migration capacity, and also because some investigators believe that better results are obtained when higher numbers of cells are delivered to the injury site. The issue is controversial, and some studies with experimental stroke models have shown that neurological recovery is obtained even when few or no cells enter the brain (Borlongan et al.,

2004; Guzman et al., 2008). The systemic routes are preferred for the administration of less mature cell types and, since less invasive, are more interesting for clinical applications. Comparisons between intraparenchymal, intracerebroventricular, intravenous and intra-arterial injections, however, are not conclusive about the best route of cell delivery and it probably depends on the cell type (mature or immature), timing of delivery (subacute or chronic) and expected mechanism of action (restoration or replacement) (Bliss et al., 2010).

Clinical studies with stroke patients have already been reported (Bliss et al., 2010). Multiple ongoing phase I and II studies are evaluating safety and effects of bone marrow-derived cells for patients in different periods after stroke. Patients within the timeframe from 3 h and up to 90 days after the vascular event, depending on the study, are usually treated with systemic cell delivery. Some clinical studies involving pre-differentiated cells locally delivered have already been completed, but most are limited to small series of patients, with modest conclusions. The largest study included 18 ischemic and hemorrhagic stroke patients at chronic phase (1–6 years after stroke), treated with stereotactic injections of human neuronal cells (Kondziolka et al., 2005). Although the results showed safety and feasibility, the study was inconclusive for effectiveness. This profile of research indicates that, although already in practice, there is still no consensus about the most adequate cell type and route of administration of cells for stroke therapy, agreeing with the status of experimental research for the disease.

Stem Cells Derived from the Endometrium

The presence of stem cells in the endometrium was described about 30 years ago, from the observation that the upper layers of this tissue shed and were renovated each month (Prianishnikov, 1978). At that time, however, it was considered that while stem cells were intact in the endometrium, all cells shed in the menstrual blood were of non-viable nature. Epithelial cells compose part of the endometrium, and are found in the surface epithelium and in the tubular glands, which extend from the surface to the interface with the myometrium. The rest of the endometrium consists of stromal cells, smooth muscle cells, endothelial cells and leukocytes (Padykula, 1991). Functionally, the endometrium can be divided in two main layers. The upper layer, named functionalis, contains mostly glands loosely held together by stromal tissue, while the lower layer, basalis, contains dense stroma and branching glands. The funcionalis is eliminated monthly, as menstruation, and the basalis persists and generates the new endometrium, under hormonal influence.

Only in the last few years, have endometrial cells been better characterized. Chan et al. (2004) isolated epithelial and stromal cells from the endometrium. Both were clonogenic and proliferated in laboratory, but the epithelial cells lost part of their phenotypic markers and needed a feeder layer as the cultures progressed. Meng et al. (2007) published a study with stem cells obtained from menstrual blood, which showed similar properties. The cells were differentiated into tissues from the three germinative layers, indicating their multipotentiality in vitro, and therefore were named endometrial regenerative cells (ERC). Shortly after, Patel et al. (2008) published a more complete study, in which stromal stem cells, again isolated from menstrual blood (MenSCs), were expanded in vitro, showed clonogenic properties and ability to differentiate into mesoderm and ectoderm derived-tissues. They also demonstrated that the MenSCs expressed markers of pluripotency, such as Oct-4, SSEA-4 and c-kit, which are frequently found in more immature cell types, including the embryonic stem cells.

Cervello et al. (2010) isolated, through flow cytometry of Hoechst-stained endometrium cells, epithelial and stromal-cell enriched side populations. The cells were characterized in vitro, and showed high proliferative potential, especially when exposed to hypoxic conditions, which mimic the endometrial environment. However, when the cells were studied in vivo, injected subcutaneously in immunodeficient mice, they showed limited proliferation and differentiation. Masuda et al. (2010) studied the same groups of cells and conducted similar research. The cells were implanted under the kidney capsule of female mice and, after estrogen stimulus, human tissue development was observed in few animals. The authors demonstrated the differentiation of the side-population cells into glandular epithelial, stromal and, for the first time, endothelial cells, since small and medium sized vessels co-expressing CD31 and human vimentin were observed. Although detectable, their differentiation capacity in vivo was considered poor and better proliferative results were obtained when the cells were combined with the remaining population (main population) of endometrial cells. These findings, taken together with existing data from literature, suggest that multiple factors derived from the endometrium, instead of a single cell type, cooperate for the therapeutic properties of this tissue.

That stem cells derived from menstrual blood can be categorized based on their phenotypic and proliferative properties has been an intensely debated topic. As an example, Murphy et al. (2008) believe that the endometrial regenerative cells (ERC) isolated by them are not the same as the endometrial stromal cells described by Taylor (2004), but may share overlapping properties cells as those reported by other studies (Meng et al., 2007; Patel et al., 2008; Patel and Silva, 2008; Wolff et al., 2010). Note though that Meng and colleagues (2007) state the cells are negative for SSEA-4 and Nanog, whereas Patel and co-workers (2008) state they are positive for SSEA-4 and Borlongan and co-investigators state the MenScs are positive for Nanog, suggesting that there are differences in reported markers. The research teams by Murphy and Meng are working together and therefore use the same harvest, processing and cell culture methods. Endometrial regenerative cells, for instance, express low concentrations of the STRO-1 marker (although Meng et al., 2007 state ERCs do not contain STRO-1) and exhibit higher proliferative capacity than other endometrial-derived cells. According to Taylor (2004), stromal cells found in the endometrium originate from the bone marrow, as observed in female recipients of allogeneic bone marrow transplantation that have donor cells detected in tissues from endometrial biopsies. The findings were later reproduced in female rats transplanted with GFP bone marrow cells, which presented GFP cells in the endometrium long after transplantation (Bratincsák et al., 2007). In practical matters, however, although endometrial-derived cells are grouped through different phenotypical and proliferative criteria, they seem to have similar effects and comparable therapeutic abilities to promote repair when applied in vivo.

Also relevant for the experimental investigations of vascular growth and remodeling, is the angiogenic potential of the endometrium-derived cells, perhaps even for designing clinical therapeutic studies, as these cells might be applied to cardiovascular diseases. Hida et al. (2008), for instance, published their experience with menstrual blood-derived stromal cells in damaged heart tissue, in which they were able to in vitro differentiate the cells into spontaneously beating cardiomyocyte-like cells. Furthermore, when menstrual blood cells were injected in the ischemic tissue of myocardial infarct rat models, functional improvement was noted, differently than what was observed when bone marrow stromal cells were used. Finally, the authors also demonstrated cell engraftment and transdifferentiation into cardiac tissue. Some authors propose to take advantage of the angiogenic potential of these cells, applying them to the treatment of chronic limb ischemia and, more recently, severe skin burns, using the cells associated to intelligent artificial films (Murphy et al., 2008; Drago et al., 2010).

Menstrual Cells in Stroke: Practical Issues

In the nervous system context, Borlongan et al. (2010), very recently published the results of menstrual blood cell transplantation in experimental stroke. Stromal-like menstrual blood stem cells were isolated, expanded and, at last, selected for CD117, a marker associated with high proliferation, migration and survival (Cho et al., 2004). In vitro studies showed that the expanded cells maintained expression of embryonic-like stem cell phenotypic markers, such as Oct4, SSEA-4 and Nanog, even when cultured up to 9 passages, as an evidence of the safety and reliability of these cells, and some were induced to express neural markers (MAP2 and Nestin). Moreover, when added to cultured rat neurons exposed to a hypoxic insult, the menstrual blood cells provided neuroprotection and when applied to rat stroke models, less neurologic deficit was observed on behavioral tests, irrespective of the injection site, i.e. systemic or local administration into the striatum. However, unlike the observations reported by Hida et al., although human cells were detected in the rat brain, some migrating to areas other than the injected, they did not show signs of differentiation, expressing their original markers.

Wolff et al. (2010) reported the use of endometrium-derived neural cells in a Parkinson's disease mouse model. The cells were differentiated in vitro into dopamine-producing cells, and were then transplanted into the brain of the animals. Migration, differentiation and production of dopamine were detected in vivo, demonstrating the therapeutic potential of these cells to functionally restore the damaged tissue, either through cell replacement or endogenous repair.

The only clinical study yet published evaluated the safety aspects of endometrial derived stromal cells administration (Zhong et al., 2009). Four patients with multiple sclerosis were treated with intrathecal injections of 16–30 million cells and one of the patients also received an additional intravenous injection. No adverse events were registered, as expected, and the authors reported stabilization of the neurological function. However, the longest follow-up reached 12 months, and any conclusions about effectiveness of the treatment seem premature in this long-term and slowly progressive illness.

Further Studies and Future Applications

Research on cell therapy for stroke has reached great proportions, due to the possibility of translational studies that may benefit patients who miss the three-hour window for thrombolytic therapy. The rescue of the penumbra area after stroke is decisive for functional outcome and a great opportunity for cell therapy. Stem cells promote neuroprotection especially through modulation of the activated immune system. Tissue repair is also described and, although cell differentiation is described in the experimental setting, its importance to the outcome of the treatment is still undefined.

Menstrual cells are a novel therapeutic option in this field and have great potential. Ease of access, availability and safety are the main arguments supporting their use in future clinical studies. Most important for effectiveness purposes, however, is the immature behavior of these cells, in which migration, pluripotentiality and trophic support circumvent the main challenges of tissue repair. In the clinic, however, some barriers must be transposed, such as the low yield and difficulty in expansion of ample supply of stem cells from this source, mainly low replication rate and risk of contamination. Additionally, the application of autologous stem cells derived from menstrual blood would be ideal to avoid graft rejection issues, however this approach is limited to the female population. Males and post-menopausal women, which are the main targets of neurovascular diseases would be excluded from the therapy. A feasible solution would be to educate the female pre-menopausal population about the potential of the menstrual cells and, therefore, stimulate the anticipated harvesting and cryopreservation of the cells, for future autologous use. For the male population, however, there remain the alternatives of using allogeneic cells and of searching for the male counterpart cell.

Despite the potential challenges still to be solved, the menstrual cells represent an important therapeutic tool that may improve the outcome of stroke and other neurodegenerative diseases, and decrease the disability of future patients. Extension of the experimental studies may increase the knowledge about the mechanisms of action of these cells, allowing optimization of their therapeutic potential.

References

Amor S, Puentes F, Baker D, van der Valk P (2010) Inflammation in neurodegenerative diseases. Immunology 129:154–169

Antonucci I, Stuppia L, Kaneko Y, Yu S, Tajiri N, Bae EC, Chheda SH, Weinbren NL, Borlongan CV (2010) Amniotic fluid as rich source of mesenchymal stromal cells for transplantation therapy. Cell Transplant. Epub ahead of print, doi: 10.3727/096368910x53907

Asplund K, Stegmayr B, Peltonen M (1998) From the twentieth to the twenty-first century: a public health perspective on stroke. In: Ginsberg MD, Bogousslavsky J (eds) Cerebrovascular disease pathophysiology, diagnosis and management. Blackwell Science, Cambridge, MA, pp 901–918

Atochin DN, Fisher D, Demchenko IT, Thom SR (2000) Neutrophil sequestration and the effect of hyperbaric oxygen in a rat model of temporary middle cerebral artery occlusion. Undersea Hyperb Med 27:185–190

Baraniak PR, McDevitt TC (2010) Stem cell paracrine actions and tissue regeneration. Regen Med 5:121–143

Bliss TM, Andres RH, Steinberg GK (2010) Optimizing the success of cell transplantation therapy for stroke. Neurobiol Dis 37:275–283

Borlongan CV, Hadman M, Sanberg CD, Sanberg PR (2004) Central nervous system entry of peripherally injected umbilical cord blood cells is not required for neuroprotection in stroke. Stroke 35:2385–2389

Borlongan CV, Kaneko Y, Maki M, Yu SJ, Ali M, Allickson JG, Sanberg CD, Kuzmin-Nichols N, Sanberg PR (2010) Menstrual blood cells display stem cell-like phenotypic markers and exert neuroprotection following transplantation in experimental stroke. Stem Cells Dev 19:439–452

Bratincsák A, Brownstein MJ, Cassiani-Ingoni R, Pastorino S, Szalayova I, Toth ZE, Key S, Nemeth K, Pickel J, Mezey E (2007) CD45-positive blood cells give rise to uterine epithelial cells in mice. Stem Cells 25:2820–2826

Centers for Disease Control and Prevention (CDC) (1999) Prevalence of disabilities and associated health conditions among adults, United States. Morb Mortal Wkly Rep 50:120–125

Cervello I, Gil-Sanchis C, Mas A, Delgado-Rosas F, Martinez-Conejero JA, Galan A, Martinez-Romero A, Martinez S, Navarro I, Ferro J, Horcajadas JA, Esteban FJ, O'Connor JE, Pellicer A, Simon C (2010) Human endometrial side population cells exhibit genotypic, phenotypic and functional features of somatic stem cells. PLoS One 5:e10964

Chan RW, Schwab KE, Gargett CE (2004) Clonogenicity of human endometrial epithelial and stromal cells. Biol Reprod 70:1738–1750

Cho NH, Park YK, Kim YT, Yang H, Kim SK (2004) Lifetime expression of stem cell markers in the uterine endometrium. Fertil Steril 81:403–407

Connolly ES, Jr., Winfree CJ, Springer TA, Naka Y, Liao H, Yan SD, Stern DM, Solomon RA, Gutierrez-Ramos JC, Pinsky DJ (1996) Cerebral protection in homozygous null ICAM-1 mice after middle cerebral artery occlusion. Role of neutrophil adhesion in the pathogenesis of stroke. J Clin Invest 97:209–216

Drago H, Marin GH, Sturla F, Roque G, Martire K, Diaz Aquino V, Lamonega R, Gardiner C, Ichim T, Riordan N, Raimondi JC, Bossi S, Samadikuchaksaraei A, van Leeuwen M, Tau JM, Nunez L, Larsen G, Spretz R, Mansilla E (2010) The next generation of burns treatment: intelligent films and matrix, controlled enzymatic debridement, and adult stem cells. Transplant Proc 42:345–349

Durukan A, Tatlisumak T (2007) Acute ischemic stroke: overview of major experimental rodent models, pathophysiology, and therapy of focal cerebral ischemia. Pharmacol Biochem Behav 87:179–197

Emsley HC, Smith CJ Tyrrell PJ, Hopkins SJ (2008) Inflammation in acute ischemic stroke and its relevance to stroke critical care. Neurocrit Care 9:125–138

Guzman R, Choi R, Gera A, De Los Angeles A, Andres RH, Steinberg GK (2008) Intravascular cell replacement therapy for stroke. Neurosurg Focus 24:E15

Hess DC, Borlongan CV (2008) Cell-based therapy in ischemic stroke. Expert Rev Neurother 8:1193–1201

Hida N, Nishiyama N, Miyoshi S, Kira S Segawa K, Uyama T, Mori T, Miyado K, Ikegami Y, Cui C, Kiyono T, Kyo S, Shimizu T, Okano T, Sakamoto M, Ogawa S, Umezawa A (2008) Novel cardiac precursor-like cells from human menstrual blood-derived mesenchymal cells. Stem Cells 26:1695–1704

Hurn PD, Subramanian S, Parker SM, Afentoulis ME, Kaler LJ, Vandenbark AA, Offner H (2007) T- and B-cell-deficient mice with experimental stroke have reduced lesion size and inflammation. J Cereb Blood Flow Metab 27:1798–1805

Jin R, Yang G, Li G (2010) Inflammatory mechanisms in ischemic stroke: role of inflammatory cells. J Leukoc Biol 87:779–789

Kim SY, Cho HS, Yang SH, Shin JY, Kim JS, Lee ST, Chu K, Roh JK, Kim SU, Park CG (2009) Soluble mediators from human neural stem cells play a critical role in suppression of T-cell activation and proliferation. J Neurosci Res 87: 2264–2272

Kleindorfer D, Lindsell CJ, Brass L, Koroshetz W, Broderick JP (2008) National US estimates of recombinant tissue plasminogen activator use: ICD-9 codes substantially underestimate. Stroke 39:924–928

Kondziolka D, Steinberg GK, Wechsler L, Meltzer CC, Elder E, Gebel J, Decesare S, Jovin T, Zafonte R, Lebowitz J, Flickinger JC, Tong D, Marks MP, Jamieson C, Luu D, Bell-Stephens T, Teraoka J (2005) Neurotransplantation for patients with subcortical motor stroke: a phase 2 randomized trial. J Neurosurg 103:38–45

Lee ST, Chu K, Jung KH, Kim SJ, Kim DH, Kang KM, Hong NH, Kim JH, Ban JJ, Park HK, Kim SU, Park CG, Lee SK, Kim M, Roh JK (2008) Anti-inflammatory mechanism of intravascular neural stem cell transplantation in haemorrhagic stroke. Brain 131:616–629

Masuda H, Matsuzaki Y, Hiratsu E, Ono M, Nagashima T, Kajitani T, Arase T, Oda H, Uchida H, Asada H, Ito M, Yoshimura Y, Maruyama T, Okano H (2010) Stem cell-like properties of the endometrial side population: implication in endometrial regeneration. PLoS One 5:e10387

Meng X, Ichim TE, Zhong J, Rogers A, Yin Z, Jackson J, Wang H, Ge W, Bogin V, Chan KW, Thebaud B, Riordan NH (2007) Endometrial regenerative cells: a novel stem cell population. J Transl Med 5:57

Murphy MP, Wang H, Patel AN, Kambhampati S, Angle N, Chan K, Marleau AM, Pyszniak A, Carrier E, Ichim TE, Riordan NH (2008) Allogeneic endometrial regenerative cells: an "Off the shelf solution" for critical limb ischemia? J Transl Med 6:45

Padykula HA (1991) Regeneration in the primate uterus: the role of stem cells. Ann N Y Acad Sci 622:47–56

Park DH, Eve DJ, Musso J 3rd, Klasko SK, Cruz E, Borlongan CV, Sanberg PR (2009) Inflammation and stem cell migration to the injured brain in higher organisms. Stem Cells Dev 18:693–702

Patel AN, Silva F (2008) Menstrual blood stromal cells: the potential for regenerative medicine. Regen Med 3:443–444

Patel AN, Park E, Kuzman M, Benetti F, Silva FJ, Allickson JG (2008) Multipotent Menstrual Blood Stromal Stem Cells: Isolation, characterization and Differentiation. Cell Transplant 17:303–311

Prianishnikov VA (1978) A functional model of the structure of the epithelium of normal, hyperplastic and malignant human endometrium: a review. Gynecol Oncol 6:420–428

Taylor HS (2004) Endometrial cells derived from donor stem cells in bone marrow transplant recipients. JAMA 292:81–85

The National Institute of Neurological Disorders (NINDS) and Stroke rt-PA Stroke Study Group (1995) Tissue plasminogen activator for acute ischemic stroke. N Engl J Med 333: 1581–1587

Wolff EF, Gao XB, Yao KV, Andrews ZB, Du H, Elsworth JD, Taylor HS (2011) Endometrial stem cell transplantation restores dopamine production in a Parkinson's disease model. J Cell Mol Med 15:747–755

Xu, J, Kochanek MA, Murphy BS, Tejada-Vera B (2010) Deaths, final data for 2007. Natl Vital Stat Rep 58:1–134

Zhong Z, Patel AN, Ichim TE, Riordan NH, Wang H, Min WP, Woods EJ, Reid M, Mansilla E, Marin GH, Drago H, Murphy MP, Minev B (2009) Feasibility investigation of allogeneic endometrial regenerative cells. J Transl Med 7:15

Chapter 21

Spontaneous Cerebral Stroke in Rats: Differentiation of New Neurons from Neural Stem Cells

Tatsuki Itoh, Kumiko Takemori, Motohiro Imano, Shozo Nishida, Masahiro Tsubaki, Shigeo Hashimoto, Hiroyuki Ito, Akihiko Ito, and Takao Satou

Abstract Stroke-prone spontaneously hypertensive rats (SHRSP) are the only animal model that suffers from spontaneous cerebral stroke. In this study, we investigated the appearance of neural stem cells (NSCs) and new neurons in the penumbra and the subventricular zone (SVZ) after cerebral stroke in SHRSP. SHRSP before cerebral stroke were intraperitoneally injected with 5-bromo-2′-deoxyuridine (BrdU). SHRSP were divided into acute and chronic phase groups after cerebral stroke. Brain sections from both groups were studied with cell-specific markers such as BrdU, a cell division and proliferation marker, SOX2, a marker of NSCs, nestin, an NSC and immature astrocyte marker, doublecortin (DCX), an immature new neuron marker, and NeuN, a marker of mature neurons. NSCs and new neurons appeared in the penumbra in the early stages after cerebral stroke, and these cells differentiated into mature neurons in the chronic phase. Furthermore, soon after being affected by a cerebral stroke, there were many new neurons and immature cells, which appear to be NSCs, in the ipsilateral SVZ. The findings of the study indicate that immature cells and new neurons from the ipsilateral SVZ might migrate into the penumbra after cerebral stroke.

Keywords Cerebral stroke · Neural stem cells · Doublecortin · Neural stem cells · Subventricular zone · Neurogenesis

Introduction

Circulatory disturbance in the brain induces neuronal degeneration and then necrosis in the penumbral areas (Rice et al., 2003). CNS disorders can be caused by widespread neuronal and axonal degeneration induced by brain insults that are aggravated by excitotoxicity and disruption to the blood-brain barrier (Xiong et al., 1997).

It was originally thought that recovery from these injuries was severely limited because neuronal loss and degeneration in the adult mammalian brain were irreversible. However, recent studies have indicated that the mammalian nervous system has the potential to replenish populations of damaged and / or destroyed neurons through proliferation of neural stem cells (NSCs)(Gage, 2000). These authors have identified NSCs in adult mammals and have the potential to differentiate into either glial or neural phenotypes. The presence of NSCs has been confirmed in two areas of the adult rodent brain. One is the subventricular zone (SVZ) of the lateral ventricles, and the other is the subgranular zone (SGZ) at the dentate gyrus-hilus interface (Parent et al., 1997). There is slow but continuous neurogenesis in these areas of the adult brain. Furthermore, we previously reported that a proportion of nestin-positive cells around a damaged area after rat traumatic brain injury (TBI) were NSCs, which can differentiate into neurons and glia, and that these nestin-expressing NSCs were involved in neurogenesis around the damaged area (Itoh et al., 2005, 2007, 2009). The appearance of NSCs and new neurons in the penumbra after rat experimental stroke has not been reported, although generation of a model of ischemic stroke by middle cerebral artery occlusion

T. Itoh (✉)
Department of Pathology, Kinki University School of Medicine, Osaka, Japan
e-mail: tatsuki@med.kindai.ac.jp

(MCAO) triggers increased NSCs and new neurons in the rat SVZ and SGZ (Itoh et al., 2010).

Stroke-prone spontaneously hypertensive rats (SHRSP) are the only animal model that has a spontaneous cerebral stroke. It appears that the mechanisms of cerebral stroke in SHRSP are similar to those of cerebral stroke in humans (Itoh et al., 2010). Moreover, and like in the human brain, neural degeneration and death are induced after cerebral stroke in SHRSP not only in the stroke lesion area but also in the penumbra (Itoh et al., 2010). However, the appearance of NSCs and new neurons in the penumbra has not been observed after a spontaneous cerebral stroke. In this study, we investigated the appearance of NSCs and new neurons in the penumbra after cerebral stroke in SHRSP.

Methods

Animals

We used 15-week old, male SHRSP, the offspring of original strains that were developed by Dr. K. Okamoto (Itoh et al., 2010) and are maintained in our laboratory.

Labeling of Dividing and Proliferating Cells

Before cerebral stroke occurred, male SHRSP (16 weeks of age) were intraperitoneally injected twice a day for two weeks with 5-bromo-2′-deoxyuridine (BrdU; 50 mg/kg, Sigma-Aldrich, St Louis, MO), which labels dividing and proliferating cells.

Experimental and Control Groups

SHRSP were divided into acute and chronic phase groups. The acute group was made up of SHRSP that displayed dyskinesia, such as tremors, rigidity and rotation, within two days of the end of the BrdU injection period (n = 6). These rats were sacrificed just after the behavioral disorder first appeared. The chronic group comprised SHRSP that had developed behavioral disorder 30 days after the last BrdU injection (n = 6). Both in the acute and chronic groups, the contralateral side in stroke-affected SHRSP was used as the control.

Brain lesions were histologically classified by gliosis (Fig. 21.1b) and glial scarring (Fig. 21.1c), using staining for glial fibrillary acidic protein (GFAP) in the penumbra after cerebral stroke. Only histologically definitive brain lesions were investigated in this study.

Immunohistochemistry

In the acute and chronic groups, all six rats were deeply anesthetized by an intraperitoneal injection of pentobarbital (150 mg/kg) and then perfused intracardially with 300 ml 0.1 M phosphate-buffered saline (PBS; pH 7.4–7.5), followed by 300 ml 4% paraformaldehyde (PFA) in PBS (pH 7.4–7.5). The brains were then removed and stored in PFA for 3 days. The stroke-lesioned area of the frontoparietal cortex was confirmed macroscopically then sliced into 10 serial coronal sections (50 μm thick) using a microslicer (Dousaka EM, Kyoto, Japan). Each section was treated with 3% H_2O_2 in Tris-buffered saline (TBS; 0.1 M Tris-HCl pH 7.5, 0.15 M NaCl) for 30 min to block endogenous peroxidase activity. Next, the sections were washed three times with TBS containing 0.1% Triton X-100 (TBS-T), blocked with 3% bovine serum albumin (BSA; Sigma, St. Louis, MO) in TBS-T (TBS-TB) for 30 min and incubated overnight at room temperature with either an anti-GFAP rabbit polyclonal antibody (1:1000 dilution in TBS-TB, DAKO, Kyoto, Japan), or an anti-DCX goat polyclonal antibody (1:1000 dilution in TBS-TB, Santa Cruz Biotechnology, CA, USA). GFAP was used as a marker of gliosis and glial scarring, and DCX was a marker of immature neurons. Following extensive washing in TBS-T, the sections were further incubated for 60 min at room temperature with a HISTIFINE Rat-PO-kit (Nichirei, Osaka, Japan) as the secondary antibody. Labeling was visualized using diaminobenzidine (DAB; Vector Peroxidase Substrate Kit; Vector Laboratories, Burlingame, CA) for 5 min, and the sections were counterstained with hematoxylin to enable counting of the positive cells.

21 Spontaneous Cerebral Stroke in Rats: Differentiation of New Neurons from Neural Stem Cells   201

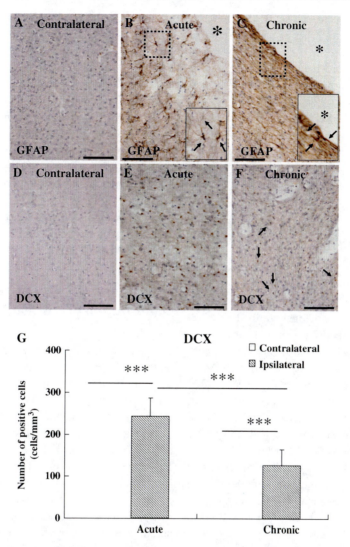

Fig. 21.1 Immunostaining for glial fibrillary acidic protein (GFAP) and doublecortin (DCX) in the penumbra after cerebral stroke in stroke-prone spontaneously hypertensive rats (SHRSP). In the contralateral cerebral cortex, there were no GFAP (a) and no DCX (d) immunopositive cells. In the acute SHRSP group, abundant GFAP immunoreactivity was present, mainly in the cytoplasm and projections around the infarct site (b). In Panel B, the *box* indicates the area depicted in the *inset* showing the gliosis. In the chronic SHRSP group, GFAP-immunopositive elongated fibers were seen around the infarct site (c). In Panel C, the *box* indicates the area depicted in the *inset* showing the glial scar. DCX immunoreactivity was present mainly in the cytoplasm and projections in the acute SHRSP group (e) and a few DCX-immunopositive cells were identified in the chronic SHRSP group (f, *arrows*). *; infarct area. Scale bars = 100 μm. (g). Graph showing the number of DCX-immunopositive cells in the penumbra after cerebral stroke. The results are shown as mean ± SD. ***$p < 0.001$, $n = 6$

Double-Immunofluorescence Staining for Nestin and Sex-Determining Region Y-Box 2 (SOX2)

The sections were washed with TBS-T, blocked with TBS-TB and incubated overnight at room temperature with an anti-rat nestin mouse monoclonal antibody (1:300 dilution in TBS-TB; BD Biosciences Pharmingen, NJ, USA). Following extensive washing in TBS-T, the sections were incubated for 80 min at room temperature with an Alexa Fluor 488-conjugated anti-mouse IgG antibody (1:300 dilution in TBS-TB, Molecular Probes, Inc.). Next, the sections were washed extensively and incubated overnight at room temperature with an anti-SOX2 goat polyclonal antibody (1:300 dilution in TBS-TB; Santa Cruz Biotechnology). SOX2 is a marker of NSCs (Komitova et al., 2005; Itoh et al., 2009). Following extensive washing, the sections were incubated for 80 min at room temperature with an Alexa Fluor 555-conjugated anti-goat IgG antibody (1:300 dilution in TBS-TB, Molecular Probes, Inc.). Subsequently, the sections were observed using a confocal laser-scanning microscope (LSM5 PASCAL; Carl Zeiss Jena GmbH, Jena, Germany).

Triple-Immunofluorescence Staining for Nestin, SOX2 and GFAP

Sections were stained as above. The sections were incubated overnight at room temperature with an anti-rat nestin mouse monoclonal antibody (1:300 dilution in TBS-TB; BD Biosciences Pharmingen). Following extensive washing, the sections were incubated for 80 min at room temperature with an Alexa Fluor 488-conjugated anti-mouse IgG antibody (1:300 dilution in TBS-TB, Molecular Probes, Inc.). Next, the sections were washed extensively and incubated overnight at room temperature with an anti-SOX2 goat polyclonal antibody (1:300 dilution in TBS-TB; Santa Cruz Biotechnology). Following extensive washing, the sections were incubated for 80 min at room temperature with an Alexa Fluor 350-conjugated anti-goat IgG antibody (1:300 dilution in TBS-TB, Molecular Probe, Inc.). Next, the sections were washed extensively and incubated overnight at room temperature with an anti-GFAP rabbit polyclonal antibody (1:300 dilution in TBS-TB; DAKO). Following extensive washing, the sections were further incubated for 80 min at room temperature with an Alexa Fluor 555-conjugated anti-rabbit IgG antibody (1:300 dilution in TBS-TB; BD Biosciences Pharmingen). Subsequently, the sections were observed using the LSM5 PASCAL confocal laser-scanning microscope. Double-Immunofluorescence Staining for BrdU and DCX or neuron-specific nuclear protein (NeuN).

Sections were stained as above. The sections were washed with TBS-T, blocked with TBS-TB and incubated overnight at room temperature with an anti-BrdU sheep polyclonal antibody (1:300 dilution in TBS-TB, Abcam Ltd., Cambridge, UK). Following extensive washing in TBS-T, the sections were incubated for 80 min at room temperature with an Alexa Fluor 488-conjugated anti-sheep IgG antibody (1:300 dilution in TBS-TB, Molecular Probes, Inc., Eugene, OR). Next, the sections were washed extensively in TBS-T then incubated overnight at room temperature with an anti-DCX antibody (1:300 dilution in TBS-TB; Santa Cruz Biotechnology) or an anti-neuron-specific nuclear protein (NeuN) mouse monoclonal antibody (1:300 dilution in TBS-TB; Chemicon, Temecula, CA). NeuN is a marker of mature neurons. Following extensive washing in TBS-T, the sections were incubated for 80 min at room temperature with an Alexa Fluor 555-conjugated anti-mouse or goat IgG antibody (1:300 dilution in TBS-TB, Molecular Probes, Inc.).

Quantitation of Positive Cells

To determine the number of DCX-positive cells, DAB-labeled cells in the penumbra around the infarct after cerebral stroke were observed and counted in three serial sections (depth 150 μm; each section 50 μm thick) under a Nikon E 1000M microscope (Nikon Corporation, Tokyo, Japan) with a 20× objective. To determine the measured area of DCX-positive cells, an image of the measured area was captured under 1× magnification on the Nikon E 1000M microscope using a CCD camera (ACT-2U; Nikon Corporation). The relevant area in each image was traced and measured using a computer (Power Macintosh G3; Apple Computers, Cupertino, CA) with NIH Image 1.6 software (NIH, Bethesda, MD). The number of DCX-positive cells was expressed as positive cells per mm^3.

Cells double-labeled with BrdU and DCX (DCX$^+$/BrdU$^+$) or NeuN (NeuN$^+$/BrdU$^+$) or triple-labeled with nestin, SOX2 and GFAP (nestin$^+$/SOX2$^+$/GFAP$^+$) were counted in the infarct penumbral region after cerebral stroke in three serial sections, using the LSM5 PASCAL confocal laser-scanning microscope with a 20× objective. The scanning area for the counted cell number was calculated automatically by the LSM5 PASCAL software. The numbers of DCX$^+$/BrdU$^+$, NeuN$^+$/BrdU$^+$ and nestin$^+$/SOX2$^+$/GFAP$^+$ cells were expressed as positive cells per mm^3. The same method was used to determine the number of DCX-positive cells in the

SVZ (+1.00, +0.95 and +0.9 mm from bregma) and the number of cells double-labeled with nestin and SOX2 (nestin$^+$/SOX2$^+$) in the SVZ (+0.85, +0.80 and +0.75 mm from bregma).

Statistical Analysis

The data were expressed as means ± SD. Statistical analysis was performed using one-way analysis of variance (ANOVA) with Fisher's post-hoc test. Values of $P < 0.05$ were considered statistically significant.

Results

Observations in the Stroke Infarct Penumbra

GFAP Immunoreactivity

The immunostaining results for GFAP expression around the infarct after cerebral stroke are shown in Fig. 21.1a–c. There were no GFAP-immunopositive cells in the contralateral cerebral cortex after cerebral stroke (Fig. 21.1a). After cerebral stroke, in the acute phase group, gliosis was evident: there were many large GFAP-positive cells in the penumbra, with GFAP staining in their cytoplasm and elongated projections (Fig. 21.1b). In the chronic phase group, there were many GFAP-immunopositive fibers that formed glial scars, and these fibers were enriched at the site of the infarct (Fig. 21.1c).

Quantification of DCX-Positive Cells Around the Infarct Penumbra Following Cerebral Stroke

The immunostaining results for DCX expression in the penumbra after cerebral stroke are shown in Fig. 21.1d–f. In the contralateral cerebral cortex after cerebral stroke, there were no DCX-positive cells (Fig. 21.1d). After cerebral stroke, in the acute phase group, there were many small DCX-positive cells with positive staining of their cytoplasm and projections in the penumbra (Fig. 21.1e). Furthermore, in the chronic phase group after cerebral stroke, there were also DCX-positive cells near the lesion, with DCX staining in their cytoplasm and projections (Fig. 21.1f).

Figure 21.1g shows the quantitation of DCX-positive cells. The contralateral cerebral cortex did not contain any DCX-positive cells. The number of DCX-positive cells was significantly higher in the acute phase group than in the contralateral control ($P < 0.001$) or the chronic phase group ($P < 0.001$).

Observation of the SVZ in SHRSP After Cerebral Stroke

The number of SOX2 and Nestin-positive cells is increased in the SVZ following cerebral stroke. In the contralateral SVZ, there were a few SOX2$^+$/nestin$^+$ double-labeled cells (Fig. 21.2a–c). In the ipsilateral SVZ, there were many SOX2$^+$/nestin$^+$ double-labeled cells in the acute (Fig. 21.2d–f) and the chronic (Fig. 21.2 g–i) phase groups.

Figure 21.3a shows the quantitation of SOX2$^+$/nestin$^+$ double-labeled cells in the contralateral and ipsilateral SVZ after cerebral stroke. The number of SOX2$^+$/nestin$^+$ double-labeled cells was significantly higher in the ipsilateral SVZ in the acute and chronic phase groups than in the contralateral SVZ ($P < 0.05$). The number of SOX2$^+$/nestin$^+$ double-labeled cells was significantly higher in the acute phase group than in the chronic phase group ($P < 0.001$).

The number of DCX-positive cells is increased in the SVZ following cerebral stroke

The immunostaining results for DCX expression in the SVZ after cerebral stroke are shown in Fig. 21.4a–c. In the contralateral SVZ, there were some small DCX-positive cells (Fig. 21.4a). In the acute and chronic phase groups after cerebral stroke, there were many small DCX-positive cells with positive staining of their cytoplasm and projections in the ipsilateral SVZ (Fig. 21.4b, c).

Figure 21.3b shows the quantitation of DCX-positive cells. The number of DCX-positive cells was significantly higher in the ipsilateral SVZ in the acute and chronic phase groups than in the contralateral SVZ ($P < 0.001$). Furthermore, the number of DCX-positive cells was significantly higher in the chronic phase group than in the acute phase group ($P < 0.05$).

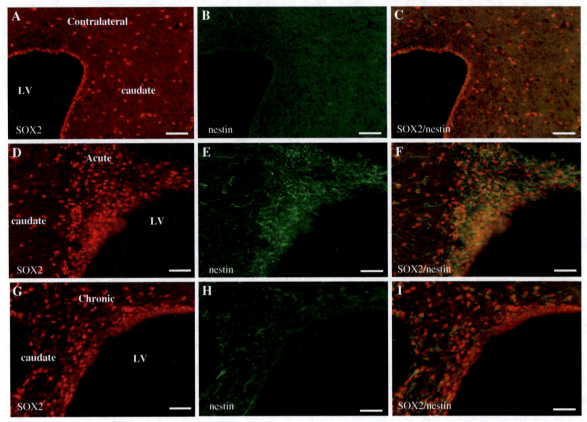

Fig. 21.2 Double-labeling fluorescence immunostaining shows SOX2 (*red*) and nestin (*green*) expression in the contralateral (**a–c**) and ipsilateral (**d–i**) subventricular zone (SVZ) of and SHRSP. In the contralateral control, there were a few SOX2$^+$/nestin$^+$ double-labeled cells in the contralateral SVZ (**a–c**). In the SHRSP acute group, there were many SOX2$^+$/nestin$^+$ double-labeled cells in the ipsilateral SVZ after stroke (**d–f**). In the SHRSP chronic group, there were SOX2$^+$/nestin$^+$ double-labeled cells in the ipsilateral SVZ after stroke (**g–i**). The merged images (**c**), (**f**) and (**i**) reveal colocalization of these proteins (*yellow*)

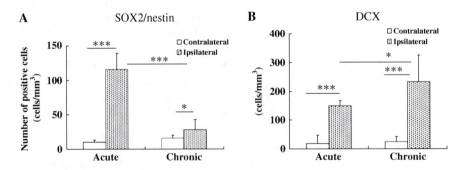

Fig. 21.3 Graph showing the number of immunopositive cells for SOX2$^+$/nestin$^+$ double-labeled (**a**) and DCX cells (**b**) in the contralateral and ipsilateral subventricular zone of SHRSP. The results are shown as mean ± SD. *$p < 0.05$, ***$p < 0.001$, $n = 5$

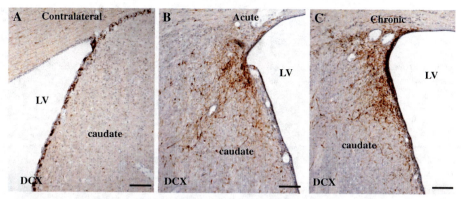

Fig. 21.4 Immunostaining for DCX in the contralateral subventricular zone (SVZ) of SHRSP (**a**) and in the ipsilateral SVZ of SHRSP (**b, c**). In the contralateral control, there were a few DCX-immunopositive cells in the SVZ (**a**). In the acute group (**b**) and the chronic group (**c**) of SHRSP, abundant DCX-immunoreactivity was present mainly in the cytoplasm and projections in the ipsilateral SVZ. Scale bars = 100 μm. *LV* lateral ventricle

Immunofluorescence Results

The number of SOX2, Nestin and GFAP-positive cells is increased in the penumbra following cerebral stroke. In the acute phase group after cerebral stroke, there were many large GFAP-positive reactive astroglial cells (GFAP$^+$/nestin$^+$) with nestin staining in their cytoplasm and long elongated projections in the penumbra (Fig. 21.4a, b). Almost all GFAP$^+$/nestin$^+$ double-labeled cells were co-localized with SOX2-immunopositivity GFAP$^+$/nestin$^+$/SOX2$^+$, Fig. 21.4c, d). However, some GFAP$^+$/nestin$^+$ double-labeled cells did not show SOX2-immunoreactivity (GFAP$^+$/nestin$^+$/SOX2$^-$, Fig. 21.4c, d). In the contralateral cerebral cortex after cerebral stroke, there were no GFAP$^+$/nestin$^+$/SOX2$^-$ double-labeled cells or GFAP$^+$/nestin$^+$/SOX2$^+$ triple-labeled cells (data not shown).

Figure 21.5e shows the quantitation of nestin$^+$/GFAP$^+$/SOX2$^+$ triple-labeled cells. The contralateral cerebral cortex after cerebral stroke did not contain any nestin$^+$/GFAP$^+$/SOX2$^+$ triple-labeled cells. The number of GFAP$^+$/nestin$^+$/SOX2$^+$ triple-labeled cells was significantly higher in the acute phase group than in the contralateral control ($P < 0.001$) or the chronic phase group ($P < 0.001$).

The number of BrdU and DCX-positive cells is increased in the penumbra following cerebral stroke. In the contralateral cerebral cortex after cerebral stroke, there were no BrdU$^+$/DCX$^+$ double-labeled cells (data not shown). In the acute and chronic phase groups, there were many BrdU$^+$/DCX$^+$ double-labeled cells in the penumbra after stroke (Fig. 21.6a–c). Figure 21.6g shows the quantitation of BrdU$^+$/DCX$^+$ double-labeled cells. The contralateral cerebral cortex after cerebral stroke did not contain any BrdU$^+$/DCX$^+$ double-labeled cells. The number of BrdU$^+$/DCX$^+$ double-labeled cells was significantly higher in the acute and chronic phase groups than in the contralateral control ($P < 0.001$). The number of BrdU$^+$/DCX$^+$ double-labeled cells was significantly higher in the acute phase group than in the chronic phase group ($P < 0.001$).

The number of NeuN and BrdU-positive cells is increased in the infarct penumbra following cerebral stroke. In the contralateral cortex in both the acute and chronic phase groups, and in the ipsilateral cerebral cortex in the acute phase group, there were no BrdU$^+$/NeuN$^+$ double-labeled cells (data not shown). In the ipsilateral cortex of the chronic phase group however, there were many BrdU$^+$/NeuN$^+$ double-labeled cells in the penumbra after stroke (Fig. 21.6d–f). Figure 21.6g shows the quantitation of BrdU$^+$/NeuN$^+$ double-labeled cells. The number of BrdU$^+$/NeuN$^+$ double-labeled cells in the chronic phase group was significantly higher than in the contralateral control or the acute phase group ($P < 0.001$).

Discussion

Because SHRSP suffer from spontaneous cerebral strokes, the exact time of the stroke is unknown. Thus, we investigated the acute and the chronic phase groups

Fig. 21.5 Triple-labeling fluorescence immunostaining shows GFAP, nestin and SOX2 expression in the penumbra after cerebral stroke in the SHRSP acute group. There were many GFAP (**a**, *red*) and nestin (**b**, *green*) immunopositive cells after stroke. There were a few SOX2-immunopositive nuclei (**c**, *blue*) after stroke. The merged image (**d**) of panels (**a**), (**b**) and (**c**) reveals colocalization of these proteins (*yellow* and *blue*). *Arrow heads* (▲) show triple-labeled (*purple*) cells (GFAP$^+$/nestin$^+$/SOX2$^+$) and *arrows* (↑) show double-labeled (*yellow*) cells without SOX2 immunopositivity (GFAP$^+$/nestin$^+$/SOX2$^-$). Scale bar = 50 μm. (**e**) Graph showing the number of triple-labeled cells (GFAP$^+$/nestin$^+$/SOX2$^+$) in the penumbra and the contralateral cerebral cortex after cerebral stroke in SHRSP. The results are shown as mean ± SD. ***$p < 0.001$, $n = 6$

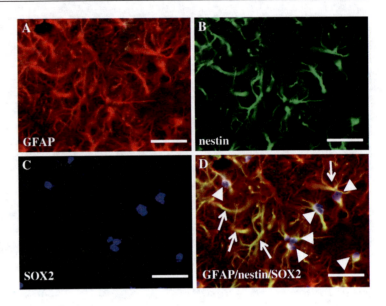

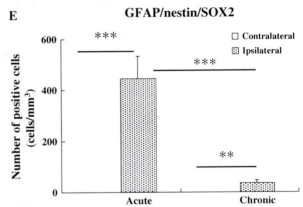

immunohistochemically, to examine and compare the degenerative and regenerative characteristics of each group.

Insult to the adult CNS results in gliosis. In the penumbra after cerebral stroke there is a rapid appearance of many reactive astrocytes with GFAP staining in their cytoplasm and elongated projections (Pekny and Nilsson, 2005). Later, the damaged infarct site becomes enriched in GFAP-immunopositive fibers that form glial scars (Pekny and Nilsson, 2005). Pathologically, gliosis has been used as an acute phase marker after brain insult, and glial scars have been used as a chronic phase marker. Thus in this study, we excluded brain lesions from the acute phase group that displayed glial scars in the penumbra. Similarly, we also excluded from the chronic phase group those brain lesions that showed gliosis.

The triple-immunofluorescence staining for nestin, GFAP and SOX2 indicated that there were nestin$^+$/GFAP$^+$/SOX2$^+$ triple-labeled cells in the penumbra after cerebral stroke. Although GFAP has been recognized as an astrocyte marker, recent studies have demonstrated that it is also expressed in pluripotent NSCs and neural precursor cells (Itoh et al., 2009). In the SVZ or SGZ after brain injury, astrocytes show blastogenesis and differentiate into neural precursor cells that are immunopositive for both nestin and GFAP. Subsequently, these cells differentiate into new immature neurons (Picard-Riera et al., 2004). Our previous data revealed the presence of nestin-positive NSCs around the damaged area after rat TBI (Itoh et al., 2005, 2007, 2009). In the SVZ or SGZ, NSCs that appeared after brain injury showed SOX2-immunopositivity (Komitova et al., 2005).

Fig. 21.6 Double-labeling fluorescence immunostaining shows BrdU plus DCX or NeuN around the infarct cerebral cortex after cerebral stroke in SHRSP. There were a few cells with BrdU-immunopositive nuclei in the acute group (**a**, *green*) and the chronic group (**d**, *green*).There were many DCX-immunopositive cells in the acute group (**b**, *red*) and NeuN-immunopositive cells in the chronic group (**e**, *red*). The merged images (**c**) and (**f**) of panels (**a** and **b**) and (**d** and **e**) respectively, reveal colocalization of these proteins (*yellow, arrows*). Scale bar = 50 μm. (**g**) Graph showing quantitation of the double-labeled cells (BrdU⁺/DCX⁺; diagonal striped column or BrdU⁺/NeuN⁺; *solid black column*) in the penumbra and the contralateral cerebral cortex after cerebral stroke in SHRSP. The results are shown as mean ± SD. ***$p < 0.001$, $n = 6$

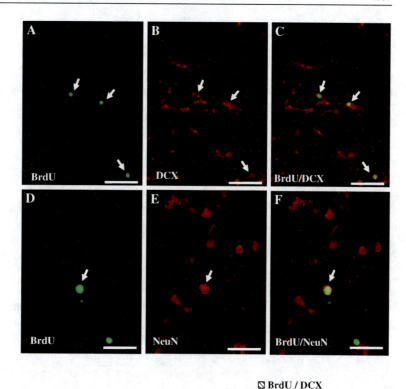

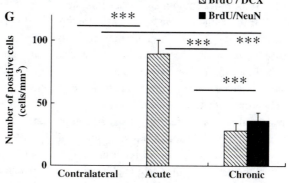

These results suggest that nestin⁺/GFAP⁺/SOX2⁺ triple- and nestin⁺/SOX2⁺ double-labeled cells that appeared in the infarct penumbral area after cerebral stroke are NSCs.

On the other hand, some reactive astrocytes also showed nestin-immunopositivity around the damaged area after TBI (Nakamura et al., 2004). Our data indicated that there were some nestin⁺/GFAP⁺ double-labeled cells without SOX2 immunoreactivity. In the SVZ or SGZ after brain injury, astrocytes differentiate into neural precursor cells and these cells differentiate into new immature neurons (Picard-Riera et al., 2004). GFAP⁺/nestin⁺ double-positive astrocytes in the SVZ differentiate into NSCs and neural precursor cells (Doetsch et al., 1999). In a recent report, we revealed that GFAP⁺/nestin⁺ double-positive astrocytes give rise to NSCs and these cells differentiate into neurons and glia in vitro (Itoh et al., 2006). These results suggest that some NSCs and new neurons appearing in the penumbra after cerebral stroke may originate from astrocytes.

In this study, there were many DCX-positive cells in the penumbral area after cerebral stroke in the acute phase. In a rat ischemic MCO model, DCX-positive cells appear within one week after stroke (Thored et al., 2006). In addition, we have reported that DCX-positive cells appear around the damaged area from 24 h after TBI in the rat (Itoh et al., 2007). These results are consistent with our present data, and indicate that DCX-positive cells appear in the early stages after cerebral stroke. These results demonstrate that new neurons and NSCs appear in the penumbra after cerebral stroke in SHRSP.

The expression of DCX is down-regulated when DCX-positive newly-formed immature neurons become mature, and the new immature neurons also co-localize with NeuN, a marker of mature neurons (Itoh et al., 2007). New, BrdU-immunopositive neurons appear after brain injury, which can divide and proliferate (Couillard-Despres et al., 2005). In the present study, there were many DCX-positive cells in the penumbra and some of these cells were DCX$^+$/BrdU$^+$-double immunopositive. Furthermore, in the chronic group, some of the NeuN-positive cells co-localized with BrdU immunopositivity (NeuN$^+$/BrdU$^+$). These results suggest that NSCs or neuroblasts newly divided and/or proliferated after cerebral stroke, and formed new immature neurons (DCX$^+$/BrdU$^+$) in the penumbra. These immature cells (DCX$^+$/BrdU$^+$) then developed into mature neurons (NeuN$^+$/BrdU$^+$). In addition, there were many DCX-positive cells in the penumbra after cerebral stroke in the chronic phase group. These results suggest that immature neurons continue to develop into mature neurons even in the chronic phase.

In the ipsilateral SVZ after cerebral stroke, the number of both nestin$^+$/SOX2$^+$ double-labeled cells and DCX-positive cells was significantly higher in the ipsilateral cortex of the acute and the chronic phase groups than in the contralateral cortex. In ischemic stroke models caused by MCO, the number of SOX2-positive NSCs and/or DCX-positive new neurons increased in the ipsilateral SVZ after cerebral stroke (Thored et al., 2006). The number of nestin-positive NSCs and/or new neurons increased in the ipsilateral SVZ after rat TBI (Salman et al., 2004).

These results are consistent with our present data, and indicate that the number of NSCs and/or new neurons increased in the ipsilateral SVZ after cerebral stroke. In addition, after rat TBI some NSCs and immature neurons from the SVZ migrate to the damaged area (Thored et al., 2006). These results indicate the possibility that a proportion of the NSCs and new neurons that appear in the infarct penumbral area after cerebral stroke may migrate from the SVZ.

Although the origin of these nestin-positive cells in the penumbra remains controversial, we previously showed that nestin-positive cells around the damaged area after TBI have the characteristics of NSCs, which can proliferate and differentiate to neurons or glia (Itoh et al., 2005). Therefore, it is considered that the generation of endogenous immature cells in the penumbra after cerebral stroke is very important for neurogenesis after brain injury.

Expression of nestin and DCX is not present in both NSCs and neurons simultaneously, because their phases of cellular differentiation differ (Brown et al., 2003; Itoh et al., 2007). Nestin-positive, pluripotent NSCs mature into neuroblasts, and these neuroblasts are positive for DCX but no longer for nestin (Brown et al., 2003). However, NSCs differentiate into not only neurons but also glial cells (Itoh et al., 2005; Itoh et al., 2006). In this study, there were fewer nestin$^+$/GFAP$^+$/SOX2$^+$-labeled cells around the infarct, and nestin$^+$/SOX2$^+$-labeled cells in the SVZ, in the chronic phase group than in the acute phase group. These results indicate that not all of the nestin-positive cells changed into DCX-positive cells. Thus it is likely that some of the nestin$^+$/GFAP$^+$/SOX2$^+$ and nestin$^+$/SOX2$^+$-labeled cells disappeared or changed into glial cells.

On the other hand, in the contralateral cerebral cortex and SVZ after cerebral stroke, there was barely any neurogenesis compared with that in the penumbra and ipsilateral SVZ after cerebral stroke. Recently, in a rat ischemic MCO model, new neurons increased and neurogenesis occurred in the penumbral area and ipsilateral SVZ, but neurogenesis barely occurred on the contralateral side (Komitova et al., 2005). In addition, activation of cell division after brain ischemia increased in the ipsilateral SVZ but not in the contralateral SVZ. These results are consistent with our data. These results suggested that NSCs and new neurons might migrate into the penumbra from the ipsilateral SVZ after cerebral stroke, but not into the contralateral SVZ.

In this model of spontaneous cerebral stroke, there were many NSCs and DCX-positive immature neurons in the penumbra very soon after the stroke event. It is unclear whether these cells originated from astrocytes or migrated from the SVZ. In the stroke-prone spontaneously hypertensive model, some of the newly formed immature neurons survive in the penumbra after cerebral stroke and become mature neurons. Our data suggest that NSCs and new neurons are present in the penumbra after a spontaneous cerebral stroke, and therefore that brain dysfunction after a spontaneous cerebral stroke may be improved by promoting the maturation and differentiation of NSCs and newly formed immature neurons in the penumbra.

Acknowledgments The authors thank Mari Machino for technical assistance.

References

Brown JP, Couillard-Despres S, Cooper-Kuhn CM, Winkler J, Aigner L, Kuhn HG (2003) Transient expression of doublecortin during adult neurogenesis. J Comp Neurol 467: 1–10

Couillard-Despres S, Winner B, Schaubeck S, Aigner R, Vroemen M, Weidner N, Bogdahn U, Winkler J, Kuhn HG, Aigner L (2005) Doublecortin expression levels in adult brain reflect neurogenesis. Eur J Neurosci 21:1–14

Doetsch F, Caille I, Lim DA, Garcia-Verdugo JM, Alvarez-Buylla A (1999) Subventricular zone astrocytes are neural stem cells in the adult mammalian brain. Cell 97:703–716

Gage FH (2000) Mammalian neural stem cells. Science 287:1433–1438

Itoh T, Satou T, Hashimoto S, Ito H (2005) Isolation of neural stem cells from damaged rat cerebral cortex after TBI. Neuroreport 16:1687–1691

Itoh T, Satou T, Hashimoto S, Ito H (2007) Immature and mature neurons coexist among glial scars after rat traumatic brain injury. Neurol Res 29:734–742

Itoh T, Satou T, Ishida H, Nishida S, Tsubaki M, Hashimoto S, Ito H (2009) The relationship between SDF-1alpha/CXCR4 and neural stem cells appearing in damaged area after traumatic brain injury in rats. Neurol Res 31:90–102

Itoh T, Satou T, Nishida S, Hashimoto S, Ito H (2006) Cultured rat astrocytes give rise to neural stem cells. Neurochem Res 31:1381–1387

Itoh T, Satou T, Takemori K, Hashimoto S, Ito H (2010) Neural stem cells and new neurons in the cerebral cortex of stroke-prone spontaneously hypertensive rats after stroke. J Mol Neurosci 41:55–65

Komitova M, Mattsson B, Johansson BB, Eriksson PS (2005) Enriched environment increases neural stem/progenitor cell proliferation and neurogenesis in the subventricular zone of stroke-lesioned adult rats. Stroke 36:1278–1282

Nakamura T, Miyamoto O, Auer RN, Nagao S, Itano T (2004) Delayed precursor cell markers expression in hippocampus following cold-induced cortical injury in mice. J Neurotrauma 21:1747–1755

Parent JM, Yu TW, Leibowitz RT, Geschwind DH, Sloviter RS, Lowenstein DH (1997) Dentate granule cell neurogenesis is increased by seizures and contributes to aberrant network reorganization in the adult rat hippocampus. J Neurosci 17:3727–3738

Pekny M, and Nilsson M (2005) Astrocyte activation and reactive gliosis. Glia 50:427–434

Picard-Riera N, Nait-Oumesmar B, Baron-Van EA (2004) Endogenous adult neural stem cells: limits and potential to repair the injured central nervous system. J Neurosci Res 76:223–231

Rice AC, Khaldi A, Harvey HB, Salman NJ, White F, Fillmore H, Bullock MR (2003) Proliferation and neuronal differentiation of mitotically active cells following traumatic brain injury. Exp Neurol 183:406–417

Salman H, Ghosh P, Kernie SG (2004) Subventricular zone neural stem cells remodel the brain following traumatic injury in adult mice. J Neurotrauma 21:283–292

Thored P, Arvidsson A, Cacci E, Ahlenius H, Kallur T, Darsalia V, Ekdahl CT, Kokaia Z, Lindvall O (2006) Persistent production of neurons from adult brain stem cells during recovery after stroke. Stem Cells 24:739–747

Xiong Y, Gu Q, Peterson PL, Muizelaar JP, Lee CP (1997) Mitochondrial dysfunction and calcium perturbation induced by traumatic brain injury. J Neurotrauma 14:23–34

Chapter 22

Neurogenesis in the Cerebral Cortex After Stroke

Yukiko Kasahara, Takayuki Nakagomi, Tomohiro Matsuyama, and Akihiko Taguchi

Abstract In the adult mammalian brain, new neurons are continuously generated at the subventricular zone of the lateral ventricles and the subgranular zone of the hippocampal dentate gyrus. In the cerebral cortex, though the generation of new neurons is rarely observed in physiological situations, induction of neurogenesis has been shown under pathological conditions, such as after cerebral ischemia. In this chapter, we introduce the injury-induced neural stem/progenitor cells in the cerebral cortex and its potential for functional recovery. We also refer to the therapeutic potential of exogenous neuronal stem cell transplantation and discuss the future of cell-based therapy for stroke patients.

Keywords Central nervous system · Neurogenesis · Cerebral cortex · Cerebral infarction · Neural stem cells

has been shown to induce neurogenesis at various brain regions, including the SVZ, SGZ, striatum, and cerebral cortex (Darsalia et al., 2005). Though most of the injury-induced neural stem/progenitor cells fail to survive after stroke (Arvidsson et al., 2002), we have shown that appropriate support of these injury-induced stem/progenitor cells can contribute to functional recovery (Taguchi et al., 2004). To develop novel therapies for patients after stroke, the leading cause of disability in developed countries, the therapeutic potential of neural stem cells has been investigated in experimental stroke models, followed by various clinical trials. In this chapter, we introduce current basic and clinical findings that focus on regeneration of the injured cerebral cortex and impaired neurological function after cerebral ischemia. We also refer to the current status and the issue of exogenous neural stem cell transplantation after cerebral infarction.

Introduction

In the central nervous system (CNS) of physiologically adult mammals, the generation of new neurons is known to be principally restricted to two regions, the subventricular zone (SVZ) of the lateral ventricles (Alvarez-Buylla and Garcia-Verdugo, 2002) and the subgranular zone (SGZ) of the hippocampal dentate gyrus (Gage, 2010). However, ischemic brain injury

A. Taguchi (✉)
Department of Cerebrovascular Disease, National Cardiovascular Center, Suita, Osaka 565-8565, Japan
e-mail: taguchi@ri.ncvc.go.jp

Neurogenesis in the Adult Brain

New neurons are continuously generated throughout life in the adult mammalian brain. In physiological situations, neurogenesis is known to be principally restricted to the SVZ of the lateral ventricle wall and the SGZ of the hippocampal dentate gyrus, where the unique niche architectures permit continuous neurogenesis (Alvarez-Buylla and Garcia-Verdugo, 2002; Gage, 2010). The presence of neural stem/progenitor cells in various regions of the adult brain has been suggested, but beside the SVZ and SGZ, neurogenesis in the intact brain is rarely observed; the percentages of generated neurons are in the range of only 0.005–0.03% of all existing neurons (Koketsu et al., 2003).

In contrast, brain injury, including cerebral ischemia, has been shown to significantly activate neurogenesis in various brain regions, such as the hippocampal cornu ammonis region (Nakatomi et al., 2002), striatum (Darsalia et al., 2005), subpial zone (Xue et al., 2009), and cerebral cortex (Leker et al., 2007). The origin of these new neurons was initially proposed to be the migration of neural stem cells from the SVZ and SGZ (Arvidsson et al., 2002), but recent studies demonstrated the presence of neural stem/progenitor cells in various regions of the brain, including the cerebral cortex (Nakagomi et al., 2009b). The exact origins of these neural stem/progenitor cells are still the subject of argument: e.g., GFAP-negative quiescent astrocytes (Buffo et al., 2008), oligodendrocyte precursor cells (Kondo and Raff, 2000), microvascular pericytes (Dore-Duffy et al., 2006), and NG2-positive glial cells (Yokoyama et al., 2006). Though the character and potential of these neural stem/progenitor cells could be heterogeneous and different from those of SVZ- or SGZ-derived neural stem cells, the injury-induced, cortex-derived neural stem/progenitor cells have been shown to have the potential to differentiate into astrocytes, oligodendrocytes, and neurons with neuronal-like electrical properties (Nakagomi et al., 2009b). Furthermore, histopathological studies in stroke patients have pointed out the presence of neural stem/progenitor cells in the post-stroke human cerebral cortex (Nakayama et al., 2010). These findings indicate the potential of a novel therapeutic strategy using injury-induced neurogenesis for functional recovery in patients with cerebral infarction.

Support Survival of Injury-Induced Neural Stem/Progenitor Cells

However, such injury-induced neural stem/progenitor cells have been shown to not survive and not contribute to functional recovery after stroke on their own (Arvidsson et al., 2002). Almost all of the injury-induced neural stem/progenitor cells cause apoptotic cell death, so appropriate support for their survival would be essential for functional recovery by endogenous neurogenesis (Taguchi et al., 2004). For the survival of injury-induced neural stem/progenitor cells, the following factors have been shown to be involved in and/or need to be addressed: a) immune responses; b) neurotrophic factors; and c) angiogenesis.

The regulation of the immune system has been proposed as one of the key factors to enhance neurogenesis and functional recovery after stroke. In our previous study, T lymphocytes, mainly CD4- but not CD8-positive lymphocytes, have been shown to lead to cell death in injury-induced neural stem/progenitor cells (Saino et al., 2010). The details of the mechanism are still under investigation, but the findings indicate that the immune system and/or enhanced inflammation induces apoptotic cell death in injury-induced neural stem/progenitor cells at the cerebral cortex though activation of CD4-positive T-lymphocytes. These findings, at least in part, would be consistent with the result that treatment with mesenchymal cells, known to suppress the immune response in graft-versus-host disease, accelerates endogenous neurogenesis after stroke (Yoo et al., 2008).

Neurotrophic factors are known to be important elements for stem cell survival, differentiation, and function. Basic fibroblast growth factor (bFGF) has beneficial effects for endogenous neurogenesis and functional recovery after cerebral ischemia (Leker et al., 2007; Nakatomi et al., 2002), though intraventricular infusion of high concentrations of bFGF causes disruption of oligodendrocyte function and myelin production at demyelinating lesions (Butt and Dinsdale, 2005). Administration of epidermal growth factor (EGF) also significantly accelerates endogenous neurogenesis and has neuroprotective effects after cerebral infarction (Nakatomi et al., 2002), though EGF has been proposed as a possible contributor to derive glioma formation from endogenous neural stem cells (Doetsch et al., 2002). Brain-derived neurotrophic factor (BDNF) has protective effects for newly generated and injured neurons after cerebral ischemia (Schabitz et al., 2007), whereas infusion of BDNF has been shown to lead to spontaneous seizure activity in treated animals (Scharfman et al., 2002). These cytokines have the potential to promote survival of newly generated neurons with accelerated functional recovery, though careful evaluation of unanticipated adverse effects should be addressed before clinical application.

Angiogenesis after stroke has been proposed as the key element for the survival of injury-induced neural stem/progenitor cells and functional recovery after cortical infarction. In the adult brain, a tight correlation between angiogenesis and neurogenesis has been shown under both physiological and pathological conditions. In the adult songbird, testosterone-induced angiogenesis leads to neuronal recruitment into the higher vocal center (Louissaint et al., 2002). In the adult rat, endogenous neurogenesis and neovascularization occur in proximity to one another in the cortex following focal ischemia (Shin et al., 2008). Moreover, angiogenesis and neurogenesis have been shown to use the same molecules for their regulation; e.g., sphongosine-1-phosphate plays a critical role in neurogenesis and angiogenesis during embryonic development (Mizugishi et al., 2005). This accumulating evidence indicates a close relationship between the vascular system and neurogenesis in the central nervous system, and recent studies that explored the therapeutic strategy focused on promotion of neurogenesis in association with angiogenesis (Nakagomi et al., 2009a).

Based on the concept that angiogenesis after stroke promotes endogenous neurogenesis and functional recovery, the therapeutic effects of angiogenic growth factors and/or cytokines have been investigated. Administration of vascular endothelial growth factor (VEGF) was initially reported to have beneficial effects for functional recovery after stroke in 1998, but most of the subsequent experiments could not reproduce its therapeutic effect, due to the enhanced permeability that causes enhanced brain edema (Zhang et al., 2000). Granulocyte colony-stimulating factor (G-CSF) has been shown to promote angiogenesis in ischemic tissue, but another effect of G-CSF, enhancement of the inflammatory response that is known to induce neural stem/progenitor cell death, negated the positive effects followed by enhanced brain damage with poorer outcomes (Taguchi et al., 2007). To achieve angiogenesis at ischemic tissue, another approach has been proposed using endothelial stem/progenitor cells (EPCs). Transplantation of EPCs has been shown to induce angiogenesis for limb and myocardial ischemia in experimental models, and clinical trials are ongoing for patients with limb and cardiac ischemia followed by promising results (Capiod et al., 2009). In the experimental stroke model, we have demonstrated that administration of EPCs supports survival and maturation of injury-induced neural stem/progenitor cells in post-stroke cerebral cortex though angiogenesis and accelerates functional recovery (Taguchi et al., 2004). This finding suggests that therapeutic angiogenesis, achieved by administration of EPCs, could be a novel therapeutic strategy for ischemic brain injury.

Exogenous Neural Stem Cell Transplantation After Cerebral Ischemia

Compared with enhancement of endogenous neurogenesis after stroke, exogenous neural stem cell transplantation might have significant advantages in the repair of damaged brain after cerebral infarction. The number of injury-induced neural stem/progenitor cells in post-stroke cortex is limited, but the number of transplanted neural stem cells could be unlimited and can be determined on demand, especially using stem cells obtained from embryonic stem cells (ESs) or induced pluripotent stem cell (iPSs). Furthermore, exogenous neural stem cell transplantation can be performed even at the chronic stage after stroke, in contrast to the limited therapeutic time window in enhancement of endogenous neurogenesis, because peak neurogenesis occurs a few weeks after onset in patients after cortical infarction (Nakayama et al., 2010). Recently, various cell sources for exogenous neural stem cell transplantation have been proposed, such as fetal brain, adult brain tissue obtained from the SVZ, notch-gene transfected bone marrow stromal cells (Dezawa et al., 2004), immortalized tumor cell lines (Saporta et al., 1999), ESs/iPSs (Buhnemann et al., 2006), and ex vivo expanded cerebral cortex-derived neural stem/progenitor cells (Nakagomi et al., 2009a, 2009b). In experimental models of stroke, increasing evidence has shown that these transplanted NSCs survive within the host, migrate into the damaged tissue, and maintain their multipotency (Darsalia et al., 2007).

In contrast to these advantages, there are some issues for clinical application of exogenous neural stem cell transplantation in patients with cerebral infarction, such as survival, safety, and suitability of transplanted cells as the cell source to repair injured adult brain. It has been shown that only a small population of grafted exogenous neural stem cells can survive in the injured brain (Toda et al., 2001). A higher survival rate can be expected by implantation of neural stem cells with possible neoplastic properties (such as ES/iPS-derived neural stem cells), but their survival is often attributed to a lack of apoptotic properties, which is directly linked to a high risk of tumorigenesis. Regarding the suitability of transplanted cells, for example, it is doubtful whether fetal neural stem cells, that are destined to form infant brain, would be able to contribute to reconstitution of injured adult brain. To achieve significant recovery of impaired neurological function, these issues should be addressed. Recently, we have reported that transplantation of neural stem/progenitor cells obtained from post-stroke cerebral cortex with endothelial cells enhances functional recovery after cortical infarction (Nakagomi et al., 2009a). Furthermore, a recent study showed that transplantation of neural stem cells with valproic acid enhanced the differentiation of transplanted stem cells to functional neurons in a spinal cord injury model (Abematsu et al., 2010). These results may indicate a possible future direction for the clinical application of exogenous neural stem cell transplantation for patients after cerebral infarction.

Clinical Trials to Enhance Neurogenesis in Patients After Stroke

The list of completed and ongoing clinical trials of exogenous stem cell transplantation is shown in Table 22.1. Results of two clinical studies have been reported. Human teratocarcinoma-derived neural stem cells were locally transplanted at the University of Pittsburgh Medical Center, and the safety and feasibility of local cell transplantation with increased metabolic activity was reported (Kondziolka et al., 2000). Group analysis revealed no significant difference in neural function recovery between patients with cell implants and the control group. Improved activities of daily living were noted in some patients undergoing cell transplantation, though no significant motor improvement was observed. A clinical trial using embryonic porcine neural stem cells was initiated at Harvard Medical School, but the study was terminated early due to reports of two serious adverse events (Savitz et al., 2005). These negative results may suggest the need for alternative cell sources and/or procedures to increase the therapeutic effect. In 2010, ReNeuron Limited announced the enrollment of the first patients in their clinical trial. The trial is designed to treat 12 patients and will measure outcomes over 24 months.

The list of major clinical trials that aim to enhance endogenous neurogenesis is shown in Table 22.2. Most of them are focused on angiogenesis to enhance neurogenesis, and 3 types of clinical trials were attempted and/or are ongoing: 1) administration of growth factors/cytokines, such as G-CSF or erythropoietin, which also have neuroprotective effects, to mobilize EPCs; 2) transplantation of autologous/allogeneic mesenchymal cells; and 3) transplantation of autologous EPCs, such as CD34-positive cells and bone marrow mononuclear cells. Though there is a report that treatment with G-CSF enhances functional recovery after stroke, the number of enrolled patients was too small ($N=3$ in the control group) to interpret the results properly (Shyu et al., 2006). Similarly, there is a report that transplantation of mesenchymal cells enhances functional recovery, but the number of enrolled patients was small, and a problem in the follow-up was noted (England et al., 2009). Clinical trials of bone marrow-derived EPC transplantation after stroke have been initiated in many countries, including the USA, England, Brazil, Spain, and Japan. Though the route of administration (intravenous or intra-arterial) and cell source (bone marrow mononuclear cells or CD34-positive cells) varied, no side effects or safety problems with

Table 22.1 Clinical trials of exogenous neural stem cell transplantation

Institute	Country	Stroke type	Cells	Administration	Status	Identifier
University of Pittsburgh Medical Center	USA	Basal ganglia infarction	Immortalized neural cells	Injection into brain	Completed	N/A
Harvard Medical School	USA	MCA infarction	Fetal porcine-derived neural stem cells	Injection into brain	Completed	N/A
ReNeuron Limited	UK	Stable ischemic stroke	CTX0E03 neural stem cells	Injection into brain	Recruiting	NCT01151124

MCA, middle cerebral artery

Table 22.2 Clinical trials for enhancement of endogenous neurogenesis after stroke

Institute	Country	Stroke type	Treatment	Administration	Status	Identifier
Clinical Institute of the Brain	Russia	Stroke in carotid area	G-CSF	Subcutaneous injection	Completed	NCT00901381
University Hospital Muenster	Germany	Chronic stroke	G-CSF and EPO	Subcutaneous injection	Completed	NCT00298597
Ajou University School of Medicine	Korea	MCA infarction	Autologous MSC	Intravenous	Completed	N/A
Federal University of Rio de Janeiro	Brazil	MCA infarction	Autologous BM	Intra-arterial or intravenous	Recruiting	NCT00473057
National Cerebral and Cardiovascular Center	Japan	Cerebral embolism	Autologous BMNC	Intravenous	Recruiting	NCT01028794
University Hospital of Grenoble	France	Stroke	Autologous MSC	Intravenous	Recruiting	NCT00875654
University of Texas Health Science Center	USA	Acute ischemic stroke	Autologous BMNC	Intravenous	Recruiting	NCT00859014
China Medical University Hospital	China	Chronic stroke	Autologous CD34+ stem cells	Injection into brain	Recruiting	NCT00950521
Hospital Universitario Central de Asturias	Spain	Acute stroke	Autologous CD34+ stem cells	Intra-arterial	Recruiting	NCT00761982
Imperial College London	UK	Acute stroke	Autologous CD34+ stem cells	Intra-arterial	Recruiting	NCT00535197

G-CSF, granulocyte-colony stimulating factor; EPO, erythropoietin; BM, bone marrow; BMNC, bone marrow mononuclear cell; MSC, mesenchymal stem cells; MCA, middle cerebral artery cell therapy have yet been reported. The results of these clinical trials are expected in several years.

Conclusion

The existence of various neural stem/progenitor cells has been shown in the cerebral cortex both in experimental stroke models and stroke patients. These injury-induced stem/progenitor cells in the cerebral cortex could be used to achieve functional recovery through enhancement of in vivo neurogenesis and neural stem/progenitor cell implantation after ex vivo expansion. Moreover, the combination of two strategies, enhancement of neurogenesis followed by exogenous neural stem cell transplantation, that may well complement each other could be expected to generate a synergistic effect. Step by step investigations will lead to establishment of novel therapies through enhancing neurogenesis for patients after stroke.

References

Abematsu M, Tsujimura K, Yamano M, Saito M, Kohno K, Kohyama J, Namihira M, Komiya S, Nakashima K (2010) Neurons derived from transplanted neural stem cells restore disrupted neuronal circuitry in a mouse model of spinal cord injury. J Clin Invest 120:3255–3266

Alvarez-Buylla A, Garcia-Verdugo JM (2002) Neurogenesis in adult subventricular zone. J Neurosci 22:629–634

Arvidsson A, Collin T, Kirik D, Kokaia Z, Lindvall O (2002) Neuronal replacement from endogenous precursors in the adult brain after stroke. Nat Med 8:963–970

Buffo A, Rite I, Tripathi P, Lepier A, Colak D, Horn AP, Mori T, Gotz M (2008) Origin and progeny of reactive gliosis: a source of multipotent cells in the injured brain. Proc Natl Acad Sci USA 105:3581–3586

Buhnemann C, Scholz A, Bernreuther C, Malik CY, Braun H, Schachner M, Reymann KG, Dihne M (2006) Neuronal differentiation of transplanted embryonic stem cell-derived precursors in stroke lesions of adult rats. Brain 129:3238–3248

Butt AM, Dinsdale J (2005) Fibroblast growth factor 2 induces loss of adult oligodendrocytes and myelin in vivo. Exp Neurol 192:125–133

Capiod JC, Tournois C, Vitry F, Sevestre MA, Daliphard S, Reix T, Nguyen P, Lefrere JJ, Pignon B (2009) Characterization and comparison of bone marrow and peripheral blood mononuclear cells used for cellular therapy in critical leg ischaemia: towards a new cellular product. Vox Sang 96:256–265

Darsalia V, Heldmann U, Lindvall O, Kokaia Z (2005) Stroke-induced neurogenesis in aged brain. Stroke 36:1790–1795

Darsalia V, Kallur T, Kokaia Z (2007) Survival, migration and neuronal differentiation of human fetal striatal and cortical neural stem cells grafted in stroke-damaged rat striatum. Eur J Neurosci 26:605–614

Dezawa M, Kanno H, Hoshino M, Cho H, Matsumoto N, Itokazu Y, Tajima N, Yamada H, Sawada H, Ishikawa H, Mimura T, Kitada M, Suzuki Y, Ide C (2004) Specific induction of neuronal cells from bone marrow stromal cells and application for autologous transplantation. J Clin Invest 113:1701–1710

Doetsch F, Petreanu L, Caille I, Garcia-Verdugo JM, Alvarez-Buylla A (2002) EGF converts transit-amplifying neurogenic precursors in the adult brain into multipotent stem cells. Neuron 36:1021–1034

Dore-Duffy P, Katychev A, Wang X, Van Buren E (2006) CNS microvascular pericytes exhibit multipotential stem cell activity. J Cereb Blood Flow Metab 26:613–624

England T, Martin P, Bath PM (2009) Stem cells for enhancing recovery after stroke: a review. Int J Stroke 4:101–110

Gage FH (2010) Molecular and cellular mechanisms contributing to the regulation, proliferation and differentiation of neural stem cells in the adult dentate gyrus. Keio J Med 59:79–83

Koketsu D, Mikami A, Miyamoto Y, Hisatsune T (2003) Nonrenewal of neurons in the cerebral neocortex of adult macaque monkeys. J Neurosci 23:937–942

Kondo T, Raff M (2000) Oligodendrocyte precursor cells reprogrammed to become multipotential CNS stem cells. Science 289:1754–1757

Kondziolka D, Wechsler L, Goldstein S, Meltzer C, Thulborn KR, Gebel J, Jannetta P, DeCesare S, Elder EM, McGrogan M, Reitman MA, Bynum L (2000) Transplantation of cultured human neuronal cells for patients with stroke. Neurology 55:565–569

Leker RR, Soldner F, Velasco I, Gavin DK, Androutsellis-Theotokis A, McKay RD (2007) Long-lasting regeneration after ischemia in the cerebral cortex. Stroke 38:153–161

Louissaint A Jr, Rao S, Leventhal C, Goldman SA (2002) Coordinated interaction of neurogenesis and angiogenesis in the adult songbird brain. Neuron 34:945–960

Mizugishi K, Yamashita T, Olivera A, Miller GF, Spiegel S, Proia RL (2005) Essential role for sphingosine kinases in neural and vascular development. Mol Cell Biol 25:11113–11121

Nakagomi N, Nakagomi T, Kubo S, Nakano-Doi A, Saino O, Takata M, Yoshikawa H, Stern DM, Matsuyama T, Taguchi A (2009a) Endothelial cells support survival, proliferation, and neuronal differentiation of transplanted adult ischemia-induced neural stem/progenitor cells after cerebral infarction. Stem Cells 27:2185–2195

Nakagomi T, Taguchi A, Fujimori Y, Saino O, Nakano-Doi A, Kubo S, Gotoh A, Soma T, Yoshikawa H, Nishizaki T, Nakagomi N, Stern DM, Matsuyama T (2009b) Isolation and characterization of neural stem/progenitor cells from post-stroke cerebral cortex in mice. Eur J Neurosci 29:1842–1852

Nakatomi H, Kuriu T, Okabe S, Yamamoto S, Hatano O, Kawahara N, Tamura A, Kirino T, Nakafuku M (2002) Regeneration of hippocampal pyramidal neurons after ischemic brain injury by recruitment of endogenous neural progenitors. Cell 110:429–441

Nakayama D, Matsuyama T, Ishibashi-Ueda H, Nakagomi T, Kasahara Y, Hirose H, Kikuchi-Taura A, Stern DM, Mori

H, Taguchi A (2010) Injury-induced neural stem/progenitor cells in post-stroke human cerebral cortex. Eur J Neurosci 31:90–98

Saino O, Taguchi A, Nakagomi T, Nakano-Doi A, Kashiwamura S, Doe N, Nakagomi N, Soma T, Yoshikawa H, Stern DM, Okamura H, Matsuyama T (2010) Immunodeficiency reduces neural stem/progenitor cell apoptosis and enhances neurogenesis in the cerebral cortex after stroke. J Neurosci Res 88:2385–2397

Saporta S, Borlongan CV, Sanberg PR (1999) Neural transplantation of human neuroteratocarcinoma (hNT) neurons into ischemic rats. A quantitative dose-response analysis of cell survival and behavioral recovery. Neuroscience 91:519–525

Savitz SI, Dinsmore J, Wu J, Henderson GV, Stieg P, Caplan LR (2005) Neurotransplantation of fetal porcine cells in patients with basal ganglia infarcts: a preliminary safety and feasibility study. Cerebrovasc Dis 20:101–107

Schabitz WR, Steigleder T, Cooper-Kuhn CM, Schwab S, Sommer C, Schneider A, Kuhn HG (2007) Intravenous brain-derived neurotrophic factor enhances poststroke sensorimotor recovery and stimulates neurogenesis. Stroke 38:2165–2172

Scharfman HE, Goodman JH, Sollas AL, Croll SD (2002) Spontaneous limbic seizures after intrahippocampal infusion of brain-derived neurotrophic factor. Exp Neurol 174:201–214

Shin HY, Kim JH, Phi JH, Park CK, Kim JE, Kim JH, Paek SH, Wang KC, Kim DG (2008) Endogenous neurogenesis and neovascularization in the neocortex of the rat after focal cerebral ischemia. J Neurosci Res 86:356–367

Shyu WC, Lin SZ, Lee CC, Liu DD, Li H (2006) Granulocyte colony-stimulating factor for acute ischemic stroke: a randomized controlled trial. CMAJ 174:927–933

Taguchi A, Soma T, Tanaka H, Kanda T, Nishimura H, Yoshikawa H, Tsukamoto, Y, Iso H, Fujimori Y, Stern DM, Naritomi H, Matsuyama T (2004) Administration of CD34+ cells after stroke enhances neurogenesis via angiogenesis in a mouse model. J Clin Invest 114:330–338

Taguchi A, Wen Z, Myojin K, Yoshihara T, Nakagomi T, Nakayama D, Tanaka H, Soma T, Stern DM, Naritomi H, Matsuyama T (2007) Granulocyte colony-stimulating factor has a negative effect on stroke outcome in a murine model. Eur J Neurosci 26:126–133

Toda H, Takahashi J, Iwakami N, Kimura T, Hoki S, Mozumi-Kitamura K, Ono S, Hashimoto N (2001) Grafting neural stem cells improved the impaired spatial recognition in ischemic rats. Neurosci Lett 316:9–12

Xue JH, Yanamoto H, Nakajo Y, Tohnai N, Nakano Y, Hori T, Iihara K, Miyamoto S (2009) Induced spreading depression evokes cell division of astrocytes in the Subpial Zone, generating neural precursor-like cells and new immature neurons in the adult cerebral cortex. Stroke 40:e606–e613

Yokoyama A, Sakamoto A, Kameda K, Imai Y, Tanaka J (2006) NG2 proteoglycan-expressing microglia as multipotent neural progenitors in normal and pathologic brains. Glia 53:754–768

Yoo SW, Kim SS, Lee SY, Lee HS, Kim HS, Lee YD, Suh-Kim H (2008) Mesenchymal stem cells promote proliferation of endogenous neural stem cells and survival of newborn cells in a rat stroke model. Exp Mol Med 40:387–397

Zhang ZG, Zhang L, Jiang Q, Zhang R, Davies K, Powers C, Bruggen N, Chopp M (2000) VEGF enhances angiogenesis and promotes blood-brain barrier leakage in the ischemic brain. J Clin Invest 106:829–838

Chapter 23
Ex Vivo Expanded Hematopoietic Stem Cells for Ischemia

Jingwei Lu, Reeva Aggarwal, Vincent J. Pompili, and Hiranmoy Das

Abstract Ischemia related diseases are on rise worldwide and have been shown to cause irreversible damage to the cells due to the blockage of blood supply to the tissue. Conventional therapies are less effective as they do not consider repair of the damaged tissues. Thus, alternative, stem cell-based therapies are currently under investigation. For example, hematopoietic stem cells (HSCs) were shown to give rise to vascular cells involved in neoangiogenesis; so, they have been tested in variety of animal models and small-scale clinical trials. Improvement in blood flow and tissue functionality was observed and adverse effects were not apparent. However, success of stem cell therapy is limited by the number of functional stem cells for clinical application. Numerous attempts are underway to address this issue via strategies that involve ex vivo expansion of stem cells preserving their stemness. This chapter outlines the mechanism of therapeutic angiogenesis, sources of HSCs, various methods of ex vivo expansion of HSCs via genetic regulators, cytokines and biomaterial scaffolds, and their preclinical and clinical applications.

Keywords Hematopoietic stem cells · Ischemia · Angiogenic · Vasculogenesis · Stromal cells · Thrombopoietin

H. Das (✉)
Cardiovascular Stem Cell Research Laboratories, Davis Heart and Lung Research Institute, Columbus, OH 43210, USA
e-mail: Hiranmoy.das@osumc.edu

Introduction

Ischemia is a pathophysiological condition, developed due to the restriction in blood flow to the tissues/organs and results in damage and dysfunction of tissues/organs. The inadequate supply of blood leads to limited supply of food, nutrition, and oxygen to the cells resulting in permanent loss of cells. Among the most sensitive organs that are being affected by restriction of blood flow are heart, limbs, brain, and kidney. Diseases developed due to ischemia include ischemic heart disease, acute limb ischemia, chronic limb ischemia, brain ischemia, ischemic colitis, mesenteric ischemia, etc. Various factors, such as hypoglycemia, tachycardia, atherosclerosis, hypotension, thromboembolism etc, are responsible for development of ischemic diseases. It has been shown that therapeutic angiogenesis mediates gradual recovery of blood flow in ischemic tissues, helps in tissue regeneration, and improves functionality of the tissue. This concept of regenerating microvasculature as part of the strategy for treating ischemic tissue originated from discovery of angiogenic growth factors (Folkman et al., 1971). Since then, various growth factors, such as vascular endothelial growth factor (VEGF)-1, VEGF-2, fibroblast growth factor (FGF)-4, hepatocyte growth factor (HGF), have been tested in variety of clinical and subclinical trials with promising results. Unfortunately, randomized controlled clinical trials failed to consistently produce conclusive evidence of benefits. It was suggested that aging and multiple comorbidities are responsible for the compromised ability of endogenous angiogenesis in patients (Gupta et al., 2009). The recent development of stem cell therapy has potential to overcome angiogenesis-related problems by providing healthy exogenous endothelial progenitor cells (EPCs) or hematopoietic stem cells (HSCs) and promote the reconstitution of microvasculature in the damaged ischemic tissue from the existing vessels of the peri-ischemic area. Promising results have been shown using cell therapy in variety of clinical trials during the past decade. However, insufficient number of isolated stem cells with biological functionality and low viability have hindered their clinical application. Therefore, it is critically important to develop a technology that will support an efficient and practical ex vivo expansion of stem cells. Stem cells should maintain their progenitor characteristics after expansion and should enhance viability after transplantation. The technology should also support the maintenance of engraftment potential of expanded-stem cells. Various approaches have been undertaken to achieve this ex vivo expansion technology. Here, we will discuss the ex vivo expansion technology for hematopoietic stem cells, and current preclinical as well as clinical application of HSCs, and ex vivo expanded HSCs for the treatment of ischemic diseases.

The Mechanism of Angiogenesis

Angiogenesis has emerged as one of the most important factors in reverting the ischemic condition of any given tissue. The process of formation of blood vessel follows two major pathways: vasculogenesis and angiogenesis. Vasculogenesis is the process by which spontaneous blood vessels are formed, which generally happens during embryogenesis. On the other hand, angiogenesis is the process that generates new blood vessels from preexisting vessels. During angiogenesis, environmental signals activate series of cascades that trigger endothelial cells to promote sprouting of new vessels. There are two types of endothelial cells involved in this processes: tips cells and stalk cells. Tips cells are located on the tip of the sprouts while stalks cells are located on the sprout following tip cells. There are other specialized endothelial cells that proliferate to form the trunk of new blood vessels. Vascular lumen is formed by the fusion of intracellular vesicles (Iruela-Arispe and Davis, 2009). The up-regulation of angiogenic factors, such as VEGF-A, after ischemia was shown to promote migration of endothelial progenitor cells (EPC), circulating EPCs, hematopoietic stem cells (HSCs), and hematopoietic progenitor cells (HPCs) to the site of injury (Rafii and Lyden, 2003). It has been shown that most circulating endothelial cells in newly formed blood originate from vessel walls and possess limited growth capability. This was determined by analyzing blood samples from bone marrow (BM) transplant recipients using in situ hybridization technique. On the other hand, bone marrow derived endothelial cells showed a delayed outgrowth but had greater proliferation rate (Lin et al., 2000). The capability of therapeutic effects of progenitor cells varied with the sources of progenitor cells.

Sources of Hematopoietic Stem Cells

The use of endothelial progenitor cells and hematopoietic stem cells is more plausible in transplantation for treatment of ischemic diseases compared to endothelial cells. The hematopoietic stem cells and endothelial progenitor cells originate from the same precursor, hemangioblast. The common origin provides the potential for transplantation of HSCs, the related descendants of EPCs, which may lead to neovascularization as efficient as direct transplantation of EPCs (Losordo and Dimmeler, 2004). The sources of these progenitor cells include BM, peripheral blood, and umbilical cord blood. Isolated $CD133^+$ or $CD34^+$ cells from either of these sources demonstrated that the progenitor cells are capable of differentiating into mature endothelial cells and contribute to the neovascularization process (Asahara et al., 1997; Peichev et al., 2000). More attention has been given to the use of umbilical cord as the source of progenitor cells for transplantation compared to BM or peripheral blood. This could be due to more primitive nature of the cord blood-derived progenitor stem cell. Also, progenitor cells isolated from aged patients resulted in a significantly reduced neovascularization process, which may compromise the therapeutic effect of the transplantation. The major benefit from transplantation of cord blood cells is the reduced development of graft-versus-host disease compared to BM cell transplantation, possibly due to the reduced maturity of immune cells, especially T cells (Mommaas et al., 2005). Even though cord blood has the advantage over the peripheral blood or BM-derived progenitor cells in preclinical as well as clinical applications (reviewed later), stem cell transplantation is limited by the insufficient number of progenitor cells. Low number of progenitor stem cells delays the engraftment and causes remission and poor recovery. To meet the necessary requirement of progenitor cells, there is an urgent need of suitable method for expanding progenitor cells, which could be used for functional engraftment and regeneration.

Ex Vivo Expansion of Hematopoietic Stem Cells

The fate of HSCs is largely regulated by intrinsic and extrinsic cues of the cells, generally governed by the HSC microenvironment in vivo. HSCs were isolated based on their surface markers (CD133 or CD34) and then expanded in vitro under different culture conditions (discussed later) and analyzed for preservation of stemness (Fig. 23.1). Several factors, such as genetic regulators, adhesion molecules, biomaterial scaffolds, and extracellular cytokines, have been shown to play a significant role in successful expansion of HSCs in vitro. Of these, genetic modification of HSCs provides an intrinsic regulator of HSCs maintenance and proliferation. Cytokines can both enhance the survival and proliferation of HSCs in an in vitro culturing condition. Biomaterial scaffolds, which mimic the in vivo extracellular matrix structure, have also been proved to be important for long-term expansion of HSCs.

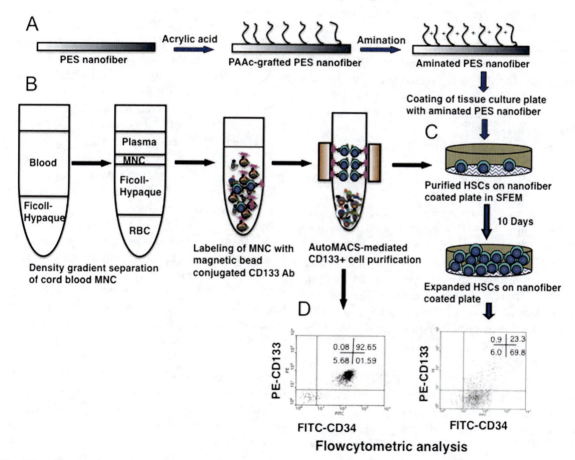

Fig. 23.1 Nanofiber-mediated ex vivo expansion of human CD133+/CD34+ HSCs. (a) Schematics of amination of PES nanofiber scaffold. (b) Schematics of autoMACS-mediated isolation of CD133+ cells. (c) Coating of tissue culture plate with PES nanofiber and plating of isolated CD133+ cells and expansion of isolated cells in serum-free media supplemented with cytokines and growth factors for 10 days. (d) Phenotypic analysis of cells right after isolation using autoMACS and after 10-days of nanofiber-mediated expansion

Cytokines and Growth Factors in Expansion of Hematopoietic Stem Cells

Early in vitro expansion of HSCs was performed using cytokines in combination with stromal cells. The BM microenvironment, containing stromal cells and extracellular matrices, plays an important role in regulating the proliferation and differentiation of hematopoietic cells by secretion of cytokines, and/or by direct cell-to-cell contact with hematopoietic cells. Stromal cells such as fibroblasts, endothelial cells, fat cells and macrophages and stromal cell lines were shown to support hematopoiesis. However, because the stromal cell culture cannot be chemically defined and stromal cell proliferation kinetics could affect the HSC self-renewal, differentiation, multipotency and subsequent transplantation, thus non-stromal and serum-free culture, supplemented with cytokines at certain concentrations was preferred for ex vivo expansion (Das et al., 2009a). Cytokines, such as interleukin (IL)-3, IL-6, IL-11, stem cell factor (SCF), thrombopoietin (TPO), and flt3-ligand (FL), were evaluated for their role in self-renewal and proliferation of HSCs. Precisely, the role of each component of the microenvironment is not fully known and this is the major limitation in the success of in vitro expansion. It was shown that combination of SF and FL alone could stimulate HSC progenitors isolated from murine BM; however, IL-11 or IL-6 was required for maintenance of stem cell functionality. Positive effects of IL-6 were mediated through gp130 expressed on HSCs derived from BM, UCB, and peripheral blood (Aggarwal et al., 2010). Also, in regards to the concentration, as high as 300 ng/ml or even more was required to reach saturated effects in proliferation of HSCs; however, requirement of IL-11 was found to be in a narrow range. Thus, optimal concentration combined with the optimum combination of cytokines is important for successful HSC proliferation in vitro. Another factor called leukemia inhibitory factor (LIF) acts in synergy with IL-3, SCF, TPO, and IL-6 to promote HSC proliferation in stromal cell supported HSC cultures and also preserved the long-term repopulating capacity of HSCs (Bryder and Jacobsen, 2000). Generally, cytokines mediate proliferation effects on HSCs via interaction with the surface receptors present on the membrane of HSCs. At genetic level, positive effect of cytokines such as TPO was linked to the activation of homeobox genes (HOXB4). Such results provide an evidence of genetic regulation of HSC proliferation via stimulation of cytokines. However, none of the cytokine cocktails was able to expand HSCs in sufficient numbers required for clinical application. On the contrary, these molecules were reported to induce HSCs differentiation after few cycles of cell divisions.

Genetic Factors Related to Expansion of Hematopoietic Stem Cells

Several genetic factors play critical role in expansion and maintenance of HSC quiescence and proliferation. Maintenance of HSC quiescence protects stem cell exhaustion, and it was shown that activation of p38 was linked to exhaustion of HSCs in vivo via upregulation of reactive oxygen species. Transcription factors such as Foxo3a and GATA-2 were shown to maintain the quiescence of HSCs in vivo and thus maintain the HSC pool. On the other hand, genetic regulators such as homeobox domain (HOX B4/ B3), Notch, Wnt, PBX-1, and CEBP were shown to have effects on self-renewal and differentiation of HSCs. HOXB4 transduced HSCs and soluble recombinant HOXB4 protein were able to induce rapid ex vivo expansion of HSCs. HOXB4 and Notch molecules were upregulated by activation of Wnt signaling pathway. Furthermore, deletion of transcriptional factor (C/EBPα) promotes HSC proliferation and blocks myeloid differentiation. Heparin binding protein, pleiotrophin, was found to cause marked increase in the umbilical cord blood-derived $CD34^+38^-$ cells in vitro compared to cytokine-supplemented cultures, via activation of P13K and Notch pathways (Himburg et al., 2010). Recently, osteoblasts (bone forming cells) were shown to express factors such as angiopoietin and osteopontin, which act as positive and negative regulators of HSCs maintenance, respectively (Arai et al., 2004). One of the key negative regulators of HSCs, TGF-β, maintains the quiescent state of HSCs by upregulation of inhibitors of cyclin D kinase (CDK) such as p21 and p57. In vitro studies suggest that immobilization of Notch ligands increased the self-renewal activity of HSCs (Blank et al., 2008). Thus, understanding genetic regulation of cell cycle and HSC proliferation due to the microenvironment could help in manipulating conditions for better outcome in expansion of HSCs.

Biomaterials in Expansion of Hematopoietic Stem Cells

Variety of biomaterials have been examined and incorporated into the stem cell culture in an effort to mimic the BM microenvironment for expansion of HSC. Most of the ideas for suitable biomaterials were derived from their usage in clinical tissue engineering for regeneration of organs such bone and musculoskeletal system (e.g., metals such as titanium, stainless steel, aluminum plates or porous matrices/ hydrogels). Numerous commercially available biomaterials were also tested for ex vivo expansion of HSCs with or without modifications with adhesive or bioactive chemical groups such as tissue culture polystyrene (TCPS), barex, titanium, stainless steel (316, 304), teflon based materials, polymethyl pentene (PMP), polyethylene (PE), high density PE (HDPE), polypropylene (PP), glass, cellulose acetate, polyether sulfones (PES), tantalum porous scaffolds, and poly-ethylene terephthalate (PET) (Li et al., 2001). In an effort to make HSC expansion suited for preclinical and clinical applications, HSC's were expanded in stromal-free and serum-free media supplemented with the cocktail of cytokines mentioned above. Materials that showed poorest expansion were PE, HDPE, acetal, teflon, stainless steel, polysulfone, and glass. CD34+ isolated from peripheral blood were shown to proliferate and survive on TCPS, PP, PMP, titanium, modified teflon, barex, and cellulose acetate. The reasons for the failure of above-mentioned materials were either attributed to toxic effects from leaching (plasticizers usually present in polymers) or poor adsorption of proteins (from media) and also due to differences in surface charge, wet ability (contact angles), and roughness (LaIuppa et al., 1997). Conjugating the biomaterial substrates with adhesion molecules supplemented with above-mentioned cytokines could enhance efficiency of in vitro expansion.

PES nanofiber with or without modifications was shown to significantly enhance HSC expansion in vitro (Chua et al., 2006). To detect the effect of various chemical cues on HSC, PES nanofiber and films were chemically conjugated with hydroxyl group, carboxyl group or amine group. PES was previously used in mammalian cell cultures and modifications with chemical groups were selected on the basis of their earlier demonstration of differential focal adhesions exhibited by mammalian cells. Amination in both the PES types was shown to have more significant expansion and was more in the PES nanofiber than in the PES film. Amine groups are positively charged, thus an electrostatic interaction with negatively charged sialyated CD34+ surface molecule was thought to cause increased proliferation by inhibiting differentiation (Chua et al., 2006; Das et al., 2009a) (Fig. 23.1). Numerous studies focused on topographical cues of scaffolds such as polyether sulfones (PES) with ethylene, butylene or hexylene spacers. The PES with hexylene spacers had minimal proliferative potential; however, displayed highest retention of CD34+45+ cells compare to PES with the other spacer molecules or tissue culture polystyrene (TCPS) (Chua et al., 2007). Engraftment potential was higher for the cell cultured on PES with either ethylene or butylene spacers reflective of effects of topographical differences on biological behavior of HSC. Micropatterned substrates were considered important for maintaining undifferentiated state of stem cells, especially in human embryonic stem cells (ESC) (Mohr et al., 2006). Besides electrostatic interactions observed with aminated PES nano fibers, integrin, selectin or CD44-mediated interaction with adhesive proteins such as fibronectin (FN) segments [RGD and cleaved segment-1 (CS-1)] were also documented. On covalently conjugated polyethylene terephthalate (PET) film with FN and CS-1, CD34+cells were cultured in serum-free media supplemented with the cocktail of cytokines (SCF, FLT-3, TPO and IL-3). Long-term repopulating cells (LT-RC) were expanded almost 3-fold, total nucleated cells were expanded almost 590-fold in 10 days and engraftment potential was higher for cells cultured on the PET film immobilized with CS-1 motif compared to immobilized with RGD motif. It has been shown that CS-1 and RGD domain of FN binds to VLA-4 and VLA-5 integrin receptors and play significant role in the survival and hematopoiesis of HSCs. Coating of maleic anhydride (MA) substrate with proteins found in the extracellular matrix (ECM) of endosteal niche in BM was evaluated for proliferation of HSC. ECM proteins such as collagen, fibronectin, heparin, and hyaluronic acid, when immobilized on MA substrates provide strong adhesions of peripheral HSCs. Adhesions were found to modulate the cell shape, trigger cell motility, and thus dictate cellular functions inducing differentiation (Franke et al., 2007). Furthermore, three-dimensional (3D) matrices were explored on the basis that 3D BM microenvironment plays a critical role in the preservation of

HSC stem cell characteristics and survival. 3D matrices such as nylon meshes, tantalum coated porous carbon lattice or fibronectin coated cellfoam matrices, supplemented with exogenous cytokines were shown to proliferate CD34$^+$ to ~ 10- to 15-fold in 3–6 weeks (Bagley et al., 1999) as compared to PES scaffolds, where we observed ~ 250-fold expansion in 10 days of culture. Nonwoven polyethylene terephthalate (PET) 3D matrices were also tested for the expansion of cord blood-derived CD34 cells, and they showed a 69-fold expansion in the first week and a decline after 3 weeks period (12.4-fold expansion) (Li et al., 2001) (Table 23.1).

Chemical and oxygen gradients are also thought to be important in modulating and mimicking the microenvironment. Exposure of cord blood-derived CD34$^+$ cells to higher oxygen gradients compromises their survival; however, engagement of α4β1 integrin substantially reduces their cell death. Similarly, calcium gradients also regulate the retention of HSCs in the BM niche. Additionally, insights from newer and less explored studies can be extended to self-renewal and proliferation of HSCs. Small synthetic pharmacological molecules such as 6-bromoindirubin-3′-oxime (BIO), potent inhibitor of GSK-3β, was shown to maintain ESC-renewal. Other small synthetic molecule, Pam3Cys, which binds to Toll-like receptors and target NF-κB signaling pathway, after addition to the culture media causes proliferation of non-hematopoietic stem cells (Ding et al., 2003). Taken together, these results suggest that many different factors need to be present in optimal proportion and orientation in 3D matrices to mimic HSC niche to obtain sufficient numbers of HSCs for transplantation.

Preclinical Applications of Hematopoietic Stem Cells in Ischemic Models

In previous decade, the therapeutic angiogenesis by of HSCs was tested in a variety of animal model and small-scale clinical trials. The underlying reasons for the development of ischemia is due to the blockade of blood supply to the tissues. Thus, neo-vascularization or therapeutic angiogenesis requires endothelial progenitor cells (EPCs) to form new blood vessels. As HSCs and EPCs originate from common ancestor hemangioblasts, neovascularization potential of HSCs was evaluated. Lin-c-kit$^+$ HSCs derived from BM have shown their ability to differentiate into ECs, smooth muscle cells SMC, and cardiomyocytes in vitro. HSCs have been investigated for their ability to regenerate or repair cardiac tissue of ischemic heart in murine and rat models. However, HSC transdifferentiation in murine model was not observed despite the elevation of the cardiac functions, rather it fused with endogeneous cardiomyocyte (Nygren et al., 2004). In the rat model of myocardial infarction, direct transplantation of CD34$^+$ cells into the infarcted zone has been shown to induce neovascularization and promote of proliferation of the existing vasculature, thereby attenuating muscle atrophy. However, total BM aspirates or total peripheral blood was shown to have severe intramyocardial calcifications after direct transplantations into syngeneic infracted mouse model. This could be due to harsh and already necrotic environment of the infarcted area favoring deposition of calcium or due to the uncontrolled proliferation of non-hematopoietic stem cells and osteoblasts (deposits calcium). Non-hematopoietic stem cells were also shown to enhance the vascular density and improve cardiac functioning in canine model of chronic myocardial ischemia (Silva et al., 2005). Hematopoietic stem cells were shown to secrete factors, which cause myogenesis, vasculogenesis, exert anti-apoptotic effects, and home to the site of infarcted areas of the heart, determined by tagging GFP with HSCs isolated from BM (Wagers et al., 2002).

Therapeutic angiogenesis induced by growth factors was shown to be critical for the treatment of MI and cardiac remodeling. Delivery of growth factors as proteins was shown to induce undesirable systemic angiogenesis due to their circulation to the whole body. Delivery of angiogenic factor such as VEGF led to immature and leaky vasculature in the system. Local gene delivery was proposed to be one option for achieving effective therapeutic effects and to overcome leakiness of the vessel. Nonviral delivery of angiogenic factors VEGF and PDGF via transient transfection of nanofiber-expanded stem cells was able to restore angiogenesis in MI models of rats, and recover the functioning of left ventricle as well as ejection fraction (volume). Genetically modified stem cells also increased capillary density, improved anterior wall motion and enhanced exercise capacity in animals treated with nanofiber-expanded stem cells compared

Table 23.1 Use of various biomaterials in ex vivo expansion of hematopoietic stem cells

Source of HSC	Type of biomaterials	Method of expansion	References
Peripheral blood (CD34)	Titanium, stainless steel-316, stainless steel-304, Glass, PMP, PE, HDPE, Acetal (PF), Teflon, PS, TCPS	Serum free, stromal free media supplemented with cytokines	Laluppa et al. (1996)
Frozen human cord blood (CD34)	PES conjugated with ethylene, butylene or hexylene spacers	Serum free, stromal free media supplemented with cytokines	Chua et al. (2007)
Fresh human cord blood (CD34)	PET conjugated with CS-1 and RGD segments of fibronectin	Serum free, stromal free media supplemented with cytokines	Chua et al. (2006)
Fresh human cord blood (CD133)	Aminated PES nanofibers	Serum free, stromal free media supplemented with cytokines	Das et al. (2009a, b)
Fresh human cord blood (CD34)	Nonwoven PET fabric and PET film	MyeloCult media supplemented with horse serum (HS) and fetal bovine serum (FBS) and hydrocortisone.	Li et al. (2001)
Human peripheral blood (CD133)	poly(ethylene-alt-maleic anhydride) (PEMA) conjugated with various adhesion molecules	Media supplemented with exogenous cytokines	Franke et al. (2007)
CD34 HSCs	3D tantalum porous scaffold	Devoid of exogenous cytokines in serum free media	Bagley et al. (1999)

HDPE high density polyethylene, *PE* polyethylene, *PEG* polyethylene glycol, *PEMA* poly(ethylene-alt-maleic anhydride), *PES* poly ether sulfone, *PF* polyformaldehyde, *PMP* polymethylenepentane, *PS* polystyrene, *TCPS* tissue culture polystyrene

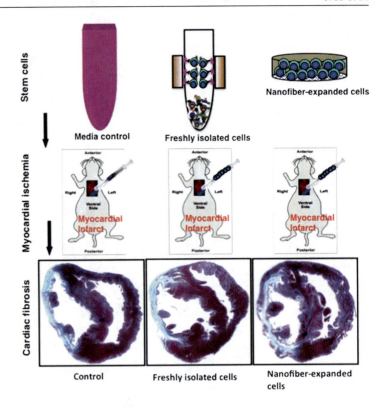

Fig. 23.2 Reduction of cardiac fibrosis in infarcted rat after stem cell therapy. Freshly isolated human CD133+ stem cells or nanofiber-expanded stem cells were used to treat myocardial infarcted tissues in an immunocompromised rat model injected via intra cardio-ventricular route. Media was used as a control. After 4 weeks of therapy, rat was sacrificed and cardiac tissue section was stained for fibrosis using Masson's trichrome staining. Reduced fibrosis was observed after nanofiber-expanded stem cells therapy

to media controls or to freshly-isolated cells treated animals (Das et al., 2009b) (Fig. 23.2) Another study conducted by our group demonstrated that with the use of nanofiber-expanded stem cells blood flow significantly increased in the hind limb vascular injury model (Das et al., 2009a). These enhancements of therapeutic effects in both cardiac infarcted model and hind limb ischemia model may be due to the elevated expression of promigratory and proadhesive molecules (CXCR4 and LFA-1). We did not find any evidence of oncogenic gene expression at the ischemic sites (Das et al., 2009b).

Clinical Applications of Hematopoietic Stem Cells

Stem cells were able to home to the infarcted heart in animal models, and these findings generated enormous interest regarding the contribution of stem cells to ventricular remodeling reduction of ischemia and improvement of cardiac function, which led to clinical application of stem cells. In one of the early trials, 10 patients were treated by intracoronary transplantation of autologous BM cells in addition to the standard therapy after myocardial infarction. Positive results were obtained for cell therapy group compared to standard therapy group. Similar results were also shown using autologous CD133+ cells, which were injected into the infarcted border zone in patients who had a myocardial infarction and undergone coronary artery bypass. Improved cardiac functions were observed within 3–9 months (Stamm et al., 2003). In a separate study, NOGA catheter was used for cell delivery, and injection was guided by electromechanical mapping. In both studies, improvements of the cardiac functions were reported (Tse et al., 2003). These and other studies encouraged the following randomized controlled clinical trials. One of the early randomized controlled clinical trial on therapeutic angiogenesis was performed by using autologous transplantation of BM cells for the treatment of limb ischemia, where 45 patients were recruited and 22 patients were injected with randomized BM mononuclear cells and peripheral blood mononuclear cells. Ischemic legs implanted with BM mononuclear cells showed significant improvement from ischemia. Improvement of ischemic status was visible after 24 weeks, which indicated that the therapeutic effect is long-term rather than short-term. In another randomized clinical trial, Transplantation of Progenitor Cells And Regeneration Enhancement in Acute Myocardial Infarction (TOPCARE-AMI), conducted by Schachinger et al. (2004) investigated the safety, feasibility, and potential therapeutic effects of myocardial function using intracoronary infusion of either circulating progenitor cells (CPCs) or BM-derived progenitor cells (BMCs) in patients with acute myocardial infarction. After 4 months, quantitative left ventricular angiography showed that left ventricular ejection fraction (LVEF) was significantly increased and end-systolic volumes significantly decreased after the stem cell therapy. The enhancement lasted up to 1 year of therapy with no delayed adverse events related to progenitor cell therapy (Schachinger et al., 2004). Various delivery methods have been used in clinical trials, including injecting progenitor cells in the infarcted border during coronary artery bypass graft surgery, in the gastrocnemius muscle in peripheral vascular disease or intracoronary infusion and intramyocardial injection.

In summary, the clinical results showed no adverse effect and autologous HSC transplantation is feasible for the treatment of ischemic patients. The therapeutic effect is long-term, which can last for years. Even though large scale double blind clinical trials are needed to further address the therapeutic effect of the efficacy of the transplantation, the promising results till now shed light on therapeutic angiogenesis and motivate the investigators to promote the efficiency of transplantation.

Conclusions and Future Directions

Numerous efforts have been directed to understand the mechanistic basis of stem cell renewal and differentiation; however, it is yet to be completely understood. It is critically important to optimize culture techniques for ex vivo expansion of stem cells and to establish their subsequent in vivo reconstitution and engraftment abilities. Ex vivo expansion techniques that employ viral proteins or viral vectors should be carefully evaluated for their bio-safety due to integration of viral genome into host's genome. Certain expansion methods that employ the use of stromal cells co-cultured with HSCs should be carefully examined for their antigenic purity before any clinical application. Therefore, it becomes of utmost importance for stem cell regenerative field to identify cytokines (because of their chemical nature and biological function) and genetic factors, biologically inert or biocompatible extracellular material, coatings and substrates, which do not cause any potential side effects to the recipient. Furthermore, owing to the limited success of ex vivo expansion, numbers of different substrate characteristics supplemented with cytokines were evaluated. Three- dimensional cultures mimicking HSC niche, surface conjugated ECM molecules, surface modifications, surface topology and pattern and oxygen concentration were shown to play a significant role in modulating HSC functionality and self -renewal ability. Development of certain universal protocols applicable to HSC harvested from the different sources is important. We reported that nanofiber-expanded stem cells were more functionally superior in restoring blood flow or cardiac functions compared to the freshly isolated stem cells in various ischemic models. These results could be due to the fact that during the ex-vivo expansion, HSCs exit the quiescent G0 phase of the cell cycle, upregulate certain surface markers or genes that have reparative functional role and undergo self-renewing symmetric divisions. Thus, when transplanted in vivo, they home to ischemic tissues and mediate repair of the infarct region via inducing neovascularization. However, further studies will be needed to address the questions such as: is the reparative effect exerted by HSCs transient, if yes, does cell dose play a role in determining downstream beneficial effects? What is the real operational mechanism of HSC mediated regeneration? Is it regulated via multiple pathways or one definitive pathway operates under a given physiological condition? To what extent does the host tissue cells and microenvironment contribute to regenerative mechanism after transplantation of HSCs? If, in vivo mechanism of HSC mediated regeneration in a pathological state depends on the microenvironment, how long do these HSCs survive in necrotic/ fibrotic areas of ischemia? If, we could address all the above questions, they will help us to better design and manipulate HSCs for effective therapeutic application in degenerative diseases such as ischemia.

Acknowledgements This work was supported in part by National Institutes of Health grants, K01 AR054114 (NIAMS), SBIR R44 HL092706-01 (NHLBI), R21 CA143787 (NCI) and The Ohio State University start-up fund. The funders had no role in study design, data collection and analysis, decision to publish or preparation of the manuscript.

References

Aggarwal R, Pompili VJ, Das H (2010) Genetic modification of ex-vivo expanded stem cells for clinical application. Front Biosci 15:854–871

Arai F, Hirao A, Ohmura M, Sato H, Matsuoka S, Takubo K, Ito K, Koh GY, Suda T (2004) Tie2/angiopoietin-1 signaling regulates hematopoietic stem cell quiescence in the bone marrow niche. Cell 118:149–161

Asahara T, Murohara T, Sullivan A, Silver M, van der Zee R, Li T, Witzenbichler B, Schatteman G, Isner JM (1997) Isolation of putative progenitor endothelial cells for angiogenesis. Science 275:964–967

Bagley J, Rosenzweig M, Marks DF, Pykett MJ (1999) Extended culture of multipotent hematopoietic progenitors without cytokine augmentation in a novel three-dimensional device. Exp Hematol 27:496–504

Blank U, Karlsson G, Karlsson S (2008) Signaling pathways governing stem-cell fate. Blood 111:492–503

Bryder D, Jacobsen SE (2000) Interleukin-3 supports expansion of long-term multilineage repopulating activity after multiple stem cell divisions in vitro. Blood 96:1748–1755

Chua KN, Chai C, Lee PC, Tang YN, Ramakrishna S, Leong KW, Mao HQ (2006) Surface-aminated electrospun nanofibers enhance adhesion and expansion of human umbilical cord blood hematopoietic stem/progenitor cells. Biomaterials 27:6043–6051

Chua KN, Chai C, Lee PC, Ramakrishna S, Leong KW, Mao HQ (2007) Functional nanofiber scaffolds with different spacers modulate adhesion and expansion of cryopreserved umbilical cord blood hematopoietic stem/progenitor cells. Exp Hematol 35:771–781

Das H, Abdulhameed N, Joseph M, Sakthivel R, Mao HQ, Pompili VJ (2009a) Ex vivo nanofiber expansion and genetic modification of human cord blood-derived progenitor/stem cells enhances vasculogenesis. Cell Transplant 18:305–318

Das H, George JC, Joseph M, Das M, Abdulhameed N, Blitz A, Khan M, Sakthivel R, Mao HQ, Hoit BD, Kuppusamy P, Pompili VJ (2009b) Stem cell therapy with overexpressed VEGF and PDGF genes improves cardiac function in a rat infarct model. PLoS One 4:e7325

Ding S, Wu TY, Brinker A, Peters EC, Hur W, Gray NS, Schultz PG (2003) Synthetic small molecules that control stem cell fate. Proc Natl Acad Sci USA 100:7632–7637

Folkman J, Bach M, Rowe JW, Davidoff F, Lambert P, Hirsch C, Goldberg A, Hiatt HH, Glass J, Henshaw E (1971) Tumor angiogenesis – therapeutic implications. New Eng J Med 285:1182

Franke K, Pompe T, Bornhauser M, Werner C (2007) Engineered matrix coatings to modulate the adhesion of CD133+ human hematopoietic progenitor cells. Biomaterials 28:836–843

Gupta R, Tongers J, Losordo DW (2009) Human studies of angiogenic gene therapy. Circ Res 105:724–736

Himburg HA, Muramoto GG, Daher P, Meadows SK, Russell JL, Doan P, Chi JT, Salter AB, Lento WE, Reya T, Chao NJ, Chute JP (2010) Pleiotrophin regulates the expansion and regeneration of hematopoietic stem cells. Nat Med 16:475–482

Iruela-Arispe ML, Davis GE (2009) Cellular and molecular mechanisms of vascular lumen formation. Dev Cell 16:222–231

LaIuppa JA, McAdams TA, Papoutsakis ET, Miller WM (1996) Culture materials affect ex vivo expansion of hematopoietic progenitor cells. J Biomed Mater Res 36:347–359

Li Y, Ma T, Kniss DA, Yang ST, Lasky LC (2001) Human cord cell hematopoiesis in three-dimensional nonwoven fibrous matrices: in vitro simulation of the marrow microenvironment. J Hematother Stem Cell Res 10:355–368

Lin Y, Weisdorf DJ, Solovey A, Hebbel RP (2000) Origins of circulating endothelial cells and endothelial outgrowth from blood. J Clin Invest 105:71–77

Losordo DW, Dimmeler S (2004) Therapeutic angiogenesis and vasculogenesis for ischemic disease: part II: cell-based therapies. Circulation 109:2692–2697

Mohr JC, de Pablo JJ, Palecek SP (2006) 3-D microwell culture of human embryonic stem cells. Biomaterials 27:6032–6042

Mommaas B, Stegehuis-Kamp JA, van Halteren AG, Kester M, Enczmann J, Wernet P, Kogler G, Mutis T, Brand A, Goulmy E (2005) Cord blood comprises antigen-experienced T cells specific for maternal minor histocompatibility antigen HA-1. Blood 105:1823–1827

Nygren JM, Jovinge S, Breitbach M, Sawen P, Roll W, Hescheler J, Taneera J, Fleischmann BK, Jacobsen SE (2004) Bone marrow-derived hematopoietic cells generate cardiomyocytes at a low frequency through cell fusion, but not transdifferentiation. Nat Med 10:494–501

Peichev M, Naiyer AJ, Pereira D, Zhu Z, Lane WJ, Williams M, Oz MC, Hicklin DJ, Witte L, Moore MA, Rafii S (2000) Expression of VEGFR-2 and AC133 by circulating human CD34(+) cells identifies a population of functional endothelial precursors. Blood 95:952–958

Rafii S, Lyden D (2003) Therapeutic stem and progenitor cell transplantation for organ vascularization and regeneration. Nat Med 9:702–712

Schachinger V, Assmus B, Britten MB, Honold J, Lehmann R, Teupe C, Abolmaali ND, Vogl TJ, Hofmann WK, Martin H, Dimmeler S, Zeiher AM (2004) Transplantation of progenitor cells and regeneration enhancement in acute myocardial infarction: final one-year results of the TOPCARE-AMI Trial. J Am Coll Cardiol 44:1690–1699

Silva GV, Litovsky S, Assad JA, Sousa AL, Martin BJ, Vela D, Coulter SC, Lin J, Ober J, Vaughn WK, Branco RV, Oliveira EM, He R, Geng YJ, Willerson JT, Perin EC (2005) Mesenchymal stem cells differentiate into an endothelial phenotype, enhance vascular density, and improve heart function in a canine chronic ischemia model. Circulation 111:150–156

Stamm C, Westphal B, Kleine HD, Petzsch M, Kittner C, Klinge H, Schumichen C, Nienaber CA, Freund M, Steinhoff G (2003) Autologous bone-marrow stem-cell transplantation for myocardial regeneration. Lancet 361:45–46

Tse HF, Kwong YL, Chan JK, Lo G, Ho CL, Lau CP (2003) Angiogenesis in ischaemic myocardium by intramyocardial autologous bone marrow mononuclear cell implantation. Lancet 361:47–49

Wagers AJ, Sherwood RI, Christensen JL, Weissman IL (2002) Little evidence for developmental plasticity of adult hematopoietic stem cells. Science 297:2256–2259

Chapter 24

Breast Cancer Risk: Role of Somatic Breast Stem Cells

John A. Eden

Abstract Somatic breast stem cells (SCs) play a critical role in normal breast formation both in fetal and post-natal life. They are oestrogen receptor negative (ER⁻) and tightly regulated within niches found along the breast duct. It seems likely that somatic SCs are a major target for carcinogenesis. Early pregnancy is known to have a markedly protective effect on the development of breast cancer in later life. The first full-term pregnancy reduces SC number and permanently induces genetic changes making the SC less vulnerable to malignant transformation. Most breast cancers contain a small population of cancer stem cells (CSCs) that appear to drive most of the malignant behaviour such as local growth and metastasis. Cancer stem cells are ER⁻ and slow-growing and so are not affected much by standard endocrine therapies, chemotherapy nor radiotherapy. It seems likely that novel cancer treatments targeting these CSCs may be clinically useful and offer new hope to women with breast cancer.

Keywords Cancer stem cells (CSCs) · Breast cancer · Risk factors · Fetus · Knockout mice · Ductal carcinoma-in-situ

Introduction

Breast cancer is the commonest tumour affecting non-smoking women and it is well established that sex-hormones, diet, and reproductive factors play a major aetiological role in the disease (Trichopoulos et al., 2008). Breast cancer incidence increases with age and yet many of the risk factors and much of the laboratory evidence indicate that the origins of breast cancer may begin in fetal life and the first two decades or so of post-natal existence. In the last decade there has been a dramatic increase in knowledge of the factors involved in breast cancer initiation and progression.

Somatic breast stem cells play an essential role in the formation of the breast and its ductal system. These SCs exist from fetal days and so are exposed to oncogenic influences for much longer than the differentiated breast ductal cells which have a short, fixed life span. Long-lived and having pleuripotential, breast SCs are a likely target for carcinogenesis.

Also, breast tumours typically show marked heterogeneity. When breast cancer tissue is examined microscopically, it is common to see within the same area abnormal ductal tissue, fat, vascularity, and so on. Currently, there are two popular theories which attempt to explain both carcinogenesis and the heterogeneity seen in breast cancer. The oldest theory is that of clonal evolution (Nowell, 1976) which states that genetic and epigenetic damage to key suppressor genes or oncogenes induce malignant transformation. Subsequently the first malignant cell will evolve, change and eventually escape the local microenvironment. Finally, clonal expansion causes the tumour to grow and eventually metastasize. According to this theory, tumour heterogeneity results from continued intratumour evolution.

More recently, the CSC theory has arisen to challenge or possibly compliment the clonal theory. As will be discussed in the following sections of this chapter, somatic breast SCs play an essential role in normal breast development, and are a likely candidate for malignant change. Most breast cancers contain cells

J.A. Eden (✉)
School of Women and Children's Health, Royal Hospital for Women, Randwick, NSW 2031, Australia
e-mail: j.eden@unsw.edu.au

with stem-like properties and as will be shown later, in many breast tumours much of the malignant behaviour appears to be driven by a small population of CSCs. These malignant SCs appear to be attempting to make a "breast within the breast." Thus, according to the CSC theory, heterogeneity results due to the activity of these CSCs.

The next section will examine the role of normal somatic breast SCs in breast formation as well as the initiation of cancer; the rest of this chapter will focus on breast CSCs, their regulation, and the molecular mechanisms involved in tumour maintenance and growth. Towards the end of the chapter, there will be a discussion of the clinical relevance of these findings.

Normal Somatic Breast Stem Cells and Breast Formation

The function of somatic breast SC in breast formation has recently been reviewed (Eden, 2010a, b c; 2011). It is clear that breast somatic SCs are responsible for the production of all cellular sub-types found within and around the breast duct. This process begins in fetal life. Somatic breast SCs, like other stem cells are slowly dividing and long lived and form microspheres in culture. They can undergo asymmetrical cell division resulting in a self-clone and a committed progenitor that may proceed down the path of differentiation. Stem cells have low or absent lineage markers ($LIN^{-/low}$) and some of the commonly expressed cell markers include ESA, CD10, CD44, CD24, cytokeratins 5/6, 14 and 19, ALDH1, Mushashi-1 and sialomucin. Breast SCs are typically ER^- and PR^-. Stem cells are tightly regulated within a stem cell niche – a specialized area found along the breast duct.

The human fetus does not seem to contain any breast cells expressing ERα until after 30 weeks of gestational age. Before this time, ER^- somatic SCs form a primitive ductal system independent of oestrogen. After 30 weeks, clearly some of the SCs progenitors acquire ER and so oestrogens begin to affect the breast ductal system. After birth and during infancy, breast growth seems to parallel the rest of the body.

At puberty, the GnRH pulse generator starts up, initially inducing unopposed low-level oestrogen pulses and so typically for about 2 years, the pubertal breast is exposed to these small pulses of oestrogen. Ovulation usually begins a couple of years after menarche and results in the breasts being exposed to cyclical progesterone. Each breast duct contains highly specialized areas called "stem cell niches." Within these niches, the ER^- SCs are tightly regulated by the cells found within the niches and many of these cells are ER^+ progenitors which retain some stem-cell properties. Thus, SC function can be indirectly regulated by oestrogen via these ER^+ progenitors in a paracrine manner using peptide signalling with compounds such as amphiregulin (LaMarca and Rosen, 2007).

During puberty, alveolar buds form around the terminal ducts and form lobules type 1 (lob1). The breast reacts to the ovulatory cycle and rates of both breast ductal cell mitosis and apoptosis are maximal in the luteal phase. The effect of progesterone on the breast depends upon many factors (Eden, 2003; Clarke and Sutherland, 1990; Horwitz, 2008), which include altering of local breast aromatase activity, ER function, and number and effects on the paracrine peptide regulation of ductal cells. It seems likely that both oestrogen and progestins can influence SC function (even though the SC is ER^-PR^-) via ER^+PR^+ progenitors.

Over the last 20 years it has become evident that the breast synthesises oestrogens locally, within the breast (Licznerska et al., 2008; Pasqualini and Chetrite, 2005). Typically, intra-breast levels of oestradiol are at least 20 times that of serum. Breast tissue not only contains aromatase but also sulphatase which is able to convert oestrone sulphate, the most abundant oestrogen in serum, into oestrone. There is some evidence that a highly specialized group of SCs that contain ER and PR might behave as sex-steroid sensors, reacting to oestrogen and progesterone and then regulating adjacent ER^-PR^- stem cells and their progenitors via peptide paracrine factors (Eden, 2010d).

Pregnancy induces marked changes to the breast (Eden, 2010c). The nulliparous breast contains mainly lobules type 1 and 2 (lob1 and lob2), but during pregnancy there is marked lengthening and branching of breast ducts and very active mitosis at the ends of the ducts. Lobule type 3 and 4 (lob3, lob4) predominate. Post lactation, marked apoptosis and breast remodelling occurs.

The first full-term pregnancy appears to reduce SC number and function. This will be discussed in more detail in the next section. Lob3 is the dominant breast lobule type until around the age of 40 years. After menopause the breast ductal system continues to atrophy and lob1 dominates. Interestingly, local breast oestrogen production rises after menopause, and so even though systemic oestrogen levels are very low at this time, the breast remains "bathed in oestrogens."

Normal Somatic Breast Stem Cells and Carcinogenesis

The cancer stem cell hypothesis postulates that it is the somatic breast SC that is the major target for carcinogenesis within the breast. As already stated, even though breast cancer is mostly a disease of women over the age of 40 years, many of the risk factors for the disease seem to indicate that the origin of cancer initiation may begin in the first 20 years of life. Having just described the role of stem cells in normal breast function and structure throughout the epochs of life, we will now examine the possible roles of somatic SCs in carcinogenesis. Some of the early life breast cancer risk factors (Eden, 2010a) include large birth weight, rapid growth during infancy resulting in a tall adult, consuming a Western diet, and large mammary gland mass (Eden, 2010a, Trichopoulos et al., 2008).

Trichopoulos et al. (2008) have suggested that the main factor linking all these risk factors together might be breast SC number. His theory has four main sections:

1. SC number is the main determinant of breast cancer risk
2. SC number is mainly determined during fetal life
3. The first full-term pregnancy reduces SC number
4. Breast stimulating hormones will affect mutations, SC number, and the expansion of initiated clones.

These authors have suggested that peptide growth factors, such as IGF1 and IGF2, may affect SC number in the fetus and during infancy and so affect breast cancer risk later in life. They have shown that cord IGF1 levels do indeed correlate with birth weight. Strohsnitter et al. (2008) have shown that haematological stem and progenitor populations in cord blood are indeed correlated with birth weight. There is also abundant evidence that the impact of diet on cancer risk is much more marked in fetal life and infancy (see references in Eden, 2010b). In contrast, changing diet late in life has little, if any impact, on cancer risk. Thus, the Women's Health Initiative (WHI) randomised dietary intervention study altered the diet of a large cohort of women, mostly over 65 years of age (Prentice et al., 2006). The study diet was low-fat and high in vegetables and grains and despite recruiting 48,835 women and following them for 8 years, they found no change in breast cancer risk.

Early first full-term pregnancy markedly reduces breast cancer risk in later life. In fact, it is one of the strongest single risk factors for breast cancer (Eden, 2010c). During a pregnancy, breast cancer risk is slightly elevated, probably because pregnancy sex-hormones may stimulate an existing tumour. However, the earlier the first pregnancy, the lower the risk of breast cancer in later life. A number of theories have been proposed to explain these facts, which include:

1. The first full-term pregnancy reduces breast SC number.
2. Breast SC function is altered, making these cells less vulnerable to malignant transformation.
3. The SC-niche environment may be altered.

There is evidence to support these concepts (Eden, 2010c, Siwko et al., 2008, Russo et al., 2005, 2007, 2008). Siwko et al. (2008) have shown that early pregnancy does permanently reduce breast SC number in a mouse model. Professor Russo's group have performed a series of experiments and shown that early full-term pregnancy induces a number of changes in the breast SC population that would be expected to reduce the risk of breast cancer in later life. The prepregnancy breast SC is quite susceptible to carcinogens. In contract, post-pregnancy breast stem cells are much less vulnerable to carcinogens. Siwko et al. (2008) have suggested that this protective effect might be mediated through HCG since they have shown that even short-term exposure of virgin rats to HCG induces a genomic change in breast SC, which is identical to that of pregnancy.

It has been known for some time that the breast stroma and microenvironment have an important role in carcinogenesis (Eden, 2010c). In rats, the stroma of parous animals is able to inhibit mammary carcinogenesis. Interestingly, these changes were mediated through oestrogen. Little is known regarding the impact of breast feeding on SC number or function.

Breast cancer incidence increases with age and after menopause, despite the fact that systemic oestrogen levels fall to extremely low levels. As mentioned earlier, intra-breast oestrogen levels remain high because of local aromatase and sulphatase activity. Asselin-Labat et al. (2010) have shown in the mouse that mouse mammary SCs are highly responsive to oestrogen despite the fact that they lack ER. As mentioned earlier this effect is probably mediated via ER$^+$ niche-progenitors that secrete paracrine factors which in turn influence the ER$^-$ SC. These authors have shown that in their mouse model, the main mediator appears to be RANK ligand.

LaMarca and Rosen (2007) have suggested that amphiregulin (AREG) is also a main paracrine regulator of breast SC. AREG is a member of the EGF family and AREG-null mice behave very much like oestrogen receptor knockout mice (ERKO) in that early fetal duct formation can occur but oestrogen dependant duct branching and terminal bud formation does not occur. They have suggested that it is the ER$^+$ progenitor that responds to oestrogen, releasing AREG which can stimulate SC and other progenitors to divide.

In summary, the seeds of carcinogenesis appear to be sown in early life and a case has been made that somatic breast SCs play an important role in initiation of oncogenesis. If SCs are more vulnerable to malignant change then SC number may well be an important risk factor for breast cancer. Early first pregnancy is a strongly protective factor against breast cancer in later life. It seems likely that this effect is mediated via a reduction in breast SC number and permanent changes to the genome of the SCs left behind making them less vulnerable to malignant transformation.

Breast Cancer Stem Cells and Tumor Progression

It is well established that ductal carcinoma-in-situ (DCIS) is the commonest premalignant breast lesion (Patani et al., 2008). Before mammographic screening, DCIS was a rare diagnosis, but now it is commonly suspected on a mammogram when abnormal microcalcifications are seen and then confirmed by biopsy. Welch and Black (1997) reviewed seven autopsy studies and found that the median prevalence of DCIS was 9% and noted that much of it was too small to be detected clinically or radiologically. It has been estimated that between 14 and 53% of DCIS will progress to invasive breast cancer over 10 years (Erbas et al., 2006).

Gene expression profiling and tumour markers have shown that there are five main subtypes of breast cancer (Eden, 2010a; Sorlie et al., 2003). In clinical practice, breast cancers are routinely tested for the presence of ER, PR and HER2. Using these tumour markers and gene profiling three major tumour subgroups and 2 minor ones can be identified. The major divisions include a HER2 group, a luminal one (ductal type, usually ER$^+$ and PR$^+$) and a basal type (the so-called "triple negative" tumour). Two luminal subtypes (A and B explained below) have been described as well as a fifth minor group which has been described as "normal breast-like."

Each of these breast cancer subtypes express different receptors and have differing gene profiles. Thus, the luminal tumours resemble the inner duct cells and express epithelial genes such as CK8 and CK18. However, the type B has less expression of ER and has a worse outcome than luminal type-A. Basal tumours typically express myoepithelial genes such as CK5, 6, and 17. Against this clinical backdrop, we will now examine the role of SCs in oncogenesis, the role of stromal regulation in tumour progression, and finally some of the intra-cellular mechanisms involved in tumour maintenance.

According to the cancer stem cell theory, because SCs are very long-lived they can acquire sufficient genomic damage to affect critical suppressor genes and/or oncogenes that they begin to escape niche-control and the malignant process begins. It is likely that breast stroma is also involved in oncogenesis. As these CECs begin to divide they produce progenitors that attempt to make an abnormal breast "within a breast." In human breast cancer, these progenitors usually acquire sex-hormone receptors early on and so will have their growth stimulated by systemic and probably more importantly, by local stroma-produced oestrogens. However, most tumours will always have a small population of rare ER$^-$ CSC to drive the malignant process.

Human breast CSCs were first identified in 2003 (Al-Hajj et al., 2003). These authors examined tissue taken from nine human cases of breast cancer. They found that each of these malignancies contained a small number of CD44$^+$ CD24$^{-/low}$ Lin$^-$ cells that exhibited malignant and SC behaviour. Very small numbers of these CSC injected into nude mice produced malignant tumours, whereas even large numbers of the other bulk tumour cells did not.

The characteristics of breast CSC have been summarised (Eden, 2010a; Ponti et al., 2006).

CSCs are long-lived, slowly dividing cells which make up <10% of the tumour mass in 78% of breast cancers. Like other stem cells a breast CSC can form microspheres and divide asymmetrically to form a clone of itself and a committed progenitor cell. Critical molecular pathways that regulate stem cell renewal (e.g., Notch) are often deregulated in CSCs and only CSCs (rather than the bulk of the non-stem tumour cells) can form tumours when transplanted into nude mice. CSCs are resistant to standard chemotherapy and radiotherapy. They nearly always express $CD44^+$ $CD24^{-/low}$ Lin^- and/or ALDH1, and often express ESA and HER2 and are usually ER^-.

CD44 is a cell adhesion molecule which is involved in binding the cell to hyaluronic acid in connective tissue. CD24 seems to have a role in metastatic spread. As breast CSCs escape control by local factors they begin to produce malignant progenitors which may then produce malignant daughter cells that will exhibit a variety of different phenotypes. For example, many of these daughter cells acquire ER early in the malignant process, but others will be ER^-. These malignant progenitors are able to produce all the heterogeneity seen in most breast cancers. They can lead to abnormal fibrous tissue, malignant fat cell or vasculature.

Another useful marker of CSCs is the expression of aldehyde dehydrogenase (ALDH; Ginestier et al., 2007). This marker has been used successfully to identify CSC in brain tumours, myeloma, and acute myeloid leukaemia. ALDH seems to play a role in cellular differentiation. Breast cancers elaborating ALDH have a worse outcome, and are more likely to be chemotherapy-resistant than ALDH-negative tumours.

If the CSC hypothesis is valid then CSCs should be found not only within invasive breast cancers but also within DCIS lesions. Espina et al. (2010) indeed found that DCIS samples contained cells that exhibit SC properties and elaborated SC markers such as CD44. Also, when these cells were implanted into athymic mice they showed malignant properties. Breast stromal cells seem to play an essential part in keeping these CSCs within the duct.

There is increasing evidence that Caveolin-1 (Cav-1) plays a major role in containing these CSC within the duct, and loss of Cav-1 is associated with progression of DCIS to malignancy (Mercier et al., 2009, Eden, 2011). Caveolae are invaginations of the cell membrane that contain many important signalling molecules. Cav-1 is the major structural protein of caveolae and is mostly found in fibroblasts, fat cells and endothelial cells. Using Cav-1 loss-of-function mice, Mercier et al. (2009) have shown that such affected mice over-express ER and develop breast lesions similar to human DCIS. Indeed it has been shown in humans that reduced or absent Cav-1 levels are associated with early breast cancer progression (Witkiewicz et al., 2009).

Stromal cells are also a major source of peptide growth factors and oestrogens which can influence tumour growth (reviewed in Eden, 2010a, 2011). Many ER^+ breast cancers are surrounded by stromal cells which over-express aromatase. High intratumoral oestrogen levels stimulate the growth of ER^+ progenitors and their offspring. Malignant fibroblasts can secrete fibroblast growth factor 2 (FGF2) and vascular endothelial growth factor (VEGF). These two growth factors recruit haematological SCs into the tumour mass. Stromal cells also secrete peptides that induce angiogenesis that is a critical process for both tumour growth and metastatic potential. Malignant fat cells not only produce oestrogens locally but also secrete VEGF, cytokines, and leptin, which all encourage new blood vessel formation.

CSCs are not very sensitive to standard chemotherapy or radiotherapy because of their slow growth and unique metabolism. Most CSCs are ER^- and so are not responsive to endocrine breast cancer treatments. If all the CSCs are removed by surgery and none has metastasized then cure is possible. However, CSCs do have some unique properties, markers, and metabolic pathways that could be targeted by novel specific CSC treatments. Some of these approaches have been recently reviewed (Eden, 2010a; Kalirai and Clarke, 2006). Several pathways involved in CSC renewal have been identified. These include LIF, Wnt, Notch, Hedgehog as well as the TGF-β and EGF family. Trastuzumab is a standard treatment for $HER2^+$ breast cancer. It has been shown that trastuzumab reduces CSC number in HER^+ breast cancer, implying that perhaps its effect, at least in part, might be mediated via its impact on CSCs. The Notch pathway is also a likely target for CSC treatments. Approximately, 40% of human breast cancers have reduced expression of the Notch inhibitor NUMB, and it has been shown that γ secretase inhibitors are able to hamper Notch signalling (Kalirai and Clarke, 2006). During embryogenesis, the Hedgehog pathway is an important regulator of many processes. Normally, the Hedgehog pathway switches off in adult life, however, it is often reactivated in many cancers. This signalling seems to be especially important in CSC renewal via a gene, Bmi-1. Interestingly, this pathway can be blocked by cyclopamine (Lui et al., 2006).

In summary, it seems likely that most breast cancers begin as DCIS. Functional CSCs have been found within DCIS lesions, and evidence has been presented that these CSCs are usually held in check by stromal regulatory factors. Loss of Cav-1 seems to be a critical early event in progression from DCIS to invasive ductal breast cancer. Stromal oestrogens and some peptide growth factors appear to encourage tumour growth and spread. Local factors are secreted, which even recruit nonbreast SCs (e.g., haematological SCs) into the tumour. Even though standard chemotherapy and radiotherapy do not much impact CSCs much, novel SC pathways such as Notch and Hedgehog have been identified, and it seems likely that in the not-too-distant future new anti-CSC therapies will be developed.

Breast Cancer Stem Cells and Clinical Medicine

Most breast cancer are diagnosed after menopause and despite the fact that normal breast somatic SCs and breast cancer SCs are usually ER⁻, it is evident that hormonal therapies, such as hormone replacement therapy (HRT) and selective-oestrogen receptor modulators (SERMs), can influence the detection and course of DCIS and invasive breast cancer (Eden, 2010a). In this section, the possible mechanisms by which sex-hormone therapies might impact SCs and their progenitors are examined.

Several excellent reviews of the impact of HRT on breast cancer risk have been published (Chen, 2009, Greiser et al., 2005). These reviews are dominated by the Women's Health Initiative (WHI) study, the largest randomised controlled trial (RCT) of HRT ever performed. There were two types of HRT-regimens tested in the WHI study – a combined oestrogen-progestin HRT and an oestrogen only HRT.

The combined oestrogen-progestin arm of WHI was stopped prematurely after 5.2 years of follow up (Writing group for WHI, 2002). 16,608 postmenopausal women aged 50–79 years (average age 63 years) with an intact uterus at baseline were recruited by 40 U.S.A. clinical centres during the years 1993–1998. Subjects were randomised to 0.625 mg conjugated equine oestrogens (CEE) and 2.5 mg medroxyprogesterone acetate (MPA) daily or placebo. The average age of the participants was 63 years (range 50–79 years). For the women taking combined HRT (cHRT), the hazard ratio (HR) for developing breast cancer was 1.26 (adjusted 95% CI 1.00–1.59; unadjusted 95% CI 0.83–1.92). The absolute increased risk of breast cancer was 8 extra cases/10,000 women/year. Interestingly, there were 6 fewer bowel cases and 2 fewer endometrial cancers/10,000 women/year in the active treatment arm.

The initial results of the oestrogen-only arm of WHI were published in 2004 (The WHI Steering Committee, 2004). This was a randomized, double-blind, placebo controlled disease prevention trial of 0.625 mg CEE versus placebo beginning in 1993. Enrolled were 10,739 postmenopausal women, aged 50–79 years (average age 64 years) with prior hysterectomy. Subjects were treated for an average of 6.8 years. The HR for developing breast cancer for the oestrogen alone HRT (ERT) group was 0.77 (adjusted 95% CI 0.57–1.06; unadjusted 95% CI 0.59–1.01). The absolute decreased risk of breast cancer was 7 fewer cases/10,000 women/year. Interestingly, in 2006, a sub-analysis of the same group was published (Stefanick et al., 2006). The incidence of ductal cancers was reduced (HR 0.71, 95% CI 0.52–0.99) and there was no significant impact of the ERT on lobular cancers.

The reduced risk of breast cancer seen in the ERT-arm of WHI would seem to be counter-intuitive and has not attracted much attention in the medical research literature. Women entering this study were screened for clinical breast cancer with mammography and breast examinations. However, as already discussed, one would expect that this study group of older women would already have a large reservoir of DCIS and even small, undetectable invasive breast cancers. Thus, to expose such a large group of older women to exogenous oestrogens for such a long period of time, one would reasonably expect an increase in ER$^+$ breast cancer compared with the placebo group.

The possible reasons for this surprising result have been summarised (Eden, 2011, 2010a, d) and some of the likely mechanisms have already been mentioned. Breast CSCs are ER$^-$ and so unlikely to be affected by ERT, although there might be indirect stimulation of CSC via ER$^+$ progenitors as mediators such as RANK-L. Local breast synthesis of oestrogens is likely to be more important than systemic oestrogens especially after menopause. Breast aromatase activity increases after natural menopause; however, breast aromatase activity is directly inhibited by oestrogen and so paradoxically allowing systemic ERT to reduce local breast-oestrogen production. The most abundant serum oestrogen is oestrone sulphate, and breast-derived sulphatase converts oestrone sulphate into oestrone. There is some evidence that within breast fat and stroma, this pathway might even be more important than aromatase. Like aromatase, breast sulphatase is directly inhibited by oestrogen. It has been postulated that some of the equine oestrogens might behave as SERMs; however, one study found that equilin and 17-α-dihydroequilin stimulated MCF-7 breast cancer cells in culture as much as oestradiol did (Mueck et al., 2003).

Taking the results of both arms of WHI together, it seems that progestins might play a more important role in breast cancer promotion than exogenous oestrogens. Horwitz (2008) have performed a series of laboratory experiments that give some insight into these clinical observations. They have shown that progesterone and progestins can influence PR$^+$ progenitors to transform back into somatic SCs rather than going down the path of differentiation. Typically, in their cell culture model, the SC population increased from 0.5 to 1% of the cellular population to 20 or 30% under the influence of progesterone and this transformation occured without cell division occurring.

As previously mentioned, normal and malignant breast tissue contains rare ER$^-$ PR$^-$ SCs that give rise to ER$^+$ PR$^+$ lineage-restricted progenitors. These breast CSCs usually express CD44$^+$, CD24$^{-/low}$. Many authors have shown that oestrogens are potent mitogens stimulating the growth of ER$^+$ PR$^+$ breast cancer cell lines (e.g., MCF-7) in culture. In contrast, when progestins are added to the same cell culture systems, the impact is minimal. Thus it was hypothesised that perhaps the effect of progestins on breast cancer risk seen in studies such as WHI was mediated through a different mechanism.

Using global gene expression profiling, it was found that one of the major progesterone-regulated genes was cytokeratin 5 (CK5), which is a protein associated with SCs and supposedly restricted to ER$^-$ PR$^-$ breast cancers. Normally, CK5 was expressed in <0.1% of the oestrogen-treated tumour cells; however, when progesterone or MPA was added to the system, the CK5-expressing SC expanded to become 5–10% of the cell population. It was demonstrated that the true breast CSCs were CD44$^+$ CD24$^{-/low}$ ER$^-$ PR$^-$ CK5$^+$ and remained rare (0.5–2% of the total tumour load). However, their progeny acquired steroid receptors. The main effect of progesterone/progestin was on the PR$^+$ progeny, which reverted back to CK5$^+$ stem cells. This transformation occurred without cell division and rapidly, often within 24 h. It was found that small, young tumours were especially susceptible to this progestin-activated process.

Thus, true breast CSCs do not elaborate sex hormone receptors, but their progeny does. Sex-hormones such as oestrogen and progesterone (either endogenous or exogenous, natural or synthetic) have no effect on these important cells, which seem likely to be the source of most breast cancers. However, if a small breast cancer is present, progesterone, not oestrogen, seems to transform the PR$^+$ breast CSC progeny back into ER$^-$PR$^-$ CSC; thus, increasing the pool of malignant SCs. Any factor that increases CSC number is likely to accelerate tumour growth and spread since it is the CSC which is responsible for much of the behaviour of the malignant tumour.

Of course, the bulk of the breast cancer is made up of daughter cells derived from ER$^+$PR$^+$ progenitor; thus, explaining why most breast cancer cells elaborate sex-hormone receptors. The cells will have their growth stimulated by oestrogens, especially those derived from adjacent stromal cells. These same ER$^+$ daughter cells will have their growth inhibited by tamoxifen or an aromatase inhibitor.

Lastly, it is well established that bilateral mastectomy and SERMs will markedly reduce the risk developing a clinically relevant breast cancer (Eden, 2011). Can these observations be explained within the CSC theory? Clearly, if all or most of the breast tissue is excised then the normal somatic breast SCs (which are likely the main site of carcinogenesis) and perhaps even some CSCs will be physically removed; thus, reducing the risk of developing invasive breast cancer.

Both tamoxifen and raloxifene have been shown in RCTs to reduce the risk of invasive breast cancer in high risk populations. As previously mentioned, the main impact of SERMs will be on the ER$^+$ progenitors and their offspring. Even though the SERM has little if any, direct impact on the ER$^-$ SC, it may delay the development of a cancer through this effect on the CSC offspring. The effect of tamoxifen on CSCs has been studied using a rat model (Ting et al., 2008). Breast cancer was induced using a known carcinogen and the rats were randomised to receiving tamoxifen or a placebo. Tamoxifen significantly reduced the premalignant changes and also reduced breast cell proliferation rates. However, the CSC pool was expanded by the carcinogens and this change was not prevented by the tamoxifen. Thus, it seems that at least in this rate model, SERMs do not prevent CSC carcinogenesis but may inhibit their malignant offspring, thus, inhibiting the development of a clinically apparent breast cancer.

Conclusions

Breast cancer is the most common tumour affecting non-smoking women. The CSC theory postulates that the somatic breast SC is the major target of carcinogenesis because of its long life and pleuripotentiality. Many of the risk factors indicate that some of the origins of the disease may occur in fetal life and infancy. It has been suggested that early life risk factors such as high birth weight and rapid growth during infancy may be linked to SC number. Early first full-term pregnancy is strongly protective of the later development of invasive breast cancer. It has been demonstrated in animal models that the first pregnancy reduces SC number and permanently alters the genome of the SCs making it less vulnerable to malignant change.

The main premalignant breast lesion is DCIS and this condition is commonly found on mammography and during autopsy studies, suggesting that only a proportion of DCIS progresses to invasive cancer. Human DCIS contains malignant SCs which appear to be kept in check by paracrine control of surrounding stromal cells. Cav-1 appears to have a significant preventive role in DCIS. Loss of Cav-1 is associated with increased risk of invasive disease and the acquisition of ER.

Studies of human breast cancers have shown that most of the growth of the tumour and metastatic tendency are mediated via the CSCs which remain slow-growing, rare and ER$^-$. The progenitors and their offspring often acquire ER. Breast stromal and fat tissues contain abundant aromatase, and so normal and malignant breast tissue levels of oestradiol are many times higher than serum. This locally-derived oestrogen is likely to stimulate the growth of the ER$^+$ daughter cells but not the ER$^-$ CSC.

Long-term combined HRT appears to slightly increase breast cancer risk by 8 extra cases/10,000 women/year. It has been shown that it is likely that the progestin is responsible for this effect rather than the oestrogen. Cell culture studies have demonstrated that addition of MPA to human breast cancers in culture results in a prompt and marked increase in CSC number from ~1 to 20% or even 30%. In contrast, SERMs have been shown clinically to reduce the risk of developing breast cancer by at least 50%. These agents appear to have little if any effect on CSCs, but rather markedly inhibit their ER$^+$ offspring.

Since the discovery of human breast CSCs in 2003, more than 400 articles have been published in this area. Breast CSC have been characterised by surface markers, unique oncogenes, and metabolic pathways. Agents that alter CSC function have been discovered and further trials are underway. It is likely that during the next few years novel CSC therapies will be offered to women with breast cancer in the hope to further improve their survival and quality of life.

References

Al-Hajj M, Wicha MS, Benito-Hernandez A, Morrison SJ, Clarke MF (2003) Prospective identification of tumorigenic breast cancer cells. Proc Natl Acad Sci USA 100:3983–3988

Asselin-Labat ML, Vaillant F, Sheridan JM, Pal B, Wu D, Simpson ER, Yasuda H, Smyth GK, Martin TJ, Lindeman GJ, Visvader JE (2010) Control of mammary stem cell function by steroid hormone signalling. Nature 465:798–803

Chen FP (2009) Postmenopausal hormone therapy and risk of breast cancer. Chang Gung Med J 32:140–147

Clarke CL, Sutherland RL (1990) Progestin regulation of cellular proliferation. Endocr Rev 11:266–301

Eden J (2003) Progestins and breast cancer risk. Am J Obstet Gynecol 188(5):1123–1131

Eden JA (2010a) Human breast cancer stem cells and sex-hormones – a narrative review. Menopause 17(4):801–810

Eden JA (2010b) Breast cancer, stem cells and sex hormones: part 1 – the impact of fetal life and infancy. Maturitas 67(2):117–120

Eden JA (2010c) Breast cancer, stem cells and sex hormones: part 2 – the impact of the reproductive years and pregnancy. Maturitas 67(3):215–218

Eden JA (2010d) Why does oestrogen-only hormone therapy have such a small impact on breast cancer risk? A hypothesis. Gynecol Endocrinol. doi:10.3109/09513590.2010.488778

Eden JA (2011) Breast cancer, stem cells and sex hormones: part 3 – the impact of the menopause and hormone replacement. Maturitas 68(2):129–136

Erbas B, Provenzano E, Armes J, Gertig D (2006) The natural history of ductal carcinoma in situ of the breast: a review. Breast Cancer Res Treat 97:135–144

Espina V, Mariani BD, Gallagher RI, Tran K, Banks S, Wiedemann J, Huryk H, Mueller C, Adamo L, Deng J, Petricoin EF, Pastore L, Zaman S, Menezes G, Mize J, Johal J, Edmiston K, Liotta LA (2010) Malignant precursor cells pre-exist in human breast DCIS and require autophagy for survival. PLoS One 5(4):e10240

Ginestier C, Hur MH, Charafe-Jauffret E, Monville F, Dutcher J, Brown M, Jacquemier J, Viens P, Kleer CG, Liu S, Schott A, Hayes D, Birnbaum D, Wicha MS, Dontu G (2007) ALDHI is a marker of normal and malignant human mammary stem cells and a predictor of poor clinical outcome. Cell Stem Cell 1:555–567

Greiser CM, Greiser EM, Dören M (2005) Menopausal hormone therapy and risk of breast cancer: a meta-analysis of epidemiological studies and randomized controlled trials. Hum Reprod Update 11(6):561–573

Horwitz KB (2008) The year in basic science: update of estrogen plus progestin therapy for menopausal hormone replacement implicating stem cells in the increased breast cancer risk. Mol Endocrinol 22:2743–2750

Kalirai H, Clarke RB (2006) Human breast epithelial stem cells and their regulation. J Pathol 208:7–16

LaMarca HL, Rosen JM (2007) Estrogen regulation of mammary gland development and breast cancer: amphiregulin takes center stage. Breast Cancer Res 9:304–307

Licznerska BE, Wegman PP, Nordenskjold B, Wingren S (2008) In situ levels of estrogen producing enzymes and its prognostic significance in postmenopausal breast cancer patients. Br Cancer Treat 112:15–23

Lui S, Dontu G, Mantle ID, Patel S, Ahn N-S, Jackson KW, Suri P, Wicha MS (2006) Hedgehog signalling and Bmi-1 regulate self-renewal of normal and malignant human mammary stem cells. Cancer Res 66:6063–6071

Mercier I, Casimiro MC, Zhou J, Wang C, Plymire C, Bryant KG, Daumer KM, Sotgia F, Bonuccelli G, Witkiewicz AK, Lin J, Tran TH, Milliman J, Frank PG, Jasmin JF, Rui H, Pestell RG, Lisanti MP (2009) Genetic ablation of caveolin-1 drives oestrogen-hypersensitivity and the development of DCIS-like mammary lesions. Am J Pathol 174(4):1172–1190

Mueck AO, Seeger H, Wallwiener D (2003) Comparison of the proliferative effects of estradiol and conjugated equine estrogens on human breast cancer cells and impact of continuous combined progestogens addition. Climacteric 6:221–227

Nowell PC (1976) The clonal evolution of tumor cell populations. Science 194:23–28

Pasqualini JR, Chetrite GS (2005) Recent insight on the control of enzymes involved in estrogen formation and transformation in human breast cancer. J Steroid Biochem Mol Biol 93:221–236

Patani N, Cutuli B, Mokbel K (2008) Current management of DCIS: a review. Breast Cancer Res Treat 111:1–10

Ponti D, Zaffaroni N, Capelli C, Daidone MG (2006) Breast cancer stem cells: an overview. Eur J Cancer 42:1219–1224

Prentice RL, Caan B, Chlebowski RT, Patterson R, Kuller LH, Ockene JK, Margolis KL, Limacher MC, Manson JE, Parker LM, Paskett E, Phillips L, Robbins J, Rossouw JE, Sarto GE, Shikany JM, Stefanick ML, Thomson CA, Van Horn L, Vitolins MZ, Wactawski-Wende J, Wallace RB, Wassertheil-Smoller S, Whitlock E, Yano K, Adams-Campbell L, Anderson GL, Assaf AR, Beresford SAA, Black HR, Brunner RL, Brzyski RG, Ford L, Gass M, Hays J, Heber D, Heiss G, Hendrix SL, Hsia J, Hubbell FA, Jackson RD, Johnson KC, Kotchen JM, LaCroix AZ, Lane DS, Langer RD, Lasser NL, Henderson MM (2006) Low-fat dietary pattern and risk of invasive breast cancer. JAMA 295:629–642

Russo J, Moral R, Balogh GA, Mailo D, Russo IH (2005) Review: the protective role of pregnancy in breast cancer. Breast Cancer Res 7:131–142

Russo J, Balogh G, Russo IH (2007) Breast cancer prevention. Climacteric 10(Suppl 2):47–53

Russo J, Balogh GA, Russo IH (2008) Full-term pregnancy induces a specific genomic signature in the human breast. Cancer Epidemiol Biomark Prev 17(1):51–66

Siwko SK, Dong J, Lewis MT, Liu H, Hilsenbeck SG, Li Y (2008) Evidence that an early pregnancy causes a persistent decrease in the number of functional mammary epithelial stem cells – implications for pregnancy-induced protection against breast cancer. Stem Cells 26:3205–3209

Sorlie T, Tibshirani R, Parker J, Hastie T (2003) Repeated observation of breast tumor subtypes in independent gene expression data sets. Proc Natl Acad Sci USA 100:8418–8423

Stefanick ML, Anderson GL, Margolis KL, Hendrix SL, Rodabough RJ, Paskett ED, Lane DS, Hubbell FA, Assaf AR, Sarto GE, Schenken RS, Yasmeen S, Lessin L, Chlebowski RT (2006) Effects of conjugated equine estrogens on breast cancer and mammography screening in postmenopausal women with hysterectomy. JAMA 295:1647–1657

Strohsnitter WC, Savarese TM, Low HP, Chelmow DP, Lagiou P, Lambe M, Edmiston K, Liu Q, Baik I, Noller KL, Adami HO, Trichopoulos D, Hsieh CC (2008) Correlation of umbilical cord blood haematopoietic stem and progenitor cell levels with birth weight: implications for a prenatal influence on cancer risk. Br J Cancer 98:660–663

The Women's Health Initiative Steering Committee (2004) Effects of conjugated equine estrogen in postmenopausal women with hysterectomy. The Women's Health Initiative randomized controlled trial. JAMA 291:1701–1712

Ting AY, Kimler BF, Fabian CJ, Petroff BK (2008) Tamoxifen prevents premalignant changes of breast, but not ovarian, cancer in rats at high risk for both diseases. Cancer Prev Res 1(7):546–553

Trichopoulos D, Adami HO, Ekbom A, Hsieh CC, Lagiou P (2008) Early life events and conditions and breast cancer risk: from epidemiology to etiology. Int J Cancer 122:481–485

Welch HG, Black WC (1997) Using autopsy series to estimate the disease "reservoir" for ductal carcinoma in situ of the breast: how much more breast cancer can we find? Ann Intern Med 127:1023–1028

Witkiewicz AK, Dasupta A, Nguyen KH, Rui HR, Lisanti M (2009) Stromal caveolin-1 levels predict early DCIS progression to invasive breast cancer. Cancer Biol Ther 8(11):1071–1079

Writing Group for the Women's Health Initiative Investigators (2002) Risks and benefits of estrogen plus progestin in healthy postmenopausal women. JAMA 288:321–333

Chapter 25

Cellular Replacement Therapy in Neurodegenerative Diseases Using Induced Pluripotent Stem Cells

Takayuki Kondo, Ryosuke Takahashi, and Haruhisa Inoue

Abstract Neurodegenerative disorders are characterized by progressive neuronal loss, resulting in clinical deficit. Several drugs can improve neural symptoms transiently but cannot halt progression or recover deficits. Stem cell transplantation is focused as upcoming regenerative treatment. After recent advances in embryonic stem cells and induced pluripotent stem cells, research is accelerating their application to neurodegerative disorders, including amyotrophic lateral sclerosis (ALS). We review the recent progress and present our future vision concerning cell replacement therapy for ALS, and we also emphasize the hurdles to be overcome before clinical trials can be begun. Basic research focusing on the safety of transplantation, besides therapeutic experiments, should lead to a beneficial outcome.

Keywords Cellular replacement therapy · Embryonic stem cells · Parkinson's disease · Huntington's disease · Amyotrophic lateral sclerosis · Central nervous system

Introduction

Resolve Limitations in Cellular Replacement Therapy

Neurodegenerative diseases, such as Alzheimer's disease (AD), Parkinson's disease (PD), Huntington's

H. Inoue (✉)
Center for iPS Cell Research and Application, Kyoto University, Kyoto, Japan
e-mail: haruhisa@cira.kyoto-u.ac.jp

disease (HD) and amyotrophic lateral sclerosis (ALS), mainly attack the central nervous system (CNS) and result in neuronal loss. A condition of decreasing numbers of neurons leads to dysfunction of the neural network, resulting in disorders such as memory loss, bradykinesia, involuntary movement or limb weakness. In the past several decades, a number of drugs have been developed to compensate at least partially for these disabilities. However, none of the drugs has been able to halt disease progression or replace neuronal loss.

To overcome these limitations of conventional drug therapy, cell replacement therapies are being prepared, step-by-step, toward clinical trials. Clinical trials using stem cells have been described for Huntington's disease, Parkinson's disease, spinal cord injury, and stroke. Several clinical trials have achieved successful improvement in neurological deficits in patients. However, most of these clinical trials were based on somatic stem cells, including fetal neural tissue, nasal mucosa progenitors, or mesenchymal stem cells. Nonetheless, the resource limitation of somatic stem cells remains a major hurdle for the universal application for cell replacement therapy.

Establishment of ESC and iPSC

In 1998 human embryonic stem cells (ESC) were first generated from the inner cell mass of the mammalian blastocyst (Thomson et al., 1998). ESC can proliferate almost indefinitely and differentiate into multiple cell-types of all three germ-layers in vivo. Additionally the molecular basis of reprogramming has been revealed by the exogenous expression of combinations of transcription factors. Four factors,

Oct3/4, Sox2, Klf4, and c-Myc, which are important for self-renewal of ESC, have been shown to reprogram both mouse and human somatic cells into ESC-like pluripotent cells, called induced pluripotent stem cells (iPSC) (Takahashi et al., 2007).

ESC and iPSC theoretically can differentiate into various cell-types of neural lineage, including dopaminergic neuron, neural crest, retina, cerebral cortex, and spinal motor neuron (Li et al., 2008). Using these differentiation methods ESC or iPSC derived neurons were applied to disease modeling (Li et al., 2008; Ebert et al., 2009; Lee et al., 2009).

Clinical Trials Using ESC-Derived Cells

The development of ESC and iPSC is attractive not only for disease mechanism research but also for cellular replacement therapy. Several clinical trials with ESC are ongoing (Table 25.1). In 2009, the Food and Drug Administration (FDA) gave the first approval for an ESC-based clinical trial, conducted by Geron Corporation. Geron planned to apply human ESC-derived oligodendrocyte progenitor cells (OPCs) to the treatment of spinal cord injury patients. In a rat model of spinal cord injury, transplantation of ESC-derived OPCs dramatically improved disability to almost a normal level (Sharp et al., 2010). The mechanism of the improvement was well assessed, demonstrating secreting nerve growth factor and remyelination. The safety of the process, especially in terms of tumorigenicity, was also evaluated. However, the FDA placed a hold on this trial because of cystic structure in animal model after transplantation. After additional safety-proving data, phase I clinical trials of ESC-derived OPCs were released in 2010 (Strauss, 2010).

Furthermore, Advanced Cell Technology, Inc. (ACT) received FDA clearance for a run of second clinical trials using ESC of age-related macular degeneration (AMD) in 2010. AMD is the most common form of macular degeneration and is intractable by existing medicine. ACT plans to transplant ESC-derived retinal pigment epithelial (RPE) cells to AMD patients and perform safety evaluation as a phase I clinical trial (Zhu et al., 2010). ACT is also approved for Stargardt's macular degeneration by transplanting ESC-derived RPE cells in 2010 November.

Regenerative Therapy for ALS

Cell replacement therapy promises to be powerful and attractive especially for CNS disorders, which are impossible to cure by conventional therapy. One of the most intractable CNS disorders is ALS.

ALS is a fatal neurodegenerative disease with late-middle age onset. ALS is clinically characterized by dysfunction of both upper and lower motor neurons, resulting in rapid progression of weakness and respiratory failure. Median survival of ALS patients without ventilators is only a few years. Numerous drugs have been attempted in clinical trials, but almost all failed to achieve even disease modification. The solely successful drug, riluzole, can only slow disease progression slightly.

The neuropathological hallmark of ALS is a massive loss of motor neurons in both the primary motor area and the anterior horn of the spinal cord. A recent study revealed that TAR DNA binding protein of 43 kDa (TDP-43) aggregates are observed not only in degenerative neurons but also in glial cells (Arai et al., 2006; Neumann et al., 2006). Unveiling the role of TDP-43 and relevant molecules would accelerate ALS research, but would still not be sufficient for a complete cure. Therefore, replacement therapy using stem cells is expected to be a potent candidate for modifying or recovering from the disease state. Here we review the recent progress and present future vision for cell replacement therapy for ALS, also emphasizing the hurdles to overcome before clinical trials can commence.

Table 25.1 Clinical trials using ESC in neurological disorders

Company	Disease	Cell type	Progress
Geron	Spinal cord injury	OPCs	Phase I 2010 October
ACT	Stargardt's macular degeneration	RPE	Phase I 2010 November
ACT	AMD	RPE	Phase I 2010 November
California stem cell	SMA type I	Motor neuron	Hold 2011 February

Transplantation Research for ALS

Before clinical trials can be initiated, basic research using animal models is necessary for evaluating their safety and efficacy. Almost all transplantation research was established using human superoxide dismutase 1 (SOD1), with G93A mutation, transgenic rats or mice. SOD1 is the most common causative gene of familial ALS, and SOD1 transgenic animals represent lower motor neuronal loss, mimicking symptoms of ALS patients (Gurney et al., 1994).

For cell resources, various kinds of stem cells are used for transplantation, e.g., rodent bone marrow cells, human mesenchymal stem cells (hMSC), neurotrophic-factor-secreting hMSC, human umbilical cord blood cells (hUCBC), neural progenitor cells (NPC), and ESC-derived glial precursors (Lepore et al., 2008; Thonhoff et al., 2009).

Transplantation routes also vary, e.g., direct injection into the spinal cord, intraperitoneal, intracerebroventricular, and intravenous injection. Direct injection into the spinal cord can localize transplanted cells and provide high survival efficacy. In contrast, intravenous injection can deliver transplanted cells widely, but it has lower efficacy of engraftment or can result in pulmonary embolism. Outcome results vary from research to research, and graft-modifying technique (e.g., molecular modification to secrete neurotrophic factors) can enhance the efficacy of engraftment (Thonhoff et al., 2009). To evaluate the optimal delivery efficacy and survival rate, Takahashi et al., (2010) compared each transplantation route (including lesion-direct, intrathecal and intravenous injection) with spinal cord injury mice model and luciferase imaging. They concluded that direct injection achieved the highest delivery efficacy and graft survival 6 weeks after injection.

Clinical Trials of Cell Transplantation for ALS

Recently, several clinical trials using somatic stem cell transplantation for ALS have been conducted. All of the published clinical trials were based on autologous MSC from bone marrow (Table 25.2). According to the published data, they successfully achieved a safety endpoint, but spinal cord swelling at the transplanted site is noted in some cases (Karussis et al., 2010). Therefore, the risk of tumorigenicity has not been excluded even in adult somatic stem cells. Emory University and Neural Stem Inc., received FDA approval in 2009, and they have already started an ALS phase I clinical trial by transplantation of fetal neural stem cells.

Hurdles in Transplantation Therapy

Basic research using animal models will help to shed light on problems needing to be overcome before clinical trials.

Ethical Issues

To obtain ESC culture, it is necessary to manipulate embryos for scientific use. However, among various moral and ethical issues involved, the catholic church identifies embryos at this stage as having the same rights as a developing human being.

Robust Supply

As described above (CLINICAL TRIALS), MCS are widely applied and are clinically easy to access from general hospitals. However, because they are not of neural lineage, their effectiveness as cell replacement is limited. Up-coming clinical trials with neural stem cells (NSC) of fetal spinal are expected to prove them as a suitable cell resource for neural replacement. However, the graft cell resource will depend on the fetal spinal cord, limiting the number of graft cells.

Somatic cells and MSC have a finite replicative lifespan, beyond which senescence will prevent division. In contrast, ESC or iPSC can proliferate indefinitely and make robust stable freeze stocks. Furthermore, transplant of ESC- or iPSC-derived NSC can provide both neuronal replacement and protective glial cells, modifying the ALS environment around remaining neurons.

Table 25.2 Clinical trials of cell transplantation in ALS

Country	Company/Center	Date	Cell source	Cell type	Route	No. enrolled	Trial	Results
Italy	Eastern Piedmont Univ.	(2010 publish)	Auto, BM	MSC	Upper Th	10	Phase I	Safe
Turkey	Akay Hospital	(2009 publish)	Auto, BM	MSC	C1-2	13?	Phase I	Safe, improved
Spain	Hospital Universitario Virgen de la Arrixaca	2007 Feb–2010 Feb	Auto, BM	MSC	Th5-6	11	Phase I	
Spain	Hospital Universitario Virgen de la Arrixaca	2010 Oct~	Auto, BM	MSC	Th5-6	63	Phase II	(Currently recruiting)
Spain	Autonomous University of Barcelona	(2010 publish)	Auto, nose/BM	OEC/MSC		20	N.A.	Safe, no effect
Israel	Hadassah Medical Organization	2010 Jan~	Auto, BM	MSC-NTF	muscle	12	Phase I	(Currently recruiting)
Israel	Hadassah Medical Organization	2010 Jan~	Auto, BM	MSC-NTF	CSF (lumbar puncture)	12	Phase II	(Currently recruiting)
U.S.A.	TCA Cellular Therapy	2010~	Auto, BM	MSC	CSF (lumbar puncture)	6	Phase I	(Currently recruiting)
U.S.A.	Emory University	2009~	Fetal Spinal Cord	NSC	Cervical/Lumbar	12	Phase I	N.A.
U.S.A.	Unknown	in plannning	hESC	Glial cells (astrocytes)	–	–	–	–

Safety

Self-renewal and plasticity features of ESC and iPSC are also characteristics of cancer cells. Sometimes graft stem cells can lose control of appropriate proliferation and develop tumor as an unacceptable side-effect. We can decrease tumorigenicity risk by (1) using well-maturated cells for transplantation or (2) characterizing and selecting ESC or iPSC that have low tumorigenicity. To achieve (1), we have to enhance the sophistication of the differentiation and purification techniques of target cells. The tumorigenic potential of ESC will be reduced after maturation. For investigating (2), Miura et al., (2009) clarified that ES and iPSC have different tendencies to form neural tumor or teratoma from clone to clone. To decrease tumorigenicity, a novel iPSC reprogramming technique, using L-Myc instead of c-Myc, was reported (Nakagawa et al., 2010). By mixing and balancing these evaluation techniques, we will be able to avoid or decrease tumorigenicity in the future.

Before transplantation, ESC and iPSC need to pass through many steps to reach an appropriate state for use. Throughout, we must prevent contamination risk by harmful components and meet the standard of "Good Manufacturing Practice". In detail, adequate screening of donor material for infectious diseases as well as possible genetic testing will be necessary. In addition, avoiding the use of nonhuman animal components (a potential source of unknown infection) will also be important.

Functional Efficacy

Even if appropriate numbers of graft-cells can survive, it is difficult to make a neural network with the remaining neurons. For example, of fetus mid-brain transplantation in PD, cell therapy could improve motor symptoms and decrease drug dosage. However, therapy cannot improve dyskinesia (inappropriate secretion of neuronal transmitter) (Barker and Kuan, 2010). This phenomenon is explained by failure to make a synchronized network with the remaining neurons around engrafting sites (Carlsson et al., 2006) or by contamination of serotonergic neurons in graft (Barker and Kuan, 2010). In the case of ALS, engrafted cells have to expand their axons to muscle (target site), far away from the spinal cord. Several researchers successfully overcame this difficulty and observed that transplanted cells (human neural stem cells) innervated host animal muscle (Gao et al., 2005; Deshpande et al., 2006).

For choosing cell type for the optimal state of ALS transplantation therapy, we can mainly list neural precursors, motor neurons, astrocytes, oligodendrocytes, and microglial cells. Simply stated, ESC- or iPSC-derived motor neurons would be a most suitable candidate for treating motor neuron disease. However, when generating or purifying motor neurons from ESC or iPSC, it is difficult to maintain moderate differentiation efficiency. Neural precursors, including various subtypes of neurons, are expected to have the most powerful ability to regenerate or protect damaged tissue. On the other hand, neural precursors generally contain immature cells and can have high tumorigenicity. In contrast to the regenerative effect of neural transplantation, glial cell transplantation can exert a neuroprotective effect via secreting neurotrophic factors and improving inflammatory damage of ALS. Then, for maintaining an all-around sufficient efficacy and safety level, matured glial cells would also be favorable candidates for clinical trials. More preclinical research will be required to approach solutions to this problem (Papadeas and Maragakis, 2009).

We utilize animal models for the evaluation of transplantation efficacy, and rodent is usually employed as disease model and recipient. However, rodent is a distinctively different species from humans. As an example of a spinal cord injury model, mice recover their motor function only a few days after injury, without any treatment. Natural recovery (or compensation), commonly observed in rodent, is never seen in humans. This difference is ascribed to the difference in upper motor neural tract between rodent and humans. Then, we have to investigate other species that are closer to humans, such as canine ALS models (Awano et al., 2009).

Difficulty of Efficient Cell-Delivery into ALS Lesions

The pathological changes of PD patients are mostly localized in midbrain or basal ganglia (striatum), and it is easy to apply direct injection of stem cells. However, pathological changes, based on TDP-43 immunostaining, are widely observed in the whole CNS (Liscic et al., 2008). ALS is contemporarily recognized as a multisystem neurodegenerative disorder. To overcome difficulties regarding the "wide-spread lesions of ALS" and the blood-brain barrier, transplantation via cerebral ventricle might be a solution (Morita et al., 2008).

For Future Clinical Trials

From the series of long discussions between the FDA and Geron, we can understand that safety is considered to be critically important for successful clinical trials. The International Society for Stem Cell Research (ISSCR) recently issued guidelines regarding threshold safety and ethical criteria for clinical transplantation therapy (Hyun et al., 2008). The ISSCR guidelines deal not only with not just ESC research but also with other pluripotent stem cells, including iPSC. ISSCR guidelines also point out the need to assess the risks of tumorigenicity. Abiding by the guidelines, stem cell transplantation is expected to win approval smoothly and to maintain a constant level of quality.

Cell Resource

We have two pluripotent stem cells, ESC and iPSC, as graft resource. Today, a few clinical or preclinical trials are mostly based on ESC or ESC-derived precursor cells, but not on iPSC. iPSC have the ability of proliferation and differentiation like ESC, and they are considered to have a similar character to that of ESC. However, recent study revealed a difference between them at the level of genome methylation or gene expression (Bock et al., 2011). We can characterize and select iPSC clones that are epigenetically identical to ESC. Then, the transplantation management of ESC is applicable to iPSC. Here we list the pros and cons of choosing ESC or iPSC in future clinical applications.

Generally, differentiation and transplantation research using ESC has a decade of history, and both usability and safety information have already accumulated to some extent. This information is a great advantage for transplantation therapy, which requires a very strict safety level (but not enough). In contrast, iPSC technology is in its nascent stages, but recent rapid advances in the field are expected to bridge the gap.

To prevent GVHD risk, recipients must continue immunosuppressant drugs after ESC transplantation. Moreover, GVHD reaction has been pointed out as raising focal inflammation at the transplant site and exacerbating degenerative progression (Kordower et al., 2008). Besides the GVHD harmful events, there is also an interesting discussion regarding GVHD possibly acting as a safety-lock against tumorigenicity, which is an intolerable side-effect. In other words, reactivated GVHD reaction, by discontinuing immunosuppressants, could eliminate "tumor" derived from ESC-graft. We need to evaluate carefully this two-sided character of GVHD mechanisms through animal model research.

In contrast, we can generate iPSC from adult somatic cells of a patient (transplantation donor) and return patient-derived iPSC-graft back to the same patient (transplantation recipient), without GHVD risk. In the future, if a quick, safe, and low-cost method for iPSC generation is developed, every patient will be able to receive his/her own iPSC-derived cells, as ultimately customized transplantation therapy. However, the reprogramming state of iPSC is known to differ from clone to clone (Miura et al., 2009). The selection of safe iPSC will be critical for safe transplantation. To overcome the described hurdles of both ESC- and iPSC based research, HLA type characterized iPSC bank will enable us to minimize the risk for GVHD and lower the dosage of immunosuppressant drugs (Nakatsuji et al., 2008). Furthermore, by using iPSC bank, we can also circumvent the ethical issue of using ESC.

In conclusion, innovations in stem cell manipulation will accelerate transplantation therapy using stem cells. Basic research focusing on the safety of transplantation, in addition to therapeutic experiments, can lead to beneficial outcome in practical use.

Acknowledgments We would like to express our sincere gratitude to all our coworkers and collaborators, and to K. Murai for editing the manuscript. This study was supported in part by a grant from the Leading Project of MEXT (HI), a grant from Yamanaka iPS cell special project (HI), JST (Japan Science and Technology Agency), CREST (Core Research for Evolutional Science and Technology) (HI), a Grant-in-Aid from the Ministry of Health and Labour (HI), a Grant-in-Aid for Scientific Research (21591079) from JSPS (HI), Grant-in-Aid for Scientific Research on Innovative Area "Foundation of Synapse and Neurocircuit Pathology" (22110007) from the Ministry of Education, Culture, Sports, Science and Technology of Japan (HI), a research grant from the Takeda Science Foundation (HI), a research grant from the Kanae Foundation for the Promotion of Medical Science (HI), and a research grant from the NOVARTIS Foundation for Gerontological Research (HI).

References

Arai T, Hasegawa M, Akiyama H, Ikeda K, Nonaka T, Mori H, Mann D, Tsuchiya K, Yoshida M, Hashizume Y, Oda T (2006) Tdp-43 is a component of ubiquitin-positive tau-negative inclusions in frontotemporal lobar degeneration and amyotrophic lateral sclerosis. Biochem Biophys Res Commun 351(3):602–611

Awano T, Johnson GS, Wade CM, Katz ML, Johnson GC, Taylor JF, Perloski M, Biagi T, Baranowska I, Long S, March PA, Olby NJ, Shelton GD, Khan S, O'Brien DP, Lindblad-Toh K, Coates JR (2009) Genome-wide association analysis reveals a sod1 mutation in canine degenerative myelopathy that resembles amyotrophic lateral sclerosis. Proc Natl Acad Sci USA 106(8):2794–2799

Barker RA, Kuan WL (2010) Graft-induced dyskinesias in parkinson's disease: What is it all about? Cell Stem Cell 7(2):148–149

Bock C, Kiskinis E, Verstappen G, Gu H, Boulting G, Smith ZD, Ziller M, Croft GF, Amoroso MW, Oakley DH, Gnirke A, Eggan K, Meissner A (2011) Reference maps of human es and ips cell variation enable high-throughput characterization of pluripotent cell lines. Cell 144(3):439–452

Carlsson T, Winkler C, Lundblad M, Cenci MA, Bjorklund A, Kirik D (2006) Graft placement and uneven pattern of reinnervation in the striatum is important for development of graft-induced dyskinesia. Neurobiol Dis 21(3):657–668

Deshpande DM, Kim YS, Martinez T, Carmen J, Dike S, Shats I, Rubin LL, Drummond J, Krishnan C, Hoke A, Maragakis N, Shefner J, Rothstein JD, Kerr D A (2006) Recovery from paralysis in adult rats using embryonic stem cells. Ann Neurol 60(1):32–44

Ebert AD, Yu J, Rose FF Jr, Mattis VB, Lorson CL, Thomson JA, Svendsen CN (2009) Induced pluripotent stem cells from a spinal muscular atrophy patient. Nature 457(7227):277–280

Gao J, Coggeshall RE, Tarasenko YI, Wu P (2005) Human neural stem cell-derived cholinergic neurons innervate muscle in motoneuron deficient adult rats. Neuroscience 131(2):257–262

Gurney ME, Pu H, Chiu AY, Dal Canto MC, Polchow CY, Alexander DD, Caliendo J, Hentati A, Kwon YW, Deng HX, et al (1994) Motor neuron degeneration in mice that express a human Cu,Zn superoxide dismutase mutation. Science 264(5166):1772–1775

Hyun I, Lindvall O, Ahrlund-Richter L, Cattaneo E, Cavazzana-Calvo M, Cossu G, De Luca M, Fox IJ, Gerstle C, Goldstein RA, Hermeren G, High KA, Kim HO, Lee HP, Levy-Lahad E, Li L, Lo B, Marshak DR, McNab A, Munsie M, Nakauchi H, Rao M, Rooke HM, Valles CS, Srivastava A, Sugarman J, Taylor PL, Veiga A, Wong AL, Zoloth L, Daley GQ (2008) New isscr guidelines underscore major principles for responsible translational stem cell research. Cell Stem Cell 3(6):607–609

Karussis D, Karageorgiou C, Vaknin-Dembinsky A, Gowda-Kurkalli B, Gomori JM, Kassis I, Bulte JW, Petrou P, Ben-Hur T, Abramsky O, Slavin S (2010) Safety and immunological effects of mesenchymal stem cell transplantation in patients with multiple sclerosis and amyotrophic lateral sclerosis. Arch Neurol 67(10):1187–1194

Kordower JH, Chu Y, Hauser RA, Freeman TB, Olanow CW (2008) Lewy body-like pathology in long-term embryonic nigral transplants in parkinson's disease. Nat Med 14(5):504–506

Lee G, Papapetrou EP, Kim H, Chambers SM, Tomishima MJ, Fasano CA, Ganat YM, Menon J, Shimizu F, Viale A, Tabar V, Sadelain M, Studer L (2009) Modelling pathogenesis and treatment of familial dysautonomia using patient-specific ipscs. Nature 461(7262):402–406

Lepore AC, Rauck B, Dejea C, Pardo AC, Rao MS, Rothstein JD, Maragakis NJ (2008) Focal transplantation-based astrocyte replacement is neuroprotective in a model of motor neuron disease. Nat Neurosci 11(11):1294–1301

Li XJ, Hu BY, Jones SA, Zhang YS, Lavaute T, Du ZW, Zhang SC (2008) Directed differentiation of ventral spinal progenitors and motor neurons from human embryonic stem cells by small molecules. Stem Cells 26(4):886–893

Liscic RM, Grinberg LT, Zidar J, Gitcho MA, Cairns NJ (2008) Als and ftld: Two faces of tdp-43 proteinopathy. Eur J Neurol 15(8):772–780

Miura K, Okada Y, Aoi T, Okada A, Takahashi K, Okita K, Nakagawa M, Koyanagi M, Tanabe K, Ohnuki M, Ogawa D, Ikeda E, Okano H, Yamanaka S (2009) Variation in the safety of induced pluripotent stem cell lines. Nat Biotechnol 27(8):743–745

Morita E, Watanabe Y, Ishimoto M, Nakano T, Kitayama M, Yasui K, Fukada Y, Doi K, Karunaratne A, Murrell WG, Sutharsan R, Mackay-Sim A, Hata Y, Nakashima K (2008) A novel cell transplantation protocol and its application to an als mouse model. Exp Neurol 213(2):431–438

Nakagawa M, Takizawa N, Narita M, Ichisaka T, Yamanaka S (2010) Promotion of direct reprogramming by transformation-deficient myc. Proc Natl Acad Sci USA 107(32):14152–14157

Nakatsuji N, Nakajima F, Tokunaga K (2008) Hla-haplotype banking and ips cells. Nat Biotechnol 26(7):739–740

Neumann M, Sampathu DM, Kwong LK, Truax AC, Micsenyi MC, Chou TT, Bruce J, Schuck T, Grossman M, Clark CM, McCluskey LF, Miller BL, Masliah E, Mackenzie IR, Feldman H, Feiden W, Kretzschmar HA, Trojanowski JQ, Lee VM (2006) Ubiquitinated tdp-43 in frontotemporal lobar degeneration and amyotrophic lateral sclerosis. Science 314(5796):130–133

Papadeas ST, Maragakis NJ (2009) Advances in stem cell research for amyotrophic lateral sclerosis. Curr Opin Biotechnol 20(5):545–551

Sharp J, Frame J, Siegenthaler M, Nistor G, Keirstead HS (2010) Human embryonic stem cell-derived oligodendrocyte progenitor cell transplants improve recovery after cervical spinal cord injury. Stem Cells 28(1):152–163

Strauss S (2010) Geron trial resumes, but standards for stem cell trials remain elusive. Nat Biotechnol 28(10):989–990

Takahashi K, Tanabe K, Ohnuki M, Narita M, Ichisaka T, Tomoda K, Yamanaka S (2007) Induction of pluripotent stem cells from adult human fibroblasts by defined factors. Cell 131(5):861–872

Takahashi Y, Tsuji O, Kumagai G, Hara CM, Okano HJ, Miyawaki A, Toyama Y, Okano H, Nakamura M (2010) Comparative study of methods for administering neural stem/progenitor cells to treat spinal cord injury in mice. Cell Transplant 20(13):727–739

Thomson JA, Itskovitz-Eldor J, Shapiro SS, Waknitz MA, Swiergiel JJ, Marshall VS, Jones JM (1998) Embryonic stem cell lines derived from human blastocysts. Science 282(5391):1145–1147

Thonhoff JR, Ojeda L, Wu P (2009) Stem cell-derived motor neurons: Applications and challenges in amyotrophic lateral sclerosis. Curr Stem Cell Res Ther 4(3):178–199

Zhu D, Deng X, Spee C, Sonoda S, Hsieh CL, Barron E, Pera M, Hinton DR (2010) Polarized secretion of PEDF from human embryonic stem cell-derived RPE promotes retinal progenitor cell survival. Invest Ophthalmol Vis Sci 52(3):1573–1585

Chapter 26

Treatment of Graft-Versus-Host Disease Using Allogeneic Mesenchymal Stem Cells

Sun U. Song

Abstract Mesenchymal stem cells (MSCs) have attracted significant attention recently because of their immunomodulatory function. Due to their immunosuppressive role, MSCs have been suggested as a novel medical therapeutic option to treat graft-versus-host disease (GVHD) and autoimmune diseases. Severe GVHD is a lethal complication of allogeneic hematopoietic stem cell transplantation (HSCT). However, there have been only a few limited therapeutic options for the treatment of GVHD. Since the initial studies and use of MSCs, density-gradient centrifugation-based isolation has been the primary conventional protocol for the isolation of clinical trial grade nonclonal MSCs in the treatment of severe GVHD and other diseases. Recently, clonal MSCs isolated by the subfractionation culturing method (SCM) have been also used in a clinical setting to treat severe GVHD. Although there are concerns about the immunogenicity of allogeneic MSCs, all the clinical trials using allogeneic nonclonal and clonal MSCs performed in the last decade have shown that no significant adverse effects or ectopic transformation were involved with allogeneic MSCs. This suggests that allogeneic MSCs can be a promising therapeutic option for the treatment of steroid- refractory acute GVHD. However, further investigations are needed to understand the exact mechanisms of the functions of MSCs and larger, well-designed human clinical trials are necessary to confirm the long-term safety and efficacy of MSCs for the treatment of GVHD and other autoimmune diseases.

Keywords Mesenchymal stem cells · Graft-versus-host disease · Hematopoietic stem cell transplantation · Multipotent stromal/stem cells · Fluorescence-activated cell sorting · Human clonal MSC

Introduction

Mesenchymal stem cells (MSCs) were first isolated from bone marrow by Friedenstein et al. in the 1960s, and while they are most prevalent in the bone marrow compartment, they are now known to be present in a variety of tissues, including adipose tissue, umbilical cord blood, and muscle (Friedenstein et al., 1968). MSCs can be readily obtained from humans and animals, purified by means of their ability to adhere to culture plates, and be expanded for many generations in culture. The culture-expanded adult MSCs appear to have multi-differentiation potential, including at least chondrogenic, osteogenic, and adipogenic differentiation under appropriate induction conditions (Pittenger et al., 1999; Phinney et al., 1999; Schwarz et al., 1999). Recently, additional differentiation potential areas, such as neurogenic, cardiogenic, myogenic, and hepatogenic differentiation have been reported (Woodbury et al., 2000; Wakitani et al., 1995; Kopen et al., 1999; Toma et al., 2002; Liechty et al., 2000; Petersen et al., 1999). Therefore, these cells are now also called multipotent stromal/stem cells (MSCs) since they are capable of differentiating to mesodermal, ectodermal and/or endodermal origin cells.

S.U. Song (✉)
Clinical Research Center, Inha University School of Medicine, Incheon, Korea 400-711
e-mail: sunuksong@inha.ac.kr

Several protocols have been developed for isolating and expanding MSCs in culture. These methods are based on density-gradient centrifugation (Rickard et al., 1996), fluorescence-activated cell sorting (FACS) (Zohar et al., 1997), specific cell-surface antibodies (Joyner et al., 1997; Waller et al., 1995), selective adhesion to laminin-coated plates (Reyes and Verfaillie, 2001), and size-sieved culture (Hung et al., 2002). Further, clonally expanded MSCs were isolated and used for the generation of myocardium (Yoon et al., 2005) and the treatment of GVHD patients (Lim et al., 2010). Despite recent extensive experimental and clinical interest, the number of stem and progenitor cell types existing in bone marrow is not known. Until recently, most preclinical and clinical studies have used a mixed (nonclonal) population of mononuclear cells. Furthermore, the benefit of using mixed populations of MSCs versus clonally expanded cells from bone marrow for clinical trials has yet to be adequately investigated.

The multilineage differentiation potential of MSCs has been under intense investigation in recent years, due to reported transplantation success in treating animal disorders and early phase human clinical trials (Lazarus et al., 1995; Koc et al., 2002; Horwitz et al., 2002; Le Blanc et al., 2004, 2006; Tse et al., 2003; Shi et al., 2005). The capacity for large-scale expansion of MSCs has facilitated the development of clinical trials aimed at assessing the safety and efficacy of MSC transplantation for a variety of pathological conditions. While the initial results are encouraging, little is known about the effect of ex vivo amplification on the growth, multi-potentiality, and homogeneity of MSCs used in clinical trials. In this chapter, isolation and production methods for clinical-grade MSCs and clinical experience in GVHD treatment using nonclonal or clonal allogeneic MSCs will be described. In addition, immunogenicity of allogeneic MSCs and effects of immunosuppressive drugs on MSC function will be briefly mentioned.

Isolation and Production Methods for Clinical-Grade Mesenchymal Stem Cells

The most popular conventional isolation method of MSCs relies on the fractionation of mononuclear cells from various tissues with or without protease treatment by gradient centrifugation and selection of fibroblast-like cells adhering to the culture plate surface by removing nonadherent floating cells (Fig. 26.1). Experimental and clinical data over the last decade have indicated that cultured adherent MSCs are heterogeneous and vary in terms of their differentiation potentials and clinical outcomes (Uccelli et al., 2008; Rosenzweig, 2006).

In order to obtain MSC populations that are more homogeneous and pure, FACS-based isolation (Zohar et al., 1997; Waller et al., 1995) and specific cell-surface antibody selection (Joyner et al., 1997) have been applied. However, although significant improvements have been made in purification techniques, these isolation methods have not yet been sufficient to isolate completely homogeneous populations of MSCs. The limiting dilution method has been the only option to generate single-cell-derived clonal MSC lines. Since the usual source for the limiting dilution method is a mononuclear cell fraction produced by gradient centrifugation or a culture-expanded population of MSCs, the possibility of losing some "real" MSCs during the isolation of mononuclear cells and culture expansion of the cells remains.

Recently, we developed a new protocol, called the subfractionation culturing method (SCM), to generate single-cell-derived clonal MSC lines from whole bone marrow aspirate without employing any centrifugation step for mononuclear cells and enzyme treatment process (Fig. 26.2). Using this method, we identified human bone marrow- and single-cell derived colony-forming fibroblastic cells as MSCs from relatively small amounts of bone marrow aspirates. This method allowed us to rapidly establish single cell-derived human clonal MSC (hcMSC) lines from raw bone marrow aspirates and to establish a library of these hcMSC lines (Song et al., 2008). The rationale behind the SCM is that different types of mesenchymal stem or stromal cells can be isolated based on their cell densities and/or adherence to a plastic culture plate after a series of transfers of the culture supernatant to subsequent dishes; thus, these low-density stem or stromal cells may have a higher proliferation and differentiation potential.

The advantages of the SCM are as follows. First, this method does not require any centrifugation step at all throughout the procedure. Second, it does not require any enzymatic process or filtering procedure. Third, it can generate single-cell-derived homogeneous

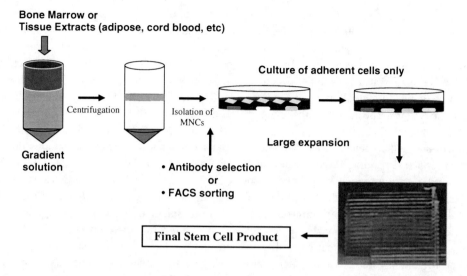

Fig. 26.1 Flow diagram of the conventional gradient centrifugation method used to isolate nonclonal MSCs, and the production of the final stem cell product for clinical trial. Briefly, bone marrow aspirates are loaded onto gradient solution and centrifuged to obtain a layer of mononuclear cells (MNCs). MNCs are plated in cell culture flasks, and then nonadherent cells are removed. Subsequently, only adherent cells are large-expanded to prepare the final MCSs for use in clinical trials

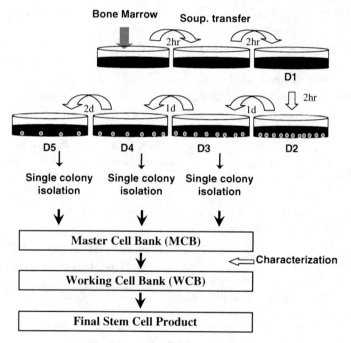

Fig. 26.2 Flow diagram of the "subfractionation culturing method" used to isolate clonal MSCs and to produce the final stem cell product for clinical trials. Briefly, 1 mL of human bone marrow aspirate is mixed with 15 mL of DMEM or α-MEM and then plated onto a 100 mm cell culture dish. After a 2-h incubation, only the supernatant is transferred to a new dish. This procedure is repeated once more and the supernatant is then transferred to subsequent cell culture dishes at 1- or 2-day intervals as shown. Each dish or plate is then incubated until single cell-derived colonies appear. When the cell colonies are sufficiently large, they are transferred to a 6-well plate and then expanded in larger flasks. At passage 5 and 9, a master cell bank (MCB) and a working cell bank (WCB) are established. Then final stem cell product is generated out of 1 or 2 frozen vials in WCB. The cells frozen in MCB are thawed and then characterized to determine they have MSC characteristics in terms of cell surface phenotypes, differentiation potential, and in vitro immunomodulatory function

clonal MSC populations. Fourth, the protocol works well for bone marrow samples from different species, including human, mouse, rat, and rabbit. These advantages suggest that the SCM can generate a homogeneous clonal population of MSCs in a simple, effective, and economical way, which may allow safer applications in therapeutic settings. The rapid establishment of clonal MSC lines and variations of the lines in phenotype, differentiation potential, gene expression, and T-cell suppression capacity encouraged us to establish a clonal MSC library of various clonal MSC lines. Such a library will be very useful for both the basic study of bone marrow-derived stem cells and for clinical studies of specific target disease treatment. For example, a clonal MSC line that exhibits a great capability to inhibit T-cell proliferation would be an excellent candidate stem cell source for the development of a stem cell product to treat GVHD. One potential concern of using clonal MSCs is their tumorigenic potential. Thus, we have tested the transformation potential of 12 hcMSC lines by in vitro-transformation assay, using the human HeLa tumor cell line as a positive control and the mouse NIH3T3 cell line as a negative control. The results showed that our hcMSC lines produced a smaller number of colonies than did the NIH3T3 negative control cells, suggesting that the hcMSC lines are not tumorigenic.

Graft-Versus-Host Disease

Graft-versus-host disease (GVHD) is a major life-threatening complication of allogeneic hematopoietic stem cell transplantation (HSCT), in which functional immune cells such as T cells in the transplanted bone marrow recognize the transplant recipient as "foreign" and attack the tissues of the recipient. T cells produce excess of cytokines, including interferon-gamma (IFN-γ) and tumor necrosis factor alpha (TNF-α). A wide range of the recipient's antigens can initiate GVHD, including human leukocyte antigens (HLAs). However, GVHD can occur even when HLA-identical siblings are the donors. There have been only a few therapeutic options for GVHD. Its incidence varies from 20 to 70%, depending on the chemotherapeutic agent used in the conditioning regimen, the intensity of the regimen, the extent of HLA match, age of the patient, and stage or status of the primary disease (Bacigalupo, 2007). At present, GVHD response rates to steroids are not consistent, and patients who do not respond to steroid therapy have a poor prognosis. Progressive steroid-refractory acute GVHD is generally considered as fatal disease (Ball et al., 2008).

GVHD is classified into acute and chronic forms. The acute form of the disease is commonly observed within the first 100 days after transplant, and it is a major challenge to transplant patients due to associated morbidity and mortality (Goker et al., 2001). The chronic form of GVHD normally occurs 100 days after transplant, although the significance of the 100th day after transplant is becoming negligible. The appearance of moderate-to-severe cases of chronic GVHD adversely affects long-term survival (Lee et al., 2003). The potential target tissues include the liver, skin, gastrointestinal tract, and lungs, among others. Regarding the treatment of GVHD, immunosuppressive drugs, such as cyclosporin, cyclophosphamide, tacrolimus, methotrexate, and mycophenolate mofetil, are the first therapeutic options commonly used. If such immunosuppressive drugs are not effective, corticosteroids, such as prednisone, are used for the standard treatment in both acute and chronic GVHD.

MSCs or multipotent mesenchymal stromal cells as defined in the International Society for Cellular Therapy (Dominici et al., 2006) are investigated and clinically used in a number of immune-mediated or inflammatory diseases such as acute GVHD. The outcomes of the recent human clinical trials of GVHD patients with autologous or allogeneic MSCs suggest that MSCs can be used as a highly effective therapeutic modality to treat GVHD.

Clinical Experiences in GVHD Treatment Using Nonclonal or Clonal Allogeneic Mesenchymal Stem Cells

Until now, MSCs used in the clinical trials were obtained mainly from bone marrow tissues of donors who were HLA-identical, haploidentical, or unrelated HLA-mismatched. Currently, a clinical trial registered in the US National Institute of Health website on clinical trials (http://clinicaltrials.gov) is using MSCs derived from either umbilical cord blood or adipose tissue (Table 26.1). As is evident from Table 26.1, acute GVHD has been the main target of allogeneic MSC therapy, since it is usually steroid-refractory, yet there

26 Treatment of Graft-Versus-Host Disease Using Allogeneic Mesenchymal Stem Cells

Table 26.1 Clinical experiences of treating GVHD with allogeneic MSCs

Disease	Patient Number	Phase Status	Outcome or Primary Outcome Measure	MSC Source, Type and Number	Start Date	Sponsor
Acute GVHD	55	Phase II Completed	30 with complete response and 9 with improvement	BM, Nonclonal, 0.4–9×10^6/kg	Oct. 2001	European group for blood and marrow transplantation (Europe)
Acute GVHD	33	Phase II Completed	77% of the patients responded Overall response (response by Day 28)	BM, Nonclonal, 2×10^6 or 2×10^8/kg	Feb. 2005	Osiris Therapeutics (USA)
Acute GVHD	30	Phase II Completed	Overall response (response by Day 28)	BM, Nonclonal	Nov. 2005	Osiris Therapeutics (USA)
Acute GVHD	240	Phase III Completed	Complete response of greater than or equql to 28 days duration	BM, Nonclonal, 2×10^6/kg	Jul. 2006	Osiris Therapeutics (USA)
Acute GVHD	30	Phase II Recruiting	Day-100 incidence of non-relapse mortality	BM, Nonclonal	Dec. 2006	University Hospital of Liege (Belgium)
Acute GVHD	15	Phase I/II Recruiting	Safety and efficacy after MSC infusion	BM, Nonclonal, 1–2×10^6/kg	Jan. 2007	University of Salamanca (Spain)
Acute GVHD	25	Phase I/II Recruiting	Control of GVHD	BM, Nonclonal, 1–2×10^6/kg	Jun. 2007	Christian Medical College (India)
Acute GVHD	100	Phase II Recruiting	Efficacy of MSC infusion	BM, Nonclonal, 2 or 4×10^6/kg	Jan. 2008	University Hospital of Liege (Belgium)
Acute GVHD	10	Phase I/II Recruiting	Day of neutrophil and platelet engraftment	UCB, Nonclonal, 1 or 2×10^6/kg	Aug. 2008	Medipost Co. Ltd (Korea)
Acute GVHD	10	Phase I/II Recruiting	Safety, toxicity, and feasibility of MSC infusion	Not available	Jan. 2009	UMC Utrecht (Netherlands)

Table 26.1 (continued)

Disease	Patient Number	Phase Status	Outcome or Primary Outcome Measure	MSC Source, Type and Number	Start Date	Sponsor
Acute GVHD	20	Phase I/II Recruiting	GVHD re-staging and/or GVHD mortality	BM, Nonclonal, $1-2 \times 10^6$/kg	Sep. 2009	Hadassah Medical Organization (Israel)
Acute GVHD	52	Phase II Recruiting	The total response rate	BM, Nonclonal, 2×10^6/kg	Sep. 2009	Guangdong General Hospital (China)
Acute GVHD	120	Phase II Recruiting	Comparison of 1-year overall survival in the 2 arms	BM, Nonclonal, $1.5-3.0 \times 10^6$/kg	Feb. 2010	University Hospital of Liege (Belgium)
Acute GVHD	30	Phase I/II Recruiting	Incidence of TE-SAE	BM, Nonclonal, 2×10^6/kg	Mar. 2010	National Heart, Lung, and Blood Institute (NHLBI) (USA)
Acute GVHD	30	Phase I/II Recruiting	Number of adverse events	AT, Nonclonal, 1 or 3×10^6/kg	Oct. 2010	Fundacion Progresoy Salud (Spain)
Acute or Chronic GVHD	10	Phase I Recruiting	Safety of clonal MSC infusion	BM, Clonal, 1×10^6/kg	Oct. 2010	HomeoTherapy Co. Ltd (Korea)

BM, bone marrow; UCB, umbilical cord blood; AT, adipose tissue; GVHD, graft-versus-host disease is no other treatment option available for such patients after steroid therapy failure.

Le Blanc et al. (2004) reported the first successful treatment of a severe steroid-refractory acute GVHD patient using ex vivo-expanded haploidentical human MSCs. The grade IV GVHD patient showed a complete response after 2 infusions of MSCs (2×10^6/kg). In a subsequent clinical trial report, Le Blanc and her co-workers demonstrated a complete response in 6 of 8 acute GVHD patients with allogeneic MSCs. A complete resolution was seen in the intestine (6 cases), liver (1 case), and skin (1 case) with no significant adverse events attributed to the cells (Le Blanc et al., 2006). These clinical results support the concept that allogeneic MSCs can be tolerated without the need for donor-recipient HLA-matching and encouraged other investigators to use allogeneic MSCs in clinical settings. These investigators later published phase II clinical trial data from 55 steroid-resistant, severe, acute GVHD patients. The average number of MSCs was 1.4×10^6 cells per kg of bodyweight, with a single dose of MSCs given to 27 patients, 2 doses to 22 patients, and 3–5 doses to 6 patients. In this study, MSCs from haploidentical donors were infused in 18 cases and third-party HLA-mismatched donors in 69 cases. Strikingly, 30 patients had a complete response and 9 showed improvement. No patients had adverse effects during or immediately after infusions of MSCs. Kebriaei et al. (2009) reported the results of another phase II clinical trial using allogeneic MSCs for the treatment of acute GVHD patients. Of the 31 patients treated, 94% of them showed initial response to MSCs, consisting of 77% with a complete response and 17% with a partial response. No infusion-related toxicities or ectopic tissue formations were observed. Two doses of allogeneic MSCs, 2×10^6 or 8×10^6 cells/kg, were tested and no significant differences were noted between the low and high doses with respect to safety or efficacy.

The recent outcomes out of larger-scale phase III human clinical trials of 192 acute GVHD patients or 260 steroid-resistant GVHD patients showed mixed results (Mills, 2009). In the study with the 192 acute GVHD patients, overall, no significant differences were found between the allogeneic MSC-treated group and the placebo control group. However, the study with the 260 steroid-resistant GVHD patients showed significant improvements in patients with gastrointestinal and liver GVHD, indicating that certain tissues affected by GVHD may be more susceptible to MSC therapy.

Allogeneic MSCs being used in current human clinical trials are nonclonal, i.e., such MSC populations may contain other types of cells in the final stem cell product. Some concerns exist about the heterogeneity of these nonclonal MSCs that are isolated and expanded by the conventional density-gradient centrifugation method. To overcome such concerns, Lim et al. (2010) have recently used single cell-derived clonal allogeneic MSCs— isolated by the SCM method as shown in Fig. 26.2—that were expanded ex vivo and tested in vivo to treat acute GVHD. After Lim et al. treated the steroid-refractory acute GVHD patients with such clonal allogeneic MSCs, they observed marked improvement of the disease in 2 GVHD patients. Derivation of clonal MSCs through SCM represents a new potential therapeutic option for the treatment of steroid-refractory acute GVHD. Phase I clinical trials using such clonal MSCs are underway for testing the safety of the cells. Next, the interesting future clinical studies would be ones in which the clonal MSCs are compared to nonclonal MSCs in a clinical setting.

The number of MSCs used in current clinical trials varies from 1×10^6 to 2×10^8 cells per patient body weight (kg), and the number of infusions varies from 1 infusion to 6 infusions. This indicates that further studies need to be performed to optimize both the MSC dose and the frequency of administration to GVHD patients. Thus far, treatment with allogeneic MSCs leads to significant improvements in patients with gastrointestinal and liver GVHD.

MSCs with an allogeneic origin might offer a number of significant advantages in a therapeutic setting. First, MSCs can be produced and frozen in bulk, providing a more economical and potentially uniform source of therapeutic cells. Second, the use of allogeneic MSCs enables cells to be available on demand, so that stem cell treatment does not have to be delayed due to culturing and characterizing the cells. Third-party human MSCs were shown to be safe and to improve clinical symptoms of acute GVHD patients. In the future, research will need to focus on elucidating the mechanisms of MSCs. In additional, larger, well-designed human clinical trials will be necessary to underscore the safety and efficacy of cMSCs in GVHD treatment.

Immunogenicity of Allogeneic Mesenchymal Stem Cells

Data from animal studies with allogeneic and xenogeneic MSCs and clinical studies with allogeneic MSCs for treating GVHD and other diseases suggest that MSCs are relatively immune privileged. However, more recent findings suggest that non-self MSCs are immunogenic: under certain conditions, the upregulation of both MHC class I and class II on MSCs has been observed (Chan et al., 2008). A few reports provide evidence that both human and mouse MSCs have the capacity to present antigens and, subsequently, to induce effector T cell responses in vitro (Stagg et al., 2006; Francois et al., 2009; Romieu-Mourez et al., 2009) and memory T cell responses in vivo (Nauta et al., 2006a, b). Nevertheless, preclinical animal models and human clinical trials using both syngeneic and allogeneic MSCs have demonstrated no adverse events associated with allogeneic MSCs (Le Blanc et al., 2008; Chen et al., 2009). In addition, data from a mouse model examining the efficacy of allogeneic MSCs in wound repair indicate that allogeneic MSCs do not evoke an immune response unlike allogeneic fibroblasts (Chen et al., 2009).

Data from the phase II clinical study of Le Blanc et al. (2008) utilizing MSCs for the treatment of acute, steroid-resistant GVHD also indicates that the administration of allogeneic MSCs does not appear to trigger an immune response. In this study, patients were infused with MSCs from HLA-identical, haploidentical, or third-party donors. Out of a total of 55 patients, 30 exhibited a "complete response" following 1 dose of MSCs; of this group, 2 patients received HLA-identical MSCs, 3 haploidentical and 24, from third-party donors (Le Blanc et al., 2008). This finding suggests that the administration of allogeneic MSCs does not induce significant immune reaction nor does it have an impact on the therapeutic outcome, at least for GVHD treatment. Therefore, it is unlikely that allogeneic MSCs will induce immune responses in vivo.

Effects of Immunosuppressive Drugs on Mesenchymal Stem Cell Function

Since all GVHD patients already received or are receiving immunosuppressive drugs at the time MSCs are administered, it would be beneficial to fully understand the extent to which these drugs may impact MSC function. A number of in vivo studies have examined the use of MSCs in combination with conventional immunosuppressive drugs. MSCs synergized the inhibition of peripheral blood mononuclear cell (PBMC) proliferation by mycophenolic acid (MPA) (Hoogduijn et al., 2008). In rat and swine models, the administration of cyclosporine A (CsA) with MSCs elongated composite skin and tissue graft (Sbano et al., 2008; Kuo et al., 2009). This complementation between MSCs and immunosuppressive drugs with regard to the suppression of T cell proliferation could be due to distinct mechanisms of action of MSCs and immunosuppressive drugs. Whether immunosuppressive drugs are required initially to create an environment in which MSCs can properly achieve their immunomodulatory action remains to be studied.

In a number of animal studies, MSCs have been injected without immunosuppressive drugs. For example, pancreatic islets transplanted to an immunocompromised mouse were not rejected when accompanied by MSCs (Ding et al., 2009). Infusion of MSCs alone delayed graft rejection in an immunocompetent allogeneic heart transplantation model (Casiraghi et al., 2008). In contrast, MSC administration alone was found to accelerate graft rejection in an animal model (Sbano et al., 2008). This result emphasizes that it is necessary to have a better understanding of the environments in which MSCs behave positively, and those in which they behave negatively. The data from animal studies and clinical experience with MSCs suggest that the effects of immunosuppressive drugs on MSC functions need to be determined after long-term observation of treated patients.

Conclusions

MSCs are a highly promising therapeutic modality to treat steroid-refractory severe GVHD. Recent clinical trial results showed a large percentage of complete response in acute GVHD patients with liver and gastrointestinal tract GVHD symptoms. Standardized isolation and production protocols for clinical-grade MSCs need to be established. The advantages and disadvantages of nonclonal and clonal MSCs also need to be further investigated. In addition, the comparative clinical efficacy of frozen versus fresh MSC product should be further studied in both animal models and human clinical trials. For acute GVHD patients, the use of a frozen allogeneic MSC source is more adequate due to the requirement of a rapid administration. However, it is not clear whether the efficacy of allogeneic MSCs improves when these are fresh. At any rate, the immunomodulatory property of MSCs will be greatly utilized to treat immune and inflammatory diseases in the future. The human clinical trials in the last decade suggest that MSC-based stem cell therapy is a very promising treatment for severe steroid-resistant acute GVHD.

References

Bacigalupo A (2007) Management of acute graft-versus-host disease. Br J Haematol 137:87–98

Ball L, Bredius R, Lankester A, Schweizer J, van den Heuvel-Eibrink M, Escher H, Fibbe W, Egeler M (2008) Third party mesenchymal stromal cell infusions fail to induce tissue repair despite successful control of severe grade IV acute graft-versus-host disease in a child with juvenile myelomonocytic leukemia. Leukemia 22:1256–1257

Casiraghi F, Azzollini N, Cassis P, Imberti B, Morigi M, Cugini D, Cavinato RA, Todeschini M, Solini S, Sonzogni A, Perico N, Remuzzi G, Noris M (2008) Pretransplant infusion of mesenchymal stem cells prolongs the survival of a semiallogeneic heart transplant through the generation of regulatory T cells. J Immunol 181:3933–3946

Chan WK, Lau ASY, Li JCB, Law HKW, Lau YL, Chan GCF (2008) MHC expression kinetics and immunogenicity of mesenchymal stromal cells after short-term IFN-gamma challenge. Exp Hematol 36:1545–1555

Chen L, Tredget EE, Liu C, Wu Y (2009) Analysis of allogenicity of mesenchymal stem cells in engraftment and wound healing in mice. PLoS One 4:e7119

Ding YC, Xu DM, Feng G, Bushell A, Muschei RJ, Wood KJ (2009) Mesenchymal stem cells prevent the rejection of fully allogenic islet grafts by the immunosuppressive activity of matrix metalloproteinase-2 and -9. Diabetes 58:1797–1806

Dominici M, Le Blanc K, Mueller I, Slaper-Cortenbach I, Marini F, Krause D, Deans R, Keating A, Prockop DJ, Horwitz E (2006) Minimal criteria for defining multipotent mesenchymal stromal cells. The International Society for Cellular Therapy position statement. Cytotherapy 8:315–317

Francois M, Romieu-Mourez R, Stock-Martineau S, Boivin MN, Bramson JL, Gailpeau J (2009) Mesenchymal stromal cells cross-present soluble exogenous antigens as part of their antigen-presenting cell properties. Blood 114:2632–2638

Friedenstein AJ, Petrakova KV, Kurolesova AI, Frolova GP (1968) Heterotopic of bone marrow. Analysis of precursor cells for osteogenic and hematopoietic tissues. Transplantation 6(2):230–247

Goker H, Haznedaroglu IC, Chao NJ (2001) Acute graft-vs-host disease: pathobiology and management. Exp Hematol 29(3):259–277

Hoogduijn MJ, Crop MJ, Korevaar SS, Peeters AMA, Eijken M, Maat LPWM, Balk AHMM, Weimar W, Baan CC (2008) Susceptibility of human mesenchymal stem cells to tacrolimus, mycophenolic acid, and rapamycin. Transplantation 86:1283–1291

Horwitz EM, Gordon PL, Koo WK, Marx JC, Neel MD, McNall RY, Muul L, Hofmann T (2002) Isolated allogeneic bone marrow-derived mesenchymal cells engraft and stimulate growth in children with osteogenesis imperfecta: implications for cell therapy of bone. Proc Natl Acad Sci USA 99:8932–8937

Hung SC, Chen NJ, Hsieh SL, Li H, Ma HL, Lo WH (2002) Isolation and characterization of size-sieved stem cells from human bone marrow. Stem Cells 20:249–258

Joyner CJ, Bennett A, Triffitt JT (1997) Identification and enrichment of human osteoprogenitor cells by using differentiation stage-specific mAbs. Bone 21:1–6

Kebriaei P, Islla L, Bahceci E, Holland K, Rowley S, McGuirk J, Devetten M, Jansen J, Herzig R, Schuster M, Monroy R, Uberti J (2009) Adult human mesenchymal stem cells added to corticosteroid therapy for the treatment of acute graft-versus-host disease. Biol Blood Marrow Transplant 15:804–811

Koc ON, Day J, Nieder M, Gerson SL, Lazarus HM, Krivit W (2002) Allogeneic mesenchymal stem cell infusion for treatment of metachromatic leukodystrophy (MLD) and Hurler syndrome (MPS-IH). Bone Marrow Transplant 30:215–222

Kopen GC, Prockop DJ, Phinney DG (1999) Marrow stromal cells migrate throughout forebrain and cerebellum, and they differentiate into astrocytes after injection into neonatal mouse brains. Proc Natl Acad Sci USA 96(19):10711–10716

Kuo YR, Goto S, Shih HS, Wang FS, Lin CC, Wang CT, Huang EY, Chen CL, Wei FC, Zheng XX, Lee WP (2009) Mesenchymal stem cells prolong composite tissue allotransplant survival in a swine model. Transplantation 87:1769–1777

Lazarus HM, Haynesworth SE, Gerson SL, Rosenthal NS, Caplan AI (1995) Ex vivo expansion and subsequent infusion of human bone marrow-derived stromal progenitor cells (mesenchymal progenitor cells): implications for therapeutic use. Bone Marrow Transplant 16:557–564

Le Blanc K, Rasmusson I, Sundberg B, Gotherstrom C, Hassan M, Uzunel M, Ringden O (2004) Treatment of severe acute graft-versus-host disease with third party haploidentical mesenchymal stem cells. Lancet 363:1439–1441

Le Blanc K, Frassoni F, Ball L, Locatelli F, Roelofs H, Lewis I, Lanina El, Sundberg B, Bernardo ME, Remberger M, Dini G, Egeler RM, Bacigalupo A, Fibbe W, Ringden O (2008) Mesenchymal stem cells for treatment of steroid-resistant, severe, acute graft-versus-host disease: a phase II study. Lancet 371:1579–1586

Lee SJ, Vogelsang G, Flowers ME (2003) Chronic graft-versus-host disease. Biol Blood Marrow Transplant 9(4):215–233

Liechty KW, MacKenzie TC, Shaaban AF, Radu A, Moseley AM, Deans R, Marshak DR, Flake AW (2000) Human mesenchymal stem cells engraft and demonstrate site-specific differentiation after in utero transplantation in sheep. Nat Med 6:1282–1286

Lim JH, Lee MH, Yi HG, Kim CS, Kim JH, Song SU (2010) Mesenchymal stromal cells for steroid-refractory acute graft-versus-host disease: a report of two cases. Int J Hematol 92:204–207

Mills CR (2009) Osiris therapeutics announces preliminary results for Prochymal phase III GVHD trials. http://investor.osiris.com/releasedetail.dfm?releaseID=407404

Nauta AJ, Kruisselbrink AB, Lurvink E, Willemze R, Fibbe WE (2006a) Mesenchymal stem cells inhibit generation and function of both CD34+-derived and monocyte-derived dendritic cells. J Immunol 177:2080–2087

Nauta AJ, Westerhuis G, Kruisselbrink AB, Lurvink E, Willemze R, Fibbe WE (2006b) Donor-derived mesenchymal stem cells are immunogenic in an allogeneic host and stimulate donor graft rejection in a nonmyeloablative setting. Blood 108:2114–2120

Petersen BE, Bowen WC, Patrene KD, Mars WM, Sullivan AK, Muras N, Boggs SS, Greenberger JS, Goff JP (1999) Bone marrow as a potential source of hepatic oval cells. Science 284:1168–1170

Phinney DG, Kopen G, Isaacson RL, Prockop DJ (1999) Plastic adherent stromal cells from the bone marrow of commonly used strains of inbred mice: variations in yield, growth, and differentiation. J Cell Biochem 72:570–585

Pittenger MF, Mackay AM, Beck SC, Jaiswal RK, Douglas R, Mosca JD, Moorman MA, Simonetti DW, Craig S, Marshak DR (1999) Multilineage potential of adult human mesenchymal stem cells. Science 284:143–147

Reyes M, Verfaillie CM (2001) Characterization of multipotent adult progenitor cells, a subpopulation of mesenchymal stem cells. Ann N Y Acad Sci 938:231–233

Rickard DJ, Kassem M, Hefferan TE, Sarkar G, Spelsberg TC, Riggs BL (1996) Isolation and characterization of osteoblast precursor cells from human bone marrow. J Bone Miner Res 11:312–324

Ringdén O, Uzunel M, Rasmusson I, Remberger M, Sundberg B, Lönnies H, Marschall HU, Dlugosz A, Szakos A, Hassan Z, Omazic B, Aschan J, Barkholt L, Le Blanc K. (2006) Mesenchymal stem cells for treatment of therapy-resistant graft-versus-host disease. Transplantation 81(10):1390–1397

Romieu-Mourez R, Francois M, Boivin MN, Bouchentouf M, Spaner DE, Gailpeau J (2009) Cytokine modulation of TLR expression and activation in mesenchymal stromal cells leads to a proinflammatory phenotype. J Immunol 182:7963–7973

Rosenzweig A (2006) Cardiac cell therapy—Mixed results from mixed cells. N Engl J Med 355(12):1274–1277

Sbano P, Cuccia A, Mazzanti B, Urbani S, Giusti B, Lapini I, Rossi L, Abbate R, Marseglia G, Nannetti G, Torricelli F, Miracco C, Bosi A, Fimiani M (2008) Use of donor bone marrow mesenchymal stem cells for treatment of skin allograft rejection in a preclinical rat model. Arch Dermatol Res 300:115–124

Schwarz EJ, Alexander GM, Prockop DJ, Azizi SA (1999) Multipotential marrow stromal cells transduced to produce L-DOPA: engraftment in a rat model of Parkinson disease. Hum Gene Ther 10:2539–2549

Shi S, Bartold PM, Miura M, Seo BM, Robey PG, Gronthos S (2005) The efficacy of mesenchymal stem cells to regenerate and repair dental structures. Orthod Craniofac Res 8:191–199

Song SU, Kim CS, Yoon SP, Kim SK, Lee MH, Kang JS, Choi GS, Moon SH, Choi MS, Cho YK, Son BK (2008) Variations of clonal marrow stem cell lines established from human bone marrow in surface epitopes, differentiation potential, gene expression, and cytokine secretion. Stem Cells Dev 17(3):451–461

Stagg J, Pommey S, Eliopoulos N, Galipeau J (2006) Interferon-gamma-stimulated marrow stromal cells: a new type of nonhematopoietic antigen-presenting cell. Blood 107:2570–2577

Toma C., Pittenger, M.F, Cahill, K.S., Byrne, B.J., and Kessler, P.D. (2002) Human mesenchymal stem cells differentiate to a cardiomyocyte phenotype in the adult murine heart. Circulation 105:93–98.

Tse, W.T., Pendleton, J.D., Beyer, W.M., Egalka, M.C., and Guinan, E.C. (2003). Suppression of allogeneic T-cell proliferation by human marrow stromal cells: implications in transplantation. Transplantation 75:389–397.

Uccelli A, Moretta L, Pistoia V (2008) Mesenchymal stem cells in health and disease. Nat Rev Immunol 8(9):726–736

Wakitani S, Saito T, Caplan AI (1995). Myogenic cells derived from rat bone marrow mesenchymal stem cells exposed to 5-azacytidine. Muscle Nerve 18:1417–1426

Waller EK, Olweus J, Lund-Johansen F, Huang S, Nguyen M, Guo GR, Terstappen L (1995) The "common stem cell" hypothesis reevaluated: human fetal bone marrow contains separate populations of hematopoietic and stromal progenitors. Blood 85:2422–2435

Woodbury D, Schwarz EJ, Prockop DJ, Black IB (2000) Adult rat and human bone marrow stromal cells differentiate into neurons. J Neurosci Res 61:364–370

Yoon YS, Wecker A, Heyd L, Park JS, Tkebuchava T, Kusano K, Hanley A, Scadova H, Qin G, Cha DH, Johnson KL, Aikawa R, Asahara T, Losordo DW (2005) Clonally expanded novel multipotent stem cells from human bone marrow regenerate myocardium after myocardial infarction. J Clin Invest 115:326–338

Zohar R, Sodek J, McCulloch CA (1997) Characterization of stromal progenitor cells enriched by flow cytometry. Blood 90(9):3471–3481

Chapter 27
Adult Neurogenesis in Etiology and Pathogenesis of Alzheimer's Disease

Philippe Taupin

Abstract The adult brain of mammals has the potential to self-repair and regenerate. Adult neurogenesis is enhanced in the hippocampus and reduced in the subventricular zone (SVZ) of patients with Alzheimer's disease (AD). Enhanced neurogenesis in the hippocampus of AD patients suggests a regenerative attempt to compensate for the neuronal loss, whereas reduced neurogenesis in the SVZ would contribute to pathological processes associated with the disease, such as anosmia. Neurogenesis has the potential to generate aneuploid neuronal cells in the adult brain. Adult neurogenesis and neural stem cells (NSCs) would thus contribute both beneficially and detrimentally to the pathology of AD. Adult neurogenesis and NSCs are as important for our understanding of the development of the nervous system and for therapy, as for our understanding of the etiology and pathogenesis of neurological diseases, particularly AD. The understanding of which will lead to novel treatments and therapies for neurological diseases and injuries.

Keywords Subventricular zone · Alzheimer's disease · Neural stem cells · Amyloid precursor protein · Dentate gyrus · Adult neurogenesis

Introduction

Alzheimer's disease is a neurodegenerative disease and the most common form of senile dementia (Burns et al., 2002). Widespread neurodegeneration, amyloid plaques, neurofibrillary tangles, aneuploidy, learning and memory deficits and impairments, and anosmia are the main landmarks of the disease (Dubois et al., 2007; Fusetti et al., 2010). There are two forms of the disease: the early onset form of AD (EOAD) and the late onset form of AD (LOAD). EOAD is a rare form of the disease. It is diagnosed before age 65 and is primarily an inherited disease. LOAD is the most common form of the disease, accounting for over 93% of all cases of AD. It is diagnosed after age 65 and is primarily a sporadic form of the disease (Querfurth and LaFerla, 2010).

Neurogenesis occurs in the adult brain of mammals, in the hippocampus and SVZ (Taupin and Gage, 2002). Hence, the adult mammalian brain may be amenable to repair. The stimulation of endogenous neural progenitor or stem cells of the adult brain and the transplantation of adult-derived neural progenitor and stem cells are proposed to repair and restore the degenerated or injured nerve pathways. Beside their potential for regeneration and repair, adult NSCs and newly generated neuronal cells of the adult brain may contribute to the development and to physiological and pathological processes of the adult brain (Duan et al., 2008). Adult neurogenesis is enhanced in the hippocampus and reduced in the SVZ of patients with AD suggesting that adult NSCs may be involved in and contribute to the pathology of the disease (Jin et al., 2004a). The understanding of the involvement and contribution of adult NSCs and newly generated neuronal cells of the adult brain to the etiology and pathogenesis of AD may not only lead to a better understanding of the disease, but also to novel treatments and therapies for AD.

P. Taupin (✉)
School of Biotechnology, Dublin City University, Dublin 9, Ireland
e-mail: philippe.taupin@dcu.ie

Alzheimer's Disease

AD is associated with neurodegeneration in areas of the brain that are vital to memory and other cognitive abilities, such as the hippocampus and the enthorhinal cortex. As the disease progresses, other regions of the brain are affected, leading to severe incapacity and death (Brun and Gustafson, 1976). Amyloid plaques and neurofibrillary tangles are the histopathological hallmarks of AD. Amyloid plaques are composed primarily of extracellular deposits of amyloid fibrils or protein beta-amyloid. Protein beta-amyloid originates from the post-transcriptional maturation of the amyloid precursor protein (APP) (Kang et al., 1987). The gene for APP, coding for a 695–770 amino acid protein, is located on chromosomes 21 (Goldgaber et al., 1987). Under certain conditions, such as the presence of specific gene mutations, in APP, presenilin 1 (PSEN1) or PSEN2, or certain risk factors, the maturation of the APP gene results in an excessive production of the 42 amino acid beta-amyloid peptide and in the formation of amyloid deposits (Nishimura et al., 1999; Newman et al., 2007; Wang et al., 2010). Amyloid plaques are present throughout the brain of patients with AD, particularly in the regions of degeneration such as the hippocampus and the entorhinal cortex, but also in the retina of patients with age-related macular degeneration (Anderson et al., 2004). Their density increases as the disease advances. Amyloid plaques may be a causative factor of AD. Neurofibrillary tangles are intracellular deposits of hyperphosphorylated tau protein, a microtubule-associated phosphoprotein. They are distributed throughout the brain of patients with AD (Fukutani et al., 1995). The hyperphosphorylation of tau protein results in their aggregation and in the breakdown of microtubules (Kim et al., 1986). This leads to the formation of neurofibrillary tangles and cell death (Iqbal et al., 2009).

Genetic mutations in the gene of APP, of PSEN1 and of PSEN2 have been identified as causative for inherited form of AD (Nishimura et al., 1999; St George-Hyslop and Petit, 2005). Genetic, acquired and environmental risk factors are the main causative factors for the sporadic form of AD. Among them, aging is the principal risk factor for LOAD. The disease affects about 3% of individuals ages 65–74 and about 50% of those 85 year old and older (Wang and Ding, 2008). Other risk factors for the sporadic form of AD include the presence of certain alleles in the genetic makeup of the individuals, particularly the presence of the apolipoprotein E varepsilon 4 allele (ApoE), hypertension, diabetes and oxidative stress (Prasher and Haque, 2000; Filipcik et al., 2006; Bertram and Tanzi, 2008). The disease for which there is no cure, leads to death within 3–9 years after being diagnosed and affects 35 million individuals worldwide (Ferri et al., 2005).

Adult Neurogenesis and Neural Stem Cells

Neurogenesis occurs in the adult mammalian brain, primarily in the hippocampus and in the SVZ, in various species including humans (Eriksson et al., 1998; Curtis et al., 2007). In the SVZ, newly generated neuronal cells migrate through the rostro-migratory stream to the olfactory bulb, where they differentiate into olfactory interneurons (Lois and Alvarez-Buylla, 1994). In the dentate gyrus (DG), newly generated neuronal cells in the subgranular zone migrate to the granule cell layer, where they differentiate into granule-like cells (Cameron et al., 1993). They extend axonal projections to the CA3 region of the Ammon's horn, where they establish synaptic contacts with their target cells (Toni et al., 2007; Taupin, 2009a). Newly generated neuronal cells of the DG establish mossy fiber-like synapses with their target cells of the CA3 region (Taupin, 2009a). The number of neuronal cells generated per day in the adult brain is relatively low, particularly in the DG. In mice, the number of neuronal cells generated per day in the DG is estimated at 9,000 cells, or about 0.1% of the granule cell population (Kempermann et al., 1997). Newly generated neuronal cells in the adult brain would originate from a population of residual stem cells. Neural stem cells (NSCs) are the self-renewing multipotent cells that generate the main phenotypes of the nervous system, nerve cells, astrocytes and oligodendrocytes (Gage, 2000). The isolation and characterization in vitro of self-renewing multipotent NSCs from the adult brain confirm that NSCs reside in the adult central nervous system (CNS) of mammals, including in humans, and provide a source of tissue that may be used for cellular therapy, for transplantation (Reynolds and Weiss, 1992; Taupin et al., 2000; Palmer et al., 2001). Neural progenitor and stem cells of the adult brain express and are characterized by molecular markers, such as the intermediate filament nestin, the transcription factors oct-3/4 and sox-2, and the RNA binding protein Musashi 1 (Lendahl et al., 1990; Kaneko et al., 2000; Komitova and Eriksson, 2004; Okuda et al., 2004). NSCs have the potential to treat and cure a broad range of neurological diseases and injuries, ranging from neurodegenerative diseases, such as AD, Huntington's disease and Parkinson's disease, cerebral strokes and spinal cord injuries.

The confirmation that adult neurogenesis occurs in the adult brain and that NSCs reside in the adult CNS reveals that the adult CNS has the potential for self-repair. The stimulation of endogenous neural progenitor or stem cells of the adult brain and the transplantation of adult-derived neural progenitor and stem cells are being considered for repairing and restoring the damaged or injured nerve pathways, and particularly for treating patients with AD. The intracerebral transplantation of adult-derived neural progenitor and stem cells may be used primarily for treating neurodegenerative diseases for which the degeneration is not widespread, such as Parkinson's disease (Brundin et al., 2010). For neurodegenerative diseases for which the degeneration is widespread, such as AD and Huntington's disease, this strategy may not be applicable, as it would require multiple sites of transplantation. Neural progenitor and stem cells migrate to sites of neurodegeneration and to diseased areas of the CNS, when administered systemically, particularly intravenously (Brown et al., 2003; Pluchino et al., 2003). Hence, the intravenous injection of adult-derived neural progenitor and stem cells may provide a strategy of choice for treating AD. It provides a non-invasive mean to deliver stem cells to the CNS. Future directions will involve improving the homing and migration of the stem cells to the diseased and injured sites of the CNS, such as the ex-vivo fucosylation of stem cells prior intravenous injection (Taupin, 2010a, b).

Adult Neurogenesis in Alzheimer's Disease

Autopsy studies report that the expression of doublecortin, a marker of immature neuronal cells, is enhanced in the hippocampus of the brain of patients with LOAD (Jin et al., 2004a). The expression of nestin and Musashi1 is reduced in the SVZ of patients with AD (Ziabreva et al., 2006). This suggests that neurogenesis is enhanced in the hippocampus of the brain of AD patients, particularly LOAD, and that it may be reduced in the SVZ of patients with AD. In animal models of AD, neurogenesis is enhanced in the hippocampus of adult transgenic mice that express the Swedish and Indiana APP mutations (Jin et al., 2004b). It is reduced in the hippocampus of adult mice deficient for APP or PSEN1 and of adult transgenic mice over expressing variants of APP or PSEN1 (Zhang et al., 2007; Rodríguez et al., 2008; Yu et al., 2009). These studies reveal data that are conflicting on the modulation of adult neurogenesis in AD in patients and in animal models, particularly in the hippocampus. Enhanced neurogenesis in the hippocampus would represent a regenerative attempt to compensate for the neuronal loss in the AD brain. In the SVZ, protein beta-amyloid stimulates neurogenesis in the SVZ of young APP/PS1 transgenic mice, but not of 12-month-old APP/PS1 transgenic models of AD (Sotthibundhu et al., 2009). Reduced neurogenesis in the SVZ of AD brain would underlie the compromised olfaction associated with the disease (Li et al., 2010). It would originate from the depletion of the pool of neural progenitor and stem cells in the SVZ of AD brains.

Bromodeoxyuridine (BrdU)-labeling combined with immunohistochemistry for markers of the neuronal lineage, immunohistochemistry for markers of the cell cycle and confocal microscopy are the paradigms and techniques the most used to study and quantify cell proliferation and neurogenesis in the adult brain of rodents and primates, including humans (Miller and Nowakowski, 1988). There are limitations and pitfalls over the use of BrdU-labeling and immunohistochemistry for markers of the cell cycle for studying cell proliferation and neurogenesis (Gould and Gross, 2002). BrdU is a thymidine analog. It is a mutagenic and toxic substance. It is a marker of DNA synthesis, not a marker of cell proliferation. Studying cell proliferation and neurogenesis using the BrdU-labeling paradigm requires distinguishing cell proliferation and neurogenesis from other events involving DNA synthesis, such as abortive cell cycle re-entry, leading to apoptosis, and gene duplication, without cell division, leading to aneuploidy (Taupin, 2007a, b). Immunohistochemistry for markers of the cell cycle indicates that the cells have reentered the cell cycle and resumed DNA synthesis, but is not indicative that the cells have completed the cell cycle (Taupin, 2007a,b).

The conflicting data reported on adult neurogenesis in the brain of patients with AD and in animal models of AD may originate from the validity of animal models, such as transgenic mice, as representative of a disease, such as AD. Transgenic mice deficient or over expressing genes, such as *APP* and *PSEN1*, are not representative models of the disease, but rather models to study the genes involved in the disease. The conflicting data reported on adult neurogenesis in the brain of patients with AD and in animal models of AD may also originate from the validity of animal models, such as transgenic mice, to study adult phenotypes such as adult neurogenesis. It may originate from the validity of the techniques and protocols used to study and quantify cell proliferation and neurogenesis and from the fact that there is no consensus on the term neurogenesis. Some studies only present data on cell proliferation, whereas others present only data on cell survival and neuronal differentiation. It may originate from the fact that in most studies, and in particular in the human post-mortem studies, only one time point along the pathology is analyzed. Neurogenesis might indeed be differentially regulated along the pathogenesis (Taupin, 2010c).

This shows that adult neurogenesis and NSCs may be involved in the pathology and pathogenesis of AD, particularly LOAD. However, the techniques and protocols primarily used in these studies are the sources of pitfalls and limitations. Hence, the involvement of adult neurogenesis and NSCs to the pathology and pathogenesis of AD not only remain to be elucidated and determined, but also validated and confirmed.

Aneuploidy and Aneuploid Newly Generated Neuronal Cells

Individuals with AD have a substantial high level of aneuploid cells, particularly lymphocytes (Migliore et al., 1999). In the brain of patients with AD, 4–10%, of nerve cells in regions of neurodegeneration, particularly the hippocampus, express proteins of the cell cycle, such as cyclin B, and are aneuploid (Busser et al., 1998; Kingsbury et al., 2006). Cells that are the most likely to generate aneuploid cells

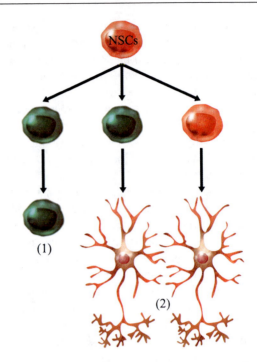

Fig. 27.1 Generation of aneuploid cells in the adult brain. The process of adult neurogenesis has the potential to generate populations of cells that are aneuploid, particularly in the neurogenic regions. The nondisjunction of chromosomes in dividing neural progenitor and stem cells of the adult brain would lead to aneuploid neural progenitor cells that may not proceed with their developmental program (1) and to aneuploid neuronal cells (2). Aneuploidy for chromosomes carrying genes involved in AD, such as the genes for ApoE, APP, PSEN1, PSEN2 and tau protein, in neural progenitor cells and newly generated neuronal cells of the adult brain would contribute to the formation of amyloid plaques and neurofibrillary tangles and neurodegeneration, particularly in the neurogenic regions of the adult brain, such as the hippocampus. Aneuploid adult neural progenitor cells and aneuploid newly generated adult neuronal cells may therefore be involved in the etiology and pathogenesis of AD. In *"orange"*, neural progenitor and stem cells; in *"green"*, aneuploid neural progenitor and stem cells

are dividing cells (Fig. 27.1). The nondisjunction of chromosomes during mitosis in stem cells or in other cell types undergoing mitosis is at the origin of aneuploid cells, such as lymphocytes, in patients with AD. Nerve cells in the adult brain are post-mitotic. Cell cycle re-entry and DNA duplication, without cell division, is at the origin of aneuploidy nerve cells in the brain, particularly of AD patients (Yang et al., 2001, 2003). These cells are fated to die; they may live in this state for months undergoing a slow death process (Herrup and Arendt, 2002; Yang and Herrup, 2007). Aneuploidy nerve cells would be an underlying of the neurodegenerative process in AD.

The genetic imbalance in aneuploid cells results in the over expression of genes. Patients with AD elicit aneuploidy particularly for chromosome 21, carrying the gene for APP (Migliore et al., 1999). Aneuploidy for chromosome 21 in individuals with AD therefore contributes to the pathogenesis of the disease by promoting the formation of amyloid plaques and neurodegeneration. Aneuploidy for chromosomes carrying other genes involved in AD, such as the genes for the ApoE, PSEN1, PSEN2 and tau protein – located on chromosomes 19, 1, 14 and 17 respectively – would contribute to the development and pathogenesis of the disease. This is by the over expression of those genes, triggering a cascade of events amplifying the development of the disease, such as the formation of amyloid plaques and neurofibrillary tangles and neurodegeneration.

The process of adult neurogenesis has the potential to generate populations of cells that are aneuploid, particularly in the neurogenic regions (Fig. 27.1) (Taupin, 2009b). The nondisjunction of chromosomes in dividing neural progenitor and stem cells of the adult brain would lead to aneuploid neural progenitor cells that may not proceed with their developmental program and to aneuploid neuronal cells (Fig. 27.1). Aneuploid adult neural progenitor cells and aneuploid newly generated adult neuronal cells may be fated to die or may survive for extended period of time. Aneuploidy for chromosomes carrying genes involved in AD, such as the genes for ApoE, APP, PSEN1, PSEN2 and tau protein, in neural progenitor cells and newly generated neuronal cells in the adult brain would contribute to the formation of amyloid plaques and neurofibrillary tangles and to neurodegeneration, particularly in the neurogenic regions of the adult brain, such as the hippocampus. Despite neurogenesis being an event of relatively low frequency in the adult brain of mammals, the contribution of aneuploid adult neural progenitor cells and aneuploid newly generated adult neuronal cells to the etiology and pathogenesis of AD may be critical. This as they are generated particularly in the hippocampus, a region involved in learning and memory and particularly affected in patients with AD.

Hence, adult neurogenesis and NSCs may be involved in the etiology and pathogenesis of AD. The generation of aneuploid adult neural progenitor cells and aneuploid newly generated adult neuronal cells remains to be demonstrated. The mutated forms of PSEN1 are detected in interphase kinetochores and centrosomes of dividing cells, the hyperphosphorylation of tau proteins, by kinases, leads to the breakdown of microtubules and the disruption in the mitotic spindle, and oxidative stress is involved in the segregation and migration of chromosomes during cells division and promotes aneuploidy (Li et al., 1997; Boeras et al., 2008; Taupin, 2010d). Causative factors of AD may promote the generation of aneuploid adult neural progenitor cells and aneuploid newly generated adult neuronal cells in the brain of individuals with AD.

Conclusion and Perspectives

Adult NSCs offer new perspectives and opportunities for treating patients with AD. Adult neurogenesis and NSCs may also lead to a better understanding of the pathology of the disease. Adult neurogenesis may be involved in regenerative attempts to compensate for neuronal cell loss in the hippocampus and in compromised olfaction in individuals with AD. Adult neurogenesis has the potential to generate aneuploid neural progenitor cells and aneuploid newly generated neuronal cells. Hence, adult neurogenesis may be both beneficial and detrimental to the disease and would contribute to the etiology and pathogenesis of AD. Future studies will aim at confirming and validating the involvement of adult neurogenesis and NSCs in the AD brain and to elucidate the role and contribution of adult neurogenesis and newly generated neuronal cells to the pathogenesis and pathology of AD. They will aim at identifying and characterizing aneuploid neural progenitor cells and aneuploid newly generated neuronal cells in the AD brain and their contribution to the etiology and pathogenesis of the disease. Such studies will not only enhance our understanding of AD, but will also lead to novel treatments and therapies for the patients.

References

Anderson DH, Talaga KC, Rivest AJ, Barron E, Hageman GS, Johnson LV (2004) Characterization of beta amyloid assemblies in drusen: The deposits associated with aging and age-related macular degeneration. Exp Eye Res 78:243–256

Bertram L, Tanzi RE (2008) Thirty years of Alzheimer's disease genetics: the implications of systematic meta-analyses. Nat Rev Neurosci 9:768–778

Boeras DI, Granic A, Padmanabhan J, Crespo NC, Rojiani AM, Potter H (2008) Alzheimer's presenilin 1 causes chromosome missegregation and aneuploidy. Neurobiol Aging 29:319–328

Brown AB, Yang W, Schmidt NO, Carroll R, Leishear KK, Rainov NG, Black PM, Breakefield XO, Aboody KS (2003) Intravascular delivery of neural stem cell lines to target intracranial and extracranial tumors of neural and non-neural origin. Hum Gene Ther 14:1777–1785

Brun A, Gustafson L (1976) Distribution of cerebral degeneration in Alzheimer's disease. A clinico-pathological study. Arch Psychiatr Nervenkr 223:15–33

Brundin P, Barker RA, Parmar M (2010) Neural grafting in Parkinson's disease: Problems and possibilities. Progr Brain Res 184:265–294

Burns A, Byrne EJ, Maurer K (2002) Alzheimer's disease. Lancet 13:163–165

Busser J, Geldmacher DS, Herrup K (1998) Ectopic cell cycle proteins predict the sites of neuronal cell death in Alzheimer's disease brain. J Neurosci 18:2801–2807

Cameron HA, Woolley CS, McEwen BS, Gould E (1993) Differentiation of newly born neurons and glia in the dentate gyrus of the adult rat. Neuroscience 56:337–344

Curtis MA, Kam M, Nannmark U, Anderson MF, Axell MZ, Wikkelso C, Holtas S, van Roon-Mom WM, Bjork-Eriksson T, Nordborg C, Frisen J, Dragunow M, Faull RL, Eriksson PS (2007) Human neuroblasts migrate to the olfactory bulb via a lateral ventricular extension. Science 315:1243–1249

Duan X, Kang E, Liu CY, Ming GL, Song H (2008) Development of neural stem cell in the adult brain. Curr Opin Neurobiol 18:108–115

Dubois B, Feldman HH, Jacova C, Dekosky ST, Barberger-Gateau P, Cummings J, Delacourte A, Galasko D, Gauthier S, Jicha G, Meguro K, O'brien J, Pasquier F, Robert P, Rossor M, Salloway S, Stern Y, Visser PJ, Scheltens P (2007) Research criteria for the diagnosis of Alzheimer's disease: Revising the NINCDS–ADRDA criteria. Lancet Neurol 6:734–746

Eriksson PS, Perfilieva E, Bjork-Eriksson T, Alborn AM, Nordborg C, Peterson DA, Gage FH (1998) Neurogenesis in the adult human hippocampus. Nat Med 4:1313–1317

Ferri CP, Prince M, Brayne C, Brodaty H, Fratiglioni L, Ganguli M, Hall K, Hasegawa K, Hendrie H, Huang Y, Jorm A, Mathers C, Menezes PR, Rimmer E, Scazufca M, Alzheimer's Disease International (2005) Global prevalence of dementia: A Delphi consensus study. Lancet 366:2112–2117

Filipcik P, Cente M, Ferencik M, Hulin I, Novak M (2006) The role of oxidative stress in the pathogenesis of Alzheimer's disease. Bratisl Lek Listy 107:384–394

Fukutani Y, Kobayashi K, Nakamura I, Watanabe K, Isaki K, Cairns NJ (1995) Neurons, intracellular and extra cellular neurofibrillary tangles in subdivisions of the hippocampal cortex in normal ageing and Alzheimer's disease. Neurosci Lett 200:57–60

Fusetti M, Fioretti AB, Silvagni F, Simaskou M, Sucapane P, Necozione S, Eibenstein A (2010) Smell and preclinical Alzheimer disease: Study of 29 patients with amnesic mild cognitive impairment. J Otolaryngol Head Neck Surg 39:175–181

Gage FH (2000) Mammalian neural stem cells. Science 287:1433–1438

Goldgaber D, Lerman MI, McBride OW, Saffiotti U, Gajdusek DC (1987) Characterization and chromosomal localization of a cDNA encoding brain amyloid of Alzheimer's disease. Science 235:877–880

Gould E, Gross GC (2002) Neurogenesis in adult mammals: some progress and problems. J Neurosci 22:619–623

Herrup K, Arendt T (2002) Re-expression of cell cycle proteins induces neuronal cell death during Alzheimer's disease. J Alzheimer's Dis 4:243–247

Iqbal K, Liu F, Gong CX, Alonso Adel C, Grundke-Iqbal I (2009) Mechanisms of tau-induced neurodegeneration. Acta Neuropathol 118:53–69

Jin K, Peel AL, Mao XO, Xie L, Cottrell BA, Henshall DC, Greenberg DA (2004a) Increased hippocampal neurogenesis in Alzheimer's disease. Proc Natl Acad Sci USA 101:343–347

Jin K, Galvan V, Xie L, Mao XO, Gorostiza OF, Bredesen DE, Greenberg DA (2004b) Enhanced neurogenesis in Alzheimer's disease transgenic (PDGF-APPSw,Ind) mice. Proc Natl Acad Sci USA 101:13363–13367

Kaneko Y, Sakakibara S, Imai T, Suzuki A, Nakamura Y, Sawamoto K, Ogawa Y, Toyama Y, Miyata T, Okano H (2000) Musashi1: an evolutionarily conserved marker for CNS progenitor cells including neural stem cells. Dev Neurosci 22:139–153

Kang J, Lemaire HG, Unterbeck A, Salbaum JM, Masters CL, Grzeschik KH, Multhaup G, Beyreuther K, Müller-Hill B (1987) The precursor of Alzheimer's disease amyloid A4 protein resembles a cell-surface receptor. Nature 325:733–736

Kempermann G, Kuhn HG, Gage FH (1997) More hippocampal neurons in adult mice living in an enriched environment. Nature 386:493–495

Kim H, Jensen CG, Rebhun LI (1986) The binding of MAP-2 and tau on brain microtubules in vitro: Implications for microtubule structure. Ann NY Acad Sci 466:218–239

Kingsbury MA, Yung YC, Peterson SE, Westra JW, Chun J (2006) Aneuploidy in the normal and diseased brain. Cell Mol Life Sci 63:2626–2641

Komitova M, Eriksson PS (2004) Sox-2 is expressed by neural progenitors and astroglia in the adult rat brain. Neurosci Lett 369:24–27

Lendahl U, Zimmerman LB, McKay RD (1990) CNS stem cells express a new class of intermediate filament protein. Cell 60:585–595

Li J, Xu M, Zhou H, Ma J, Potter H (1997) Alzheimer presenilins in the nuclear membrane, interphase kinetochores, and centrosomes suggest a role in chromosome segregation. Cell 90:917–927

Li W, Howard JD, Gottfried JA (2010) Disruption of odour quality coding in piriform cortex mediates olfactory deficits in Alzheimer's disease. Brain 133:2714–2726

Lois C, Alvarez-Buylla A (1994) Long-distance neuronal migration in the adult mammalian brain. Science 264:1145–1148

Migliore L, Botto N, Scarpato R, Petrozzi L, Cipriani G, Bonuccelli U (1999) Preferential occurrence of chromosome 21 malsegregation in peripheral blood lymphocytes of Alzheimer disease patients. Cytogenet Cell Genet 87:41–46

Miller MW, Nowakowski RS (1998) Use of bromodeoxyuridine-immunohistochemistry to examine the proliferation, migration and time of origin of cells in the central nervous system. Brain Res 457:44–52

Newman M, Musgrave FI, Lardelli M (2007) Alzheimer disease: amyloidogenesis, the presenilins and animal models. Biochim Biophys Acta 1772:285–297

Nishimura M, Yu G, St George-Hyslop PH (1999) Biology of presenilins as causative molecules for Alzheimer disease. Clin Genet 55:219–225

Okuda T, Tagawa K, Qi ML Hoshio M, Ueda H, Kawano H, Kanazawa I, Muramatsu M, Okazawa H (2004) Oct-3/4 repression accelerates differentiation of neural progenitor cells in vitro and in vivo. Brain Res Mol Brain Res 132:18–30

Palmer TD, Schwartz PH, Taupin P, Kaspar B, Stein SA, Gage FH (2001) Cell culture. Progenitor cells from human brain after death. Nature 411:42–43

Pluchino S, Quattrini A, Brambilla E, Gritti A, Salani G, Dina G, Galli R, Del Carro U, Amadio S, Bergami A, Furlan R, Comi G, Vescovi AL, Martino G (2003) Injection of adult neurospheres induces recovery in a chronic model of multiple sclerosis. Nature 422:688–694

Prasher VP, Haque MS (2000) Apolipoprotein E, Alzheimer's disease and Down's syndrome. Br J Psychiatry 177:469–470

Querfurth HW, LaFerla FM (2010) Alzheimer's disease. N Engl J Med 362:329–344

Reynolds BA, Weiss S (1992) Generation of neurons and astrocytes from isolated cells of the adult mammalian central nervous system. Science 255:1707–1710

Rodríguez JJ, Jones VC, Tabuchi M, Allan SM, Knight EM, LaFerla FM, Oddo S, Verkhratsky A (2008) Impaired adult neurogenesis in the dentate gyrus of a triple transgenic mouse model of Alzheimer's disease. PLoS One 3:e2935

Sotthibundhu A, Li QX, Thangnipon W, Coulson EJ (2009) Abeta(1-42) stimulates adult SVZ neurogenesis through the p75 neurotrophin receptor. Neurobiol Aging 30:1975–1985

St George-Hyslop PH, Petit A (2005) Molecular biology and genetics of Alzheimer's disease. C R Biol 328:119–130

Taupin P (2007a) Protocols for studying adult neurogenesis: Insights and recent developments. Regener Med 2:51–62

Taupin P (2007b) BrdU immunohistochemistry for studying adult neurogenesis: Paradigms, pitfalls, limitations, and validation. Brain Res Rev 53:198–214

Taupin P (2009a) Characterization and isolation of synapses of newly generated neuronal cells of the adult hippocampus at early stages of neurogenesis. J Neurodegener Regener 2: 9–17

Taupin P (2009b) Adult neurogenesis, neural stem cells and Alzheimer's disease: Developments, limitations, problems and promises. Curr Alzheimer Res 6:461–470

Taupin P (2010a) Ex vivo fucosylation to improve the engraftment capability and therapeutic potential of human cord blood stem cells. Drug Discov Today 15:698–699

Taupin P (2010b) Transplantation of cord blood stem cells for treating hematologic diseases and strategies to improve engraftment. Therapy 7:703–715

Taupin P (2010c) Adult neurogenesis and neural stem cells as a model for the discovery and development of novel drugs. Expert Opin Drug Discov 5:921–925

Taupin P (2010d) A dual activity of ROS and oxidative stress on adult neurogenesis and Alzheimer's disease. Central Nervous SystAgents Med Chem 10:16–21

Taupin P, Gage FH (2002) Adult neurogenesis and neural stem cells of the central nervous system in mammals. J Neurosci Res 69:745–749

Taupin P, Ray J, Fischer WH, Suhr ST, Hakansson K, Grubb A, Gage FH (2000) FGF-2-responsive neural stem cell proliferation requires CCg, a novel autocrine/paracrine cofactor. Neuron 28:385–397

Toni N, Teng EM, Bushong EA, Aimone JB, Zhao C, Consiglio A, van Praag H, Martone ME, Ellisman MH, Gage FH (2007) Synapse formation on neurons born in the adult hippocampus. Nat Neurosci 10:727–734

Wang JF, Lu R, Wang YZ (2010) Regulation of β cleavage of amyloid precursor protein. Neurosci Bull 26:417–427

Wang XP, Ding HL (2008) Alzheimer's disease: Epidemiology, genetics, and beyond. Neurosci Bull 24:105–109

Yang Y, Herrup K (2007) Cell division in the CNS: Protective response or lethal event in post-mitotic neurons? Biochim Biophys Acta 1772:457–466

Yang Y, Geldmacher DS, Herrup K (2001) DNA replication precedes neuronal cell death in Alzheimer's disease. J Neurosci 21:2661–2668

Yang Y, Mufson EJ, Herrup K (2003) Neuronal cell death is preceded by cell cycle events at all stages of Alzheimer's disease. J Neurosci 23:2557–2563

Yu Y, He J, Zhang Y, Luo H, Zhu S, Yang Y, Zhao T, Wu J, Huang Y, Kong J, Tan Q, Li XM (2009) Increased hippocampal neurogenesis in the progressive stage of Alzheimer's disease phenotype in an APP/PS1 double transgenic mouse model. Hippocampus 19:1247–1253

Zhang C, McNeil E, Dressler L, Siman R (2007) Long-lasting impairment in hippocampal neurogenesis associated with amyloid deposition in a knock-in mouse model of familial Alzheimer's disease. Exp Neurol 204:77–87

Ziabreva I, Perry E, Perry R, Minger SL, Ekonomou A, Przyborski S, Ballard C (2006) Altered neurogenesis in Alzheimer's disease. J Psychosom Res 61:311–316

Part IV
Tissue Repair (Regeneration)

Chapter 28

Generating Human Cardiac Muscle Cells from Adipose-Derived Stem Cells

Rodney Dilley, Yu Suk Choi, and Gregory Dusting

Abstract Therapies using stem cells and tissue engineering for cardiovascular regeneration aim to repair damaged cardiac tissue by delivering stem cells with biomaterials and biomolecules to support cell survival and differentiation. When implanted in undifferentiated states, stem cells recognize the cues around them to adopt a variety of cell fates. However, disease processes (e.g., myocardial infarcts) alter the microenvironment, and differentiation is often misdirected. For this reason it is best to differentiate stem cells into cardiomyocyte specific lineages in vitro prior to implantation. Stem cells can form mature cardiac muscle cells by employing various differentiation methods, including epigenetic modification, differentiation media, and co-culture with neonatal cardiomyocytes. Here we discuss adipose tissue-derived stem cells and how they may be directed into cardiomyocytes for tissue engineering.

Keywords Cardiomyocyte · Myocardial regeneration · Bone marrow stem cell (BMSC) · Adipogenic unipotency · 5-Azacytidine · GATA4

Introduction

Human left ventricle is made up of approximately 4×10^9 cardiomyocytes (Olivetti et al., 1990). The loss of 25% of the ventricle following myocardial

R. Dilley (✉)
O'Brien Institute, Fitzroy, VIC 065, Australia
e-mail: rdilley@unimelb.edu.au

infarction compromises ventricular function and leads to heart failure (Caulfield et al., 1976). To regenerate infarcted left ventricle tissue we may need to deliver sustainably more than 1 billion functional cardiomyocytes which can integrate and contract synchronously with the host myocardium (Murry et al., 2006). Over the past decade, several donor cell sources have been studied in an effort to find an optimal solution for cardiac regeneration by cell therapy or tissue engineering. Fully differentiated mature cells, progenitor cells, and stem cells obtained from different sources offer unique promises and hurdles for therapeutic cardiac repair (Murry et al., 2006). An optimal cell source for an engineered myocardial tissue is required to be easy to harvest, nonimmunogenic (autologous), highly proliferative, and able to differentiate into mature and functional cardiomyocytes. Table 28.1 describes some advantages and limitations of prominent candidate cell populations.

Cardiac Muscle-Derived Cells

Intuitively, autologous cardiomyocytes are the ideal cell source for cardiac cell and tissue therapy. Clearly, however, they have severe limitations including low availability, are difficult to isolate and have a very low potential for expansion. It was long held that cardiomyocytes were terminally matured soon after birth and growth was restricted to cellular hypertrophy, but evidence now shows that a fraction of younger myocytes (15–20%) may be derived from cardiac stem cells during adult life and retain capacity to replicate (Anversa and Nadal-Ginard, 2002; Kajstura et al., 2010). Recent quantitative analyses of cardiomyocyte

Table 28.1 Advantages and disadvantages of various cell source candidates for myocardial regeneration

Cells	Easy accessibility	High expandability	Cardiac differentiation	Autologous
Cardiomyocyte	No	No	Yes	No
Skeletal myoblast	Yes (w/pain)	No	No	Yes
Cardiac stem cell (CSC)	No	Yes	Yes	Yes
Embryonic stem cell (ESC)	No	Yes	Yes	No
Induced pluripotent stem cell (iPS cell)	Yes	Yes	Yes	Yes
Umbilical cord blood-derived stem cells	No	Yes	Yes	Yes
Bone marrow stem cell (BMSC)	Yes (w/pain)	Yes	Yes	Yes
Adipose-derived stem cell (ASC)	Yes	Yes	Yes	Yes

turnover have produced controversial results, with at least a modest renewal capacity throughout life, from 1% annually at the age of 25 to 0.45% at the age of 75 from one study (Bergmann et al., 2009), and more than an order of magnitude higher turnover rates from another study (Kajstura et al., 2010). Whichever of these views proves correct, application of cardiomyocytes or precursors to regenerative therapies is promising and awaits progress in methods for harvesting, expanding and delivering autologous cells from patients who already have heart failure, where the endogenous regenerative capacity of cardiomyocytes has not been sufficient for repair.

Stem Cells

Of the stem cells with potential to contribute to cardiac tissue engineering (Table 28.1), some are currently hampered by ethical (ESC) and safety concerns (myoblast, ESC, iPS) or not preferred due to potential immunological issues (ESC, UCB). The use of autologous stem cell populations may be restricted by their low numbers (cardiac, BMSC) or technically difficult extraction protocols (cardiac, BMSC). One attractive option comes from autologous adipose tissue. Unlike many other tissues, adipose tissue has the ability to undergo a dramatic change in volume in the adult human. While cellular hypertrophy accounts for some of this plasticity, large increases in volume are associated with an increased number of adipocytes and expansion of the microvasculature (Fraser et al., 2006). The hyperplastic response is derived from a population of progenitor cells, which show multipotential beyond adipogenic unipotency (Choi et al., 2005, 2006; Kim et al., 2006; Zuk et al., 2001). These cells, now referred to as adipose-derived stem cells (ASC), have extensive self-renewal capacity and multipotency. The main benefit of ASC is that they can be easily harvested from patients by the simple, minimally invasive method of liposuction (Nakagami et al., 2006). Adipose tissue can be harvested in relatively large quantities (from 100 ml to several litres) using liposuction, which is a low morbidity procedure that is widely performed (more than 340,000 elective cosmetic procedures in U.S. in 2008; The-American-Society-for-Aesthetic-Plastic-Surgery 2008). Moreover, cultured populations of ASC can maintain long-term multipotency (Nakagami et al., 2006). Animal studies show that these cells may be particularly useful in cardiac tissue engineering for they can differentiate into cardiomyocytes (Planat-Benard et al., 2004a), endothelial cells, and smooth muscle cells as well as expressing angiogenic and antiapoptotic factors (Planat-Benard et al., 2004b). Furthermore, several studies have reported that these in vitro activities may act in vivo after myocardial infarction to improve cardiac function in animals treated with these cells (Miyahara et al., 2006). These findings, together with the especially high yield of cells from adipose tissue compared with bone marrow, as well as the relative ease of obtaining moderately large volumes with minimal pain, suggest that ASC can be a clinically relevant source of cells for cardiac tissue engineering.

In Vitro Cardiac Differentiation

There is no definitive cardiomyocyte 'specific' cell surface marker, so a range of nuclear and cytoplasmic markers have been used to establish the cardiac phenotype including (1) positive staining for cardiac transcription factors, GATA4 and Nkx2.5, and cardiac proteins including sarcomeric α-actin, cardiac troponin

I and T, desmin, and cardiac myosin heavy chain, (2) expression of cardiac messenger ribonucleic acid (mRNA) including cardiac transcription factors and proteins, (3) contractility in culture by video recording or pharmacological test, (4) calcium transients, and (5) electrophysiological analysis (Choi et al., 2010a). The differentiation toward cardiomyocytes from ASC has been promoted by three main methods: epigenetic modification, differentiation media, and co-culture with neonatal cardiomyocytes.

Epigenetic Modification

Cellular differentiation involves massive alterations of the genome-wide epigenetic status of multiple gene loci, with changes in both de novo methylation and demethylation of DNA and in various histone modifications. 5-azacytidine is a nucleoside inhibitor of DNA methyltransferases that can be incorporated into DNA. 5-azacytidine may then act to demethylate DNA to produce an open opportunity for RNA polymerase to bind onto gene promoter regions. A cardiomyogenic mouse cell line has been established from immortalized BMSC by repetitive treatments of 5-azacytidine and colony screenings for spontaneously beating cells (Makino et al., 1999). This observation was confirmed by Tomita et al. (1999) who showed that after exposure to 5-azacytidine for 24 h, BMSC could also differentiate into cardiomyocytes. In contrast, other studies failed to reproduce cardiac differentiation from BMSC using 5-azacytidine. Only passage 4 (P4) but not P1 and P8 rat BMSC showed expression of cardiac markers including Nkx2.5 and troponin I (Zhang et al., 2005). Rat BMSC could not be expanded extensively in vitro nor could they be induced to differentiate into cardiomyocyte-like cells using various concentrations of 5-azacytidine with single or repeated treatment (Liu et al., 2003). Moreover, spontaneously and synchronously pulsating cardiomyocyte-like cells were not observed after 8 weeks in culture. In addition, repeated exposure of 5-azacytidine to ASC significantly inhibited cell growth (Lee et al., 2008). Lee et al. also failed to observe the conversion of human ASC into beating cardiomyocyte-like cells (they neither formed myotubes nor produced spontaneously beating cells after 8 weeks). Similarly, in our hands the use of 5-azacytidine on human ASC cultures (Choi et al., 2010a) did not increase cardiac gene expression and no contraction was observed. We further showed a lack of methylation of cardiomyocyte-specific gene promoters in human ASC as determined by MeDIP-chip microarray analysis.

In previous studies, the histone deacetylase inhibitor trichostatin A has shown cardiomyogenic-inducing effects on stem cells, including mouse ESC, cardiac side population cells and P19 embryonic carcinoma stem cells (Illi et al., 2005; Karamboulas et al., 2006; Kawamura et al., 2005; Oyama et al., 2007). Histone modifications were enhanced by shear stress in murine ESC and activated cardiac lineage gene expression (Illi et al., 2005). Treatment of embryonic stem cells with trichostatin A induced acetylation of histone-3/4 near GATA sites within the atrial natriuretic peptide (ANP) promoter. In addition, trichostatin augmented the increase in an acetylated form of GATA4 and its DNA binding during ESC differentiation (Kawamura et al., 2005). Trichostatin A treatment of human ASC increased cardiac actin mRNA expression 11-fold after 1 week (Choi et al., 2010a) and could be sustained for 2 weeks by culturing cells in cardiomyocyte culture medium. Trichostatin A treated cells also stained positively with cardiac myosin heavy chain, sarcomeric α-actin, troponin I and connexin43 antibodies. Despite this evidence for cardiac gene regulation, such treatments did not produce beating cells and therefore suggested only partial cardiomyogenic differentiation.

The interplay between epigenetic status modifiers, gene expression and differentiation potential of stem cells clearly plays an important role (Azuara et al., 2006). Attempting to differentiate ASC with broad spectrum epigenetic modification may only influence some parts of the cardiac differentiation program and may also induce differentiation into other lineages, requiring sorting protocols to enrich for cardiomyocytes.

Differentiation Media

A small number of studies have been performed using non-epigenetic approaches and several interesting results have been obtained utilizing two main methods. One is to use media with differentiating growth factor combinations (Planat-Benard et al., 2004a) and the other uses cardiomyocyte extracts (Gaustad et al., 2004). Murine ASC cultured in methylcellulose-based culture media enriched with recombinant mouse stem cell factor, interleukin-3 and -6 showed various cell morphologies after 6 days of culture (Planat-Benard et al., 2004a). Some rounded cells began to contract spontaneously at days 11–14. These beating cells expressed several cardiomyocyte-related mRNA, such as GATA4, Nkx2.5, myosin light chain 2v, and ANP. Antibodies to MEF2c, sarcomeric α-actinin, beta myosin heavy chain, and connexin 43 also stained the cells and they behaved like pacemaker cells, as characterized electrophysiologically. Rat ASC were differentiated into cells expressing cardiomyocyte markers after 2 weeks of culture with TGF beta 2: troponin I mRNA, myosin heavy chain and sarcomeric α-actin proteins were expressed after 2 weeks, but there was no evidence of contraction. Shim et al. (2004) showed that human BMSC differentiated towards cardiomyocyte-like cells using a simple culture medium consisting of 60% Dulbecco's modified Eagle's medium-low glucose (DMEM-lg)/28% MCDB-201, 1 mg/ml bovine insulin, 0.55 mg/ml human transferrin, 0.5 mg/ml sodium selenite, 50 mg/ml bovine serum albumin (BSA), 0.4 mg/ml linoleic acid, 10^{-4} M ascorbate phosphate, 10^{-9} M dexamethasone, 100 U/ml penicillin G, 100 mg/ml streptomycin sulfate, and 10% fetal calf serum (FCS). Dexamethasone and ascorbic acid included in this medium were shown to promote sarcomeric myosin and cardiac myosin heavy chain expression in adult and embryonic stem cells, respectively (Takahashi et al., 2003). Cardiomyocytes were isolated from 4 to 6 week-old rats and homogenized by pulse-sonication. After 3 weeks of exposure to extracts, ASC expressed several cardiac markers, including sarcomeric α-actin, desmin, cardiac troponin I, and connexin 43. Moreover, whole-heart protein extracts showed the additional capacity to induce differentiation into endothelial-like and smooth muscle-like cells. The mechanism underlying cardiac differentiation in cardiomyogenic media is not clear, but stem cells were partially or fully differentiated into cardiomyocytes. To use growth factors can be very costly for large-scale application, and non-autologous cardiomyocyte extracts can cause immune rejection in human studies. Clearly these promising approaches need further development.

Co-culture with Cardiomyocytes

The evidence for cardiomyogenic differentiation of BMSC after implantation in vivo suggests the existence of environmental differentiating factors (Orlic et al., 2001). The nature of these factors is not known because they are in vivo phenomena, making investigation difficult. Possible contributors include soluble factors secreted from cardiomyocytes or transmitted through cell-to-cell interactions, cell fusion, electrical or mechanical stimulation or as yet unknown cell signals. Rangappa et al. (2003) have demonstrated that human BMSC have the potential to differentiate into cardiomyocytes under the appropriate microenvironment. Soluble factors alone were not sufficient to induce cardiomyogenic differentiation of human BMSC and physical contact between the BMSC and cardiomyocytes was required. Similar results were obtained with rodent BMSC (Fukuhara et al., 2003; Wang et al., 2006). BMSC contracted synchronously with cardiomyocytes from 2 days of co-culture and 2.5% of cells were myosin heavy chain positive cells and 1.9% troponin I positive. In contrast, there was no cardiomyogenic phenotype from co-culture with cells in culture well inserts, which had no direct cell-to-cell interaction. Wang and his colleagues also obtained similar data with rat BMSC. In their study, rat BMSC exhibited characteristics of cardiomyocytes when cultured in direct co-culture with adult rat cardiomyocytes (Wang et al., 2006). To clarify whether physical contact or soluble chemical factors are dominant in the differentiation of BMSC, they used a semi-permeable membrane culture system, which only permits chemical factors to diffuse, but not cells. They found that there was no expression of sarcomeric α-actin, desmin, cardiac troponin T in BMSC. This implies that soluble chemical factors released from cardiomyocytes were not sufficient to differentiate BMSC into cardiomyocytes. However, direct cell-to-cell contact between BMSC and cardiomyocytes did induce cardiac differentiation of BMSC.

Recently, we have also demonstrated that human ASC differentiated into cardiomyocytes in a direct contact co-culture setting with neonatal rat cardiomyocytes in vitro (Choi et al., 2010a). Human ASC in non-contact co-culture showed no evidence for cardiac differentiation, but ASC co-cultured in direct contact with rat cardiomyocytes exhibited

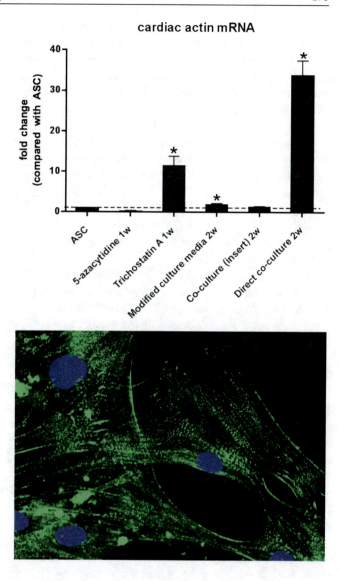

Fig. 28.1 *Upper panel*: A bar graph showing basal levels of cardiac actin mRNA observed in human adipose-derived stem cell cultures by real-time quantitative polymerase chain reaction. Significant increases in expression were found after exposure of cultures to the epigenetic modifier Trichostatin, in modified culture media or in direct contact co-culture with neonatal rat cardiomyocytes. * = significantly different from ASC (Choi et al., 2010a). *Lower panel*: A fluorescence micrograph showing alpha-actinin immunostaining in human adipose-derived stem cells after coculture with rat cells for 2 weeks. Human cells had been labeled with DiI prior to coculture then were purified by flow cytometry after coculture

a time-dependent increase in cardiac actin mRNA expression (up to 34-fold; Fig. 28.1) between days 3 and 14. Immunocytochemistry revealed co-expression of GATA4 and Nkx2.5, sarcomeric α-actin, a-actinin (Fig. 28.1), troponin I, and cardiac myosin heavy chain in CM-DiI labeled ASC. Most importantly, many of these cells showed spontaneous contractions which were accompanied by synchronous transient changes in cell calcium levels in culture. Human ASC showed Ca^{2+} transients and contractions synchronous with the surrounding rat cardiomyocytes (up to 106 beats/min). Functional gap junctions also formed between them as observed by dye transfer (Choi et al., 2010a). The precise mechanisms involved in the induction of differentiation remains to be determined but this model may ultimately provide tools to identify an effective strategy for human cardiomyocyte differentiation from autologous stem cells.

In Vivo Cardiac Differentiation

In order to test this coculture differentiation model in vivo, human ASC have also been implanted into a vascularised tissue engineering chamber with rat cardiomyocytes (rCM) to examine the cardiomyogenic differentiation of ASC in vivo (Choi et al., 2010b). In this vascularised cardiac tissue engineering model constructs up to 2 mm thickness form and contract spontaneously within weeks of implantation. When ASC were coimplanted at a 1:10 ratio with neonatal rat cardiomyocytes, constructs were formed that contracted at up to 140 beats/min. The rats containing ASC (ASC-rCM and ASC groups) grew bigger tissues in the chamber than the rCM group (55% and 26% larger respectively). Morphometric analysis of tissue composition showed that ASC implanted alone generated a small amount of spontaneously differentiated muscle tissue (1.3 ± 0.5 µl). The ASC-rCM and rCM groups generated a larger volume of cardiac muscle (14.5 ± 4.8 and 18.5 ± 2.6 µl). The ASC-rCM group also grew nearly twice as much vascular tissue in the engineered construct than the rCM group constructs. Immunostaining using human specific nuclear antibody and cardiac markers revealed various fates for ASC implanted in the chamber; (1) differentiation into cardiac muscle cells and integration with co-implanted rat cardiomyocytes; (2) differentiation into smooth muscle cells and recruitment into vascular structures as well as probable paracrine recruitment of endogenous endothelial cells; (3) differentiation into adipocytes.

In conclusion, cell-to-cell interaction with cardiomyocytes was found to promote cardiomyogenic differentiation of human ASC in vivo. This method indicates potential for a cardiomyogenic differentiation system to progress applications for human cardiac cell therapy or tissue engineering once the animal-based elements are substituted out. We also generated highly vascularised cardiac tissue by co-culturing human ASC with rat cardiomyocytes in the tissue engineering chamber. The ASC were shown to survive and differentiated into new vasculature, cardiac muscle and adipose tissue. Implantation of ASC into the tissue engineering chamber also appeared to substantially increase the vascularity of the cardiac construct and show a substantial supporting role for tissue regenerative approaches.

Conclusion and Future Direction

Thus several stem cell sources have shown capacity for cardiomyogenesis after applying epigenetic modification, differentiation media, and co-culture techniques. None of these methods is sufficiently mature to produce functioning human cardiomyocytes at a scale suitable for clinical application. The optimization of existing strategies and the exploration of new approaches (e.g., matrix biology to control stem cell fate, direct reprogramming) to differentiate stem cells into functional cardiomyocytes will eventually offer new possibilities for treatment of cardiovascular diseases, particularly if applied through cardiac tissue engineering.

References

Anversa P, Nadal-Ginard B (2002) Myocyte renewal and ventricular remodelling. Nature 415:240–243

Azuara V, Perry P, Sauer S, Spivakov M, Jorgensen HF, John RM, Gouti M, Casanova M, Warnes G, Merkenschlager M, Fischer AG (2006) Chromatin signatures of pluripotent cell lines. Nat Cell Biol 8:532–538

Bergmann O, Bhardwaj RD, Bernard S, Zdunek S, Barnabe-Heider F, Walsh S, Zupicich J, Alkass K, Buchholz BA, Druid H, Jovinge S, Frisén J (2009) Evidence for cardiomyocyte renewal in humans. Science 324:98–102

Caulfield JB, Leinbach R, Gold H (1976) The relationship of myocardial infarct size and prognosis. Circulation 53:I141–I144

Choi YS, Park SN, Suh H (2005) Adipose tissue engineering using mesenchymal stem cells attached to injectable PLGA spheres. Biomaterials 26:5855–5863

Choi YS, Cha SM, Lee YY, Kwon SW, Park CJ, Kim M (2006) Adipogenic differentiation of adipose tissue derived adult stem cells in nude mouse. Biochem Biophys Res Commun 345:631–637

Choi YS, Dusting GJ, Stubbs S, Arunothayaraj S, Han XL, Collas P, Morrison WA, Dilley RJ (2010a) Differentiation of human adipose-derived stem cells into beating cardiomyocytes. J Cell Mol Med 14:878–889

Choi YS, Matsuda K, Dusting GJ, Morrison WA, Dilley RJ (2010b) Engineering cardiac tissue in vivo from human adipose-derived stem cells. Biomaterials 31:2236–2242

Fraser JK, Schreiber R, Strem B, Zhu M, Alfonso Z, Wulur I, Hedrick MH (2006) Plasticity of human adipose stem cells toward endothelial cells and cardiomyocytes. Nat Clin Pract Cardiovasc Med 3(Suppl 1):S33–S37

Fukuhara S, Tomita S, Yamashiro S, Morisaki T, Yutani C, Kitamura S, Nakatani T (2003) Direct cell-cell interaction of cardiomyocytes is key for bone marrow stromal cells to go into cardiac lineage in vitro. J Thorac Cardiovasc Surg 125:1470–1480

Gaustad KG, Boquest AC, Anderson BE, Gerdes AM, Collas P (2004) Differentiation of human adipose tissue stem cells using extracts of rat cardiomyocytes. Biochem Biophys Res Commun 314:420–427

Illi B, Scopece A, Nanni S, Farsetti A, Morgante L, Biglioli P, Capogrossi MC, Gaetano C (2005) Epigenetic histone modification and cardiovascular lineage programming in mouse embryonic stem cells exposed to laminar shear stress. Circ Res 96:501–508

Kajstura J, Urbanek K, Perl S, Hosoda T, Zheng H, Ogórek B, Ferreira-Martins J, Goichberg P, Rondon-Clavo C, Sanada F, D'Amario D, Rota M, Del Monte F, Orlic D, Tisdale J, Leri A, Anversa P (2010) Cardiomyogenesis in the adult human heart. Circ Res 107:305–315

Karamboulas C, Swedani A, Ward C, Al-Madhoun AS, Wilton S, Boisvenue S, Ridgeway AG, Skerjanc IS (2006) HDAC activity regulates entry of mesoderm cells into the cardiac muscle lineage. J Cell Sci 119:4305–4314

Kawamura T, Ono K, Morimoto T, Wada H, Hirai M, Hidaka K, Morisaki T, Heike T, Nakahata T, Kita T, Hasegawa K (2005) Acetylation of GATA-4 is involved in the differentiation of embryonic stem cells into cardiac myocytes. J Biol Chem 280:19682–19688

Kim M, Choi YS, Yang SH, Hong HN, Cho SW, Cha SM, Pak JH, Kim CW, Kwon SW, Park CJ (2006) Muscle regeneration by adipose tissue-derived adult stem cells attached to injectable PLGA spheres. Biochem Biophys Res Commun 348:386–392

Lee WC, Sepulveda JL, Rubin JP, Marra KG (2008) Cardiomyogenic differentiation potential of human adipose precursor cells. Int J Cardiol 133:399–401

Liu Y, Song J, Liu W, Wan Y, Chen X, Hu C (2003) Growth and differentiation of rat bone marrow stromal cells: does 5-azacytidine trigger their cardiomyogenic differentiation? Cardiovasc Res 58:460–468

Makino S, Fukuda K, Miyoshi S, Konishi F, Kodama H, Pan J, Sano M, Takahashi T, Hori S, Abe H, Hata J, Umezawa A, Ogawa S (1999) Cardiomyocytes can be generated from marrow stromal cells in vitro. J Clin Invest 103:697–705

Miyahara Y, Nagaya N, Kataoka M, Yanagawa B, Tanaka K, Hao H, Ishino K, Ishida H, Shimizu T, Kangawa K, Sano S, Okano T, Kitamura S, Mori H (2006) Monolayered mesenchymal stem cells repair scarred myocardium after myocardial infarction. Nat Med 12:459–465

Murry CE, Reinecke H, Pabon LM (2006) Regeneration gaps: observations on stem cells and cardiac repair. J Am Coll Cardiol 47:1777–1785

Nakagami H, Morishita R, Maeda K, Kikuchi Y, Ogihara T, Kaneda Y (2006) Adipose tissue-derived stromal cells as a novel option for regenerative cell therapy. J Atheroscler Thromb 13:77–81

Olivetti G, Capasso JM, Sonnenblick EH, Anversa P (1990) Side-to-side slippage of myocytes participates in ventricular wall remodeling acutely after myocardial infarction in rats. Circ Res 67:23–34

Orlic D, Kajstura J, Chimenti S, Jakoniuk I, Anderson SM, Li B, Pickel J, McKay R, Nadal-Ginard B, Bodine DM, Leri A, Anversa P (2001) Bone marrow cells regenerate infarcted myocardium. Nature 410:701–705

Oyama T, Nagai T, Wada H, Naito AT, Matsuura K, Iwanaga K, Takahashi T, Goto M, Mikami Y, Yasuda N, Akazawa H, Uezumi A, Takeda S, Komuro I (2007) Cardiac side population cells have a potential to migrate and differentiate into cardiomyocytes in vitro and in vivo. J Cell Biol 176:329–341

Planat-Benard V, Menard C, Andre M, Puceat M, Perez A, Garcia-Verdugo JM, Penicaud L, Casteilla L (2004a) Spontaneous cardiomyocyte differentiation from adipose tissue stroma cells. Circ Res 94:223–229

Planat-Benard V, Silvestre JS, Cousin B, Andre M, Nibbelink M, Tamarat R, Clergue M, Manneville C, Saillan-Barreau C, Duriez M, Tedgui A, Levy B, Pénicaud L, Casteilla L (2004b) Plasticity of human adipose lineage cells toward endothelial cells: physiological and therapeutic perspectives. Circulation 109:656–663

Rangappa S, Entwistle JW, Wechsler AS, Kresh JY (2003) Cardiomyocyte-mediated contact programs human mesenchymal stem cells to express cardiogenic phenotype. J Thorac Cardiovasc Surg 126:124–132

Shim WS, Jiang S, Wong P, Tan J, Chua YL, Tan YS, Sin YK, Lim CH, Chua T, Teh M, Liu TC, Sim E (2004) Ex vivo differentiation of human adult bone marrow stem cells into cardiomyocyte-like cells. Biochem Biophys Res Commun 324:481–488

Takahashi T, Lord B, Schulze PC, Fryer RM, Sarang SS, Gullans SR, Lee RT (2003) Ascorbic acid enhances differentiation of embryonic stem cells into cardiac myocytes. Circulation 107:1912–1916

The-American-Society-for-Aesthetic-Plastic-Surgery (2008) Liposuction turns 20. http://www.surgery.org/media/news-releases/liposuction-turns-20

Tomita S, Li RK, Weisel RD, Mickle DA, Kim EJ, Sakai T, Jia ZQ (1999) Autologous transplantation of bone marrow cells improves damaged heart function. Circulation 100:II247–II256

Wang T, Xu Z, Jiang W, Ma A (2006) Cell-to-cell contact induces mesenchymal stem cell to differentiate into cardiomyocyte and smooth muscle cell. Int J Cardiol 109:74–81

Zhang FB, Li L, Fang B, Zhu DL, Yang HT, Gao PJ (2005) Passage-restricted differentiation potential of mesenchymal stem cells into cardiomyocyte-like cells. Biochem Biophys Res Commun 336:784–92

Zuk PA, Zhu M, Mizuno H, Huang J, Futrell JW, Katz AJ, Benhaim P, Lorenz HP, Hedrick MH (2001) Multilineage cells from human adipose tissue: implications for cell-based therapies. Tissue Eng 7:211–228

Chapter 29

Mesenchymal Stem Cells and Mesenchymal-Derived Endothelial Cells: Repair of Bone Defects

Jian Zhou and Jian Dong

Abstract It is a major clinical challenge for reconstructive surgeons to repair the bone defects caused by trauma, infection, tumor resection and other reasons. Bone tissue engineering is a promising method for repairing bone defects, and mesenchymal stem cells (MSCs) from adult tissues are an attractive stem cell source for bone tissue engineering. The vascularization is critical for the performance of a tissue-engineered bone. Endothelial cells (ECs) can be used to promote vascularization in the tissue-engineered bone since transplanted ECs can create a blood vessel network in the graft before implantation. This blood vessel network connects to the host vasculature, thus establishing a vascular supply much faster. MSCs and ECs can accelerate the vascularization of the tissue-engineered bone and enhance the effectiveness of osteogenesis by complementing the functions of each other.

Keywords Autogenous bone grafts · Mesenchymal stem cells · Endothelial cells · Extracellular matrix · HUVEC · Mononuclear cells (MNCs)

Introduction

It is a major clinical challenge for orthopedic surgeons to manage the segmental bone defects caused by trauma, infection, tumor resection and other reasons.

Autogenous bone grafts are considered as the gold standard as repair material. However, autogenous bone grafts have limitations, such as the requirement of additional surgical procedure, the limited amount and size, and the associated donor site morbidities. Bone tissue engineering, as one of the most promising alternative approach, has been widely used in developing biological bone substitutes, which restore and maintain bone tissue function. Mesenchymal stem cells (MSCs) from adult tissues are an attractive source of stem cells for bone tissue engineering (Kim et al., 2005). MSCs are characterized as undifferentiated and self-renewable cells with a high proliferative capacity, and they possess a mesodermal differentiation potential. These cells have been used to generate tissue-engineered bone in a combination with three-dimensional (3-D) porous biomaterial carriers. After implantation, the tissue-engineered bone undergoes osteogenesis and contributes to the direct repair of a number of site-specific bone defects. However, the clinical application of bone tissue engineering is still restricted, and more and more researches have demonstrated that the vascularization is the key factor (Kawamura et al., 2006). When the tissue-engineered bone is implanted, MSCs have a limited capacity either in uptaking substrate molecules, including oxygen, glucose and amino acids, or in clearing byproducts of metabolism. MSCs can die quickly because of insufficient nutrition and hypoxia if the blood supply is not established in time. Therefore, the rate and range of vascular growth determine the efficiency of new bone formation. Several strategies for enhancing vascularization have been extensively investigated (Lovett et al., 2009). Regardless of the approach adopted to accelerate vascularization, endothelial cells (ECs) are involved in all of these strategies directly or indirectly.

J. Dong (✉)
Department of Orthopaedic Surgery, Zhongshan Hospital,
Fudan University, Shanghai 200032, China
e-mail: Dong.jian@zs-hospital.sh.cn

In our present review, we focused on the application of MSCs and Mesenchymal-derived ECs in the repair of bone defects.

Mesenchymal Stem Cells

MSCs are first described by Friedenstein, which form the units of fibroblasts (Friedenstein et al., 1966). MSCs are isolated due to their capacity to adhere to plastic culture flasks and then to expand via colony forming unit-fibroblasts. Furthermore, they possess the potential to differentiate into bone, cartilage, adipose and muscle. To date, MSCs have been isolated from bone marrow of a variety of mammalian species, including humans (Ouyang et al., 2004), as well as other tissues including blood, adipose tissue, trabecular bone, umbilical cord blood and placenta. Bone marrow, umbilical cord blood, muscle and adipose tissue are the most common sources for MSCs used in bone tissue engineering (Seong et al., 2010). In order to differentiate MSCs into osteogenic lineage in vitro, it is necessary to supplement the cell growth medium with specific compounds, including β-glycerophosphate, ascorbic acid and dexamethasone. In addition to those commonly used osteogenic supplements, it has been reported that other exogenic factors, such as recombinant human BMP-2 (rhBMP-2) (Yamagiwa et al., 2001), parathyroid hormone (PTH)-related peptide (Miao et al., 2001) and FK506 (Dai et al., 2008) can be used to facilitate osteogenic proliferation and MSCs differentiation in both in vitro and in vivo.

Currently, autologous bone graft is the main therapy in repairing the site-specific bone defect. However, it is restricted by donor site morbidity and limited availability. Allografts have also been applied but accompanying with limited supply and increased the risk of disease transmission. Bone tissue engineering is a promising alternative approach for bone regeneration. MSCs have been seeded on 3-D porous biomaterials, and they undergo osteogenesis and contribute to the direct repair of bone defects after implantation. These biomaterials include hydroxyapatite and tricalcium phosphate ceramics, synthetic polymers consisting of polyglycolic and polylactic acid, and natural polymers, such as silk fibroin and demineralized bone composites. Ideal synthetic scaffold must be capable of providing temporary mechanical support to the affected area, and it contains a porous architecture and is made from biocompatible materials with controlled biodegradability or bioresorbability, osteoinduction, osteointegration (Mistry and Mikos, 2005). The 3-D scaffolds greatly improve the efficiency of tissue regeneration of bone. The porosity of the scaffolds enhances the conductivity for cells. Furthermore, the culture medium containing growth factors promotes the proliferation and distribution of cells through the connected pores of the scaffolds, and accelerates the degradation of biomaterials. However, not many cells in the inner parts of the scaffolds are found as anticipated, and the regenerated tissue only presents in the superficial layer of the scaffolds. In addition, cell distribution throughout the scaffolds is far from uniform, and few cells are found in the center area of the scaffolds (Roh et al., 2007). Various methods have been investigated to improve cell seeding efficiency and uniform distribution, including perfusion, centrifugation, low pressure and the combination of these methods.

Two primary tissue engineering strategies using MSCs in scaffolds have been applied as the most promising approaches (Langer and Vacanti, 1993). First, MSCs have been loaded into the scaffolds in vitro, and then the cell-scaffold composites are implanted after a short incubation to insure attachment (Solchaga et al., 2000). Second, MSCs are isolated, expanded *ex vivo* and seeded onto a scaffold before implantation, and then the cell-scaffold composites are incubated in differentiation medium to stimulate MSCs progression into an osteogenic lineage. After 7–14 days, extracellular matrix (ECM) is allowed to produce on the scaffold, and finally it is implanted into the osseous defects (Ohgushi et al., 2005). In order to promote the rapid development of cell-scaffold composite, a variety of novel *ex vivo* culture techniques have been developed, which promote both MSC osteogenic differentiation and bonelike matrix deposition in vitro before in vivo incorporation. Protein therapy, gene therapy and bioreactor systems are the three predominant in vitro culture techniques utilized in bone tissue engineering. Protein therapy has demonstrated the most practical promise, mainly incorporating osteoinductive growth factors, such as bone morphogenetic proteins (Bessa et al., 2008), transforming growth factor beta-1 (Sun et al., 2003) and transforming growth factor beta-2 (Moursi et al., 2003). Although the conjunction of signaling molecules with a scaffold is a very promising tool in bone tissue engineering, the requirement of large amount instable protein is its main limitation. Gene therapy aims to eliminate problems from direct protein therapy by genetically modifying cells to produce an increased amount of selective protein in a sustained manner in vivo or *ex vivo*. Genetically modified MSCs are seeded and cultured on a scaffold in vitro before implantation. The 3-D porous scaffolds seeded with MSCs producing osteogenic proteins have been tested in large animal models, and promising results have been obtained (Cancedda et al., 2007). Various bioreactors, including spinner flasks (Meinel et al., 2004), rotating vessels (Qiu et al., 1998), perfusion systems (Sikavitsas et al., 2003) and four-point bending systems (Mauney et al., 2004), have been utilized in improving the in vitro culture conditions. Consequently, it promotes the proliferation and osteogenic differentiation of scaffold-incorporated MSCs before implantation, leading to improved structure and function of the engineered tissue.

Mesenchymal-Derived Endothelial Cells

Bone tissue engineering with MSCs seeded on 3-D porous scaffolds has been tested in animal models, and promising results have been obtained. However, its clinical application remains limited. Within the body, most cells locate no more than 100 μm from the nearest capillary, and sufficient diffusion of oxygen, nutrients and waste products can be provided to support and maintain viable tissue with this distance (Lee et al., 2006). After MSCs-scaffolds composite implantation, if the blood supply is not established in time, nutrient transport only supplies the cells on the superficial area of scaffold. Therefore, those cells growing in the center of the construct die quickly due to the insufficient nutrition and hypoxia. There is a strong association between bone formation and angiogenesis in bone development, healing and in formation of tissue-engineered bone (Akita et al., 2004). It has been identified that poor vascularization in the MSCs-scaffolds composite is the culprit for implant failure, and it is the major challenge in current bone tissue engineering.

Several strategies have been employed for enhancing vascularization in the tissue-engineered bone, including scaffold design, angiogenic factor delivery, in vivo prevascularization and in vitro prevascularization (Santos and Reis, 2010). Regardless of the approach adopted to accelerate vascularization, ECs are involved in all of these strategies directly or indirectly. ECs can be used to promote vascularization in the tissue-engineered bone since transplanted ECs can create a blood vessel network in the graft before implantation. This blood vessel network connects to the host vasculature, thus establishing a vascular supply much faster (Kannan et al., 2005). Besides their contribution to better vascularization and bone graft survival, ECs support osteogenesis. Co-culture of ECs and MSCs has a positive influence on osteogenic differentiation and bone formation (Fedorovich et al., 2010). Three types of ECs have been utilized in promoting vascularization in tissue engineering, including mature ECs, endothelial progenitor cells (EPCs) and MSCs-derived ECs.

Mature ECs can be isolated from a great variety of sources, such as the umbilical cord, kidney vascular, skin, fat tissue and saphenous vein. Rouwkema et al. (Rouwkema et al., 2006) has reported that a 3-D prevascular network is found within 10 days from the in vitro co-culture of human umbilical vein ECs (HUVECs) with human MSCs. Furthermore, the pre-vascular network develops further, and structures including lumen can be seen regularly upon implantation. Sun et al. (2007) has reported a co-culture of rat bone marrow MSCs and kidney vascular ECs (VEC) with polylactide-glycolic acid scaffolds. in vivo implantation of MSCs and VEC co-culture into rats results in a pre-vascular network-like structure. These structures develop into vascularized tissue and increase the amount and size of the new bone compared with the control group. These results suggest that mature ECs can efficiently stimulate the in vitro proliferation and differentiation of osteoblast-like cells and promote osteogenesis. Moreover, mature ECs can form a 3-D pre-vascular network in vitro in the bone tissue engineering setting. However, the low availability and proliferation capacity are the major drawbacks of using these cells (Kim and Von Recum, 2008).

If one wants to implement in vitro prevascularization in clinical applications, sufficient ECs should be readily isolated from adult patients within an acceptable time frame. An alternative source of autologous ECs to promote vascularization in tissue engineering is EPCs. EPCs can be identified through three cell markers (CD133, CD34 and vascular endothelial growth factor receptor 2), and they are enriched from mononuclear cells (MNCs) of bone marrow, peripheral blood and umbilical cord blood. EPCs are highly proliferative and exhibit a stable endothelial phenotype. Yu et al. (Yu et al., 2009) co-seeded EC-derived EPCs and MSCs in the polycaprolactone-hydroxyapatite scaffolds. They found a widely distributed capillary network and improved osteogenesis. Pre-seeding scaffold with EPCs can effectively promote neovascularization in grafts, prevent the ischemic necrosis, and improve osteogenesis.

If MSCs can be induced to differentiate into ECs, these ECs derived from this cell source are ideal for prevascularized bone tissue engineering. It suggests that a prevascularized bone tissue engineering construct can be prepared from a single, easily accessible, bone marrow biopsy. This exciting concept has recently been demonstrated in many researches (Liu et al., 2007). Oswald et al. (Oswald et al., 2004) induced MSCs to differentiate into ECs and showed that these ECs have more proliferative potential than the terminally differentiated ECs, and they form an angiogenic microenvironment with other bone marrow cells. Valarmathi et al. (Valarmathi et al., 2008) seeded bone marrow-derived MSCs onto a 3-D tubular scaffold engineered from aligned type I collagen strands and cultured them in osteogenic medium. They found that the MSCs simultaneously mature and differentiate into osteoblastic and vascular cell lineages. Zhou et al. (2010) constructed a vascularized tissue-engineered bone with MSCs and MSC-derived ECs co-cultured in porous β-tricalcium phosphate ceramic (β-TCP), and they repaired critical sized ulnar defects in the rabbit with this vascularized tissue-engineered bone. They found that the rabbits treated with vascularized tissue-engineered bone demonstrate more extensive osteogenesis and good vascularization. Therefore, one effective approach to promote repair of bone defects is the vascularized tissue-engineered bone constructed by co-culture of MSCs and MSC-derived ECs in porous scaffold.

References

Akita S, Tamai N, Myoui A, Nishikawa M, Kaito T, Takaoka K, Yoshikawa H (2004) Capillary vessel network integration by inserting a vascular pedicle enhances bone formation in tissue-engineered bone using interconnected porous hydroxyapatite ceramics. Tissue Eng 10:789–795

Bessa PC, Casal M, Reis RL (2008) Bone morphogenetic proteins in tissue engineering: the road from the laboratory to the clinic, part I (basic concepts). J Tissue Eng Regen Med 2:1–13

Cancedda R, Giannoni P, Mastrogiacomo M (2007) A tissue engineering approach to bone repair in large animal models and in clinical practice. Biomaterials 28:4240–4250

Dai WD, Dong J, Fang TL, Uemura T (2008) Stimulation of osteogenic activity in mesenchymal stem cells by FK506. J Biomed Mater Res A 86A:235–243

Fedorovich NE, Haverslag RT, Dhert WJA, Alblas J (2010) The role of endothelial progenitor cells in prevascularized bone tissue engineering: development of heterogeneous constructs. Tissue Eng Part A 16:2355–2367

Friedenstein AJ, Shapiro-Piatetzky II, Petrakova KV (1966) Osteogenesis in transplants of bone marrow cells. J Embryol Exp Morphol 16:381

Kannan RY, Salacinski HJ, Sales K, Butler P, Seifalian AM (2005) The roles of tissue engineering and vascularizationin the development of micro-vascular networks: a review. Biomaterials 26:1857–1875

Kawamura K, Yajima H, Ohgushi H, Tomita Y, Kobata Y, Shigematsu K, Takakura Y (2006) Experimental study of vascularized tissue-engineered bone grafts. Plast Reconstr Surg 117:1471–1479

Kim H, Suh H, Jo SA, Kim HW, Lee JM, Kim EH, Reinwald Y, Park SH, Min BH, Jo I (2005) In vivo bone formation by human marrow stromal cells in biodegradable scaffolds that release dexamethasone and ascorbate-2-phosphate. Biochem Biophys Res Commun 332:1053–1060

Kim S, Von Recum H (2008) Endothelial stem cells and precursors for tissue engineering: cell source, differentiation, selection, and application. Tissue Eng Part B Rev 14: 133–147

Langer R, Vacanti JP (1993) Tissue engineering. Science 260:920–926

Lee SH, Coger RN, Clemens MG (2006) Antioxidant functionality in hepatocytes using the enhanced collagen extracellular matrix under different oxygen tensions. Tissue Eng 12: 2825–2834

Liu JW, Dunoyer-Geindre S, Serre-Beinier V, Mai G, Lambert JF, Fish RJ, Pernod G, Buehler L, Bounameaux H, Kruithof EK (2007) Characterization of endothelial-like cells derived from human mesenchymal stem cells. J Thromb Haemost 5:826–834

Lovett M, Lee K, Edwards A, Kaplan DL (2009) Vascularization strategies for tissue engineering. Tissue Eng Part B 15: 353–370

Mauney JR, Sjostorms S, Blumberg J, Horan R, O'Leary JP, Vunjak-Novakovic G, Volloch V, Kaplan DL (2004) Mechanical stimulation promotes osteogenic differentiation of human bone marrow stromal cells on 3-D partially demineralized bone scaffolds in vitro. Calcif Tissue Int 74: 458–468

Meinel L, Karageorgiou V, Fajardo R, Snyder B, Shinde-Patil V, Zichner L, Kaplan D, Langer R, Vunjak-Novakovic G (2004) Bone tissue engineering using human mesenchymal stem cells: effects of scaffold material and medium flow. Ann Biomed Eng 32:112–122

Miao D, Tong XK, Chan GK, Panda D, McPherson PS, Goltzman D (2001) Parathyroid hormone-related peptide stimulates osteogenic cell proliferation through protein kinase C activation of the ras/mitogen-activated protein kinase signaling pathway. J Biol Chem 276:32204–32213

Mistry AS, Mikos AG (2005) Tissue engineering strategies for boneregeneration. Adv Biochem Eng Biotechnol 94:1–22

Moursi AM, Winnard PL, Fryer D, Mooney MP (2003) Delivery of transforming growth factor-beta2-perturbing antibody in a collagen vehicle inhibits cranial suture fusion in calvarial organ culture. Cleft Palate Craniofac J 40:225–232

Ohgushi H, Kotobuki N, Funaoka H, Machida H, Hirose M, Tanaka Y, Takakura Y (2005) Tissue engineered ceramic artifical joint-ex vivo osteogenic differentiation of patient mesenchymal cells on total ankel joints for treatment of osteoarthritis. Biomaterials 26:4654–4661

Oswald J, Boxberger S, Jorgensen B, Feldmann S, Ehninger G, Bornhauser M, Werner C (2004) Mesenchymal stem cells can be differentiated into endothelial cells in vitro. Stem Cells 22:377–384

Ouyang HW, Goh JC, Lee EH (2004) Use of bone marrow stromal cells for tendon graft-to-bone healing: histological and immunohistochemical studies in a rabbit model. Am J Sports Med 32:321–327

Qiu Q, Ducheyne P, Gao H, Ayyaswamy P (1998) Formation and differentiation of three-dimensional rat marrow stromal cell culture on microcarriers in a rotating wall vessel. Tissue Eng 4:19–34

Roh JD, Nelson GN, Udelsman BV, Brennan MP, Lockhart B, Fong PM, Lopez-Soler RI, Saltzman WM, Breuer CK (2007) Centrifugal seeding increases seeding efficiency and cellular distribution of bone marrow stromal cells in porous biodegradable scaffolds. Tissue Eng 13:2743–2749

Rouwkema J, De Boer J, Van Blitterswijk CA (2006) Endothelial cells assemble into a 3-dimensional prevascular network in a bone tissue engineering construct. Tissue Eng 12:2685–2693

Santos MI, Reis RL (2010) Vascularization in bone tissue engineering: physiology, current strategies, major hurdles and future challenges. Macromol Biosci 10:12–27

Seong JM, Park JH, Kwon IK, Mantalaris A, Hwang YS (2010) Stem cells in bone tissue engineering. Biomed Mater 5:1–15

Sikavitsas VI, Bancroft GN, Holtorf HL, Jansen JA, Mikos AG (2003) Mineralized matrix deposition by marrow stromal osteoblasts in 3D perfusion culture increases with increasing fluid shear forces. Proc Natl Acad Sci USA 100: 14683–14688

Solchaga LA, Yoo JU, Lundberg M, Dennis JE, Huibregtse BA, Goldberg VM, Caplan AI (2000) Hyaluronan-based polymers in the treatment of osteochondral defects. J Orthop Res 18:773–780

Sun HC, Qu Z, Guo Y, Zang GX, Yang B (2007) In vitro and in vivo effects of rat kidney vascular endothelial cells on osteogenesis of rat bone marrow mesenchymal stem cells growing on polylactide-glycoli acid (PLGA) scaffolds. Biomed Eng Online 6:41

Sun JS, Lin FH, Wang YJ, Huang YC, Chueh SC, Hsu FY (2003) Collagen-hydroxyapatite/tricalciumphosphate microspheres as a delivery system for recombinant human transforming growth factorbeta1. Artif Organs 27:605–612

Valarmathi MT, Yost MJ, Goodwin RL, Potts JD (2008) A three-dimensional tubular scaffold that modulates the osteogenic and vasculogenic differentiation of rat bone marrow stromal cells. Tissue Eng 14:491–U17

Yamagiwa H, Endo N, Tokunaga K, Hayami T, Hatano H, Takahashi HE (2001) In vivo bone-forming capacity of human bone marrow-derived stromal cells is stimulated by recombinant human bone morphogenetic progein-2. J Bone Miner Metab 19:20–28

Yu HY, VandeVord PJ, Mao L, Matthew HW, Wooley PH, Yang SY (2009) Improved tissue-engineered bone regeneration by endothelial cell mediated vascularization. Biomaterials 30:508–517

Zhou J, Lin H, Fang TL, Li XL, Dai WD, Uemura T, Dong J (2010) The repair of large segmental bone defects in the rabbit with vascularized tissue engineered bone. Biomaterials 31:1171–1179

Chapter 30

Omentum in the Repair of Injured Tissue: Evidence for Omental Stem Cells

Ignacio García-Gómez

Abstract The omentum is a fatty peritoneal fold with an apron-like structure that extends from the greater curvature of the stomach to cover most abdominal organs. Its unique biological properties in healing and regeneration have long been noted in surgical practice. In particular, the use of the omentum in a number of pathological conditions has demonstrated its capacity to revascularize ischemic areas, to absorb large amounts of edema fluids and to limit the formation of scar tissue at the site of injury. However, despite its clinical importance, the mechanisms underlying its role in healing and regeneration remain poorly understood. The current knowledge of stem cells could shed some light on these reparative properties of the omentum, first observed by surgeons a relatively long time ago, as recent studies provide evidence for the presence of stem cells in omentum. This fact has drawn attention to the omentum as a possible source of stem cells for use in cell therapies. For this purpose it is necessary to develop a deeper understanding of omentum biology and to learn from the results obtained using the omentum in surgical practice.

Keywords Omentum · Gastroepiploic arteries · Moyamoya disease · Amyloid plaques · Arachnoid membrane · Lumbosacral arachnoiditis · GM-CSF

I. García-Gómez (✉)
Laboratory of Cell Therapy, Autonoma University-La Paz University Hospital (idiPAZ), P.C. 28046, Madrid, Spain
e-mail: biogarc@yahoo.es

Introduction

Stem cell research in general has generated growing optimism during the last decade based on the promising results obtained in in vitro and in vivo studies. However, the potential of the omentum as a source of adult stem cells remains understudied even though its regenerative properties have been exploited by surgeons for over a century. For a long time the omentum was widely thought to have no specific functions. Nonetheless, a few surgeons recognized its remarkable ability to facilitate wound healing and prevent infections after surgical procedures. During the 19th century, De Lamballe, who was physician to Napoleon III, was the first to draw attention to the greater omentum as an interesting structure. He reported that the omentum formed adhesions around injured bowels and postulated that it prevented the development of peritonitis in injured soldiers (Liebermann-Meffert, 2000). Since that early description, many surgeons have taken advantage of the unique biological properties of the omentum.

In 1908, the British surgeon Morison called the omentum "the policeman of the abdomen" in recognition of its properties to protect the abdominal cavity against infection. There followed several reports of detaching the omentum to use it as a piece of autologous tissue for vesicovaginal fistula repair or as a source of new blood vessels to revascularize areas damaged by ischemia (O'Shaughnessy, 1937). Later in 1948, Cannaday tailored the omentum into a long intact pedicle, by cutting its attachment to the stomach without disrupting its vascular supply, for distant reconstruction and revascularization using microsurgical techniques (Cannaday, 1948). Indeed, this was a natural progression, with the development of better reconstructive techniques. The omental pedicle is used extensively for application to various different sites for treating large ischemic defects. Further development of this procedure has allowed the omental pedicle to be used in novel ways, such as, for the treatment of traumatic spinal cord injuries and chronic brain disorders (Goldsmith, 2007, 2009).

Although these benefits of omental transposition to various areas of the body are well documented, the mechanisms underlying its role in healing and regeneration remain poorly understood. To date, it is known that the native omentum contains high concentrations of vascular endothelial growth factor (VEGF) and basic fibroblast growth factor (bFGF) and even higher levels of these growth factors are induced when the omentum is activated by injury (Zhang et al., 1997). Notably, the omentum was found to contain a 10- to 100-fold higher concentration of VEGF than other adult tissues (Litbarg et al., 2007). Moreover, in recent years it has been reported that large amounts of these angiogenic growth factors and other chemotactic factors are produced due to the presence of stem cells in the omentum (Singh et al., 2008). These factors promote cell growth and recruit other progenitor cells in order to bring about repair and regeneration. This new evidence of stem cells in the omentum opens the possibility of using the omentum as a source of stem cells for regenerative medicine. Indeed, the use of omentum in tissue engineering has been suggested as an in vivo culture system and to generate bioengineered tissue with specific attributes, such as that used for bypass grafts (Suh et al., 2004; Song et al., 2010). As we move towards a broader use of omentum in stem cell therapy, a deeper understanding of the morphology, physiology and cellular composition of this tissue is needed.

Omentum Anatomy, Structure and Embryology Overview

The omentum is a visceral, peritoneal fold that is divided into the lesser omentum and the greater omentum. The greater omentum arises from the greater curvature of the stomach. It crosses the transverse colon, to which it is attached and descends in front of the viscera down to the pubic symphysis. The anterior and posterior surfaces face the parietal and visceral peritoneum respectively. On the right side, the lesser omentum hangs from the pyloric region, duodenum, anterior surface of the pancreas, and ascending colon to form the hepatogastric ligament and a mesentery for the gallbladder. On the left side, the greater omentum extends to the fundus, in some cases up to the intra-abdominal esophagus. It forms the gastrosplenic ligament between the stomach and spleen, which attaches the spleen to the posterior abdominal wall. The gastrocolic ligament, also usually considered part of the greater omentum, connects the stomach to colon. Dorsal to this ligament and to the stomach lies the omental bursa. This cavity communicates through the epiploic foramen (also known as the foramen of Winslow) with the main peritoneal cavity. The surface area of the omentum has been found to vary from 300 to 500 cm^2, its length ranging from 14 to 36 cm in length and width from 20 to 46 cm. There is no clear relationship between the weight of the patient and that of the omentum. However, obese individuals may have extensive omental fat deposits (Liebermann-Meffert, 2000).

Human and murine omenta have a similar structure and both are composed of two structurally distinct tissue types: thin translucent membranes and adipose-rich areas. The translucent region is poorly vascularized and is composed of two closely-spaced mesothelial cell layers, which do not appear to rest on a basement membrane but enclose collagen fibers and occasional fibroblast-like cells. These translucent membranes are randomly arranged in omentum as fenestrations which make it resemble a net-like mesh. In contrast, the adipose-rich area is predominately composed of adipocytes embedded in well-vascularized connective tissue. This region of the omentum is covered by a single mesothelial cell layer that does have a basement membrane but is interrupted by opaque patches called "milky spots" (Wilkosz et al., 2005). These milky spots play a role in the clearance of particles, bacteria, and tumor cells from the peritoneal cavity. The milky spots contain numerous macrophages, mast cells, and lymphocyte aggregates, and are seems to be the main source of peritoneal macrophages (Krist et al., 1997). It has been found that the number of milky spots is highest in infancy and gradually decreases with age, while their size ranges between microscopic and macroscopic dimensions but increases significantly under pathological conditions in the abdominal cavity (i.e., a hypertrophic response to inflammatory stimuli);

in this way, it seems that the milky spots becomes activated (Shimotsuma et al., 1989).

The arterial vascularization of the omentum is provided by the right and left gastroepiploic arteries. Both receive their blood supply from the celiac trunk, the left by the splenic artery and the right by the gastroduodenal artery. The two gastroepiploic arteries wind around the greater curvature of the stomach and decrease in diameter as gastric and epiploic vessels branch off. Finally, the gastroepiploic arteries anastomose to the left of the midline of the greater curvature of the stomach on the exterior or interior of the gastric wall forming an arterial arcade. They descend through the trabecula mostly at right angles to the greater curvature and bifurcate close to the omental margin, where they eventually anastomose through small branches with adjacent epiploic vessels. The venous drainage of the omentum parallels the arterial supply and drains into the portal system. On the other hand, the lymphatics of the omentum form a delicate, interconnecting network. The lymph channels begin as blind endothelial sacculations within the milky spots or as a network of endothelial channels within the omental stroma. Subsequently, they converge to form collecting vessels that contain valves but the overall increase in their caliber is relatively small. Though in the omentum itself there do not seem to be any true lymph nodes, these vessels course laterally in the trabeculae and drain to the right towards the subpyloric lymph nodes and to the left towards the splenic lymph nodes (Liebermann-Meffert, 2000).

The development of the omentum is closely related to adjacent structures, in particular the stomach and spleen. In most modern embryology textbooks the greater omentum is said to be of mesodermal origin and develops following rotation of the stomach and subsequent folding and fusion of the dorsal mesentery. However, there are studies of the embryology of the stomach which contradict this traditional picture (Liebermann-Meffert, 2000). In humans, primitive omental tissue can be distinguished from the stomach as early as the 7th or 8th week of gestation by cell criteria. Then the mesenchymal cells between the stomach and the caudal portion of the spleen become slightly elongated and arrange to form a vessel-containing bulge. Subsequently, the omentum continues in the shape of a small, delicate fringe along the enlarged greater curvature of the stomach. In the 12th to 14th week of gestation, this omental fringe slightly increases in length but is still floating freely in the abdominal cavity. At the end of this stage, the omentum fuses with the transverse colon close to the hepatic flexure, the region of the spleen, and in the middle of the transverse colon. In full-term newborns, the omentum is usually in the form of a thin, transparent membrane with no fat deposits covering a quarter of the small bowel but already with the specific vascular pattern of adults (Liebermann-Meffert, 2000). Milky spots appear in the 26th week of gestation, are well developed at birth, reach their maximum number at the end of the first year of life, and tend to decrease in number with age (Shimotsuma et al., 1989). At 3 or 4 months of age, the greater omentum of the infant covers two-thirds of the small bowel and contains small islands of fatty tissue where the vessels branch. At 5 years of age, most of the intestines are covered by the omentum, which also extends beyond the flexures of the colon. The fat deposits form large, confluent plaques along the vessels, leaving thin translucent membranes. By age 11, the omentum resembles that of adults (Liebermann-Meffert, 2000).

The Omentum in Reparative Medicine: Surgical Applications

The applications of the omentum in reparative medicine have long been noted. Indeed, this tissue has been widely used in surgical practice in particular for the procedure of free omental transfer or to provide a lengthened and intact pedicle, an operation known as omental transposition (OT). The procedure involves the separation of omental connections to the transverse colon and the omentum's proximal attachments to the greater curvature of the stomach, leaving the gastroepiploic vessels intact within the omental apron. After the left gastroepiploic vessels are divided, the blood supply of the omental apron comes entirely from the right gastric and right gastroepiploic vessels. The omental apron is then surgically tailored to create a long pedicle with arterial and venous connections remaining intact. Importantly in this context, the omentum has the capacity to develop vascular connections with adjacent and subjacent tissues. Therefore, OT allows the omentum to deliver angiogenic and neurotrophic growth factors and stem cells, increasing the blood flow to any injured area of the body. The development of microvascular surgery, the introduction of new techniques in plastic surgery and organ reconstruction, and the possibility of harvesting the omentum as a vascular pedicle by laparoscopic techniques have presented promising new surgical possibilities. The omentum has been widely applied in surgery, in particular, in the fields of gastrointestinal, plastic and reconstructive, cardiothoracic, urological and genital, vascular and gynecological surgery (Alagumuthu et al., 2006). In addition, applications are being developed in neurosurgery for some pathological conditions; these are of special interest and will be described in more detail below.

Omental Placement on the Brain

The omentum has been placed on the human brain for a variety of pathological conditions. Some of the indications for this have included strokes, moyamoya disease, encephalitis, and Alzheimer's disease (AD). Placing the omentum on the brain has been shown to deliver large volumes of blood to the human brain over an extended period of time (Goldsmith et al., 1990). In moyamoya disease, the omentum develops multiple vascular vessels that penetrate into the brain, thus allowing an increase in cerebral blood flow which can account for the clinical improvement seen in these patients (Karasawa, 2010). Comparative clinical success has also been achieved by increasing cerebral blood flow in patients who have suffered a stroke. The penumbral cells surrounding a cerebral infarct remain neurophysiologically and neuroelectrically depressed but still remain viable. Therefore, increasing the blood flow and neurochemical factors by OT can lead to increased biological activity within the penumbral cells. This would be expected to include increased dendritic growth, greater synaptic activity and new nerve pathways that ultimately result in considerable neurological benefit. Of particular interest today is the use of the omentum in treating AD. There is a growing body of evidence suggesting that amyloid plaques are not the underlying cause of AD but rather that decreased cerebral blood flow may be the basis for the development of the disease (Goldsmith, 2007). For many years it has been thought that a decrease in cerebral blood flow in this disease is the result of neuronal degeneration. However, one might look at this in a different way; namely, that it is a decrease in cerebral blood flow which in turn causes neuronal degeneration. This concept has led to increasing interest in the idea that cerebral hypoperfusion could be the cause of the disease. Placing the omentum directly on the brain has been shown to increase cerebral blood flow and may be the reason why several studies have shown that OT to the brain is able to improve the cognitive ability of such patients (Shankle and Hara, 2010; Goldsmith, 2007).

Recently, in China several hundred cerebral palsy patients have been operated on for this condition by performing OT to the brain. The most common cause of cerebral palsy is oxygen deprivation associated with fetal distress during a difficult delivery. Oxygen deprivation at that time can result in lasting speech difficulties, decreased mental activity, and varying degrees of motor dysfunction. In addition to performing OT in order to increase cerebral blood flow, a further step in the operation is the partial detachment of the thickened arachnoid membrane which has been found in all cerebral palsy patients. The thickness of the arachnoid membrane seems to be related to the degree of oxygen deprivation at birth; the greater the anoxia, the thicker the membrane. Removing pieces of the constrictive arachnoid membrane combined with placing the omentum on the brain enables cerebral blood flow to be increased in a progressive and sustained manner. This has been found to result in improvement in a significant number of patients in terms of improvements in mental capacity, motor function, and speech, many years after the cerebral anoxia (Wu et al., 2010a).

Omental transposition to the brain also has been used for treating the sequelae of viral encephalitis. Epidemic encephalitis B, commonly called Japanese B encephalitis, is an acute inflammatory disease caused either by direct viral invasion of the brain or by hypersensitivity of the brain initiated by the virus. The sequalae usually involve movement, speech, and mental disorders. Until 1980 there was no known treatment for this disease but, recently, a Chinese group has been successful in treating the disease by transposing a pedicle graft of the omentum to the brain (Wu et al., 2010b). The degree of improvement seen in these patients appeared to be directly related to the degree of cerebral damage observed at surgery that had been caused by the previous viral infection. It is very interesting that many of the clinical improvements seen in these patients occurred within a few days following surgery even though their encephalitic attacks occurred many years earlier. The authors believe that this early improvement resulted from biochemical changes originating at the omental-cerebral interface.

Omental Placement on the Spinal Cord

Omental placement on the spinal cord has been used in traumatic spinal cord injury and for lumbosacral arachnoiditis. Placing the omentum on the spinal cord has the ability to absorb enormous amounts of edema fluids (Goldsmith et al., 1967) and limit scar tissue (Goldsmith et al., 1985). From the moment a spinal cord injury (SCI) occurs, there is post-traumatic edema and a deposition of blood at the injury site. This is the result of leakage through the porous endothelial lining of damaged capillaries located mainly in the central grey matter of the spinal cord. The mixture of edema fluid, blood and fibrinogen that is subsequently activated produces fibrin deposits which lead to post-injury scar formation (Goldsmith, 2009). It has been known since the time of Ramon y Cajal, over 100 years ago, that it is post-injury scar tissue which inhibits the ability of axons to grow through a scar. Consequently, the axons cannot make connections with critical neurological structures in the distal spinal cord. When the omentum is placed directly on an SCI site, a dynamic equilibrium appears to be established between the presence of edema and blood originating from the injured spinal cord and the known ability of the overlying omentum to absorb such material. The absorption of fibrinogen present in the blood limits the subsequent formation of scar tissue which normally develops within days following an SCI. These findings strongly suggest that the surgical treatment of a spinal cord injury should begin by omental placement on the SCI site as soon as it is clinically possible following an injury.

Omental placement on the spinal cord also has been used for the treatment of lumbosacral arachnoiditis. One of the most difficult orthopedic problems today is dealing with patients who have this condition, namely, inflammation of their arachnoid membrane in the lumbosacral region. Various forms of trauma can lead to this situation including, in addition to accidents, lumbar myelography, meningitis, and spinal anesthesia. All of these events may lead to the formation of fibrous arachnoid bands followed by calcium deposition around the cauda equina which results in varying degrees of ischemia. This hypoperfusion due to the scar tissue leads to pain in the area. When patients are later operated on to remove the scar, there can be temporary cessation of pain, but within a short period of time, scars reform and pain recurs. It is a vicious cycle: repeated operations always reveal further scar formation in the area to be removed, but repeated operations are always followed by subsequent scar reformation. A promising treatment for this condition appears to be the removal of scar tissue followed immediately by the application of an intact omental pedicle on the site of the cauda equina. The success of OT in patients with chronic arachnoiditis has been attributed to the ability of the omentum to prevent the recurrence of scar tissue (Ferguson et al., 2010).

Omental Stem Cells

The benefits observed using the omentum in surgical practice have shown its unique biological properties such as its capacity for revascularization, and its ability to absorb enormous amounts of edema fluids and to limit scar tissue formation after injury among others. The current development of stem cell research could shed some light on the role of omentum in healing and regeneration.

It is known that the stromal vascular fraction of subcutaneous adipose tissue is a source of mesenchymal stem cells (MSC) with the surface antigen expression pattern $CD73^+CD90^+CD105^+CD34^-CD45^-CD11b^-CD14^-CD19^-CD79a^-HLA-DR^-$ (Dominici et al., 2006). Since Zuk et al. demonstrated this in 2001 (Zuk et al., 2001), stem cell groups have become increasingly interested in fatty tissue. One of the main questions that researchers have asked is whether the different human fat depots are also a source of MSCs. However, it is to be noted that although omentum and subcutaneous adipose tissue are both fat depots, they are anatomically separate, differ in size, structure, and function, as well as their contribution to pathological conditions, such as metabolic syndrome. This is confirmed studying depot-specific human cell progenitors in terms of their distinct expression profiles and developmental gene patterns, and it can be concluded that fat is not a homogeneous organ (Tchkonia et al., 2007). The various fat depots appear to be, in effect, separate mini-organs.

Some studies have explored the possibility of human omentum being a potential source of MSCs with varying outcomes (van Harmelen et al., 2004; Maiorana et al., 2009; Baglioni et al., 2009). However, when the comparison between the stromal vascular fraction of human adipose tissue derived cells from subcutaneous and omental tissue is not focused only on MSCs, the presence of an undefined cell population has been reported, solely in omental adipose tissue, with the following surface antigen expression pattern CD34$^+$CD45$^-$CD90$^-$CD105$^-$CD146$^-$CD31$^-$ (Toyoda et al., 2009). A previous report has described an analogous CD34$^+$ stem cell population in human omentum with a spindle-like morphology and a high rate of proliferation in vitro (García-Gómez et al., 2005). An interesting characteristic of this CD34$^+$ population is its ability to synthesize angiogenic growth factors, such as bFGF and VEGF. The capacity to produce these factors confers to omental cells the potential to promote angiogenesis when implanted into a tissue by creating an environment that favors new vessel formation. This potential was demonstrated when these omental stem cells were loaded onto gelatin sponges and implanted subcutaneously into immunosuppressed Sprague-Dawley rats. The results observed in that study showed neovascularization in the area of the sponges and the localization of the CD34$^+$ omental stem cells in the endothelium of some neo-vessels (García-Gómez et al., 2005). Unfortunately, so far, there has been little research investigating the use of omental stem cells in humans.

It is important to remember that the omentum has the innate property of sensing injured sites in the abdominal cavity and of firmly adhering to them. It likewise reacts to foreign bodies present in the abdomen (Luijendijk et al., 1996). On sensing a foreign body, the omentum rapidly extends and expands encapsulating the object as if to protect the adjoining internal organs from coming into contact with it. Therefore, the study of this reaction to foreign bodies and the factors produced in the process might be relevant to understanding the way that omental fusion brings about healing and regeneration. Once the omentum becomes activated, it greatly increases in size and in mass (>20 fold increase) by producing new tissue that consists mainly of stromal and interstitial cells, and blood vessels. Fat cells in the omentum, which in the native state amount to 95% of the total tissue, decrease to less than 30%, with stromal cells representing more than 70% of the total omental mass. In this expanded state, there are large increases in the densities of blood vessels and lymphatic vessels, in blood volume, in the level of the angiogenesis factor VEGF, and in other growth and chemotactic factors in the omentum. An experimental study that mimicked the effects of intraperitoneal injury by injecting polydextran gel particles intraperitoneally (Litbarg et al., 2007) found that non-fat stromal cells in expanded omental tissue, especially those immediately surrounding the polydextran particles, express markers of stem cell activity, such as stromal-cell-derived factor (SDF-1α), chemokine receptor 4 (CXCR4), and Wilms' tumor antigen 1 (WT-1), and also express pluripotent embryonic markers, such as Nanog, Oct-4 and the stage-specific embryonic antigen 1 (SSEA-1) (Singh et al., 2008). The chemokines/chemokine receptor axis SDF-1α/CXCR-4 is particularly important in embryogenesis and tissue repair (Kayali et al., 2003). Specifically, SDF-1α, which usually occurs in developing and injured organs but not in adult tissues, is present in the milky spots of native omentum and, more abundantly, in activated omentum. The presence of SDF-1α may create an environment in which progenitor cells from injured tissue or bone marrow are attracted to the injured site. In accordance with this, another experimental study that reported the presence in the omentum of early bipotent hematopoietic progenitors throughout life, showed that omental stromal cells constitutively express IL-7, Flt3 ligand, granulocyte-macrophage colony stimulating factor (GM-CSF), macrophage colony stimulating factor (M-CSF), and SDF-1α and offer the required physical contact and growth stimulation to pro-B cells during the early stage of differentiation. Moreover, omental stromal cells are able to sustain long-term B lymphopoiesis from bone marrow progenitor cells (Pinho et al., 2005). Consistent with these reports, the omentum stroma, especially after its activation following injury, becomes a reservoir of stromal cells that express stem cell markers (SDF-1α, CXCR-4, WT-1, Nanog, Oct-4, SSEA-1). Currently, these omental stem cells from the omentum stroma have been cultured and continue to exhibit stem-cell like properties. When disperse 7-day activated omental tissue is placed in culture, cells that have originally clustered around the polydextran particles start to attach to the dish and multiply by day 4–5. The morphology and phenotype of these cells resemble that of smooth muscle cells in that they are positive for α-smooth muscle actin but negative for cytokeratin-17 (epithelial marker) and von Willebrand factor (endothelial marker). These cells synthesize VEGF at a rate 10–20 times higher than primary mesangial cells and glomerular epithelial cells in culture and retain the adult stem cell markers WT-1, CXCR4, and SDF-1α, Nanog and Oct-4 (Singh et al., 2008).

In in vivo experiments it has been shown that these omental stem cells specifically migrate to injured tissues. When they are injected in the vicinity of subcutaneous granulation tissue, they appear to migrate and integrate into the growing granulation tissue within 24 h. Indeed, when they are injected systemically into rats with unilateral ischemic injured kidney (3 days after injury), the cells migrate into the injured tubules and appear to attach to them, again suggesting their participation in the healing process (Singh et al., 2008).

In conclusion, the activation of the omentum by contact with injured tissue increases its content of stromal stem cells and of growth, angiogenesis and chemotactic factors, all of which promote the healing and regeneration of the injured tissue. The isolation and expansion of stromal stem cells derived from the omentum could be used to repair and possibly regenerate damaged tissue, and all this suggests that the omentum may well be a convenient source of adult stem cells.

References

Alagumuthu M, Das BB, Pattanayak SP, Rasananda M (2006) The omentum: a unique organ of exceptional versatility. Indian J Surg 68:136–141

Baglioni S, Francalanci M, Squecco R, Lombardi A, Cantini G, Angeli R, Gelmini S, Guasti D, Benvenuti S, Annunziato F, Bani D, Liotta F, Francini F, Perigli G, Serio M, Luconi M (2009) Characterization of human adult stem-cell populations isolated from visceral and subcutaneous adipose tissue. FASEB J 23:3494–3505

Cannaday J (1948) Some uses of undetached omentum in surgery. Am J Surg 76:502–505

Dominici M, Le Blanc K, Mueller I, Slaper-Cortenbach I, Marini F, Krause D, Deans R, Keating A, Prockop D, Horwitz E (2006) Minimal criteria for defining multipotent mesenchymal stromal cells. The International Society for Cellular Therapy position statement. Cytotherapy 8:315–317

Ferguson RL, Luken MG, Gettleman RA (2010) Pedicled omental lumbar grafts for lumbosacral adhesive arachnoiditis. In: sGoldsmith HS (ed) The omentum: basic research and clinical applications. Cine-Med, Woodbury, CT, pp 103–109

García-Gómez I, Goldsmith HS, Angulo J, Prados A, López-Hervás P, Cuevas B, Dujovny M, Cuevas P (2005) Angiogenic capacity of human omental stem cells. Neurol Res 27:807–811

Goldsmith HS (2007) Omental transposition in treatment of Alzheimer disease. J Am Coll Surg 205:800–804

Goldsmith HS (2009) Treatment of acute spinal cord injury by omental transposition: a new approach. J Am Coll Surg 208:289–292

Goldsmith HS, de los Santos R, Beattie EJ (1967) The relief of chronic lymphedema by omental transposition. Ann Surg 166:571–585

Goldsmith HS, Steward E, Duckett S (1985) Early application of pedicled omentum to the acutely traumatized spinal cord. Paraplegia 23:100–112

Goldsmith HS, Bacciu P, Cossu M, Pau A, Rodriguez G, Rosadini G, Ruju P, Viale ES, Turtas S, Viale GL (1990) Regional cerebral blood flow after omental transposition to the ischaemic brain in man. A five year follow-up study. Acta Neurochir (Wien) 106:145–152

Karasawa JTH (2010) Application of omental transplantation to moyamoya disease. In: Goldsmith HS (ed) The omentum: basic research and clinical applications. Cine-Med, Woodbury, CT, spp 111–127

Kayali AG, Van Gunst K, Campbell IL, Stotland A, Kritzik M, Liu G, Flodström-Tullberg M, Zhang YQ, Sarvetnick N (2003) The stromal cell-derived factor-1alpha/CXCR4 ligand-receptor axis is critical for progenitor survival and migration in the pancreas. J Cell Biol 163:859–869

Krist LFG, Koenen H, Calame W, van der Harten JJ, van der Linden JC, Eestermans IL, Meyer S, Beelen RHJ (1997) Ontogeny of milky spots in the human greater omentum: an immunochemical study. Anat Rec 249:399–404

Liebermann-Meffert D (2000) The greater omentum: anatomy, embryology, and surgical applications. Surg Clin North Am 80:275–293

Litbarg N, Gudehithlu K, Sethupathi P, Arruda J, Dunea G, Singh A (2007) Activated omentum becomes rich in factors that promote healing and tissue regeneration. Cell Tissue Res 328:487–497

Luijendijk RW, de Lange DC, Wauters CC, Hop WC, Duron JJ, Pailler JL, Camprodon BR, Holmdahl L, van Geldorp HJ, Jeekel J (1996) Foreign material in postoperative adhesions. Ann Surg 223:242–248

Maiorana A, Fierabracci A, Cianfarani S (2009) Isolation and characterization of omental adipose progenitor cells in children: a potential tool to unravel the pathogenesis of metabolic syndrome. Horm Res Paediatr 72:348–358

O'Shaughnessy L (1937) Surgical treatment of cardiac ischaemia. Lancet 229:185–194

Pinho MdFB, Hurtado SP, El-Cheikh MC, Borojevic R (2005) Haemopoietic progenitors in the adult mouse omentum: permanent production of B lymphocytes and monocytes. Cell Tissue Res 319:91–102

Shankle WR, Hara J (2010) Omentum transposition for treatment of Alzheimer's disease: clinical outcome and future therapeutic interpretation. In: Goldsmith HS (ed) The omentum: basic research and clinical applications. Cine-Med, Woodbury, CT, pp 199–207

Shimotsuma M, Kawata M, Hagiwara A, Takahashi T (1989) Milky spots in the human greater omentum. Cells Tissues Organs 136:211–216

Singh A, Patel J, Litbarg N, Gudehithlu K, Sethupathi P, Arruda J, Dunea G (2008) Stromal cells cultured from omentum express pluripotent markers, produce high amounts of VEGF, and engraft to injured sites. Cell Tissue Res 332:81–88

Song L, Wang L, Shah PK, Chaux A, Sharifi BG (2010) Bioengineered vascular graft grown in the mouse peritoneal cavity. J Vasc Surg 52:994–1002

Suh S, Kim J, Shin J, Kil K, Kim K, Kim H, Kim J (2004) Use of omentum as an in vivo cell culture system in tissue engineering. ASAIO J 50:464–467

Tchkonia T, Lenburg M, Thomou T, Giorgadze N, Frampton G, Pirtskhalava T, Cartwright A, Cartwright M, Flanagan J, Karagiannides I, Gerry N, Forse RA, Tchoukalova Y, Jensen MD, Pothoulakis C, Kirkland JL (2007) Identification of depot-specific human fat cell progenitors through distinct expression profiles and developmental gene patterns. Am J Physiol Endocrinol Metab 292:E298–E307

Toyoda M, Matsubara Y, Lin K, Sugimachi K, Furue M (2009) Characterization and comparison of adipose tissue-derived cells from human subcutaneous and omental adipose tissues. Cell Biochem Funct 27:440–447

van Harmelen V, Röhrig K, Hauner H (2004) Comparison of proliferation and differentiation capacity of human adipocyte precursor cells from the omental and subcutaneous adipose tissue depot of obese subjects. Metabolism 53:632–637

Wilkosz S, Ireland G, Khwaja N, Walker M, Butt R, de Giorgio-Miller A, Herrick SE (2005) A comparative study of the structure of human and murine greater omentum. Anat Embryol 209:251–261

Wu WL, Xu SQ, Liu M, Hua XM, Jiang F (2010a) Omental transposition following arachnoid excision to treat post-cerebral anoxia (cerebral palsy). In: Goldsmith HS (ed) The omentum: basic research and clinical applications. Cine-Med, Woodbury, CT, pp 167–172

Wu WL, Xu SQ, Liu M, Hua XM, Zhong J (2010b) Omental transposition for treating the sequelae of viral encephalitis: a long term follow-up of 54 cases. In: Goldsmith HS (ed) The omentum: basic research and clinical applications. Cine-Med, Woodbury, CT, pp 159–165

Zhang QX, Magovern CJ, Mack CA, Budenbender KT, Ko W, Rosengart TK (1997) Vascular endothelial growth factor is the major angiogenic factor in omentum: mechanism of the omentum-mediated angiogenesis. J Surg Res 67:147–154

Zuk PA, Zhu M, Mizuno H, Huang J, Futrell JW, Katz AJ, Benhaim P, Lorenz HP, Hedrick MH (2001) Multilineage cells from human adipose tissue: implications for cell-based therapies. Tissue Eng 7:211–228

Chapter 31

Human Embryonic Stem Cells Transplanted into Mouse Retina Induces Neural Differentiation

Akira Hara, Hitomi Aoki, Manabu Takamatsu, Yuichiro Hatano, Hiroyuki Tomita, Toshiya Kuno, Masayuki Niwa, and Takahiro Kunisada

Abstract Embryonic stem (ES) cells and induced pluripotent stem (iPS) cells can be transplanted and integrated into the retinas of adult mice as well-differentiated retinal cells. Thus these cells have the potential to be used to repair or regenerate diseased retina as cell replacement therapy in the future. The major concern with the possible transplantation of human ES (hES) or iPS cells in retinal diseases is, however, their ability to form tumors including mature and immature teratoma. In this review, we discuss the differentiation to retinal cells, including photoreceptor cells, and ganglion cells from hES or iPS cells transplanted into mouse retina. We also discuss possible strategies to overcome the major concern of potential teratoma formation and improve cell integration into host retina. Finally, we consider the future retinal cell therapy that may be used as a therapeutic strategy to treat retinal diseases.

Keywords Embryonic stem (ES) cells · Induced pluripotent stem (iPS) cells · Teratoma · CNS · Glaucoma · Retinal transplantation · Methotrexate

Introduction

Various cell sources for possible cell replacement in retinal transplantation have been identified (Aoki et al., 2009; Baker and Brown, 2009; Bhatia et al., 2010; Comyn et al., 2010; Dahlmann-Noor et al., 2010; Jin et al., 2009; Lamba et al., 2009; Meyer et al., 2009; Osakada et al., 2009; Wang et al., 2010), including embryonic stem (ES) cells, adult ciliary margin stem cells, neural stem/progenitor cells derived from central nervous system (CNS), other lineage stem cells such as mesenchymal stem cells, and induced pluripotent stem (iPS) cells, which are genetically reprogrammed to an embryonic stem cell-like state. Recent advances in stem cell and progenitor cell research have raised the possibility that these cells have the potential to be used to repair or regenerate mammalian damaged retina (Baker and Brown, 2009; Comyn et al., 2010; Jin et al., 2009; Lamba et al., 2009). Furthermore, continuous intraocular delivery of a neurotrophic factor itself (Parrilla-Reverter et al., 2009), or through transplanted stem cells releasing neurotrophic factors (Levkovitch-Verbin et al., 2010), may also rescue photoreceptor cell and retinal ganglion cell loss in experimental models of retinal degeneration. Retina and the optic nerve originate as outgrowths of the developing brain, so the retina is essentially a neural compartment and may be used experimentally for understanding the development of the CNS (Marquardt and Gruss, 2002; Shatz, 1996). As the retina itself is a multi-layered structure, with various neurons interconnected by synapses, the transplantation and cultivation of stem cells in the adult mouse eye may provide an in vivo model for future neural cell transplantation in other areas of the CNS.

Age-related macular degeneration, glaucoma, and diabetic retinopathy are common causes of visual impairment and blindness in people in developed countries (Bunce and Wormald, 2006). In these diseases, there are progressive losses of the retinal cells, such as photoreceptors, retinal ganglion cells and interneurons,

A. Hara (✉)
Department of Tumor Pathology, Gifu University Graduate School of Medicine, 1-1 Yanagido, Gifu 501-1194, Japan
e-mail: ahara@gifu-u.ac.jp

as well as retinal pigment epithelium, essential supporting cells of the retina. Cell replacement for retinal degeneration has been shown to be feasible in animal models of these diseases, but any cell-replacement strategy will require suitable cell sources that can differentiate to each of the specific retinal cell type. Among recent advances in stem cell and progenitor cell research, use of hES cells raises hope for successful cell-replacement therapies, and recent advances in somatic cell reprogramming to iPS cells has provided a potential method by which patient-specific cells may be generated for regenerative medicine. Importantly, the major concern and limitation to the possible transplantation of hES cells or iPS cells as cell replacement therapies is their potential to form tumors, including mature and immature teratomas (Hara et al., 2004, 2010; Prokhorova et al., 2009). The transplanted ES and iPS cells have not only pluripotent potential but also tumorigenic activity. Thus, these cells may develop into a teratoma, which contains a variety of differentiated or undifferentiated tissue types, as they have the ability for multipotent differentiation to various tissues. It is essential that the proliferation as well as the differentiation potential of ES cells is controlled, and the teratogenic risk of the ES cells is eliminated (Hara et al., 2004, 2006, 2008).

This review will focus on the following targets: cell types for retinal transplantation, retinal regeneration by hES/iPS cells, teratomas derived from hES/iPS cells, stem cells and cancer stem cells, and strategies for teratoma suppression.

Cell Types for Retinal Transplantation

Various cell types that are potential candidates for use in retinal transplantation are summarized in Table 31.1. Human ES cells, which are genetically normal, self-renewing, pluripotent cells, are isolated from the inner cell mass of blastocysts, a developmental stage at 5 days after fertilization (Donovan and Gearhart, 2001; Hochedlinger and Jaenisch, 2006). Although hES cells have the full differentiation potential, differentiation consists of a complicated process and is difficult to standardize. The accessibility of hES cells not only offers hope for cell replacement therapies, but also provides a system for understanding the mechanisms of embryonic development and disease mechanism.

However, there are important ethical issues that need to be resolved before the use of the stem cells in clinical practice (Sugarman, 2008). Animal ES cells have also been derived from animal blastocysts and have been used mostly in in vivo animal studies.

Recently, it was shown that adult somatic cells such as human fibroblasts can be reprogrammed to behave like hES cells by ectopic expression of four genes, Oct4, Sox2, c-Myc and Klf4 (Takahashi et al., 2007; Yu et al., 2007). Thus, by using human iPS cells, researchers for cell replacement therapies can easily obtain pluripotent stem cells without ethical issues about the destruction of human embryos. In contrast to the use of hES cells, use of iPS cells avoids the potential of graft-versus-host disease and immune rejection, because they can be derived from the patient own tissues. However, while there are still concerns regarding their safety, including the possibility of tumorigenesis (e.g., teratoma formation), use of iPS cells is an attractive option as it avoids the ethical issues associated with use of hES cells.

iPS cells were originally reprogrammed by the forced overexpression of the four key transcription factors by using viral vectors. Using this approach, these genes are randomly integrated into the genome, and may create artificial mutations. The use of retroviral and lentiviral vectors for expressing the reprogramming transcription factors involves the risk of insertional mutagenesis, which would be a significant risk if the cells were used in cell replacement therapies. Recent adenoviral and plasmid-based strategies have revealed that insertional integration into the genome is not required for the reprogramming process (Stadtfeld et al., 2008). However, even without viral integrations into the genome, the potential of genetic changes occurring during the reprogramming process cannot be completely ruled out. Recently, human iPS cells from human fibroblasts were generated by directly delivering four reprogramming proteins, Oct4, Sox2, Klf4, and c-Myc (Kim et al., 2009). These protein-induced human iPS cells exhibited similarities to hES cells in regard to their morphology, proliferation, and expression of characteristic pluripotency markers (Kim et al., 2009). Taken together, it is now possible to generate safer iPS cells by eliminating the potential risks associated with the use of viruses, DNA transfection, and potentially harmful chemicals. However, even safer iPS cells created by non-genetic methods and the techniques associated with iPS have been

Table 31.1 Summary of the cell types of stem/progenitor cells for retinal transplantation

	Engraftment rate	Neuro-network formation	Teratoma tumorigenesis	Availability	Ethical problems
ES/iPS cells					
Undiff.	++/++	++/++	++/++	++/++	+/−
Mod. diff.	+/+	+/+	+/+	++/++	+/−
Well diff.	±/±	±/±	±/±	++/++	+/−
Retinal SC/PC	+/±	+/±	±/±	±/±	±/±
Neural SC/PC	+/±	+/±	±/±	±/±	±/±
Other lineage SC	±	±	±	±	−

ES, embryonic stem; iPS, induced pluripotent stem; undiff., undifferentiated; mod. diff., moderately differentiated; well diff., well differentiated; SC, stem cells; PC, progenitor cells
++, Strongly Yes; +, Yes; ±, Neutral; −, No

improved for the purpose of clinical trials, human iPS cells as well as hES cells still possess the possibility of tumor generation because of their pluripotent potentials.

Various populations of stem cells and progenitor cells derived from the mammalian neural retina and ciliary body seems to be the most successful cell type demonstrating differentiation into retina-specific cells (Bhatia et al., 2010; Dahlmann-Noor et al., 2010). These cells can be isolated at different stages of mammalian development. But at present, there are not enough cell population to complete cell replacement of damaged retina because of low proliferation activities and limited reproducibility in mammalian retinal stem cells. In some vertebrates, however, retina continue to have the ability to self-renew and to generate differentiated cell component (Amato et al., 2004). The amphibian and fish retinas, which are known to contain stem cell populations, are leading models for stem cell research and provide key developmental cues that guide the reliable differentiation of mammalian retinal stem cells towards specific retinal cells.

Neural stem cells and progenitor cells have been isolated from the adult CNS. Adult neural precursor cells are derived from the dentate gyrus of the hippocampus, which is an area of continuous neuron renewal even in adult animals. In this context, neural stem cells, which are obtained from the adult mammalian brain, have also been shown to be able to integrate into the host retina when they are transplanted, but have failed to express retinal-specific markers (Young et al., 2000).

Mesenchymal stem cells can be derived from bone marrow and human umbilical cord blood and have the advantage of allowing autologous transplantation. Neuroprotective effect of intravitreal injections of neurotrophic factors-secreting mesenchymal stem cells on the survival of retinal ganglion cells was shown in rat eyes after optic nerve transection (Levkovitch-Verbin et al., 2010).

Retinal Regeneration by hES/iPS Cells

Among retinal cell replacement, photoreceptors, which are unidirectional sensory neuron, might be less difficult to replace with stem cells than that of retinal ganglion cell, which have complex afferent inputs and long axons with distant synapses. Photoreceptor cells are connected in only one direction (toward inside of eye ball) and does not require complex dendritic synapses to generate afferent inputs, because it responds to light as a simple sensory receptor. Recently hES cells have be used for photoreceptor replacement therapies in an animal model of photoreceptor degeneration (Lamba et al., 2009). The transplanted hES-derived retinal progenitor cells migrate into the appropriate layers in the retina following intravitreal transplantation in newborn mice, express markers consistent with retinal neuron and rod and cone photoreceptor differentiation, and show a synaptic marker in the outer plexiform layer. However, migration was restricted to the early time points within postnatal day 1, as intravitreal transplants from postnatal day 2 onward resulted in absence of migration of cells into retina (Lamba et al., 2009). In an adult mouse photoreceptor-degeneration model, hES cells labeled with GFP-expressing virus injected into the subretinal space failed to extend into inner and outer segments, either due to the lack of supporting host photoreceptors or to the inability to establish a healthy interaction with host retinal pigment epithelium, important factors in their maintenance (Lamba et al., 2009). Recent studies have demonstrated that an undifferentiated cell is the ideal candidate for transplant strategies to replace photoreceptors, because more differentiated donor cells do not migrate or integrate well into the host retina. Furthermore, it has been observed that hES cell transplantation into retina is successful only in neonatal recipients.

Retinal ganglion cells, located in the most inner layer of the retina, integrate information from photoreceptors and project axons into the brain, where they make synapses at the thalamus, the hypothalamus and the superior colliculus. They are vulnerable to ischemia and excitatory amino acids like *N*-methyl-D-aspartate (NMDA), a glutamate receptor agonist (Hara et al., 2006), and their loss is a hallmark of many ophthalmic diseases, including retinal ischemia and glaucoma. In contrast to photoreceptor transplantation, retinal ganglion cell replacement in diseased retina may present a far more difficult goal. This is because ganglion cells require remodeling of complex afferent inputs within the retina, reconnection over long distances to downstream targets and complex navigation (MacLaren, 1999). In this context, there are few reports showing in vivo transplantation of retinal ganglion cells, and ganglion cell transplantation produces an incomplete cellular network compared with normal network of ganglion cell layer of the retina (Hara et al., 2004). Furthermore, only undifferentiated ES cells are able to generate a neural network, with incomplete structure, in the adult mouse retina. However, recent studies using ex vivo or three-dimensional cell culture system successfully demonstrated that regeneration of retinal ganglion cell-resembling neural network differentiated from mouse ES cells (Aoki et al., 2007; Hara et al., 2008).

Teratomas Derived from hES/iPS Cells

Undifferentiated cells are the best transplant candidate for optimal engraftment and migration of the transplanted cells, because differentiated donor cells do not migrate or integrate well within the host retinal structure. This means that too much differentiation prior to transplantation reduced specific neural morphology and function of the hES cells after transplantation. On the other hand, in vivo application of undifferentiated hES or iPS cells into immune-deficient mice produces teratomas composed of many cell types, since these cells have both pluripotent potential and tumorigenic activity. In fact, while many promising cell types such as neurons, cardiomyocytes, hepatocytes, pancreatic beta cells, and blood cells have been successfully derived from ES cells in vitro, it is still difficult to control the risk of teratogenic tissue occurrence associated with in vivo-transplanted ES cells. Although ES cells may be attractive candidates for cell-replacement therapy of various degenerative diseases in the future, the major limitation of its application to the therapy is teratoma formation. For example, even neuro-progenitor cells derived from ES cells show unlimited self-renewal and high differentiation potential and have the risk of tumor induction after engraftment (Arnhold et al., 2004). In this report, teratoma formation was demonstrated in 50% of the eyes evaluated at 8 weeks after transplantation of neuro-progenitor cells derived from ES cells, although no morphologic tumorigenesis was detected in eyes at 2 and 4 weeks after transplantation. Furthermore, in long-term culture hES cells have recurrent genomic instability associated with oncogenic transformation (Lefort et al., 2008). Even for successful retinal incorporation and differentiation of neural precursors derived from hES cells, proliferation of transplanted precursors (analyzed by Ki-67 expression) was observed throughout the 16-week follow-up period, with neuro-progenitor cells occasionally forming rosette structures; histopathologically, such cells expressing Ki-67 within large clusters of grafted cells with rosette-like formations are usually regarded as a part of immature teratoma.

Stem Cells and Cancer Stem Cells

Recent reports suggest that many types of cancer contain their own stem cells, called as cancer stem (CS) cells in a same way as normal stem cell or progenitor cell development (Bomken et al., 2010). These specific tumor cells exhibit the ability to self-renew as well as give rise to various subtype of original cancer cells. The concept of CS cells, similar to normal stem cells, has developed in leukemia. Human acute myeloid leukemia is organized as a hierarchy that originates from a primitive hematopoietic cell. The cancer, or leukemic clone, is also organized as a hierarchy in which only a rare subset of cancer cells possess the ability to initiate new tumor growth and recapitulate the tumor heterogeneity. Thus, the CS cell model has great implications for understanding of oncogenesis and treatment for cancer, however, their characteristics are still unknown.

OCT-4 is a key regulator of self-renewal in ES cells. The existence of a small subpopulation of self-renewing CS cells that are capable of expressing the pluripotent marker, OCT-4 are suggested in some human cancer. Interestingly, in vivo transplanted ES cells often produce immature teratoma or teratocarcinoma with small subpopulations of undifferentiated OCT-4 expressing cell clusters. This means that OCT-4 positive ES cells may have a potential to be CS cells. Thus, we should pay attention to the fact that ES cells after in vivo transplantation have the potential to transform by themselves into CS cells, which possess ability to form immature teratoma or teratocarcinoma. In fact, there are some OCT-4 expressing cells in surgically resected human immature teratoma.

Teratomas have tumor characteristics, but also show differentiated organization in various tissues. Undifferentiated OCT-4 expressing cells in surgically resected human teratoma are regarded as stem cells, forming various tissues in the teratoma. This means histological analysis of teratoma provides us some information about stem cell differentiation in vivo. While each tissue observed in human teratoma is usually located randomly, there are some rules about histological localization and tissue polarity. Thus observation and analysis of the teratoma can provide some clues in applying the stem cells to the regenerative medicine.

Strategies for Teratoma Suppression

The proliferation as well as the differentiation potential of in vivo-transplanted ES cells need to be controlled, and the risk associated with the growth of teratogenic tissues needs to be eliminated. Several trials of in vivo application of cell-replacement therapy avoiding uncontrolled cell proliferation have been reported recently (Choo et al., 2008; Hara et al., 2006, 2008, 2010).

Cytotoxic monoclonal antibodies directed against undifferentiated hES cells is one approach that has been investigated to reduce the risk of teratoma formation by contaminating undifferentiated hES cells (Choo et al., 2008). Specific monoclonal antibody recognizing a cell surface marker may be useful in eliminating residual undifferentiated hES cells from differentiated cells populations for clinical applications in the future.

In our studies using mouse ES cells (Hara et al., 2006) and hES cells (Hara et al., 2010) transplanted in the adult mouse retina (injected intravitreally with the glutamate analog, NMDA to produce a retinal ganglion cell damage), we have demonstrated that the folate antagonist, methotrexate (MTX) induces neural differentiation of the transplanted ES cells and decrease their proliferative activity. Figure 31.1 shows representative microphotograph of hES cells transplanted into the vitreous cavity of BALB/C (nu/nu) nude mice at 5 weeks after transplantation. The retinal structure is destroyed by the immature teratoma in non-treated mice (Fig. 31.1a). Following intraperitoneal MTX treatment (1 mg/kg once per day), started at 4 days after hES cell injection for 15 days, ganglion-like cells are observed as a monolayer structure along the inner surface of retina (Fig. 31.1b). The monolayer structure shows vesicular glutamate transporter 1 (VGLUT1), which is preferentially associated with the membranes of synaptic vesicles (Fig. 31.1j). MTX is used clinically for its anti-inflammatory actions in the treatment of rheumatoid arthritis, and is also used as a chemotherapeutic agent, where it can induce clinical remission of intraocular malignant lymphoma and other intraocular malignancies. Furthermore, MTX is considered relatively safe even when used as an intrathecal chemotherapy as well as in children with leukemia and lymphoma and in some brain tumors. These characteristics of MTX indicate that MTX could control proliferation of undifferentiated stem cells and promote their neural differentiation because of its safety to nervous system in the case of tumor chemotherapy. In these studies, induction of neural differentiation and decrease of the tumorigenic activity of MTX on mouse ES or hES cells transplanted into mouse retina implicated the pathophysiology of human glaucoma as a model for cell-replacement therapy of retina.

In another study of ours, selective ablation of undifferentiated mouse ES cells expressing herpes simplex virus-thymidine kinase (HSV-tk) gene under the control of Oct-4 promoter was achieved by treatment with

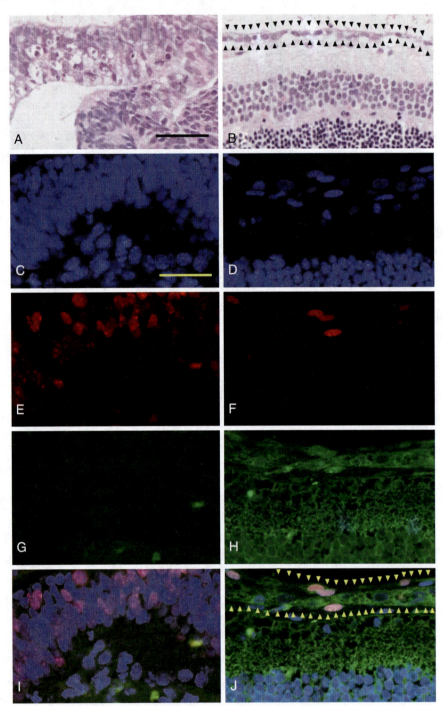

Fig. 31.1 Representative microphotograph of transplanted hES cells treated by intraperitoneal administration of MTX (**a, c, e, g, i**) and non-treated hES cells (**b, d, f, h, j**) in mouse retina. Conventional HE staining (**a, b**) and immunofluorescence images (**c–j**) are presented. (**a**) The retinal structure of host mouse is destroyed by the immature teratoma. (**b**) Following MTX treatment, ganglion-like cells are observed (between *black arrowheads*). Vesicular glutamate transporter 1 (VGLUT1) positive neuron-like cells are recognized as a monolayer structure covering inner surface of retina and some of them express human Ki-67 antigen (between *yellow arrowheads* in **j**). However, undifferentiated hES cell forming multilayer structure composed of high density cells expressing Ki-67 do not show VGLUT1 (**i**). (**a, b**) HE staining; (**c, d**) DAPI (*blue*); (**e, f**) human Ki-67 (*red*); (**g, h**) vesicular glutamate transporter 1 (*green*); (**i, j**) merge. Scale bar in (**a**) 50 μm and (**c**) 40 μm

the antiviral agent, ganciclovir (Hara et al., 2008). By using a three-dimensional cell culture system allowing a multilayer cell construct, ES cells containing HSV-tk transgene for a suicide gene expression under the control of the Oct-4 promoter was used for ablation of undifferentiated ES cells, which may produce teratomas. Thus, only the undifferentiated ES cells expressing Oct-4 actively produce HSV-tk, which metabolizes ganciclovir to cytotoxic nucleotide analogs, while differentiated ES cells do not produce HSV-tk and are therefore not sensitive to ganciclovir. Finally, a HSV-tk/ganciclovir system induces neuron-like differentiation, and decreases the number of Oct-4-positive cells as well as proliferative activity of ES cells.

For cell replacement in CNS, it is quite common that neural precursor cells derived from hES cell do not migrate or integrate into the host neural network. Moreover, the migration of the transplanted cells could have been prevented by a glial scar, which has been reported to form around the transplant site in ischemic brain. Similarly, Müller glia in the retina are believed to be responsible for the reactive gliosis observed in some retinal lesions, and consequently retinal progenitor cells derived from hES cells may potentially be prevented from complete integration into retina by such gliosis. It is possible that excessive differentiation of the progenitor cells derived from hES cells may prevent the migration and integration activity to the host retina as a neural network.

It is still unclear if it is better to induce differentiation of undifferentiated hES cells in vitro and then transplant the differentiated cells into retina, or to transplant undifferentiated cells and then differentiate them spontaneously in the target microenvironment. While undifferentiated mouse ES cells possessed potential to migrate and integrate into the host neural network, these cells also have the potential to generate teratogenic tumors. Moderately differentiated hES cells may be better, because more differentiated donor cells do not migrate or integrate well into the host retina. Further studies are needed to optimize the in vivo conditions necessary for pluripotent cell transplantation in future clinical trials of cell replacement therapies, while ensuring the prevention of tumor formation.

References

Amato MA, Arnault E, Perron M (2004) Retinal stem cells in vertebrates: parallels and divergences. Int J Dev Biol 48: 993–1001

Aoki H, Hara A, Niwa M, Motohashi T, Suzuki T, Kunisada T (2007) An in vitro mouse model for retinal ganglion cell replacement therapy using eye-like structures differentiated from ES cells. Exp Eye Res 84:868–875

Aoki H, Hara A, Niwa M, Yamada Y, Kunisada T (2009) In vitro and in vivo differentiation of human embryonic stem cells into retina-like organs and comparison with that from mouse pluripotent epiblast stem cells. Dev Dyn 238:2266–2279

Arnhold S, Klein H, Semkova I, Addicks K, Schraermeyer U (2004) Neurally selected embryonic stem cells induce tumor formation after long-term survival following engraftment into the subretinal space. Invest Ophthalmol Vis Sci 45:4251–4255

Baker PS, Brown GC (2009) Stem-cell therapy in retinal disease. Curr Opin Ophthalmol 20:175–181

Bhatia B, Singhal S, Jayaram H, Khaw PT, Limb GA (2010) Adult retinal stem cells revisited. Open Ophthalmol J 4: 30–38

Bomken S, Fiser K, Heidenreich O, Vormoor J (2010) Understanding the cancer stem cell. Br J Cancer 103: 439–445

Bunce C, Wormald R (2006) Leading causes of certification for blindness and partial sight in England & Wales. BMC Public Health 6:58

Choo AB, Tan HL, Ang SN, Fong WJ, Chin A, Lo J, Zheng L, Hentze H, Philp RJ, Oh SK, Yap M (2008) Selection against undifferentiated human embryonic stem cells by a cytotoxic antibody recognizing podocalyxin-like protein-1. Stem Cells 26:1454–1463

Comyn O, Lee E, MacLaren RE (2010) Induced pluripotent stem cell therapies for retinal disease. Curr Opin Neurol 23:4–9

Dahlmann-Noor A, Vijay S, Jayaram H, Limb A, Khaw PT (2010) Current approaches and future prospects for stem cell rescue and regeneration of the retina and optic nerve. Can J Ophthalmol 45:333–341

Donovan PJ, Gearhart J (2001) The end of the beginning for pluripotent stem cells. Nature 414:92–97

Hara A, Niwa M, Kunisada T, Yoshimura N, Katayama M, Kozawa O, Mori H (2004) Embryonic stem cells are capable of generating a neuronal network in the adult mouse retina. Brain Res 999:216–221

Hara A, Niwa M, Kumada M, Aoki H, Kunisada T, Oyama T, Yamamoto T, Kozawa O, Mori H (2006) Intraocular injection of folate antagonist methotrexate induces neuronal differentiation of embryonic stem cells transplanted in the adult mouse retina. Brain Res 1085:33–42

Hara A, Aoki H, Taguchi A, Niwa M, Yamada Y, Kunisada T, Mori H (2008) Neuron-like differentiation and selective ablation of undifferentiated embryonic stem cells containing suicide gene with Oct-4 promoter. Stem Cells Dev 17:619–627

Hara A, Taguchi A, Aoki H, Hatano Y, Niwa M, Yamada Y, Kunisada T (2010) Folate antagonist, methotrexate induces neuronal differentiation of human embryonic stem cells transplanted into nude mouse retina. Neurosci Lett 477:138–143

Hochedlinger K, Jaenisch R (2006) Nuclear reprogramming and pluripotency. Nature 441:1061–1067

Jin ZB, Okamoto S, Mandai M, Takahashi M (2009) Induced pluripotent stem cells for retinal degenerative diseases: a new perspective on the challenges. J Genet 88:417–424

Kim D, Kim CH, Moon JI, Chung YG, Chang MY, Han BS, Ko S, Yang E, Cha KY, Lanza R, Kim KS (2009) Generation of human induced pluripotent stem cells by direct delivery of reprogramming proteins. Cell Stem Cell 4:472–476

Lamba DA, Gust J, Reh TA (2009) Transplantation of human embryonic stem cell-derived photoreceptors restores some visual function in Crx-deficient mice. Cell Stem Cell 4:73–79

Lefort N, Feyeux M, Bas C, Feraud O, Bennaceur-Griscelli A, Tachdjian G, Peschanski M, Perrier AL (2008) Human embryonic stem cells reveal recurrent genomic instability at 20q11.21. Nat Biotechnol 26:1364–1366

Levkovitch-Verbin H, Sadan O, Vander S, Rosner M, Barhum Y, Melamed E, Offen D, Melamed S (2010) Intravitreal injections of neurotrophic factors secreting mesenchymal stem cells are neuroprotective in rat eyes following optic nerve transection. Invest Ophthalmol Vis Sci 51:6394–6400

MacLaren RE (1999) Re-establishment of visual circuitry after optic nerve regeneration. Eye (Lond) 13(Pt 3a):277–284

Marquardt T, Gruss P (2002) Generating neuronal diversity in the retina: one for nearly all. Trends Neurosci 25:32–38

Meyer JS, Shearer RL, Capowski EE, Wright LS, Wallace KA, McMillan EL, Zhang SC, Gamm DM (2009) Modeling early retinal development with human embryonic and induced pluripotent stem cells. Proc Natl Acad Sci USA 106:16698–16703

Osakada F, Ikeda H, Sasai Y, Takahashi M (2009) Stepwise differentiation of pluripotent stem cells into retinal cells. Nat Protoc 4:811–824

Parrilla-Reverter G, Agudo M, Sobrado-Calvo P, Salinas-Navarro M, Villegas-Perez MP, Vidal-Sanz M (2009) Effects of different neurotrophic factors on the survival of retinal ganglion cells after a complete intraorbital nerve crush injury: a quantitative in vivo study. Exp Eye Res 89:32–41

Prokhorova TA, Harkness LM, Frandsen U, Ditzel N, Schroder HD, Burns JS, Kassem M (2009) Teratoma formation by human embryonic stem cells is site dependent and enhanced by the presence of Matrigel. Stem Cells Dev 18:47–54

Shatz CJ (1996) Emergence of order in visual system development. J Physiol Paris 90:141–150

Stadtfeld M, Nagaya M, Utikal J, Weir G, Hochedlinger K (2008) Induced pluripotent stem cells generated without viral integration. Science 322:945–949

Sugarman J (2008) Human stem cell ethics: beyond the embryo. Cell Stem Cell 2:529–533

Takahashi K, Tanabe K, Ohnuki M, Narita M, Ichisaka T, Tomoda K, Yamanaka S (2007) Induction of pluripotent stem cells from adult human fibroblasts by defined factors. Cell 131:861–872

Wang NK, Tosi J, Kasanuki JM, Chou CL, Kong J, Parmalee N, Wert KJ, Allikmets R, Lai CC, Chien CL, Nagasaki T, Lin CS, Tsang SH (2010) Transplantation of reprogrammed embryonic stem cells improves visual function in a mouse model for retinitis pigmentosa. Transplantation 89:911–919

Young MJ, Ray J, Whiteley SJ, Klassen H, Gage FH (2000) Neuronal differentiation and morphological integration of hippocampal progenitor cells transplanted to the retina of immature and mature dystrophic rats. Mol Cell Neurosci 16:197–205

Yu J, Vodyanik MA, Smuga-Otto K, Antosiewicz-Bourget J, Frane JL, Tian S, Nie J, Jonsdottir GA, Ruotti V, Stewart R, Slukvin, II, Thomson JA (2007) Induced pluripotent stem cell lines derived from human somatic cells. Science 318:1917–1920

Chapter 32

Stem Cells to Repair Retina: From Basic to Applied Biology

Muriel Perron, Morgane Locker, and Odile Bronchain

Abstract Loss of photoreceptors, the sensory cells of the retina, occurs in several genetic and sporadic retinal diseases, resulting in visual disturbance or blindness. Stem-cell based therapies could represent effective approaches to cure these neurodegenerative pathologies. A pivotal issue in this context is to unravel the gene regulatory network that drives multipotent progenitors towards retinal cell types in vivo in order to devise in vitro procedures for stem cell directed differentiation. We will therefore briefly present the current knowledge on mechanisms underlying cell specification during retinogenesis. We will then discuss the rapidly evolving field aiming at generating photoreceptors from stem cells of various origins, and the attempts to restore sight in animal models for retinal diseases. Success, failures and future prospects are reviewed.

Keywords Retina · Neural stem cells · ES/iPS cells · Photoreceptors · Regenerative medicine

Introduction

The vertebrate retina is a layered structure at the back of the eye that converts light detection into electric signals. It contains three nuclear layers separated by synaptic or "plexiform" layers (Fig. 32.1a, b). The two classes of photoreceptors, rods and cones, lie in the outer nuclear layer and closely interact with the pigmented retinal epithelium (RPE). The inner nuclear layer contains horizontal, bipolar, and amacrine interneurons, as well as Müller cells, the only intrinsic glial cell of the retina. The ganglion cell layer mainly consists of retinal ganglion cells (RGC) that project their axons through the optic nerve to various regions in the brain. Many eye diseases such as age-related macular degeneration (AMD), retinitis pigmentosa (RP), Leber's congenital amaurosis (LCA), diabetic retinopathy (DR) or glaucoma, are associated with retinal neuron degeneration (Fig. 32.1c). AMD and RP, which ultimately lead to the irreversible loss of photoreceptors, are prominent causes of human blindness in the world. Although gene therapy is investigated to cure patients with inherited diseases such as RP and LCA, a more general strategy able to restore sight in a wide range of genetic as well as sporadic retinal dystrophies would be a better option. Cell-based therapy represents a promising approach, as the retina offers some unique advantages compared to other areas of the central nervous system (CNS). Its accessibility facilitates cell transplantation and subsequent monitoring through noninvasive procedures. Additionally, the eye constitutes one of the immunologically privileged sites of the human body, allowing for allograft survival for extended periods of time without rejection. Finally, photoreceptors can be considered as the easiest neuron to be replaced in the CNS, since they establish unidirectional connections due to their afferent stimulation by light.

Researchers have put great expectations in stem cells as a source for cell transplantation, with the idea that their plasticity would sustain their integration and differentiation in the diseased retina. A variety of embryonic or adult neural stem cells

M. Perron (✉)
Laboratory of Neurobiology and Development, UPR CNRS 3294, Université Paris-Sud, Orsay, France
e-mail: Muriel.perron@u-psud.fr

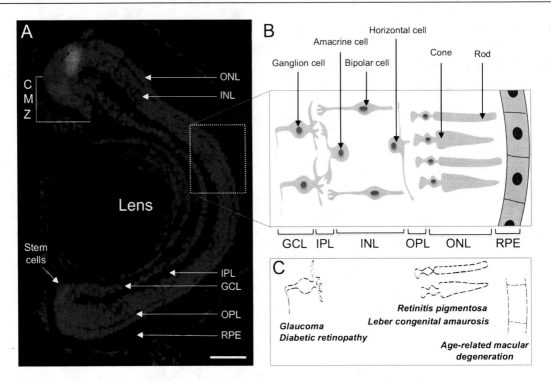

Fig. 32.1 Retina structure and retinal cell types. (**a**) Cross section of a *Xenopus* tadpole retina labeled with EdU (*red*), which stains dividing cells, and counterstained with Hoechst (nuclei in *blue*). Three nuclear layers can be distinguished, surrounded by the retinal pigment epithelium (RPE): the ganglion cell layer (GCL) composed of ganglion cells; the inner nuclear layer (INL) that comprises amacrine, bipolar and horizontal neurons as well as Müller glial cells; the outer nuclear layer (ONL) with cone and rod photoreceptors. The inner and the outer plexiform layers (IPL and OPL) lie between the nuclear layers. EdU labeling reveals the ciliary marginal zone (CMZ), which is responsible for continuous retinal growth in adult amphibians (Perron et al., 1998). Stem cells reside at the extreme periphery of the CMZ. Given their low division rate, EdU incorporation is reduced in these cells compared to progenitor cells. Note that in the adult, vitreous humor fills the space between the lens and the retina. This latter thus ends as a thin sheet at the back of the eye (see Fig. 32.2e). (**b**) Schematic of retinal cell neurons present in the three nuclear layers. (**c**) Examples of retinal dystrophies in human. The retinal cell type whose loss or dysfunction is the primary cause of the disease is illustrated with *dotted lines*. Age-macular degeneration results from RPE cell damages and subsequently leads to photoreceptor death; Retinitis pigmentosa is associated with degenerescence of rods while Leber's congenital amaurosis involve cone photoreceptor loss; Glaucoma and diabetic retinopathy involves apoptosis of retinal ganglion cells. Scale bar: 40 μm

have thus been tested for their potential in retinal repair and will be discussed below (Fig. 32.2). More recently, major advances in directing embryonic (ES) or induced (iPS) pluripotent stem cells towards retinal fates have been achieved. These could represent expandable sources from which to derive photoreceptors for transplantation. Importantly, the design of such protocols relies in part on our basic knowledge of the molecular mechanisms underlying cell type specification under physiological conditions. A brief update on this field is therefore presented first.

Generating Cell Diversity in the Retina

Formation of the eye field primarily requires the adoption by anterior neural plate cells of a retinal identity. This occurs in response to a series of inductive events involving in particular FGF, Wnt and BMP signaling modulation (reviewed in Esteve and Bovolenta, 2006). These specification steps eventually lead to the upregulation of the neural patterning gene *Otx2* (*Orthodenticle homeobox 2*) and a group of "eye field transcription factors" (EFTF), namely *tbx3*, *Rx1*, *Pax6*, *Six3*, *Lhx2*, *nr2e1* and *Six6*, which turned out to be

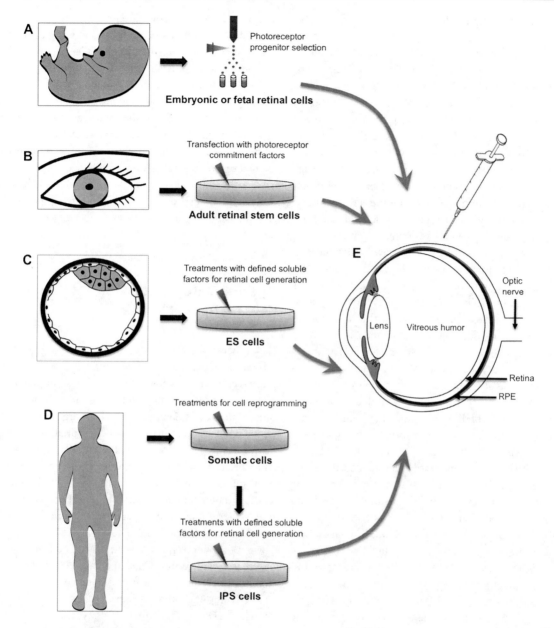

Fig. 32.2 Illustration of stem cell sources and associated assays that have been successfully assessed in mice for their potential in retinal repair. (**a**) Transplantation of cone or rod precursors isolated by fluorescence activated cell sorting from fetal or postnatal retina, revealed an efficient strategy to replace lost photoreceptors in model mice (MacLaren et al., 2006; Lakowski et al., 2010). (**b**) Human adult retinal stem cells harvested from the ciliary body epithelium and genetically induced towards a photoreceptor fate proved efficient functional integration into neonatal animal eyes (Inoue et al., 2010). (**c**) ES cell-derived retinal cells can differentiate into functional photoreceptors and improve light response in model mice following transplantation (Lamba et al., 2009). (**d**) IPS cell-derived photoreceptors can integrate into the retina and express photoreceptor markers after transplantation in normal mice (Lamba et al., 2010). (**e**) Cell grafts are generally attempted into the subretinal space (between the retina and the RPE) or in the vitreous cavity of the adult eye

essential and sufficient for eye formation. Strikingly indeed, pluripotent embryonic stem cells misexpressing this set of genes formed ectopic eye-like structure following their transplantation in the flank of developing *Xenopus* embryos (Viczian et al., 2009).

Basically, early retinal morphogenesis consists in separation of the eye field into two primordia, followed by evagination of the optic vesicles. Cells located in different positions within the optic vesicle then give rise to three morphologically and functionally different compartments: presumptive optic nerve, RPE and neural retina. Within the later, multipotent progenitors generate retinal cell types in a defined temporal sequence, conserved in all vertebrates: ganglion cells are the first to be born (i.e. withdrawn from the cell cycle and committed to the ganglion cell lineage), followed by amacrine, cone, horizontal, rod, bipolar cells and eventually Müller glia. Understanding how these different cell types are generated in the appropriate proportions and order during retinogenesis has been an attractive issue for neurobiologists. Two decades of research led to the discovery of many transcription factors involved in the specification of retinal cell types. A widely accepted model stipulates that basic helix-loop-helix (bHLH) activators and homeodomain factors function in a combinatorial mode to generate cell diversity in the retina. As most human retinal degenerative diseases primarily or secondarily affect photoreceptors, researchers have paid much attention on the transcriptional network sustaining cone and rod specification (Hennig et al., 2008; Swaroop et al., 2010). The core of the network includes two members of the *Orthodenticle* family: *Otx2* and *Crx (Cone-rod homeobox)* genes. *Otx2* specifies the photoreceptor lineage by regulating the expression of *Crx*, which in turn controls photoreceptor differentiation. Transcription factors of the Retinal homeobox (Rx) family were recently proposed to cooperate with Crx to regulate photoreceptor specific genes such as *rhodopsin*, *red cone opsin* or *rod arrestin* (Pan et al., 2010). Besides, the maintenance of the photoreceptor fate was shown to require the repression of genes involved in bipolar cell fate specification, like *Chx10* (Brzezinski et al., 2010; Katoh et al., 2010). Factors responsible for the choice between rod *versus* cone pathways have also started to be uncovered. The neural retina leucine zipper protein (Nrl), a transcription factor belonging to the Maf subfamily, proved to play an instructive role in determining the rod lineage. The orphan nuclear receptor Nr2e3 acts downstream Nrl to reinforce the rod phenotype establishment by suppressing cone specific gene expression. Mutations in *Crx*, *Nrl* or *Nr2e3* are the cause of various inherited retinal diseases in human, such as autosomal dominant forms of RP (Hennig et al., 2008). The cone differentiation pathway is far less understood and the main candidates identified so far include thyroid hormone receptor β2 (Trβ2), retinoid-related orphan receptor Rorβ, and retinoid-related receptor Rxrγ. As we will see below, such basic knowledge have paved the way for establishing rational in vitro procedures for photoreceptor differentiation and purification from stem cells of various origin.

Optimal Ontogenetic Stage of Donor Cells for Retinal Repair

Key processes for effective cellular therapy include migration, integration and eventual differentiation of grafted cells into the host retina. Neural stem/precursor cells were thus initially viewed as appropriate candidates for transplantation as they are intrinsically endowed with migratory and differentiation properties. Several studies were conducted in rodent models using brain-derived as well as embryonic, fetal or postnatal retinal stem/progenitor cells (West et al., 2009). These studies generated variable data but as a whole highlighted rather limited levels of integration and/or photoreceptor differentiation. Procedure efficiency was however shown to be enhanced in traumatized or diseased recipient retina (Chacko et al., 2003). Trials in human have consisted in transplantation of fetal retinal cells into the subretinal space of patients with RP or AMD (Das et al., 1999; Humayun et al., 2000). Although the results indicated an apparent high tolerance of the host retina for the graft, a positive effect on visual function could not be demonstrated. Altogether, these studies suggested that the mature retina is not permissive to integration and differentiation of exogenous multipotent stem/progenitor cells. MacLaren and collaborators then raised the hypothesis that transplantation of committed progenitors might be more efficient (MacLaren et al., 2006; Fig. 32.2a). Indeed, *Nrl*-expressing postmitotic rod precursors displayed better engraftment ability compared to immature progenitor cells. In addition, such precursors transplanted into the eyes of RP model mice differentiated along the rod lineage, formed synaptic connections and, most importantly, improved visual function. Along the same line, the importance of ontogenetic stage of donor cells for cone cell replacement was recently demonstrated in a genetic model of LCA (Lakowski et al., 2010). These major data highlighted that the mature retina is receptive to integrate new photoreceptors into pre-existing circuitry and thus offered hope for further studies aiming at restoring vision through cell-replacement strategies. However, apart from ethical issues, the limited availability of human embryonic or fetal cells constitutes a major limitation for clinical translation of these procedures. Besides, although the eye is considered immune-privileged, a recent study suggested the need for immune suppression of recipient animals for long-term survival of integrated cell. This data reinforced the idea that autologous transplants might be more suitable for therapeutic approaches of retinal repair (West et al., 2010).

The Adult Retina as a Potential Source for Autologous Transplantation

A potential autologous source of donor cells revealed to be the retina itself, with the discovery in 2000 of putative stem cells in the murine eye. The rational of looking for stem cells in the mammalian retina, which is devoid of tissue renewal, repair or regenerating capacities, came from evolutionary considerations. Adult retinas of fish and amphibians are indeed known to contain a population of neural stem cells, located in a peripheral region called the ciliary marginal zone (CMZ, Fig. 32.1a). These cells allow for continuous retinal growth and contribute to regeneration processes following eye injury (reviewed in Locker et al., 2010). Although mammalian retinas lack a CMZ, it was hypothesized that some peripheral cells might have retained stemness features along evolution. Cells able to clonally expand in vitro were indeed identified in mammals, including humans, within the ciliary body, a structure derived from the optic cup and located between the retina and the iris (Tropepe et al., 2000; Coles et al., 2004). It was thus assumed that the adult mammalian ciliary body harbored a population of retinal stem cells (RSC), yet in a mitotically quiescent state in vivo. Although both their proliferation and differentiation potentials appear limited (reviewed in Locker et al., 2010), their discovery prompted many researchers to investigate their therapeutic relevance as sources for autologous transplantation.

As a proof of concept, upon transplantion into diseased retina, murine adult RSC were shown to integrate the different cell layers and accordingly express specific retinal cell markers, noticeably photoreceptor ones (Chacko et al., 2003). Human adult RSC subsequently proved similar abilities when transplanted vitreously into neonatal animal eyes (Coles et al., 2004). The integration efficiency and the proportion of new photoreceptor-like cells however remained very low. In line with the work by MacLaren et al. (2006; see above), Inoue and colleagues recently demonstrated the advantage of directing human RSC towards a photoreceptor fate prior to transplantation (Fig. 32.2b). The procedure consisted in the combined overexpression of *Otx2* and *Crx*, together with the inhibition of the bipolar cell inducing activity of CHX10. Such genetically modified RSC progeny exhibited greatly enhanced survival and photoreceptor differentiation following their transplantation into mouse eyes (Inoue et al., 2010). Importantly, they were also shown to promote functional recovery in mutant mice with defective rod photoreceptors. Despite these promising data, the use of adult RSC for stem cell-based therapies is presently limited by the shortage of donor cells.

A New Turn in the Field of Retinal Repair: The iPS Era

The establishment of human ES cell lines in 1998 offered tremendous hope for their use in regenerative medicine. Their pluripotency and ability to proliferate indefinitely makes them a potential inexhaustible source for various human cell types production. ES cell-based therapy however presents three major downsides. The first one resides in the oncogenicity of ES cells that may be responsible for the formation of teratomas and thus requires high cell sorting purification of differentiated progenies. The second is linked to their embryonic origin that raises ethical concerns. Finally, even by using established cell lines limiting destruction of human embryos, ES cells can only be considered for allografts. The two latter issues have recently been substantially alleviated with the demonstration in 2006–2007 in mouse and human, that somatic cells can be reprogrammed into an ES-like state. These induced pluripotent cells (iPS) were initially obtained through retroviral delivery of four key stem cell transcription factors (Takahashi and Yamanaka, 2006). Importantly, these past 2 years, the reprogramming method has been considerably optimized, making the process more efficient and safer with regards to putative therapeutic applications (reviewed in Stadtfeld and Hochedlinger, 2010). Thus, in contrast to human ES cells, iPS cells avoid ethical dilemmas and offer the possibility of autologous transplantation. Importantly, an additional step of gene correction should nevertheless be considered for patients with identified mutations causing rapid photoreceptor degeneration.

A major difficulty for exploiting embryonic or induced pluripotent stem cells is to direct them univocally along a chosen lineage at high frequency. Rational for setting up in vitro procedures relies on the fact that differentiation of pluripotent cells mimics the time course and processes of embryonic development. A recent milestone was the selective generation from mouse and human ES cells of progenies exhibiting features of retinal precursors, as inferred notably by the expression of EFTF such as *Pax6* and *Rx* (Ikeda et al., 2005; Lamba et al., 2006). Basically, such a retinal-restricted identity could be obtained using biological compounds inhibiting Wnt and BMP/Nodal pathways, a known requirement for eye field formation in vivo. These studies then provided the basis for subsequent establishment of stepwise protocols aiming at specifically inducing RPE, photoreceptor or even ganglion cell fate from "retinalized" ES or iPS (Jin et al., 2009; Bharti et al., 2010).

RPE defects constitute the primary cause of several retinal degenerative diseases including AMD. Autologous RPE grafts have been carried out in the last 20 years but the overall visual outcomes remained poor and the surgical intervention challenging (da Cruz et al., 2007). IPS cell-derived RPE may thus be a better option for autologous transplantation. RPE-like cells revealed seemingly easy to generate in vitro (reviewed in Bharti et al., 2010). In addition, several studies reported that transplantation of ES- or iPS-derived RPE cells exerted a protective effect on photoreceptors and improved visual functions in Royal College of Surgeons rats, a model of retinal degeneration caused by RPE dysfunction.

Interestingly, it was recently demonstrated that some human iPS cell lines reprogrammed from RPE cells exhibit a marked preference for redifferentiation into RPE, likely due to epigenetic memory of their parental tissue (Hu et al., 2010). The iPS cell of origin may thus be a crucial element to consider in the future, in order to optimize the generation of retinal cell types.

In contrast to RPE, directing photoreceptor differentiation proved to be more elusive. This was accomplished first by Takahashi's group, who reported an efficient stepwise procedure for producing large numbers of photoreceptors from ES cells (Osakada et al., 2008). The method was then successfully adapted to iPS cells (Hirami et al., 2009). Based on their previously published protocol (Ikeda et al., 2005), they first generated *Rx*-positive retinal progenitors and next established conditions for efficient conversion into post-mitotic *Crx*-expressing photoreceptor progenitors. These could spontaneously further differentiate into cone-like cells or be induced towards putative rod photoreceptors. It should however be stressed out that the whole procedure requires several months and is technically difficult. Importantly, Osakada and colleagues recently reported that recombinant proteins (a potential source of infection or immune rejection), previously used to "retinalize" human ES/iPS cells, could be successfully replaced by chemical compounds (Osakada et al., 2009), allowing safer conditions with regards to potential clinical translation. Finally, proof of principle that ES/iPS cell-derived photoreceptor precursors could integrate the retina and differentiate into functional photoreceptors following their transplantation in adult murine eyes was recently achieved in T. Reh's laboratory (Lamba et al., 2009, 2010; Fig. 32.2c, d). Lamba and collaborators additionally showed that ES-derived photoreceptors could restore some light response in *Rx* deficient mice, a model of LCA (Lamba et al., 2009).

Future Prospects

As a whole, it appears that tremendous advancements in the field have been made in just a few years, widening the prospects of cell-based therapies, in particular through the use of iPS cells. However, several issues have yet to be solved before they can be considered as an option in human trials for the treatment of retinal neurodegenerative diseases. Regarding photoreceptor replacement, improvement of differentiation procedures is noticeably required. This includes obtaining pure neuronal populations at higher frequency and in a shorter time and guarantying safety through limited use of animal derivatives and elimination of oncogenic pluripotent cells. Another angle of research, that could be of much interest in the future, relates to the induction of endogenous repair processes (reviewed in Karl and Reh, 2010; Locker et al., 2010). Non-mammalian vertebrates, like frog or fish, have the remarkable ability to regenerate their retina following damage, a property that has been lost in mammals. Accumulating evidences however suggest that, although quiescent or barely active, mammalian stem cells could have retained remnants of repair capacities and could thus be amenable to drive regeneration following appropriate stimulation. Further knowledge on the molecular cues controlling retinal stem cell behavior in various animal models might thus allow foreseeing novel therapeutic strategies based on endogenous stem cell mobilization in patients with retinal dystrophies.

Acknowledgements This work is supported by grants from the CNRS, University Paris Sud, ARC, Retina France and ANR. We thank C. Borday for providing us the immunostaining image.

References

Bharti K, Miller SS, Arnheiter H (2010) The new paradigm: retinal pigment epithelium cells generated from embryonic or induced pluripotent stem cells. Pigment Cell Melanoma Res 24:21–34

Brzezinski JAt, Lamba DA, Reh TA (2010) Blimp1 controls photoreceptor versus bipolar cell fate choice during retinal development. Development 137:619–629

Chacko DM, Das AV, Zhao X, James J, Bhattacharya S, Ahmad I (2003) Transplantation of ocular stem cells: the role of injury in incorporation and differentiation of grafted cells in the retina. Vision Res 43:937–946

Coles BL, Angenieux B, Inoue T, Del Rio-Tsonis K, Spence JR, McInnes RR, Arsenijevic Y, van der Kooy D (2004) Facile isolation and the characterization of human retinal stem cells. Proc Natl Acad Sci USA 101:15772–15777

da Cruz L, Chen FK, Ahmado A, Greenwood J, Coffey P (2007) RPE transplantation and its role in retinal disease. Prog Retin Eye Res 26:598–635

Das T, del Cerro M, Jalali S, Rao VS, Gullapalli VK, Little C, Loreto DA, Sharma S, Sreedharan A, del Cerro C et al (1999) The transplantation of human fetal neuroretinal cells in advanced retinitis pigmentosa patients: results of a long-term safety study. Exp Neurol 157:58–68

Esteve P, Bovolenta P (2006) Secreted inducers in vertebrate eye development: more functions for old morphogens. Curr Opin Neurobiol 16:13–19

Hennig AK, Peng GH, Chen S (2008) Regulation of photoreceptor gene expression by Crx-associated transcription factor network. Brain Res 1192:114–133

Hirami Y, Osakada F, Takahashi K, Okita K, Yamanaka S, Ikeda H, Yoshimura N, Takahashi M (2009) Generation of retinal cells from mouse and human induced pluripotent stem cells. Neurosci Lett 458:126–131

Hu Q, Friedrich AM, Johnson LV, Clegg DO (2010) Memory in induced pluripotent stem cells: reprogrammed human retinal-pigmented epithelial cells show tendency for spontaneous redifferentiation. Stem Cells 28:1981–1991

Humayun MS, de Juan E Jr, del Cerro M, Dagnelie G, Radner W, Sadda SR, del Cerro C (2000) Human neural retinal transplantation. Invest Ophthalmol Vis Sci 41:3100–3106

Ikeda H, Osakada F, Watanabe K, Mizuseki K, Haraguchi T, Miyoshi H, Kamiya D, Honda Y, Sasai N, Yoshimura N et al (2005) Generation of Rx+/Pax6+ neural retinal precursors from embryonic stem cells. Proc Natl Acad Sci USA 102:11331–11336

Inoue T, Coles BL, Dorval K, Bremner R, Bessho Y, Kageyama R, Hino S, Matsuoka M, Craft CM, McInnes RR et al (2010) Maximizing functional photoreceptor differentiation from adult human retinal stem cells. Stem Cells 28:489–500

Jin ZB, Okamoto S, Mandai M, Takahashi M (2009) Induced pluripotent stem cells for retinal degenerative diseases: a new perspective on the challenges. J Genet 88:417–424

Karl MO, Reh TA (2010) Regenerative medicine for retinal diseases: activating endogenous repair mechanisms. Trends Mol Med 16:193–202

Katoh K, Omori Y, Onishi A, Sato S, Kondo M, Furukawa T (2010) Blimp1 suppresses Chx10 expression in differentiating retinal photoreceptor precursors to ensure proper photoreceptor development. J Neurosci 30:6515–6526

Lakowski J, Baron M, Bainbridge J, Barber AC, Pearson RA, Ali RR, Sowden JC (2010) Cone and rod photoreceptor transplantation in models of the childhood retinopathy Leber congenital amaurosis using flow-sorted Crx-positive donor cells. Hum Mol Genet 19:4545–4559

Lamba DA, Karl MO, Ware CB, Reh TA (2006) Efficient generation of retinal progenitor cells from human embryonic stem cells. Proc Natl Acad Sci USA 103:12769–12774

Lamba DA, Gust J, Reh TA (2009) Transplantation of human embryonic stem cell-derived photoreceptors restores some visual function in Crx-deficient mice. Cell Stem Cell 4:73–79

Lamba DA, McUsic A, Hirata RK, Wang PR, Russell D, Reh TA (2010) Generation, purification and transplantation of photoreceptors derived from human induced pluripotent stem cells. PLoS One 5:e8763

Locker M, El Yakoubi W, Mazurier N, Dullin JP, Perron M (2010) A decade of mammalian retinal stem cell research. Arch Ital Biol 148:59–72

MacLaren RE, Pearson RA, MacNeil A, Douglas RH, Salt TE, Akimoto M, Swaroop A, Sowden JC, Ali RR (2006) Retinal repair by transplantation of photoreceptor precursors. Nature 444:203–207

Osakada F, Ikeda H, Mandai M, Wataya T, Watanabe K, Yoshimura N, Akaike A, Sasai Y, Takahashi M (2008) Toward the generation of rod and cone photoreceptors from mouse, monkey and human embryonic stem cells. Nat Biotechnol 26:215–224

Osakada F, Jin ZB, Hirami Y, Ikeda H, Danjyo T, Watanabe K, Sasai Y, Takahashi M (2009) In vitro differentiation of retinal cells from human pluripotent stem cells by small-molecule induction. J Cell Sci 122:3169–3179

Pan Y, Martinez-De Luna RI, Lou CH, Nekkalapudi S, Kelly LE, Sater AK, El-Hodiri HM (2010) Regulation of photoreceptor gene expression by the retinal homeobox (Rx) gene product. Dev Biol 339:494–506

Perron M, Kanekar S, Vetter ML, Harris WA (1998) The genetic sequence of retinal development in the ciliary margin of the Xenopus eye. Dev Biol 199:185–200

Stadtfeld M, Hochedlinger K (2010) Induced pluripotency: history, mechanisms, and applications. Genes Dev 24:2239–2263

Swaroop A, Kim D, Forrest D (2010) Transcriptional regulation of photoreceptor development and homeostasis in the mammalian retina. Nat Rev Neurosci 11:563–576

Takahashi K, Yamanaka S (2006) Induction of pluripotent stem cells from mouse embryonic and adult fibroblast cultures by defined factors. Cell 126:663–676

Tropepe V, Coles BL, Chiasson BJ, Horsford DJ, Elia AJ, McInnes RR, van der Kooy D (2000) Retinal stem cells in the adult mammalian eye. Science 287:2032–2036

Viczian AS, Solessio EC, Lyou Y, Zuber ME (2009) Generation of functional eyes from pluripotent cells. PLoS Biol 7:e1000174

West EL, Pearson RA, MacLaren RE, Sowden JC, Ali RR (2009) Cell transplantation strategies for retinal repair. Prog Brain Res 175:3–21

West EL, Pearson RA, Barker SE, Luhmann UF, Maclaren RE, Barber AC, Duran Y, Smith AJ, Sowden JC, Ali RR (2010) Long-term survival of photoreceptors transplanted into the adult murine neural retina requires immune modulation. Stem Cells 28:1997–2007

Chapter 33

Heterogeneous Responses of Human Bone Marrow Stromal Cells (Multipotent Mesenchymal Stromal Cells) to Osteogenic Induction

Hideaki Kagami, Hideki Agata, Yoshinori Sumita, and Arinobu Tojo

Abstract Tissue engineering is a novel technology developed for the regeneration of tissue using cultured cells, scaffolds, and osteogenic inductive signals. Bone marrow stromal cells (also designated as multipotent mesenchymal stromal cells, mesenchymal stem cells, or MSCs) have been the most commonly used cell source for bone tissue engineering. For efficient bone tissue engineering, the cells must be expanded in vitro and induced into osteogenic cells with an osteoinductive reagent such as dexamethasone. Recently, physiological factors such as bone morphogenetic proteins have been shown to induce the osteogenic lineage of bone marrow stromal cells. Osteogenic reagents have been widely used in both basic and clinical studies. However, it is apparent that the cellular responses to those reagents have been heterogeneous in human cells compared with animal cells, which possess a more uniform genetic background. Since the clinical use of those factors will increase further in the cases of orthopaedic applications and in the context of tissue engineering, these responses could be a serious problem in the future. In this chapter, the heterogeneous response of human bone marrow stromal cells to those inductive factors is discussed with reference to possible underlying mechanisms.

Keywords Tissue engineering · Mesenchymal stem cells · Osteogenic reagents · BMSCs · Dexamethasone · Chondrogenesis · TGF-β

Introduction

In the field of regenerative medicine, the use of biological materials in place of artificial substrates and chemical reagents is gaining acceptance. Growth factors are now in the pharmaceutical market and have attracted much attention. However, one of the ultimate biological materials is cells that can supply a variety of biological reagents such as growth factors and cytokines. More importantly, cells can produce matrices, may repair and moderate cell functions and play important roles during tissue regeneration.

Cultured cells have been used to treat various diseases including severe burns, joint cartilage degeneration, and bone defects. Since the cells can be expanded in vitro, those treatments require only a small amount of donor tissue and even autologous transplantation is feasible. Accordingly, this concept is considered a future therapeutic option in the treatment of various pathologic conditions. Tissue engineering, one of the most well recognized technologies, focuses on the regeneration of lost or damaged tissues using cultured cells, biodegradable scaffold materials, and biological factors. The initial clinical application of cultured cells was the skin substitute for severe burn cases. Subsequently, cultured cells from cartilage have been applied to repair cartilage defects of arthritis patients. Those cells were committed to specific lineages such as keratinocytes or chondrocytes. More recently, the presence of multipotent stem/progenitor cells in adults has been reported. The potential of those stem/progenitor cells for tissue engineering has been explored, since those cells possess higher proliferating capability and can differentiate into various cell lineages.

H. Kagami (✉)
Tissue Engineering Research Group, Division of Molecular Therapy, The Advanced Clinical Research Center, The Institute of Medical Science, The University of Tokyo, Tokyo 108-8639, Japan
e-mail: kagami@ims.u-tokyo.ac.jp

In terms of tissue engineering, one of the most important differences between committed (differentiating/differentiated) cells and multipotent (undifferentiated) stem/progenitor cells is the requirement for induction during cell culture. Multipotent stem/progenitor cells usually require induced differentiation to a specific lineage to regenerate a specific tissue. On the other hand, committed cells only require expansion prior to transplantation. Although cultured cells have been used clinically for more than 20 years, clinical application of multipotent stem/progenitor cells has a shorter history and information is still limited. Bone marrow stromal cells (BMSCs) are one of the most widely used cell types for this purpose. Although the results from preliminary clinical studies using BMSCs show the usefulness of this population, the heterogeneity of the population is a shortcoming (Phinney et al., 1999; Mendes et al., 2002; Mizuno et al., 2010). The heterogeneity of human BMSCs was much broader than that of animal cells and may affect the efficacy of the treatment.

In this chapter, we focus on BMSCs and their heterogeneity, which was noted from basic and clinical studies using human cells. In particular, we focus on the response to osteogenic induction using dexamethasone and BMP-2 with reference to possible underlying mechanisms.

Bone Marrow Stromal Cells (BMSCs)

BMSCs are fibroblast-like cells that can be cultured as an adherent cell fraction from bone marrow aspirates (Friedenstein et al., 1970). BMSCs possess high proliferating potential and include osteogenic stem/progenitor cells. Since BMSCs differentiate into various mesenchymal tissues, BMSCs have also been designated as multipotent mesenchymal stromal cells, mesenchymal stem cells or simply MSCs. Although BMSCs likely contain multipotent stem/progenitor cells, the population is heterogeneous. In fact, only a small portion of cells can form a secondary (osteogenic) colony (Sacchetti et al., 2007) and self-renewal capability, an essential criterion for stem cells, is difficult to confirm. Accordingly, we prefer to use the term "bone marrow stromal cells" (BMSCs).

Although various specific markers for BMSCs have been suggested, there is still no established marker to define BMSCs. The minimum criteria for MSCs were proposed by The International Society for Cellular Therapy as follows: positive for CD105, CD73 and CD90 and negative for CD34, CD45, CD11a, CD19, and HLA-DR (Dominici et al., 2006). More recent studies suggested that MCAM/CD146$^+$, CD271, mesenchymal stem cell antigen-1 (MSCA-1), CD56, SSEA-4, STRO-1, and platelet-derived growth factor receptor-beta (PDGF-RB; CD140b) might be used to enrich the stem/progenitor cells in culture (reviewed by Salem and Thiemermann, 2010).

Osteogenic Induction of BMSCs for Bone Tissue Engineering

As stated above, one of the major differences between committed (or relatively differentiated) and multipotent (or less differentiated) stem/progenitor cells is the requirement for induction. However, cultures of multipotent stem/progenitor cells such as BMSCs contain some differentiated cells (Mendes et al., 2002; Mizuno et al., 2010). Accordingly, the induction process is not always mandatory for bone regeneration, but considered favorable, especially in cases of BMSCs with relatively low osteogenic ability (e.g., elderly patients) (Mendes et al., 2002). Furthermore, the ability of BMSCs to differentiate into osteoblast-like cells diminishes during culture and passage (Agata et al., 2010). Thus, osteogenic induction might be important to increase the probability of in vivo bone formation. The steroid dexamethasone has been widely used for osteogenic induction for human and most other mammalian BMSCs. More recently, members of the TGF-super family, the bone morphogenetic proteins (BMP), have been used as potent inducers of osteogenesis.

Effect of Dexamethasone on Human BMSCs

Glucocorticoids, small lipophilic hormones that are secreted from the adrenal gland, are important regulators of various physiological functions such as carbohydrate and lipid metabolism, immune function and stress responses in mammals. Because of their strong anti-inflammatory and immunosuppressive properties, synthetic glucocorticoids such as dexamethasone have been widely used as therapeutic reagents for a variety of diseases (McCulloch and Tenenbaum, 1986; Harrison et al., 2002). However, excessive exposure to glucocorticoids, such as long-term usage of dexamethasone or Cushing's syndrome (hypercorticism) results in the disruption of physiological functions and may lead to osteoporosis (McCulloch and Tenenbaum, 1986; Harrison et al., 2002; Tamura et al., 2004). Accordingly, the inhibitory effects of glucocorticoids on bone formation have been investigated for more than 40 years (Birkenhäger et al., 1967).

It has been shown that glucocorticoids have bimodal effects on bone formation (Harrison et al., 2002). The pharmacological dose ($>10^{-6}$ M) of glucocorticoid suppresses the generation and survival of osteoblasts, while physiological doses (10^{-8} to 10^{-7} M) selectively stimulate proliferation and differentiation of osteoprogenitors, suggesting that the effect of glucocorticoid on bone formation is dose- and target-specific (McCulloch and Tenenbaum, 1986; Weinstein et al., 1998; Harrison et al., 2002). To support this interpretation, previous studies have shown that the physiological dose of dexamethasone can efficiently induce osteogenic differentiation of human and other mammalian BMSCs (Kadiyala et al., 1997; Diefenderfer et al., 2003; Osyczka et al., 2004), while a similar dose suppresses the activities of mature osteoblasts (Harrison et al., 2002). For these reasons, physiological doses of dexamethasone treatment have become the current gold standard for the induction of osteogenic differentiation of human BMSCs (Phinney et al., 1999; Siddappa et al., 2007; Agata et al., 2010).

Alkaline phosphatase (ALP) activity is an early marker for osteogenic differentiation and is required for the initiation of matrix mineralization (Fedde et al., 1999). Accordingly, ALP activity analysis is frequently performed to investigate the osteogenic ability of BMSCs. When non-human BMSCs are exposed to a physiological dose of dexamethasone, they differentiate into the osteogenic lineage with elevated levels of ALP activity (McCulloch and Tenenbaum, 1986; Kadiyala et al., 1997; Aubin, 1999). Human BMSCs are also responsive to dexamethasone. The results from our own experiments showed that the levels of ALP activity increased among all five volunteer donors after exposure to dexamethasone (Fig. 33.1a, b). However, it is noteworthy that huge differences in the basal levels were already present among the donors (ALP activity of non-induced cells). Similarly, the ALP activity levels in induced BMSCs (after exposure to dexamethasone) also showed significant variations (Fig. 33.1a, b). Consequently, these variations led to differences in average ALP activity between induced and non-induced cells, which failed to achieve statistical significance (Fig. 33.1c). Similarly, several groups reported that the responses of human BMSCs to dexamethasone varied significantly among donors (Phinney et al., 1999; Siddappa et al., 2007). On the other hand, it may not be true in non-human BMSCs, such as rat BMSCs, which show relatively consistent responses to dexamethasone regardless of the origin of donor animals (Diefenderfer et al., 2003; Osyczka et al., 2004). Thus, significant donor variation in dexamethasone-responsiveness might be a specific problem for human BMSCs. Therefore, it is quite important to take the influence of donor variation into account when evaluating the osteogenic ability of human BMSCs when using dexamethasone. As suggested elsewhere (Siddappa et al., 2007), compensation for donor variations in basal ALP activity by calculating the rising ratio of ALP activity (ALP activity of induced/non-induced cells) might be a better approach to evaluate the osteogenic ability of human BMSCs.

It has been suggested that human BMSCs are composed of a heterogeneous mixture of cells at various stages of differentiation and that the proportions of non-osteogenic, osteoprogenitors, and committed osteogenic cells vary significantly among donors (Phinney et al., 1999). At least two classes of osteoprogenitor cells are present in BMSC populations: those differentiating without glucocorticoid and those requiring glucocorticoid to differentiate (Aubin, 1999). Thus, there may be differences in the proportions of dexamethasone-responsive osteoprogenitors in human BMSC populations among donors. These differences might explain the significant donor variations in dexamethasone-responsiveness of human BMSCs. To better understand the heterogeneous responses of human BMSCs to dexamethasone, specific markers of dexamethasone-responsive osteoprogenitors and differences in the proportion of dexamethasone-responsive osteoprogenitors among donors should be further investigated.

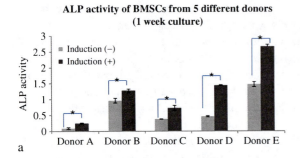
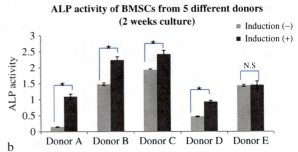
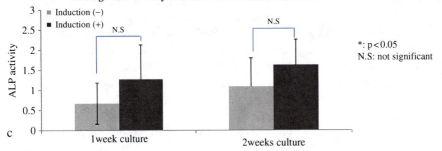

Fig. 33.1 Heterogeneous responses of human BMSCs to dexamethasone. Each graph shows the ALP activity of human BMSCs from five different donors after 1 or 2 weeks of osteogenic induction with 10 nM dexamethasone, 100 μM ascorbic acid, and 10 mM β-glycerophosphate (**a**, **b**). Graph (**c**) shows the average ALP activity of human BMSCs after 1 or 2 weeks of osteogenic induction, which were compared with that of the control without induction. *$p < 0.05$

Effect of Recombinant Bone Morphogenetic Protein-2 on Human Bone Marrow Stromal Cells

Bone morphogenetic proteins (BMPs) constitute a group of conserved signaling molecules, which belong to the transforming growth factor-β (TGF-β) superfamily. BMPs were originally identified by their capacity to induce ectopic bone formation, which naturally exists within the bone matrix (Urist, 1965). Subsequent studies have shown that BMPs have a variety of functions as pleiotropic regulators for chemotaxis, mitosis, differentiation, stimulation of extracellular matrix synthesis, binding to matrix components, maintenance of phenotype, and apoptosis. The general role of BMPs in the process of bone formation during the development, regulation of bone volume and repair of fractures has been well established (Reddi, 1998). However, only selected BMPs can induce bone formation in ectopic sites.

Although more than 20 BMPs have been discovered, only BMP-2, -4, -6, -7, and -9 have been proven capable of driving multipotent cells into osteoblastic phenotypes in culture (De Biase and Capanna, 2005). Among them, BMP-2 is considered the most potent osteoinductive agent in the TGF-β superfamily. Since the expression of BMP-2 is correlated with the differentiation of osteoblasts and chondroblasts from mesenchymal stem cells, it is considered a strong inducer of bone formation and chondrogenesis (Reddi, 1998). However, the exact cellular and molecular mechanisms of BMP-2 are not fully understood.

The osteoinductive property of BMP-2 has been clearly shown with animal cells (Chen et al., 2002). BMP-2 target genes include several homeodomain proteins, the bone-related runt homology domain factor *RUNX2* (*CBFA1/AML3*), and an SP1 family member, *OSTERIX*, which may co-operatively work to promote cell differentiation into osteoblasts (Li et al., 2011). When rodent BMSCs were treated with BMP-2, they committed to the osteogenic lineage, produced bone matrix proteins and expressed ALP (Reilly et al., 2007;

Difenderfer et al., 2003). For human BMSCs, BMP-2 upregulates bone matrix proteins and mineralization, and enhances dexamethasone-induced osteogenic differentiation (Lecanda et al., 1997). However, the efficacy of rhBMP-2 on human BMSCs might be less consistent than that observed with rodent cells and limited and/or conflicting effects have also been reported (Diefenderfer et al., 2003; Osyczka et al., 2004; Reilly et al., 2007; Mizuno et al., 2010) (Fig. 33.2). Among donors from more than a dozen patients, only the cells from one donor showed significantly elevated alkaline phosphatase activity after exposure to BMP-2 (Difenderfer et al., 2003). Interestingly, the responsiveness was partially affected by the choice of serum. When five different sera were used for cultivation and induction with rhBMP-2, ALP activities increased in two of them, but not in the others (Mizuno et al., 2010). Although the reason for those controversial results is not clear, it may reflect the heterogeneous responsiveness of human BMSCs to rhBMP-2.

The in vivo efficacy of rhBMP-2 was also evaluated using animal models. RhBMP-2-coated natural bone mineral (NBM) accelerates regeneration in a rat calvarial defect model (Schwarz et al., 2009). When rhBMP-2 was applied to critical sized craniotomy defects in rhesus macaque, it facilitated the osseointegration of rectangular bone flaps. After 6 months, the BMP-2-treated craniotomy defects were on average 71% covered with calcified material versus an average of 28% coverage in empty control defects (Sheehan et al., 2003). Thus, BMP-2 has been shown as a strong osteogenic inducer in vivo. In clinical studies, rhBMP-2 combined with allograft dowels increased the rate of interbody fusion in patients who have undergone anterior lumbar fusion surgery (Burkus et al., 2003). The addition of rhBMP-2 to the treatment of type-III open tibial fractures reduced the frequency of bone-grafting procedures and other secondary interventions (Swiontkowski et al., 2006). Currently, rhBMP-2 is commercially available as an osteoinductive material (Infuse, Medtronic, Sofamar Danek, TN, USA). Although most of the results from clinical studies showed the usefulness of rhBMP-2, high doses of the factor are required for in vivo efficacy. Some researchers reported that the efficacy in human study

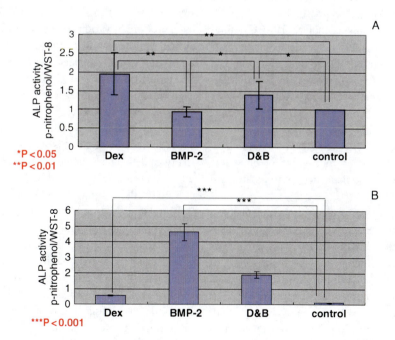

Fig. 33.2 Effects of osteogenic induction media on ALP activities of human and murine MSCs. Graph (**a**) shows the average ALP activity from six human samples after 1 week of osteogenic induction with Dex (D), BMP-2 (B), or D + B. Control represents the results from hMSCs without induction. Graph (**b**) shows the average ALP activity from mouse MSCs after 1 week of osteogenic induction with D, B, or D + B, which were compared with that of the control without induction. In hMSCs, Dex significantly upregulated ALP activity. On the other hand, BMP-2 showed no effect and even reduced the ALP activity of hMSCs with Dex. In mouse cells, BMP-2 significantly upregulated ALP activity (From Mizuno et al., 2010 with permission)

was less remarkable than that from animal studies, which may also imply species differences (Kwong and Harris, 2008).

Factors that Might Affect Responsiveness to Recombinant Bone Morphogenic Protein-2

Although the results from previous studies on the responsiveness of human MSCs to rhBMP-2 were variable, the reasons for these discrepancies are not well understood. Several studies including our own have tried to show underlying mechanisms for the lack of responsiveness.

It was possible that differences in the use of BMP receptors affected the downstream actions of BMP signaling. Although rat BMSCs and differentiated human osteoblasts express mRNA for one of the type I BMP receptors (ALK-6), human BMSCs lack this BMP receptor (Osyczka et al., 2004). However, forced expression of this receptor did not enhance ALP activity. This result suggests that the lack of ALK-6 is not a major reason for the limited response.

Other possible mechanisms include BMP-2 antagonists, since the expression of various antagonists against BMPs has been reported in animal and human cells. It was shown that *noggin* expression was upregulated in most of the samples after exposure to BMP-2, thus the application of exogenous BMP-2 may induce *noggin* expression in hMSCs in a serum-containing environment (Diefenderfer et al., 2003; Mizuno et al., 2010). Although the effect of noggin is plausible, the effects of other antagonists such as follistatin and chordin were not clear.

Other than antagonists, receptor modifications have also been suggested. Since TGF-β treatment causes rapid translocation of BMPR-IB from the cytoplasm to the cell surface (Singhatanadgit et al., 2008), it is possible that serum TGF-β plays some role in the responsiveness of human MSCs to rhBMP-2. It has been reported that BMP activates ERK signaling, which in turn decrease nuclear translocation of BMP-activated Smads, thus affecting the responsiveness of MSCs to BMP-2 (Osyczka and Leboy, 2005). However, the results from experiments using the same ERK inhibitor were not consistent and may require further clarification (Mizuno et al., 2010). So far, a simple explanation of the heterogeneous response of human BMSCs to rhBMP-2 is not available. The responsiveness might be determined as a balance of positive stimuli (rhBMP-2) and inhibitory factors, which may include some unknown mechanisms.

Heterogenicity of Human Cells for Therapeutic Use

Interestingly, the heterogenic response to osteogenic induction was observed not only for rhBMP-2 but also for dexamethasone. Since BMP receptors are located on the cell membrane while glucocorticoid receptors are located in the nucleus, the major reason for this heterogeneous responsiveness might not be environmental factors but may depend on the cells themselves.

There is no doubt that human cells are more heterogeneous than those from laboratory animals since various factors (age, gender, general condition, and also genetic background) could affect the properties of BMSCs (Phinney et al., 1999) (Fig. 33.3a). As mentioned above, cultured BMSCs vary in their responsiveness. First, BMSCs are not a uniform population but a mixture of various types of cells. The results from clonal analyses showed that not all BMSC-colonies were osteogenic (Kuznetsov et al., 1997) (Fig. 33.3b). Second, various levels of differentiation were observed even in a single culture flask (or even in one colony) (Ylöstalo et al., 2008) (Fig. 33.3c). Since flow cytometry showed relatively uniform cell surface marker expression by BMSCs, this second hypothesis is more likely and the heterogeneous responsiveness may be due to varying levels of differentiation (stemness) of cultured cells. In support of this interpretation, rhBMP-2 stimulated ALP activities in undifferentiated cells (fresh bone marrow cells and colony-forming units fibroblasts) but not in differentiated osteoblastic cells (Kim et al., 1997). Although the detailed mechanisms require further investigation, those characteristic features of BMSCs as well as human cells should be kept in mind when clinical use of these somatic cells or growth factors are planned.

Preliminary clinical studies have shown the usefulness of somatic cells such as BMSCs for various diseases including bone tissue engineering. It will be important to understand the mechanisms of heterogeneous response, which may contribute to the further

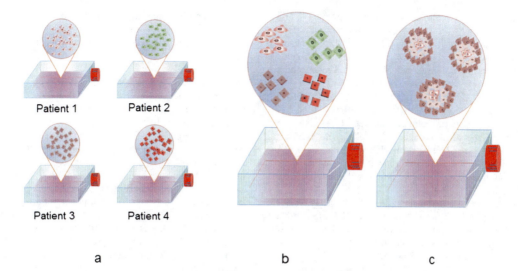

Fig. 33.3 Schematic illustration of the potential heterogeneity in human BMSCs. Various factors (age, gender, general condition and also genetic background) differ among individuals, which should affect the heterogeneity of BMSCs from donors (**a**). The nature of BMSC culture is heterogeneous and BMSC culture consists of a mixture of various types of cells. It is noteworthy that not all BMSC-colonies are osteogenic (**b**). Even in one culture flask (and in one colony), various levels of differentiation can be observed, which may explain another type of heterogeneity (**c**)

development of bone tissue engineering as well as clinical use of BMP-2.

Acknowledgement The authors with to thank Ms. Sachiko Sawada for the technical assistance.

References

Agata H, Asahina I, Watanabe N, Ishii Y, Kubo N, Ohshimam S, Yamazaki M, Tojo A, Kagami H (2010) Characteristic change and loss of in vivo osteogenic abilities of human bone marrow stromal cells during passage. Tissue Eng Part A 16:663–673

Aubin JE (1999) Osteoprogenitor cell frequency in rat bone marrow stromal populations: role for heterotypic cell-cell interactions in osteoblast differentiation. J Cell Biochem 72:396–410

Birkenhäger JC, van der Heul RO, Smeenk D, van der Sluys Veer J, van Seters AP (1967) Bone changes associated with glucocorticoid excess. Proc R Soc Med 60:1134–1136

Burkus JK, Dorchak JD, Sanders DL (2003) Radiographic assessment of interbody fusion using recombinant human bone morphogenetic protein type 2. Spine 28:372–377

Chen X, Kidder LS, Lew WD (2002) Osteogenic protein-1 induced bone formation in an infected segmental defect in the rat femur. J Orthop Res 20:142–150

De Biase P, Capanna R (2005) Clinical applications of BMPs. Injury 36:S43–S46

Diefenderfer DL, Osyczka AM, Reilly GC, Leboy PS (2003) BMP responsiveness in human mesenchymal stem cells. Connect Tissue Res 44:305–311

Dominici M, Le Blanc K, Mueller I, Slaper-Cortenbach I, Marini F, Krause D, Deans R, Keating A, Prockop Dj, Horwitz E (2006) Minimal criteria for defining multipotent mesenchymal stromal cells. The International Society for Cellular Therapy position statement. Cytotherapy 8:315–317

Fedde KN, Blair L, Silverstein J, Coburn SP, Ryan LM, Weinstein RS, Waymire K, Narisawa S, Millán JL, MacGregor GR, Whyte MP (1999) Alkaline phosphatase knock-out mice recapitulate the metabolic and skeletal defects of infantile hypophosphatasia. J Bone Miner Res 14:2015–2026

Friedenstein AJ, Chailakhjan RK, Lalykina KS (1970) The development of fibroblast colonies in monolayer cultures of guinea-pig bone marrow and spleen cells. Cell Tissue Kinet 3:393–403

Harrison JR, Woitge HW, Kream BE (2002) Genetic approaches to determine the role of glucocorticoid signaling in osteoblasts. Endocrine 17:37–42

Kadiyala S, Young RG, Thiede MA, Bruder SP (1997) Culture expanded canine mesenchymal stem cells possess osteochondrogenic potential *in vivo* and *in vitro*. Cell Transplant 6:125–134

Kim KJ, Itoh T, Kotake S (1997) Effects of recombinant human bone morphogenetic protein-2 on human bone marrow cells cultured with various biomaterials. J Biol Chem 35:279–285

Kuznetsov SA, Krebsbach PH, Satomura K, Kerr J, Riminucci M, Benayahu D, Robey PG (1997) Single-colony derived strains of human marrow stromal fibroblasts form bone after transplantation *in vivo*. J Bone Miner Res 12:1335–1347

Kwong FN, Harris MB (2008) Recent developments in the biology of fracture repair. J Am Acad Orthop Surg 16:619–625

Lecanda F, Avioli LV, Cheng SL (1997) Regulation of bone matrix protein expression and induction of differentiation of human osteoblasts and human bone marrow stromal cells by bone morphogenetic protein-2. J Cell Biochem 67:386–396

Li J, Khavandgar Z, Lin SH, Murshed M (2011) Lithium chloride attenuates BMP-2 signaling and inhibits osteogenic differentiation through a novel WNT/GSK3-independent mechanism. Bone 48:321–331

McCulloch CAG, Tenenbaum HC (1986) Dexamethasone induces proliferation and terminal differentiation of osteogenic cells in tissue culture. Anat Rec 215:397–402

Mendes SC, Tibbe JM, Veenhof M, Bakker K, Both S, Platenburg PP, Oner FC, de Bruijn JD, van Blitterswijk CA (2002) Bone tissue-engineered implants using human bone marrow stromal cells: Effect of culture conditions and donor age. Tissue Eng 8:911–920

Mizuno D, Agata H, Furue H, Kimura A, Narita Y, Watanabe N, Ishii Y, Ueda M, Tojo A, Kagami H (2010) Limited but heterogeneous osteogenic response of human bone marrow mesenchymal stem cells to bone morphogenetic protein-2 and serum. Growth Factors 28:34–43

Osyczka AM, Leboy PS (2005) Bone morphogenetic protein regulation of early osteoblast genes in human marrow stromal cells is mediated by extracellular signal-regulated kinase and phosphatidylinositol 3-kinase signaling. Endocrinology 146:3428–3437

Osyczka AM, Diefenderfer DL, Bhargave G, Leboy PS (2004) Different effects of BMP-2 on marrow stromal cells from human and rat bone. Cell Tissues Organs 176:109–119

Phinney DG, Kopen G, Righter W, Webster S, Tremain N, Prockop DJ (1999) Donor variation in the growth properties and osteogenic potential of human marrow stromal cells. J Cell Biochem 75:424–436

Reddi AH (1998) Initiation of fracture repair by bone morphogenetic proteins. Clin Orthop Relat Res 355S:s66–s72

Reilly GC, Radin S, Chen AT, Ducheyne P (2007) Differential alkaline phosphatase responses of rat and human bone marrow derived mesenchymal cells to 45S5 bioactive glass. Biomaterials 28:4091–4097

Sacchetti B, Funari A, Michienzi S, Di Cesare S, Piersanti S, Saggio I, Tagliafico E, Ferrari S, Robey PG, Riminucci M, Bianco P (2007) Self-renewing osteoprogenitors in bone marrow sinusoids can organize a hematopoietic microenvironment. Cell 131:324–336

Salem HK, Thiemermann C (2010) Mesenchymal stromal cells: current understanding and clinical status. Stem Cells 28:585–596

Schwarz F, Ferrari D, Sager M, Herten M, Hartig B, Becker J (2009) Guided bone regeneration using rhGDF-5- and rhBMP-2-coated natural bone mineral in rat calvarial defects. Clin Oral Implants Res 1219–1230

Sheehan JP, Sheehan JM, Seeherman H, Quigg M, Helm GA (2003) The safety and utility of recombinant human bone morphogenetic protein-2 for cranial procedures in a nonhuman primate model. J Neurosurg 98:125–130

Siddappa R, Licht R, van Blitterswijk C, de Boer J (2007) Donor variation and loss of multipotency during in vitro expansion of human mesenchymal stem cells for bone tissue engineering. J Orthop Res 25:1029–1041

Singhatanadgit W, Mordan N, Salih V, Olsen I, (2008) Changes in bone morphogenic protein receptor-IB localization regulate osteogenic responses of human bone cells to bone morphogenic protein-2. Int J Biochem Cell Biol 40:2854–2864

Swiontkowski MF, Aro HT, Donell S, Esterhai JL, Goulet J, Jones A, Kregor PJ, Nordsletten L, Paiement G, Patel A (2006) Recombinant human bone morphogenetic protein-2 in open tibial fractures. A subgroup analysis of data combined from two prospective randomized studies. J. Bone Joint Surg Am 88:1258–1265

Tamura Y, Okinaga H, Takami H (2004) Glucocorticoid-induced osteoporosis. Biomed Pharmacother 58:500–504

Urist MR (1965) Bone formation by autoinduction. Science 150:893–899

Weinstein RS, Jilka RL, Parfitt AM, Manolagas SC (1998) Inhibition of osteoblastogenesis and promotion of apoptosis of osteoblasts and osteocytes by glucocorticoids. Potential mechanisms of their deleterious effects on bone. J Clin Invest 102:274–282

Ylöstalo J, Bazhanov N, Prockop DJ (2008) Reversible commitment to differentiation by human multipotent stromal cells in single-cell-derived colonies. Exp Hematol 36:1390–1402

Chapter 34

Adipose-Derived Stem Cells and Platelet-Rich Plasma: Implications for Regenerative Medicine

Natsuko Kakudo, Satoshi Kushida, and Kenji Kusumoto

Abstract Adipose-derived stem cells (ASCs) are equally capable of differentiating into multiple lineages compared with bone marrow-derived stem cells. Because human adipose tissue can be easily obtained in large quantities under local anesthesia with little patient discomfort, it may provide an alternative source of stem cells for mesenchymal tissue regeneration and engineering. On the other hand, platelet-rich plasma (PRP) contains a high concentration of thrombocytes. In α-granules of platelets, there are platelet-released growth factors that include molecules such as platelet-derived growth factor (PDGF) and transforming growth factor (TGF)-β, which stimulate cell proliferation and differentiation, including those of ASCs for tissue regeneration. ASCs and PRP can be used for clinical cases without concerns for infection and immunological rejection because these are autologous tissue and blood. The efficacy of combination therapy using these has been increasingly recognized in the fields of wound healing, fat grafting, and periodontal tissue regeneration.

Keywords Adipose-derived stem cells · Platelet-rich plasma · Thrombocytes · TGF-β · DMEM · Adipogenesis

N. Kakudo (✉)
Department of Plastic and Reconstructive Surgery, Kansai Medical University, Moriguchi 570-8506, Japan
e-mail: kakudon@takii.kmu.ac.jp

Introduction

Recently, adipose tissue has been confirmed as one source of multipotent adult stem cells, and these stem cells are called adipose-derived stem cells (ASCs). Platelet-rich plasma (PRP) is a concentration of platelets in a small volume of plasma. Platelet α-granules contain growth factors such as platelet-derived growth factor (PDGF) and transforming growth factor (TGF)-β. Autologous platelet-rich plasma has gained in popularity as a clinical treatment in a wide variety of soft- and hard-tissue applications in surgery, particularly in problematic wound, maxillofacial bone defect, and cosmetic surgeries. Both ASCs and PRP have been shown to be simply prepared from autologous tissue and blood and exhibit marked effects on tissue regeneration, being expected to play important roles in regenerative medicine in the future. In this chapter, the isolation method and molecular characterization of ASCs and PRP are described. Furthermore, animal studies on combination therapy using ASCs and PRP and prospects for clinical application are described.

Availability of Adipose-Derived Stem Cells

A cell population that is similar to bone-marrow stem cells has been demonstrated to exist within human adipose tissue (Zuk et al., 2001, 2002). Because adipose tissue can be obtained under local anesthesia more easily than bone marrow in humans, making the procedure less invasive to the donor, adipose tissue is considered

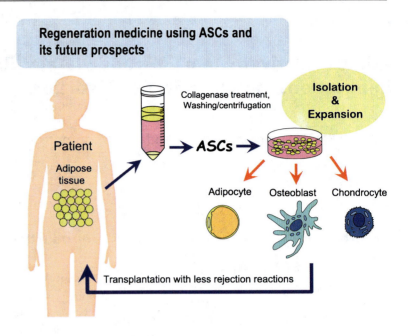

Fig. 34.1 Schema of application of adipose-derived stem cells for regenerative medicine

a suitable source for collection of stem cells for clinical application. One gram of adipose tissue yields approximately 5×10^3 stem cells, which is 500-fold greater than the number of bone-marrow stem cells in 1 g of bone marrow (Fraser et al., 2006). Therefore, ASCs are now expected as an alternative source of autologous adult stem cells that can be obtained repeatedly in large quantities with a minimum of patient discomfort. Because of their convenient isolation, extensive proliferative capacities in vitro, and differentiation potential, ASCs are a promising source of human stem cells for regenerative medicine (Fig. 34.1).

The Isolation of Adipose-Derived Stem Cells

In previous studies, we established a standard protocol for the isolation of ASCs from adipose tissue using collagenase enzymatic digestion (Kakudo et al., 2007). This method was partially modified from the method reported by Zuk et al. (2001). Briefly, adipose tissue was washed extensively with 20 ml of phosphate-buffered saline (PBS) three times, cut into small pieces, and the extracellular matrix was digested with 0.1% collagenase solution with shaking at 37°C for 40 min. After adding medium consisting of Dulbecco's modified Eagle's medium (DMEM), 10% fetal bovine serum (FBS), and 1% penicillin, it was centrifuged at 1,500 rpm for 3 min and washed using DMEM with FBS 3 times. Since prolonged digestion with collagenase and insufficient washing reduce cell viability and influence proliferation and differentiation, these processes should be carefully performed. The supernatant was discarded and the pellet resuspended and filtered through a 100-μm cell strainer to remove undigested tissue fragments. The cells were pelleted and then resuspended in cell culture medium, consisting of DMEM, 10% FBS, and 1% penicillin. The adhered ASCs were maintained until passage 3 in the medium, and nearly all cells formed fibroblast-like cells.

Devices that automatically isolate and recover stem cells from aspirated adipose tissue have recently been developed Hicok and Hedrick (2011). The development and utilization of automated processes and instrumentation to reduce the variability and increase the quality of the recovered cells are required for clinical use because of an automated, closed processing platform for isolation and concentration of ASCs. However, most of such devices have not been approved for use for treatment, and physicians have to take responsibility for health damage caused by such devices, since it would be regarded that the decision to use devices and agents not approved for healthcare use was their own.

The Differentiation Capacity of Adipose-Derived Stem Cells

We and other researchers have demonstrated the ability of ASCs to undergo differentiation along classic multiple lineages: adipogenesis, osteogenesis, chondrogenesis, and myogenesis (Zuk et al., 2001; Kakudo et al., 2008b). Non-mesenchymal lineages, such as nerve and blood cells, have also been investigated and confirm the transdifferentiation ability of ASCs (Safford et al., 2002; Planat-Benard et al., 2004). Of classic lineages, adipogenesis, osteogenesis, and chondrogenesis are described in this report.

Adipogenesis

ASCs incubated in adipogenic medium for 2 weeks exhibited intracellular lipid accumulation, which was stained positively with Oil red O. Lipid droplets expanded in the cytosol, which is consistent with the phenotype of mature adipocytes. The expressions of several adipocytic genes, such as lipoprotein lipase, aP2, PPARγ2, leptin, and Glut4, as well as the development of lipid-laden intracellular vacuoles, the definitive marker of adipogenesis, were observed (Strem et al., 2005; Zuk et al., 2001, 2002). These results indicate that ASCs undergo adipogenic differentiation. Furthermore, we clarified that FGF-2 promotes not only ASC proliferation but also differentiation into fat by enhancing PPARγ expression (Kakudo et al., 2007), suggesting a possibility of mass preparation of stem cells with differentiation ability to fat (ASCs) from a small amount of donor tissue (adipose tissue) using FGF-2-supplemented medium. The in vivo capacity of ASCs to differentiate into cells of the adipocytic lineage has also been demonstrated in studies involving implantation of cell-seeded collagen (von Heimburg et al., 2001), and hyaluronic (Halbleib et al., 2003) or polyglycolic acid (Patrick et al., 1999).

Osteogenesis

Under osteogenic conditions, similar to those used for bone marrow-derived stem cells, ASCs are observed to express genes and proteins associated with an osteoblastic phenotype, including alkaline phosphatase, type I collagen, osteopontin, osteonectin, osteocalcin, bone sialoprotein, Runx-1, BMP-2, BMP receptors I and II, and PTH receptor (Zuk et al., 2001, 2002; Halvorsen et al., 2001). Furthermore, ASCs incubated in osteogenic medium for 2–4 weeks formed monolayered calcified extracellular matrix stained positively for von Kossa. These findings strongly suggested that ASCs are capable of osteogenesis. ASCs are also able to form mineralized matrix in vivo in both 2-D and 3-D long-term osteogenic cultures. We reported the possibility of using honeycomb collagen scaffold to culture ASCs in bone tissue engineering (Kakudo et al., 2008b). The histological data showed that the scaffold was filled with the grown ASCs, and calcification, stained black with von Kossa, was confirmed. These results suggest that this carrier is a suitable scaffold for ASCs and will be useful as a three-dimensional bone tissue engineering scaffold in vitro and in vivo. In addition, other researchers reported polyglycolic acid (Lee et al., 2003) and hydroxyapatite/tricalcium phosphate (Hicok et al., 2004) as candidate scaffold for bone regeneration.

Chondrogenesis

Under high-density micromass cultures, ASCs and bone marrow-derived stem cells differentiate chondrogenic nodules that produce a large amount of cartilage-related extracellular matrix molecules, including sulfated proteoglycans, collagen II and IV, and aggrecan (Zuk et al., 2001, 2002; Huang et al., 2004). Moreover, ASCs seeded onto alginate discs and implanted into immunodeficient mice exhibit prolonged (12 weeks) synthesis of cartilage matrix molecules including collagen II and IV, and aggrecan (Erickson et al., 2002). These results strongly suggested that ASCs possess the capability of differentiation toward the chondrogenic lineage.

The Molecular Characterization of Adipose-Derived Stem Cells

The cell surface phenotype of human ASCs is quite similar to that of bone marrow-derived stem cells. For example, CD105, CD166 (ALCAM), and STRO-1 are common markers used to identify cells with multi-lineage differentiation potential and are consistently expressed on ASCs and bone marrow-derived stem cells (BMSC) (Strem et al., 2005). In addition, CD117 (the stem cell factor receptor) has been shown to be expressed on an array of totipotent or pluripotent stem cells including embryonic stem cells, hematopoietic stem cells, BMSC, and ASCs. In addition, ASCs and BMSC express CD9, CD10, CD13, CD29, CD44, CD49e, CD54, CD55, CD59, CD90, CD105, CD117, and CD146. Surface markers absent on both cell types include CD34 and CD45 (Strem et al., 2005), but it has been reported that fresh ASCs exhibited the phenotype of CD31(–), CD34(+), CD45(–), CD90(+), CD105(–), and CD146(–), and strongly expressed CD105 in culture (Yoshimura et al., 2006). Changes in the ASC markers due to culture conditions and number of passages have been pointed out as causes of this inconsistency.

Characteristics of Platelet-Rich Plasma

Platelet-rich plasma (PRP) is enriched with platelets collected by centrifugation of autologous blood. Platelets in PRP are collected without coagulation, and cytokines contained at a high concentration in α-granules can be applied by administration of PRP activated by adding autologous thrombin and calcium to tissue-defective regions.

PDGF, TGF-β, vascular endothelial growth factor (VEGF), insulin-like growth factor (IGF), epidermal growth factor (EGF), platelet factor-4, interleukin (IL)-1, osteocalcin, osteonectin, fibrinogen, vitronectin, and fibronectin have been reported to be peptides and proteins contained in platelet α-granules (Harrison and Cramer, 1993; Smith and Roukis, 2009). These growth factors play important roles in various stages of wound healing. For example, PDGF is involved in proliferation of fibroblasts, smooth muscle cells, and chondrocytes, vascularization, and macrophage activation. In wound healing, white blood cells migrate upon stimulation by PDGF released from the wound and secondarily produce other cytokines, promoting wound-healing reactions. TGF-β promotes production of extracellular matrix components, such as collagen and fibronectin, regulates cell differentiation and proliferation, and promotes fibroblast migration. VEGF promotes vascular endothelial cell proliferation and vascular permeability. EGF promotes proliferation of fibroblasts, epidermal cells, vascular smooth muscle cells, and various epithelial cells. It is considered that, when platelets are activated, these cytokines are released from α-granules and act in concert to promote wound healing. Approximately 10 min after platelet aggregation/clotting, platelets begin to actively secrete these proteins to the extent that, within 1 h, approximately 95% of a granule's contents have been secreted (Marx, 2004).

The use of PRP for regenerative medicine has attracted attention since Marx et al. reported its application for bone grafting in the dental field in 1998 (Marx et al., 1998); now, superior efficacy in reconstructive, traumatic, and esthetic surgeries and antiaging medical care has been shown, such as efficacy for healing of skin and soft-tissue wounds including chronic ulcers, such as diabetic and ischemic lower limb ulcers and bed sores, bone regeneration, and improvement of facial and hand wrinkles. PRP is markedly safe because it is autologous, blood sampling is not very invasive, allowing repeated application, and it contains several cytokines, for which a synergistic effect can be expected.

Collection and Processing Technique of Platelet-Rich Plasma

The first step of PRP preparation is concentration of platelets in whole blood samples. The concentration factor of PRP is presented as a platelet concentration, and reportedly, the factor is generally about 2–10 times the platelet concentration in whole blood. A pioneer of PRP, Marx, reported that $1 \times 10^6/\mu l$ or a 4–6 times greater platelet count is clinically effective (Marx, 2004).

Centrifugal separation methods of PRP are roughly divided into single- and double-spin methods:

Single-spin method: PRP is prepared by a single centrifugation. Although it is simple, only 358%, that is, 3.58 times, has been reported as a high concentration factor (Eby, 2002). Moreover, errors are likely to occur in the PRP recovery step, and control of the concentration factor is difficult.

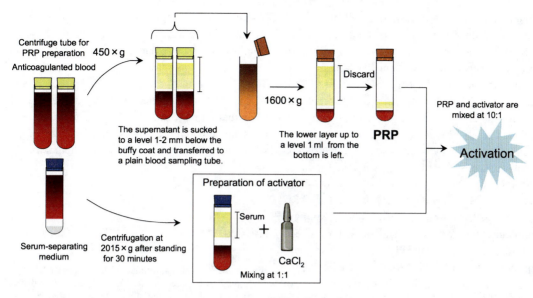

Fig. 34.2 Collection and processing technique of platelet-rich plasma

Double-spin method: PRP is prepared by 2 centrifugations. The preparation process becomes slightly complex, but reliability is higher because the platelet layer can be macroscopically confirmed and the concentration factor is controllable. The platelet concentration factor obtained by the double-spin method is reported to be generally about 2–8 times (Marx, 2004; Kakudo et al., 2008a, 2009). We normally prepare PRP employing the double-spin method for clinical use and experiments. The preparation protocol established by us is as follows.

PRP was prepared using a PRP kit (JP200) (Japan Paramedic Co., Ltd., Tokyo, Japan), as previously described (Kakudo et al., 2008a). Briefly, blood was collected into tubes containing acid-citrate-dextrose solution formula A (ACD-A; 1:4 vol/vol) anticoagulant. The citrated blood was centrifuged in a standard laboratory centrifuge for 7 min at $450 \times g$. Subsequently, the yellow plasma with buffy coat (containing platelets, leukocytes, and a few erythrocytes) was taken up into a monovette with a long cannula. The second centrifugation was performed for 5 min at $1,600 \times g$. The platelet pellet accumulated at the bottom, and the thrombocyte pellet in 1.0 ml of plasma was used as PRP. A 1:1 (v/v) mixture of 0.5 M $CaCl_2$ and autologous thrombin was prepared in advance as an activator. A 10:1 (v/v) mixture of PRP and the activator was incubated for 5 min at room temperature, and this mixture was regarded as activated (Fig. 34.2). For clinical application, PRP should be used as soon as possible after activation. For the experiment, activated PRP is centrifuged at $2,015 \times g$ for 15 min and the supernatant is stored at $-20°C$.

Adipose-Derived Stem Cell/Platelet-Rich Plasma Combination Therapy

We reported the potential of PRP on human ASCs and human dermal fibroblasts in vitro (Kakudo et al., 2008a). Activated and nonactivated PRP and platelet-poor plasma (PPP) were prepared and applied to cultures of human ASCs and human dermal fibroblasts and cultured for 7 days. The application of activated PRP and PPP resulted in significant proliferation of both cell types compared with their nonactivated forms, with activated PRP having the strongest proliferative effect. Furthermore, we observed a dose-dependent relationship with the effect of PRP on proliferation, with 1–5% having a maximal effect, and a decreasing effect observed with higher concentrations of 10–20% (Kakudo et al., 2008a).

Animal studies using PRP and ASCs have also recently been reported. Tobita et al. (2008) reported that ASCs isolated from Wistar rats were mixed with PRP obtained from inbred rats, and implanted into a periodontal tissue defect in rats. A small amount of alveolar bone regeneration was observed 2 and 4 weeks after ASC/PRP implantation. Moreover, 8 weeks after implantation, a periodontal ligament-like structure was observed along with alveolar bone. Tobita et al. (2008) concluded that ASCs with PRP can promote periodontal tissue regeneration in rats.

Niemeyer et al. (2010) compared the osteogenic potentials of ASCs and bone marrow-derived mesenchymal stem cells (BMSC), and evaluated the influence of PRP on the osteogenic capacity in sheep tibia. Ovine BMSC (BMSC group) and ASCs (ASC group) were seeded on mineralized collagen sponges and implanted into a critical size defect of sheep tibia. In an additional group, PRP was used in combination with ASCs (ASC/PRP group). Radiographic evaluation revealed a significantly higher amount of newly formed bone in the BMSC group than in the ASC group. Radiographic level showed superior bone formation of the ASC/PRP group versus the empty control group, but not for the ASC group.

Del Bue et al. (2008) reported on cell therapy of tendonitis using ASCs and PRP in horse. Expanded visceral ASCs were inoculated into damaged tendon after their dispersal in activated PRP, a biological scaffold that plays an important role in maintaining cells in defective sites and contributes to tissue healing.

Blanton et al. (2009) examined the efficacy of adipose stem cells, when supplied either alone or in platelet-rich fibrin gels, to improve wound healing in pigs. There was no significant difference in the re-epithelialization rate, but treatments containing adipose stem cells demonstrated increased microvessel densities compared with those for groups without adipose stem cells. Furthermore, wound cosmesis was improved in the adipose stem cell plus PRP group compared with the outcomes in other treatment groups.

Hadad et al. (2010) examined the capacity of ASCs, either alone or in PRP fibrin gels, to promote wound healing in pigs. The combination of ASCs and PRP was superior to all other treatments in accelerating the rate of wound contraction. Furthermore, there was a significant increase in the microvessel density of healed wounds treated with the combination of ASCs and PRP compared with that for saline solution. They documented that a combination of ASCs and PRP improves the healing rates of perfusion-depleted tissues, possibly through enhancing local levels of growth factors.

As described above, PRP/ASC combination therapy may be clinically applied in the fields of wound healing and tissue regeneration in the future. Through this combination, growth factors contained in PRP may promote the proliferation and differentiation of ASCs. Aiming at clinical application, the elucidations of mutual influences between ASCs and PRP and their mechanism as well as investigation of the effect and safety using a large animal experimental model are necessary.

References

Blanton MW, Hadad I, Johnstone BH, Mund JA, Rogers PI, Eppley BL, March KL (2009) Adipose stromal cells and platelet-rich plasma therapies synergistically increase revascularization during wound healing. Plast Reconstr Surg 123:56S–64S

Del Bue M, Ricco S, Ramoni R, Conti V, Gnudi G, Grolli S (2008) Equine adipose-tissue derived mesenchymal stem cells and platelet concentrates: their association in vitro and in vivo. Vet Res Commun 32 Suppl 1:S51–S55

Eby BW (2002) Platelet-rich plasma: harvesting with a single-spin centrifuge. J Oral Implantol 28:297–301

Erickson GR, Gimble JM, Franklin DM, Rice HE, Awad H, Guilak F (2002) Chondrogenic potential of adipose tissue-derived stromal cells in vitro and in vivo. Biochem Biophys Res Commun 290:763–769

Fraser JK, Wulur I, Alfonso Z, Hedrick MH (2006) Fat tissue: an underappreciated source of stem cells for biotechnology. Trends Biotechnol 24:150–154

Hadad I, Johnstone BH, Brabham JG, Blanton MW, Rogers PI, Fellers C, Solomon JL, Merfeld-Clauss S, DesRosiers CM, Dynlacht JR, Coleman JJ, March KL (2010) Development of a porcine delayed wound-healing model and its use in testing a novel cell-based therapy. Int J Radiat Oncol Biol Phys 78:888–896

Halbleib M, Skurk T, de Luca C, von Heimburg D, Hauner H (2003) Tissue engineering of white adipose tissue using hyaluronic acid-based scaffolds. I: in vitro differentiation of human adipocyte precursor cells on scaffolds. Biomaterials 24:3125–3132

Halvorsen YD, Franklin D, Bond AL, Hitt DC, Auchter C, Boskey AL, Paschalis EP, Wilkison WO, Gimble JM (2001) Extracellular matrix mineralization and osteoblast gene expression by human adipose tissue-derived stromal cells. Tissue Eng 7:729–741

Harrison P, Cramer EM (1993) Platelet alpha-granules. Blood Rev 7:52–62

Hicok KC, Hedrick MH (2011) Automated isolation and processing of adipose-derived stem and regenerative cells. Methods Mol Biol 702:87–105

Hicok KC, Du Laney TV, Zhou YS, Halvorsen YD, Hitt DC, Cooper LF, Gimble JM (2004) Human adipose-derived adult stem cells produce osteoid in vivo. Tissue Eng 10:371–380

Huang JI, Zuk PA, Jones NF, Zhu M, Lorenz HP, Hedrick MH, Benhaim P (2004) Chondrogenic potential of multipotential cells from human adipose tissue. Plast Reconstr Surg 113:585–594

Kakudo N, Shimotsuma A, Kusumoto K (2007) Fibroblast growth factor-2 stimulates adipogenic differentiation of human adipose-derived stem cells. Biochem Biophys Res Commun 359:239–244

Kakudo N, Minakata T, Mitsui T, Kushida S, Notodihardjo FZ, Kusumoto K (2008a) Proliferation-promoting effect of platelet-rich plasma on human adipose-derived stem cells and human dermal fibroblasts. Plast Reconstr Surg 122:1352–1360

Kakudo N, Shimotsuma A, Miyake S, Kushida S, Kusumoto K (2008b) Bone tissue engineering using human adipose-derived stem cells and honeycomb collagen scaffold. J Biomed Mater Res A 84:191–197

Kakudo N, Kushida S, Kusumoto K (2009) Platelet-rich plasma: the importance of platelet separation and concentration. Plast Reconstr Surg 123:1135–1136, author reply 1136–1137

Lee JA, Parrett BM, Conejero JA, Laser J, Chen J, Kogon AJ, Nanda D, Grant RT, Breitbart AS (2003) Biological alchemy: engineering bone and fat from fat-derived stem cells. Ann Plast Surg 50:610–617

Marx RE (2004) Platelet-rich plasma: evidence to support its use. J Oral Maxillofac Surg 62:489–496

Marx RE, Carlson ER, Eichstaedt RM, Schimmele SR, Strauss JE, Georgeff KR (1998) Platelet-rich plasma: growth factor enhancement for bone grafts. Oral Surg Oral Med Oral Pathol Oral Radiol Endod 85:638–646

Niemeyer P, Fechner K, Milz S, Richter W, Suedkamp NP, Mehlhorn AT, Pearce S, Kasten P (2010) Comparison of mesenchymal stem cells from bone marrow and adipose tissue for bone regeneration in a critical size defect of the sheep tibia and the influence of platelet-rich plasma. Biomaterials 31:3572–3579

Patrick CW Jr, Chauvin PB, Hobley J, Reece GP (1999) Preadipocyte seeded PLGA scaffolds for adipose tissue engineering. Tissue Eng 5:139–151

Planat-Benard V, Silvestre JS, Cousin B, Andre M, Nibbelink M, Tamarat R, Clergue M, Manneville C, Saillan-Barreau C, Duriez M, Tedgui A, Levy B, Penicaud L, Casteilla L (2004) Plasticity of human adipose lineage cells toward endothelial cells: physiological and therapeutic perspectives. Circulation 109:656–663

Safford KM, Hicok KC, Safford SD, Halvorsen YD, Wilkison WO, Gimble JM, Rice HE (2002) Neurogenic differentiation of murine and human adipose-derived stromal cells. Biochem Biophys Res Commun 294:371–379

Smith SE, Roukis TS (2009) Bone and wound healing augmentation with platelet-rich plasma. Clin Podiatr Med Surg 26:559–588

Strem BM, Hicok KC, Zhu M, Wulur I, Alfonso Z, Schreiber RE, Fraser JK, Hedrick MH (2005) Multipotential differentiation of adipose tissue-derived stem cells. Keio J Med 54:132–141

Tobita M, Uysal AC, Ogawa R, Hyakusoku H, Mizuno H (2008) Periodontal tissue regeneration with adipose-derived stem cells. Tissue Eng Part A 14:945–953

von Heimburg D, Zachariah S, Heschel I, Kuhling H, Schoof H, Hafemann B, Pallua N (2001) Human preadipocytes seeded on freeze-dried collagen scaffolds investigated in vitro and in vivo. Biomaterials 22:429–438

Yoshimura K, Shigeura T, Matsumoto D, Sato T, Takaki Y, Aiba-Kojima E, Sato K, Inoue K, Nagase T, Koshima I, Gonda K (2006) Characterization of freshly isolated and cultured cells derived from the fatty and fluid portions of liposuction aspirates. J Cell Physiol 208:64–76

Zuk PA, Zhu M, Mizuno H, Huang J, Futrell JW, Katz AJ, Benhaim P, Lorenz HP, Hedrick MH (2001) Multilineage cells from human adipose tissue: implications for cell-based therapies. Tissue Eng 7:211–228

Zuk PA, Zhu M, Ashjian P, De Ugarte DA, Huang JI, Mizuno H, Alfonso ZC, Fraser JK, Benhaim P, Hedrick MH (2002) Human adipose tissue is a source of multipotent stem cells. Mol Biol Cell 13:4279–4295

Chapter 35

Skeletal Muscle-Derived Stem Cells: Role in Cellular Cardiomyoplasty

Tetsuro Tamaki

Abstract Skeletal muscle-derived myoblasts were initially considered to be a potential source for cardiomyoplasty. These cells were expected to be able to trans-differentiate into cardiomyocytes after transplantation in the cardiac muscle environment. However, several studies have shown differentiation into multinucleated myotubes, and no differentiation into cardiomyocytes has been observed. Complete differentiation of murine skeletal muscle interstitium-derived multipotent stem cells (SKMI-DMSCs) into cardiomyocytes was recently demonstrated following engraftment into the infarcted heart muscle (left ventricle). Engrafted SKMI-DMSCs showed typical formation of gap-junctions, as well as intercalated discs and desmosomes, between donor and recipient and/or donor and donor cells in vivo. When SKMI-DMSCs were co-cultured with embryonic cardiomyocytes on a glass slide, cells typically formed sphere-like cell aggregations together in vitro. These mixed cell aggregations showed spontaneous synchronous contractions with the formation of gap-junctions between aggregated cells. Cardiomyocyte differentiation was also confirmed by the expression of cardiomyogenic transcription factors, such as GATA-4, Nkx2-5, Isl-1, Mef2 and Hand2. Vigorous expression of these factors in the SKMI-DMSCs was seen after co-culture, and lower expression of these factors was also observed in their clonal cell culture. These results indicate that SKMI-DMSCs are a potential source for practical cellular cardiomyoplasty, and that they should be isolated and transplanted in a more primitive state for milieu-dependent differentiation of stem cells.

Keywords SKMI-DMSCs · Cardiomyoplasty · Teratoma · Cardiomyocytes · Desmosomes · Connexion

Introduction

Cardiac dysfunction induced by myocardial infarction is a leading cause of morbidity and mortality in humans because of the limited regenerative capacity of injured cardiomyocytes. Therefore, the idea of cellular cardiomyoplasty, based on transplantation of various cell types has been proposed as follows. Fetal or neonatal cardiomyocyte transplantation (Reinecke et al., 1999) may certainly provide cardiomyocytes, but allogenic transplantation raises two major concerns: (1) graft rejection and subsequent immunosuppression; and (2) considerable ethical issues. Similar issues are also raised in the case of embryonic stem cell (ESC)-derived cardiomyocytes (Laflamme et al., 2007; van Laake et al., 2007) and/or ESCs themselves (Min et al., 2002), with the latter approach also raising the risk of teratoma formation due to their totipotency (Murry and Keller, 2008; Odorico et al., 2001). The recent discovery of inducible pluripotent stem (iPS) cells (Takahashi et al., 2007), which are derived from genetic reprogramming of somatic stem cells may resolve the ethical and immunogenic issues. However, the risk of teratoma and/or malignant tumor formations remains. Therefore, autologous somatic stem cell transplantation is the most practical solution to overcome the above issues.

T. Tamaki (✉)
Muscle Physiology and Cell Biology Unit, Division of Basic Clinical Science, Department of Regenerative Medicine, School of Medicine, Tokai University, Isehara, Kanagawa 259-1143, Japan
e-mail: tamaki@is.icc.u-tokai.ac.jp

Transplantation of bone marrow-derived stem cells (Orlic et al., 2001), dermal fibroblasts (Hutcheson et al., 2000) and skeletal myoblasts (Ghostine et al., 2002; Pouzet et al., 2000; Reinecke et al., 2002; Taylor et al., 1998) has been attempted, with the expectation that such cells differentiate and/or trans-differentiate into cardiomyocytes. Among these cell types, transplantation of bone marrow-derived stem or mesenchymal stem cells has been most actively attempted, but the results were somewhat contradictory (reviewed by Joggerst and Hatzopoulos, 2009).

In contrast, skeletal myoblast transplantation has shown several advantages as an attractive source of stem cells, including relatively easy access to donor cells, as autologous myoblasts are readily available from patients without immunosuppression and the skeletal muscle system accounts for a substantial proportion of total body mass. The most commonly used skeletal myoblasts are often called satellite cells, and are located beneath the basal lamina of muscle fiber. Skeletal myoblasts show an inherent resistance to ischemia in injured myocardium (Pagani et al., 2003), and improve left ventricular function with decreased remodelling and matrix breakdown (Ghostine et al., 2002; Taylor et al., 1998). However, it has been concluded that complete trans-differentiation into cardiomyocytes does not occur (Reinecke et al., 2002). Indeed, multinucleated myotube formations that are able to contract develop, but they do not operate in synchrony with the surrounding myocardium (Leobon et al., 2003; Reinecke et al., 2002). Therefore, there has been considerable concern regarding the potential for arrhythmias (Fouts et al., 2006; Reinecke et al., 2002).

Stem cell populations showing complete differentiation into cardiomyocytes distinct from myoblasts and/or satellite cells have recently been identified in the skeletal muscle (Tamaki et al., 2008a, 2010). This review will focus on the localization, isolation and cardiac differentiation of skeletal muscle-derived stem cells.

Localization and Isolation of Skeletal Muscle Interstitium-Derived Multipotent Stem Cells (SKMI-DMSCs)

In this section, we would like to re-define the characteristics of skeletal muscle interstitium-derived multipotent stem cells (SKMI-DMSCs), including differences in isolation method, expression of putative cell markers at initial isolation and cellular multipotency, for comparison with other reported stem cells in the skeletal muscle.

Firstly, SKMI-DMSCs were identified in the interstitial spaces of skeletal muscle as $CD34^+/45^-$ cells (Tamaki et al., 2002), designated as Sk-34 cells. These cells are located in the interstitium, outside of muscle fiber basal lamina, and are distinct from satellite cells. Therefore, for their isolation, it is important to minimize contamination by satellite cells. For this purpose, intact whole muscle must be prepared for enzymatic digestion. In other words, the muscles are not minced prior to enzymatic digestion. This allows SKMI-DMSC isolation with minimum contamination by other cell types, such as committed endothelial cells. In fact, there are no $CD31^+$ cells present among Sk-34 cells (Tamaki et al., 2002), nor are there CD133- or NCAM-expressing cells (Tamaki et al., 2008a).

After collagenase digestion and separation from debris, extracted cells were stained with CD34 and CD45, and $CD34^+/45^-$ (Sk-34) and $CD34^-/45^-$ (designated Sk-DN) cells were sorted by fluorescence activating cell sorting (FACS) method (Tamaki et al., 2002, 2003). These two cell populations showed myogenic, vasculogenic, and adipogenic differentiation potential on culture in vitro. Using these methods, Sk-DN cells are the negatively selected fraction, and cellular characteristics thus remain uncertain.

We recently found that both Sk-34 and Sk-DN cells were wholly positive for CD29 as anti-integrin β-1 (95.2 and 92.1%), and can therefore be positively sorted as Sk-DN/29^+ ($CD34^-/45^-/29^+$) cells (Tamaki et al., 2011). However, possible contamination of satellite cells among enzymatically extracted cells could not be completely eliminated. To clarify this point, we examined the relationship between Sk-34, Sk-DN and Pax7 expression, as a marker for satellite cells (Seale et al., 2000). The results clearly indicated that there were no $Pax7^+$ cells among Sk-34 cells, and that $Pax7^+$ cells accounted for <1% of the Sk-DN cell fraction immediately after sorting (Tamaki et al., 2008b). This was thought to be the result of contamination by satellite cells in the Sk-DN cell fraction. Therefore, a small number of contaminating $Pax7^+$ satellite cells (<1% for total) were $CD34^-$ in this analysis, as we have consistently reported before (Tamaki et al., 2002, 2008b), in contrast to other reports (Beauchamp et al., 2000).

As Sk-34 and Sk-DN cells are not derived from bone marrow (Tamaki et al., 2005, 2007a), they are different from bone marrow-derived myogenic cells, although it appears that bone marrow-derived myogenic cells are preferentially detected in the satellite cell niche beneath the parent fiber basal lamina (LaBarge and Blau, 2002). Similarly, Sk-34 and Sk-DN cells included less than 0.1% side population (SP) cells, and were thus 99.9% main-population (MP) cells (Tamaki et al., 2003). Irrespective, for stem cell isolation, 5–10% FCS should be included in the digestive collagenase solution in order to reduce protease activity and minimize damage to isolated cells. This will further affect stem cell differentiation capacity, as recent findings strongly indicate the importance of cell isolation method, particularly when using enzymatic digestion that lowers proteolytic contamination, in conserving stem cell function in skeletal muscle (Collins et al., 2005).

Differentiation Potential of SKMI-DMSCs

Sk-34 cells form colonies and have the potential to differentiate into mesodermal cells, such as endothelial cells (ECs), myogenic cells and adipocytes in vitro and in vivo (Tamaki et al., 2002). Freshly isolated Sk-34 cells were also found to give rise to ectodermal lineage cells (Schwann cells) after transplantation into severely damaged tibialis anterior muscle, with significant functional recovery (Tamaki et al., 2005). Sk-DN cells, as putative immature stem cells, typically form spherical colonies with high (about 10–40%) colony-forming activity in collagen-based cell culture containing bFGF and EGF (Tamaki et al., 2003, 2007a, b; 2008b).

Therapeutic bulk cell transplantation of 5-day cultured Sk-DN cells results in the synchronized reconstitution of muscular, vascular and peripheral nervous systems (Tamaki et al., 2007a), as is seen with freshly isolated Sk-34 cell transplantation (Tamaki et al., 2005). Furthermore, this apparent multipotent capacity was confirmed to be clonal by cell transplantation and RT-PCR analysis for single cell-derived spheres (Tamaki et al., 2007b). Subsequently, it was found that Sk-DN cells are highly immature stem cells situated upstream of Sk-34 cells in the same lineage and that they are potentially capable of self-renewal (Tamaki et al., 2008b). Thus, Sk-34 and Sk-DN cells are of the same lineage, and can give rise to mesodermal cells (skeletal muscle cells, vascular cells, vascular smooth muscle cells, pericytes and ECs) and ectodermal cells (Schwann cells and perineurium), and have synchronized reconstitution capacity of the muscular, vascular and peripheral nervous systems.

Interestingly, this synchronous multipotent nerve-muscle-blood vessel formation by Sk-34 and Sk-DN cells is also seen in non-muscle tissue environments (beneath the kidney capsule) (Tamaki et al., 2005, 2007a), thus confirming their intrinsic multipotent capacity and muscle fiber formation. These observations strongly indicate that myogenic cells are also present in the interstitial spaces of skeletal muscle. It is important to note that SKMI-DMSC-derived myogenic cells are primary myoblasts that can form satellite cells during new fiber formation in the damaged skeletal muscle and even in a non-muscle environment (Tamaki et al., 2005, 2007a). This is also supported by the fact that Pax7$^+$ cells are produced by Pax7$^-$ Sk-34 and Sk-DN cells after asymmetric cell division during clonal cell culture (Tamaki et al., 2008b). Differentiation of SKMI-DMSCs is summarized in Fig. 35.1.

Complete Differentiation of SKMI-DMSCs into Cardiomyocytes In Vivo

When these SKMI-DMSCs (Sk-34 and Sk-DN cells) were obtained from green fluorescence protein transgenic (GFP-Tg) mouse muscle and exposed to the cardiac environment, complete differentiation into cardiomyocytes was observed (Tamaki et al., 2008a, 2010), and this shows the additional differentiation potential of SKMI-DMSCs. Freshly isolated Sk-34 cells were directly transplanted into a myocardial infarction (MI) zone induced by coronary ligations. At 4 weeks after transplantation, donor cells were able to give rise to cardiomyocytes having desmosomes and intercalated discs associated with gap-junctions after therapeutic bulk-cell transplantation, significantly contributing to the functional recovery of the left ventricle (Tamaki et al., 2008a).

Physiological assessment of LV function was evaluated using echocardiography and a micro-tip conductance catheter as measured end-diastolic and end-systolic dimensions, fractional shortening at the mid-papillary muscle level. Regional wall motion score

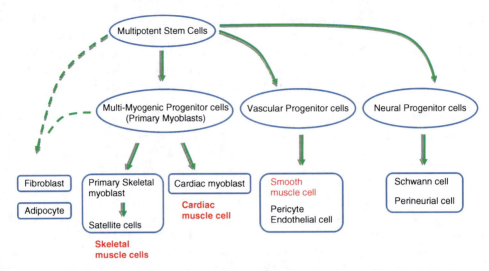

Fig. 35.1 Differentiation potential of skeletal muscle interstitium-derived stem cells. There are mainly obtained from in vivo cell transplantation studies

(RWMS) was evaluated as per published criteria. Formation of desmosomes, intercalated discs and gap-junctions between donor and recipient and/or donor and donor cells were confirmed by immunohistochemistry (anti-connexin43) and immunoelectron microscopy (anti-GFP). Cardiomyogenic differentiation potential of SKMI-DMSCs was also confirmed by clonal transplantation of Sk-DN cells, which are hierarchically situated upstream of Sk-34 cells (Tamaki et al., 2010). Cell fusion-independent differentiation was confirmed by fluorescence in situ hybridization (FISH, mouse to rat), Cre- and loxP systems, and electron microscopy (mononucleated cells). Interestingly, in this SKMI-DMSC transplantation, the multinucleated myotube formation that was consistently seen in the skeletal myoblast transplantation (Hagege et al., 2003; Horackova et al., 2004; Menasche, 2007; Reinecke et al., 2002) was not observed, while blood vessels having GFP$^+$ endothelial cells were observed (Tamaki et al., 2008a).

The above observations confirm that differentiation into skeletal myogenic lineage in SKMI-DMSCs was inhibited after transplantation into the cardiac milieu. Thus, early exposure (such as freshly isolated state) to a specific tissue environment apparently leads to preferential commitment and/or differentiation of SKMI-DMSCs by receiving several damaged tissue-releasing factors. In addition, both Sk-34 and Sk-DN cells are considered to be highly immature cells, similarly to epiblastic-like cells, because of their differentiation into mesodermal and ectodermal cell lineages. Differentiation into cardiomyocytes might therefore occur as a result of milieu-dependent differentiation rather than trans-differentiation.

Immature cells receive differentiation signals from their microenvironment, such that the topobiological location of a cell leads to expression of a specific phenotype. Therefore, SKMI-DMSCs are thought to be stem cells remaining in the interstitium of skeletal muscle from the developmental stage and possessing epiblast-like capacity. This milieu-dependent differentiation is also supported by the fact that complete formation of gap-junctions was mainly observed at the border zone of the MI, and spot-like connexin43$^+$ reactions, indicating the early stages of gap-junction formation, were distributed toward the central zone of the MI (Tamaki et al., 2008a). Thus, formation of gap-junctions began at the border zones and spread to the central zone. This indicates that the topobiological effects are stronger in the border zones of the MI than in the central zone.

Formation of Gap-Junctions and Spontaneous Synchronous Contraction In Vitro

The cardiac differentiation potential of Sk-34 cells was also examined in normal culture and in co-culture with embryonic cardiomyocytes. Embryonic cardiomyocytes obtained from DsRED-Tg mice (E14–16) and freshly isolated Sk-34 cells from GFP-Tg mice were scattered together in glass-slide chambers at an appropriate cell density. Sphere-like cell aggregations then formed after 3–5 days of culture. The process was as follows: (1) after 1–2 h in culture, mouse embryonic cardiomyocytes began to plate-down on the glass slide; (2) synchronous contractions were observed after 1 day of culture; (3) plate-down cellular confluency increased toward 2–3 days of culture, and was associated with vigorous synchronous contraction; (4) aggregating cell-sheets then began to detach from the glass-slide due to their continuous and rhythmic contractions, with the help of the lower cell-holding capacity of the glass surface, and form sphere-like cardiomyocytes aggregations (Tamaki et al., 2008a).

Under fluorescence microscopy, there were several GFP+ Sk-34-derived cells in the DsRED cardiomyocyte spheres after 6 days of culture. These cardiomyocyte spheres showed vigorous spontaneous and synchronous contraction (supplemental movies on web-site in Tamaki et al., 2008a). When these spheres were stained with anti-connexin-43 and observed by confocal laser scanning microscopy, dot-like staining for gap-junctions was similarly evident around the red cells and green cells supporting the synchronous contraction of the spheres. This evidence suggests that skeletal muscle interstitium-derived Sk-34 cells can form gap-junctions with cardiomyocytes and work synchronously (contraction) with host cardiomyocytes in vitro; thus, they probably differentiate into cardiomyocytes.

Myocardial differentiation of Sk-34 cells in vitro was confirmed by RT-PCR analysis after 5 days of co-culture with normal SD rat embryonic cardiomyocytes (E10–12), as compared with solo culture of Sk-34 cells. After 5 days of co-culture when spontaneous synchronous contractions were evident, cells were harvested and separated, and then GFP+ cells were sorted by FACS, and analyzed by RT-PCR using putative skeletal myogenic, smooth myogenic, ion channel, vascular cell, cardiomyogenic and cell proliferation markers. In this case, primers were designed as detectable mouse mRNAs. The freshly isolated Sk-34 cell fraction (before culture) primarily expressed mRNAs for several ion channel-, vascular- and proliferation-related mRNAs. Thus, skeletal and cardio myogenic commitment is unlikely, whereas smooth myogenic and vascular commitment are seen. However, expression of both skeletal myogenic (such as MyoD, Pax7) and cardio myogenic (except for Nkx2.5) markers can be seen after solo Sk-34 cell culture, and expression of all 6 cardio myogenic markers (Nkx2.5, GATA-4, Mef2c, Hand2, isl-1 and Cacn-1b) was seen after co-culture with rat embryonic cardiomyocytes. Interestingly, vascular marker expression decreased after culture.

In order to further analyze the cardiomyogenic commitment of Sk-34 cells, we performed RT-PCR of single and 2–8 clonal cells after 3 days of culture. In this analysis, single cell refers to the stage before cell division, 2 cells refers to the stage after the first cell division, 3–4 cells refers to the second cell division, and 5–8 cells refers to the stage after the third division. The results suggested that cardiac differentiation of Sk-34 cells is not sufficiently induced by clonal cell culture, while skeletal and smooth myogenic differentiation progressed.

Essential Qualification for Cardiac Differentiation

SKMI-DMSCs are able to give rise to cardiac muscle cells for several reasons. First, gentle isolation of the cells appears to be important, including the use of lower concentrations of collagenase (0.1%) in the digestive solution compared to previous studies (1–2%), the addition of 5–10% FBS to minimize contaminating protease activity and to protect isolated cells, and not mincing donor muscle before enzymatic digestion, which is advantageous for cell isolation and reducing contamination by other cell types. It is likely that these are minimum requirements for isolating SKMI-DMSCs.

Second, for therapeutic use of SKMI-DMSCs for cardiomyoplasty, it is important to maintain cells in an immature state, even after expansion culture. Our previous data show that the myogenic potential of Sk-34 cells reduces markedly after culture because of undesired differentiation into fibroblast-like cells and/or adipocytes in severely damaged skeletal muscle, whereas Sk-DN cells can be expanded while maintaining cardiomyogenic potential (Tamaki et al., 2010), and thus Sk-34 cells should be transplanted in a freshly isolated state. Thus, early exposure (such as freshly isolated state) to the specific tissue environment apparently leads to preferential commitment and/or differentiation of SKMI-DMSCs by receiving several damaged tissue-releasing factors.

The default differentiation potential of SKMI-DMSCs may be set to skeletal muscle, vascular and peripheral nerve cells. This was supported by in vitro data that cardiac differentiation was only induced in co-culture with cardiomyocytes, and not in solo and/or clonal cell culture of SKMI-DMSCs. Thus, early exposure to the cardiac environment is the most important factor in the cardiomyogenesis of SKMI-DMSCs.

In conclusion, based on the mouse studies, it is certain that the SKMI-DMSCs are cardiomyogenic somatic stem cells that can use autologous cell transplantation therapy. To the best of our knowledge, these SKMI-DMSCs are the only somatic stem cells demonstrating complete cardiomyogenic differentiation associated with the formation of desmosomes and gap-junctions in a mononucleated state, and incorporating alignment between recipient cardiomyocytes and/or transplanted donor cells. These results are reflected by the significant functional recovery (LV function) after transplantation. Therefore, the potential of SKMI-DMSCs is clearly different from that of skeletal myoblasts with regard to use in cardiomyoplasty, while both are derived from skeletal muscle.

Other Studies Using Skeletal Muscle-Derived Stem Cells

As mentioned above, a large number of experimental cardiomyoplasty studies using skeletal myoblasts have been reported, with most showing robust engraftment and several beneficial effects, such as paracrine effects for surrounding myocardium and attenuation of left-ventricular remodelling, whereas complete trans-differentiation into cardiomyocytes was not observed (Menasche, 2007). In contrast, few studies have examined cardiomyoplasty using skeletal muscle-derived stem cells. Recently, skeletal muscle-derived stem cells (MDSCs) obtained by the pre-plate culture system were applied to the repair of MI (Drowley et al., 2009). MDSCs improved cardiac regeneration and repair through the promotion of angiogenesis without differentiation into the cardiac lineage.

Similarly, it was reported that adult murine skeletal muscle contains cells that can differentiate into beating cardiomyocytes in vitro. That paper described cells showing $CD34^-/CD45^-/C\text{-}kit^-/Sca\text{-}1^-$ at initial isolation, and showing round shape, floating and/or weakly attaching behavior, sphere-colony formation and spontaneous beating (contracting) in culture, and that these cells may be different from satellite cells, referring to them as Spoc (skeletal-based precursors of cardiomyocytes) cells (Winitsky et al., 2005). Spontaneous beating (contracting) in culture is a typical behavior of the present Sk-34 cells (Tamaki et al., 2002), but these cells are $CD34^+/45^-/C\text{-}kit^-/Sca\text{-}1^+$ at initial isolation. Thus, Spoc cells and Sk-34 cells appear to be different. However, Sk-DN cells comprise $CD34^-/45^-/C\text{-}kit^-/Sca\text{-}1^+$ (25%) and $Sca\text{-}1^-$ (75%) cells (Tamaki et al., 2003, 2008b). Thus, Spoc cells correspond 75% of Sk-DN cells. However, the number of Sk-DN cells is small when compared to Sk-34 cells (1:16–20) (Tamaki et al., 2002, 2003, 2005) at initial isolation. Thus, simultaneous isolation of Sk-34 and Sk-DN cells showed 16–20-fold higher efficiency for isolation of potential cardiomyocyte precursors from skeletal muscle than Spoc cells.

In summary, non-adherent and/or loosely attached, round and spontaneously beating characteristics in culture are a key feature of skeletal muscle-derived stem cells that can differentiate into cardiomyocytes. This is also supported by the fact that primary myoblasts (see Fig. 35.1) distinct from satellite cells are present in non-adherent cell population in culture (Tamaki et al., 2011).

Perspective

In order to obtain sufficient numbers of engrafting SKMI-DMSCs for therapeutic usage, expansion cell culture is necessary. Therefore, expansion of SKMI-DMSCs, while maintaining their immature state, is the next issue to be resolved. In addition, to clarify whether the same kind of cardiomyogenic SKMI-DMSCs are present in human skeletal muscle is currently being investigated.

References

Beauchamp JR, Heslop L, Yu DS, Tajbakhsh S, Kelly RG, Wernig A, Buckingham ME, Partridge TA, Zammit PS (2000) Expression of CD34 and Myf5 defines the majority of quiescent adult skeletal muscle satellite cells. J Cell Biol 151:1221–1234

Collins CA, Olsen I, Zammit PS, Heslop L, Petrie A, Partridge TA, Morgan JE (2005) Stem cell function, self-renewal, and behavioral heterogeneity of cells from the adult muscle satellite cell niche. Cell 122:289–301

Drowley L, Okada M, Payne TR, Botta GP, Oshima H, Keller BB, Tobita K, Huard J (2009) Sex of muscle stem cells does not influence potency for cardiac cell therapy. Cell Transplant 18:1137–1146

Fouts K, Fernandes B, Mal N, Liu J, Laurita KR (2006) Electrophysiological consequence of skeletal myoblast transplantation in normal and infarcted canine myocardium. Heart Rhythm 3:452–461

Ghostine S, Carrion C, Souza LC, Richard P, Bruneval P, Vilquin JT, Pouzet B, Schwartz K, Menasche P, Hagege AA (2002) Long-term efficacy of myoblast transplantation on regional structure and function after myocardial infarction. Circulation 106:I131–I136

Hagege AA, Carrion C, Menasche P, Vilquin JT, Duboc D, Marolleau JP, Desnos M, Bruneval P (2003) Viability and differentiation of autologous skeletal myoblast grafts in ischaemic cardiomyopathy. Lancet 361:491–492

Horackova M, Arora R, Chen R, Armour JA, Cattini PA, Livingston R, Byczko Z (2004) Cell transplantation for treatment of acute myocardial infarction: unique capacity for repair by skeletal muscle satellite cells. Am J Physiol Heart Circ Physiol 287:H1599–H1608

Hutcheson KA, Atkins BZ, Hueman MT, Hopkins MB, Glower DD, Taylor DA (2000) Comparison of benefits on myocardial performance of cellular cardiomyoplasty with skeletal myoblasts and fibroblasts. Cell Transplant 9:359–368

Joggerst SJ, Hatzopoulos AK (2009) Stem cell therapy for cardiac repair: benefits and barriers. Expert Rev Mol Med 11:e20

LaBarge MA, Blau HM (2002) Biological progression from adult bone marrow to mononucleate muscle stem cell to multinucleate muscle fiber in response to injury. Cell 111:589–601

Laflamme MA, Chen KY, Naumova AV, Muskheli V, Fugate JA, Dupras SK, Reinecke H, Xu C, Hassanipour M, Police S, O'Sullivan C, Collins L, Chen Y, Minami E, Gill EA, Ueno S, Yuan C, Gold J, Murry CE (2007) Cardiomyocytes derived from human embryonic stem cells in pro-survival factors enhance function of infarcted rat hearts. Nat Biotechnol 25:1015–1024

Leobon B, Garcin I, Menasche P, Vilquin JT, Audinat E, Charpak S (2003) Myoblasts transplanted into rat infarcted myocardium are functionally isolated from their host. Proc Natl Acad Sci USA 100:7808–7811

Menasche P (2007) Skeletal myoblasts as a therapeutic agent. Prog Cardiovasc Dis 50:7–17

Min JY, Yang Y, Converso KL, Liu L, Huang Q, Morgan JP, Xiao YF (2002) Transplantation of embryonic stem cells improves cardiac function in postinfarcted rats. J Appl Physiol 92:288–296

Murry CE, Keller G (2008) Differentiation of embryonic stem cells to clinically relevant populations: lessons from embryonic development. Cell 132:661–680

Odorico JS, Kaufman DS, Thomson JA (2001) Multilineage differentiation from human embryonic stem cell lines. Stem Cells 19:193–204

Orlic D, Kajstura J, Chimenti S, Jakoniuk I, Anderson SM, Li B, Pickel J, McKay R, Nadal-Ginard B, Bodine DM, Leri A, Anversa P (2001) Bone marrow cells regenerate infarcted myocardium. Nature 410:701–705

Pagani FD, DerSimonian H, Zawadzka A, Wetzel K, Edge AS, Jacoby DB, Dinsmore JH, Wright S, Aretz TH, Eisen HJ, Aaronson KD (2003) Autologous skeletal myoblasts transplanted to ischemia-damaged myocardium in humans. Histological analysis of cell survival and differentiation. J Am Coll Cardiol 41:879–888

Pouzet B, Vilquin JT, Hagege AA, Scorsin M, Messas E, Fiszman M, Schwartz K, Menasche P (2000) Intramyocardial transplantation of autologous myoblasts: can tissue processing be optimized? Circulation 102:III210–III215

Reinecke H, Zhang M, Bartosek T, Murry CE (1999) Survival, integration, and differentiation of cardiomyocyte grafts: a study in normal and injured rat hearts. Circulation 100:193–202

Reinecke H, Poppa V, Murry CE (2002) Skeletal muscle stem cells do not transdifferentiate into cardiomyocytes after cardiac grafting. J Mol Cell Cardiol 34:241–249

Seale P, Sabourin LA, Girgis-Gabardo A, Mansouri A, Gruss P, Rudnicki MA (2000) Pax7 is required for the specification of myogenic satellite cells. Cell 102:777–786

Takahashi K, Tanabe K, Ohnuki M, Narita M, Ichisaka T, Tomoda K, Yamanaka S (2007) Induction of pluripotent stem cells from adult human fibroblasts by defined factors. Cell 131:861–872

Tamaki T, Akatsuka A, Ando K, Nakamura Y, Matsuzawa H, Hotta T, Roy RR, Edgerton VR (2002) Identification of myogenic-endothelial progenitor cells in the interstitial spaces of skeletal muscle. J Cell Biol 157:571–577

Tamaki T, Akatsuka A, Okada Y, Matsuzaki Y, Okano H, Kimura M (2003) Growth and differentiation potential of main- and side-population cells derived from murine skeletal muscle. Exp Cell Res 291:83–90

Tamaki T, Uchiyama Y, Okada Y, Ishikawa T, Sato M, Akatsuka A, Asahara T (2005) Functional recovery of damaged skeletal muscle through synchronized vasculogenesis, myogenesis, and neurogenesis by muscle-derived stem cells. Circulation 112:2857–2866

Tamaki T, Okada Y, Uchiyama Y, Tono K, Masuda M, Wada M, Hoshi A, Akatsuka A (2007a) Synchronized reconstitution of muscle fibers, peripheral nerves and blood vessels by murine skeletal muscle-derived CD34(-)/45 (-) cells. Histochem Cell Biol 128:349–360

Tamaki T, Okada Y, Uchiyama Y, Tono K, Masuda M, Wada M, Hoshi A, Ishikawa T, Akatsuka A (2007b) Clonal multipotency of skeletal muscle-derived stem cells between mesodermal and ectodermal lineage. Stem Cells 25:2283–2290

Tamaki T, Akatsuka A, Okada Y, Uchiyama Y, Tono K, Wada M, Hoshi A, Iwaguro H, Iwasaki H, Oyamada A, Asahara T (2008a) Cardiomyocyte formation by skeletal muscle-derived multi-myogenic stem cells after transplantation into infarcted myocardium. PLoS One 3:e1789

Tamaki T, Okada Y, Uchiyama Y, Tono K, Masuda M, Nitta M, Hoshi A, Akatsuka A (2008b) Skeletal muscle-derived CD34+/45- and CD34-/45- stem cells are situated hierarchically upstream of Pax7+ cells. Stem Cells Dev 17:653–667

Tamaki T, Uchiyama Y, Okada Y, Tono K, Masuda M, Nitta M, Hoshi A, Akatsuka A (2010) Clonal differentiation of skeletal muscle-derived CD34(-)/45(-) stem cells into cardiomyocytes in vivo. Stem Cells Dev 19:503–512

Tamaki T, Tono K, Uchiyama Y, Okada Y, Masuda M, Soeda S, Nitta M, Akatsuka A (2011) Origin and hierarchy of basal lamina-forming and -non-forming myogenic cells in mouse skeletal muscle in relation to adhesive capacity and Pax7 expression in vitro. Cell Tissue Res 344:147–168

Taylor DA, Atkins BZ, Hungspreugs P, Jones TR, Reedy MC, Hutcheson KA, Glower DD, Kraus WE (1998) Regenerating functional myocardium: improved performance after skeletal myoblast transplantation. Nat Med 4:929–933

van Laake LW, Passier R, Monshouwer-Kloots J, Verkleij AJ, Lips DJ, Freund C, den Ouden K, Ward-van Oostwaard D, Korving J, Tertoolen LG, van Echteld CJ, Doevendans PA, Mummery CL (2007) Human embryonic stem cell-derived cardiomyocytes survive and mature in the mouse heart and transiently improve function after myocardial infarction. Stem Cell Res 1:9–24

Winitsky SO, Gopal TV, Hassanzadeh S, Takahashi H, Gryder D, Rogawski MA, Takeda K, Yu ZX, Xu YH, Epstein ND (2005) Adult murine skeletal muscle contains cells that can differentiate into beating cardiomyocytes in vitro. PLoS Biol 3:e87

Chapter 36

Cardiac Regenerative Medicine Without Stem Cell Transplantation

Carlo Ventura and Vincenzo Lionetti

Abstract Heart diseases are a leading cause of adult and childhood mortality. The underlying pathology is typically loss of cardiomyocytes progressing towards heart failure, or improper development of cardiomyocytes during embryogenesis leading to congenital heart malformations. Although stem cells may hold promise for cardiac regenerative medicine, a number of obstacles, such as the control of stem cell fate, low-yield commitment, and limited cell survival during differentiation must be overcome before their therapeutic potential can be realized. Moreover, the need for ex vivo cell expansion involves a substantial delay in transplantation after the onset of heart attack. It is now increasingly becoming evident that a novel chemistry, based on the development of multicomponent/multitarget agents, may afford rapid and sustained cardiac repair without stem cell transplantation. The rescuing effect is achieved after direct delivery of these molecules into the heart and results from in vivo epigenetic/transcriptional activation of angiogenic, prosurvival and antifibrotic patterning. Other major fields of investigation are the induction of cell cycle reentry in cardiac-resident cardiomyocytes, or the direct reprogramming of endogenous myocardial fibroblasts into functional cardiomyocytes. To this end, great expectations ensue from the identification of naturally occurring molecules or the development of synthetic compounds avoiding the use of cumbersome and potentially harmful gene delivery by viral vectors to afford efficient somatic cell reprogramming or cardiomyocyte proliferation. Future developments in these fields may pave to way to a cardiac regenerative medicine without stem cell transplantation.

Keywords Antifibrotic patterning · Cardiomyocyte proliferation · Myocardial infarction · Cardiomyopathies · Cardiogenesis · Neurogenin1 · HGF · von Willebrand factor

Introduction

Acute myocardial infarction (MI) and inherited cardiomyopathies, due to extensive loss of cardiomyocytes, may progress toward heart failure despite revascularization procedures and pharmacological treatments. Initial studies supported the concept that bone marrow cells may hold the promise of rebuilding the injured heart from its component elements, offering a valid alternative to the ultimate resort of heart transplantation (Orlic et al., 2001). However, stem cell biology turned out to be considerably more complex than initially expected. Different stem cell populations, including mesenchymal stem cells, adipose- and amniotic fluid-derived stem cells, and cardiac-resident stem cells have been progressively characterized. It is also evident that growth factor secretion from transplanted stem cells may activate angiogenic, antiapoptotic and antifibrotic paracrine patterning, playing a major role in cardiac repair (Ventura et al., 2007). Stem cell growth and differentiation may be subjected to autocrine regulation by secreted growth factors or

C. Ventura (✉)
Laboratory of Molecular Biology and Stem Cell Engineering, Cardiovascular Department, National Institute of Biostructures and Biosystems, S.Orsola-Malpighi Hospital (Pavilion 21), University of Bologna, 40138 Bologna, Italy
e-mail: Carlo.ventura@unibo.it

it may be orchestrated in an "intracrine" fashion by growth regulatory peptides acting within their cell of synthesis through nuclear receptors and signaling (Ventura et al., 2003; Ventura and Branzi, 2006). Indeed, cardiovascular commitment and secretion of trophic mediators are extremely low-yield processes in both adult and embryonic stem (ES) cells. Cell-based phenotypic- and pathway-specific screens of natural and synthetic compounds are on the way to provide a number of molecules achieving selective control of stem cell growth and differentiation (Ventura et al., 2007). Recent achievements in the area of stem cell research have been boosted by an increasing understanding of transcriptional regulation and epigenetic modifications, including histone acetylation, DNA methylation and chromatin remodeling. The development of molecules affording high-throughput of cardiogenesis from pluripotent cells would have obvious therapeutic potential and is an emerging new field in regenerative medicine. To this end, we have synthesized a hyaluronan mixed ester of butyric and retinoic acids (HBR), acting as a multicomponent-multitarget molecule harboring both differentiating and paracrine "logics" for cardiovascular repair. The rationale for the synthesis of this novel glycoconjugate is discussed in detail elsewhere (Ventura et al., 2004). Briefly, the CD44 hyaluronan (HA) receptor is highly expressed by cardiogenic cells (Wheatley et al., 1993) and cardiogenesis is abrogated by disruption of HA synthase-2 (Camenisch et al., 2000). HA-binding proteins translocate to the nucleus, priming cell growth and differentiation (Savani et al., 2001). Hence, HA may regulate cardiovascular commitment, acting as a carrier for HA-grafting synthetic compounds, such as butyrate (BU) and retinoic acid (RA). BU inhibits histone deacetylases, increasing transcription factor accessibility to target *cis*-acting regulatory sites, and drives both endothelial and cardiac fates (Illi et al., 2005). Grafting of RA into HBR is supported by the occurrence of abnormal heart development following RXRα gene inactivation and by RA-mediated increase in ES cardiogenesis (Wobus et al., 1997) and mammalian vascular development (Lai et al., 2003). Notably, histone deacetylase inhibitors enhanced RXR/RAR heterodimer action, and major developmental patterns in stem cells (Dilworth et al., 2000).

In mouse ES cells, HBR remarkably increased the expression of the cardiac lineage-promoting genes GATA4, Nkx2.5, and prodynorphin, as well as the synthesis and secretion of dynorphin B, leading to a consistent increase in the yield of spontaneously beating ES-derived cardiomyocytes (Ventura et al., 2004). HBR also proved effective in inducing a high-throughput of cardiac and endothelial commitment in human mesenchymal stem cells (hMSCs) isolated from the bone marrow and alternative sources, including the dental pulp and fetal membranes of term placenta (Ventura et al., 2007). Nuclear run-off transcription analyses indicated that the activation of a cardio-vasculogenic program of gene expression by HBR occurred at the transcriptional level. HBR failed to affect the transcription rate of MyoD and neurogenin1 (Ventura et al., 2004, 2007), two genes involved in skeletal myogenesis and neuronal determination, respectively, indicating that a novel generation of mixed esters of HA may be proposed to selectively organize lineage patterning in stem cells. Interestingly, transplantation of hMSCs preconditioned ex vivo with HBR into the hearts of rats subjected to acute MI by coronary ligation led to complete normalization of myocardial performance and dramatic reduction in scar formation (Ventura et al., 2007). This effect not only involved the persistence in vivo of the cardiovascular lineages acquired by hMSCs through the mixed ester, but encompassed the secretion of trophic mediators, such as Vascular Endothelial Growth Factor (VEGF) and Hepatocyte Growth Factor (HGF), affording a paracrine rescuing circuitry within the recipient tissue.

Despite these promising results, it is now evident that an extremely limited percentage of stem cells will engraft and survive within the recipient myocardium following intracoronary infusion or transendocardial injection (Bonaros et al., 2008). Moreover, the use of injectable scaffolds to augment stem cell engraftment is not devoid of harmful decrease in myocardial perfusion. Most important, the timing for cell culture, ex vivo expansion, and eventual chemical preconditioning prior to intracardiac delivery will involve a substantial delay (several weeks) in autologous stem cell transplantation with respect to the acute phase of a heart attack. Meanwhile, the hostile environment of the damaged tissue will progress towards fibrous scarring, fibroblast to myofibroblast transition, and myocardial stiffness, a process of "remodeling" that nullifies most of beneficial effects of stem cell-based therapy.

In this chapter, we will focus on the possibility to use the same chemistry developed to coax stem cells into cardiovascular fate as a tool to directly afford a rapid and sustained rescue of the infarcted heart without stem cell transplantation. Within this context, we will also discuss a different approach in providing a source of new cardiomyocytes based on the idea of targeting adult cardiomyocytes to cell cycle reentry, or the possibility of achieving direct cardiac reprogramming of endogenous myocardial fibroblasts into functionally competent cardiomyocytes.

Lesson from Clinical Trials

Most of clinical trials involving bone marrow for myocardial repair have been uncontrolled or have used non-randomized controls for comparison, being focused on bone marrow mononuclear cells, a heterogeneous population of hematopoietic and hMSCs containing less than 0.1% stem cells. Cells have both been delivered intracoronary to patients with recent MI or subjected to catheter-based intramyocardial injection into patients with chronic ischemic disease and old infarcts. Interestingly, these trials indicated that cell delivery was feasible and devoid of significant complications. However, while several studies reported improved ventricular function and perfusion, recent double-blind, randomized, placebo-controlled trials in patients receiving intracoronary unfractionated bone marrow cells within 24 h of acute infarction reported modest (Cleland et al., 2006) or no improvement in ejection fraction (Janssens et al., 2006; Lunde et al., 2005). Nevertheless, enhanced infarct shrinkage was detected with magnetic resonance imaging, suggesting that several degree of cardiac repair might have occurred (Janssens et al., 2006). An important cautionary note was raised by a recent randomized clinical trial showing that an increase in cardiac performance following bone marrow cell transfer in patients with acute MI was short-lived, and that the difference with the control group receiving optimal post-infarction therapy was significant after 6 months but not after 18 months (Meyer et al., 2006).

On the whole, the results from these clinical studies indicate that (i) additional randomized, controlled clinical trials should be warranted to explore the efficacy of stem cell transplantation as a novel therapy for MI and heart failure, and (ii) a paradigm shift in the current view of cardiovascular regenerative medicine should be envisioned.

A Role for Chemistry to Drive a Rapid and Sustained Cardiovascular Repair

Based on the above reported challenges, and the inherent chemical/mechanistic logics behind the HBR action, we hypothesized that this ester may also prove effective in triggering cardiovascular repair without the needs of stem cell transplantation. To verify this hypothesis, we directly injected HBR into the myocardium of infarcted rat hearts, and provided evidence that the mixed ester afforded substantial structural repair and functional recovery of myocardial performance (Lionetti et al., 2010a). No adverse reactions were observed during and after intra-myocardial injection of HBR in healthy rats. Within 4 weeks, the animals exhibited no cardiovascular complications, such as arrhythmias, pulmonary edema, ascites, or thrombosis. Animal behavior was normal. Histological analysis did not show interstitial edema and inflammatory infiltrates.

MRI analysis showed a marked recovery of cardiac performance in infarcted rats treated with HBR, compared to untreated animals (Lionetti et al., 2010b). The ejection fraction and cardiac output remarkably recovered in infarcted rats receiving HBR, with significant reduction in left ventricle (LV) end-diastolic volume 4 weeks after MI. LV end-systolic wall thickening, an index of regional contractile function, and LV end-diastolic thickness, an index of regional mass, were preserved in LV border zone of infarcted HBR-treated hearts. Cardiac MRI was also performed to detect scar tissue, which appears hyper-intense, and for infarct size assessment. Noteworthy, we found a significant reduction in the extension of the delayed contrast enhancement of LV infarct zone in HBR-injected hearts, compared with the untreated group (Lionetti et al., 2010a). In this study, Small Animal PET (mPET) analysis of ^{18}F-FDG uptake, an index of myocardial viability, revealed that glucose metabolism was also preserved in the border and remote regions of infarcted, HBR-treated hearts. Gross pathologic examination of ischemic myocardium after nitro blue tetrazolium staining confirmed that HBR injection substantially decreased the percentage of LV occupied by fibrosis. Picro-Mallory trichrome staining and quantitative analyses showed that the infarct scarring was significantly smaller in animals receiving HBR than in the untreated group, being mainly confined to a limited area in the subendocardial zone, which also exhibited regions of viable tissue. Moreover, HBR-treated hearts exhibited a decreased number of apoptotic cardiomyocytes when compared to untreated hearts.

Immunohistochemical analysis showed that the density of capillary vessels was significantly increased at the infarct border zone of animals injected with HBR. This "vascular front" extended from the subepicardial ventricular myocardium and spread into adjacent clusters of "viable" cardiomyocytes (Lionetti et al., 2010b). Immunohistochemistry also revealed an increased number of perivascular Stro-1-positive cells nearby newly formed capillaries in HBR-treated hearts after 4 weeks, significantly exceeding the few Stro-1-positive cells detected in the non-injected group. Interestingly, most of the Stro-1-positive cells lacked staining with von Willebrand Factor (vWF), an endothelial marker. On the contrary, some Stro-1-positive cells coexpressed cardiac-specific α-sarcomeric actinin. Differently from the Stro-1 expressing elements, the number of c-kit-positive cells did not differ significantly among treated and untreated animals, suggesting that Stro-1 resident perivascular mesenchymal cells, but not c-kit bone marrow-derived mononuclear cells, were selectively embedded in the site of tissue repair following HBR injection. Analysis of early tissue responses occurring 24 h after HBR injection indicated a significant increase in cycling, Ki-67 positive cells. The Ki-67 nuclear antigen was markedly expressed by perivascular spindle- and round-shaped stromal cells located between cardiomyocytes. These cells expressed NG2, and PDGF-Rβ, a set of markers that represent a phenotype indicator of pericyte/perivascular identity. The same cells lacked expression of hematopoietic cell markers. Other Ki-67-positive cytotypes included endothelial cells and polymorphonuclear leukocytes. VEGF cytoplasmic expression also significantly increased in the cardiomyocytes following HBR injection.

In vitro exposure to HBR of both rat cardiomyocytes (RCm) and rat Stro-1-positive stem cells significantly enhanced the gene expression of VEGF, KDR (encoding a major VEGF receptor), HGF, Akt, and Pim-1 (Lionetti et al., 2010a). The HBR treatment also enhanced the secretion of VEGF and HGF in the culture medium from both RCm and Stro-1 cells. These factors have been shown to possess angiogenic, antifibrotic and antiapoptotic properties (Nakamura et al., 2000), significantly contributing to the establishment of a rescuing "paracrine milieu" within the infarcted myocardium. Accordingly, a remarkable increase in capillarogenesis was observed when either human umbilical vein endothelial cells or rat aortic endothelial cells were cultured with medium obtained from RCm or Stro-1-positive cells previously exposed to the mixed ester (Lionetti et al., 2010b). Cumulatively, these findings suggest the activation of prominent paracrine effects by HBR on both cell populations, enhancing the expression of cytokines and genes with a crucial role in cell survival and angiogenesis.

Nuclear run-off experiments indicated that the action of HBR was mediated at the transcriptional level, and that while the transcription rate of VEGF and Pim-1 was unaffected following nuclear exposure to HBR, it was conversely enhanced by BU and RA with superimposable time courses and additive effects. These results also prompt the hypothesis that, at least at nuclear level, HBR may have acted following the hydrolysis of its grafted moieties.

Western blot and immunohistochemical analyses revealed that early after HBR injection (6 h), the acetyl-histone H4 signal rose in the border zone, progressively increasing up to 16 h, as compared with the untreated group. After 24 h, histone H4 acetylation increased both in border and remote zone of infarcted HBR-injected hearts. In vitro experiments provided evidence that acetyl-H4 immunoreactivity was also higher in HBR-exposed RCm and Stro-1-positive cells, as compared with unexposed cells. These results indicate that the transcriptional responses elicited by HBR in vivo may be mediated, at least in part, by epigenetic modifications and chromatin remodeling likely attributable to a decrease in HDAC activity due to the BU moiety of the mixed ester.

The finding that a synthetic glycoconjugate afforded effective cardiac repair in the acute phase of MI may have several biomedical implications. In fact, the rescuing effect: (i) was obtained without the needs of viral vector mediated approaches, (ii) did not require stem cell transplantation, (iii) was rapid and long lasting, and (iv) significantly reduced the extent of myocardial fibrosis and scarring. Moreover, the cardiac repair and functional normalization afforded by a myocardial injection of HBR may serve as first aid to rescue a damaged heart. This intervention may be followed by delayed transplantation of autologous stem cells, eventually preconditioned to a cardiovascular fate ex vivo with the same molecule, to enhance a long-term potential for cardiovascular cell therapy.

Resuming Cardiomyocyte Proliferation

Enabling proliferation of cardiomyocytes may represent an alternative area of inquiry in cardiac reparative/regenerative medicine and may also involve a paradigm shift in the current view(s) of cardiac cell therapy. Compelling evidence indicate that adult cardiomyocytes still harbor signaling circuits capable of efficiently resuming their proliferative potential. P38 MAP kinase inhibition enabled proliferation of adult mammalian cardiomyocytes, and FGF1/p38 MAPKinase inhibitor therapy after acute MI in rats increased cardiomyocyte mitosis in vivo and resulted in reduced scarring and wall thinning with markedly improved cardiac function (Engel et al., 2006). A relevant mechanism controlling proliferation in adult cardiomyocytes involves the growth factor neuregulin1 (NRG1) and its tyrosine kinase receptor, ErbB4 (Bersell et al., 2009). NRG1 induced mononucleated, but not binucleated, cardiomyocytes to divide. In vivo, genetic inactivation of ErbB4 reduced cardiomyocyte proliferation, whereas increasing ErbB4 expression enhanced it. Injecting NRG1 in adult mice induced cardiomyocyte cell-cycle activity and promoted myocardial regeneration, leading to improved function after MI.

Periostin was also found to stimulate mononucleated cardiomyocytes to go through the full mitotic cell cycle (Kuhn et al., 2007). Periostin activated alphaV, beta1, beta3 and beta5 integrins located in the cardiomyocyte cell membrane. Activation of phosphatidylinositol-3-OH kinase was required for periostin-induced reentry of cardiomyocytes into the cell cycle and was sufficient for cell-cycle reentry in the absence of periostin. After MI, periostin-induced cardiomyocyte cell-cycle reentry and mitosis were associated with improved ventricular remodeling and myocardial function, reduced fibrosis and infarct size, and increased angiogenesis.

These data indicate that adult cardiomyocytes and a number of cell signaling pathways may provide a target for innovative molecular strategies to promote myocardial regeneration and treat heart failure. This issue has been further dissected by investigating the effects elicited by TNF-related weak inducer of apoptosis (TWEAK) on post-natal rat cardiomyocytes (Novoyatleva et al., 2010). TWEAK, a member of the TNF-α family regulates proliferation in multiple cell types including liver oval cells, salivary epithelial cells, skeletal muscle myoblasts, kidney mesangial cells, podocytes, and tubular cells. TWEAK is produced as a Type II transmembrane glycoprotein and is processed into a 156 amino acid soluble cytokine. Its biological processes involve inflammation, angiogenesis, and cell survival, and are mediated through the fibroblast growth factor-inducible molecule 14 (FN14) receptor, a finely tuned, inducible receptor encompassing multiple downstream signaling cascades. Stimulation of neonatal rat cardiomyocytes with TWEAK recombinant protein resulted in a remarkable, dose-dependent increase in DNA synthesis (Novoyatleva et al., 2010). TWEAK also increased the expression of the proliferative markers Cyclin D2 and Ki67, while downregulating the cell cycle inhibitor p27KIP1. The promitotic action of TWEAK was further supported by the observation that it enhanced the number of H3P-positive cardiomyocytes. Evidence that TWEAK led to effective cardiomyocyte division was provided by the finding that the cytokine also increased the number of myocardial cells concomitantly stained for Aurora B, a marker of the central spindle and the mid-body, and Troponin I. Loss-of-function experiments using the ITEM-2 antibody blocking the interaction between TWEAK and FN14, or FN14 siRNA, revealed that re-induction of proliferation was dependent on FN14 signaling (Novoyatleva et al., 2010). Assessment of the phosphorylated form of targeted kinases and the use of specific kinase inhibitors indicated that the TWEAK/FN14-mediated patterning involved the activation of ERK, and PI3K, as well as inhibition of GSK-3β which in turn led to stabilization and accumulation of total β-catenin and accumulation of dephosphorylated β-catenin in the nucleus. TWEAK did not affect proliferation of adult rat cardiomyocytes. This different behavior resulted from progressive downregulation of FN14 gene and protein expression after birth. Accordingly, adenoviral expression of FN14 enabled efficient induction of cell cycle reentry in adult cardiomyocytes after TWEAK stimulation. To this end, overexpression of FN14 receptor alone induced DNA synthesis in adult cardiomyocytes, owing to the presence of endogenous TWEAK protein in these cells (Novoyatleva et al., 2010).

Direct functional approaches should then be designed in experimental models of MI or heart failure to further assess whether selective or merged activation of defined signaling patterning in vivo may contribute to replenish lost cardiomyocytes and improve myocardial performance. Indeed, efficient induction of proliferation in resident adult cardiomyocytes may represent a rapid, first aid to rescue a failing heart. Further efforts should also attempt at identifying chemical compounds that functionally replace viral vector-mediated overexpression of signaling players affording proliferation of adult cardiomyocytes in vitro and in vivo.

Direct Cardiac Reprogramming of Endogenous Fibroblasts Within the Infarcted Tissue

The ability to reprogram fibroblasts into induced pluripotent stem cells (iPSCs) with three or four defined factors might address the fundamental issue of providing an alternative source of embryonic-like stem cells (Takahashi and Yamanaka, 2006). However, generating sufficient iPSC-derived cardiomyocytes that are pure and mature and that can be delivered safely has long remained challenging. Intriguingly, cardiac fibroblasts comprise over 50% of all the cells in the heart (Baudino et al., 2006), as compared with cardiomyocytes, and vascular cells. Cardiac fibroblasts are fully differentiated somatic cells that provide support structure, secrete signals, and contribute to scar formation upon cardiac damage. Fibroblasts arise from an extracardiac source of cells known as the proepicardium, and do not normally have cardiogenic potential. The large population of endogenous cardiac fibroblasts is a potential source of cardiomyocytes for regenerative therapy, theoretically avoiding transplantation of exogenous pluripotent cells, if it were possible to directly reprogram the resident fibroblasts into beating cardiomyocytes. The iPSC story suggests that a specific combination of defined factors, rather than a single factor, could epigenetically alter the global gene expression of a cell and allow greater plasticity of cell type than previously appreciated. Consistent with this, a specific combination of three transcription factors, Gata4, Mef2c, and Tbx5, was found to be sufficient in generating functional beating cardiomyocytes directly from mouse postnatal cardiac or dermal fibroblasts (Ieda et al., 2010). The induced cardiomyocytes (iCMs) were reprogrammed to adopt a global cardiomyocyte-like gene expression profile, expressing cardiac-specific marker proteins, including α-sarcomeric actinin, cTnT, and ANF. iCMs also expressed defined sarcomeric structures similar to neonatal cardiomyocytes, lacking expression of both smooth muscle and endothelial markers. Most of iCMs originated from a c-kit negative population and could also be obtained from mouse tail-tip dermal fibroblasts. Moreover, iCMs were not first reprogrammed to cells expressing Isl1, an early cardiac progenitor marker that is transiently expressed before cardiac differentiation (Ieda et al., 2010). Cumulatively, these observations exclude an origin of iCMs from rare cardiac progenitors.

Comparative analysis of the enrichment of trimethylated histone H3 of lysine 27 (H3K27me3) and lysine 4 (H3K4me3), which mark transcriptionally inactive or active chromatin, respectively, was performed in cardiac fibroblasts, iCMs, and neonatal cardiac cells. These studies revealed that after reprogramming, H3K27me3 was significantly depleted at the promoters of all the genes analyzed in iCMs, reaching levels comparable to those in cardiac cells, whereas H3K4me3 increased on the promoter regions of Actn2 and Tnnt2 in iCMs, as compared with cardiac fibroblasts (Ieda et al., 2010). Ryr2 had similar levels of H3K4me3 in iCMs as in fibroblasts, suggesting that its activation reflects the resolution of a "bivalent" chromatin mark. These results suggested that cardiac fibroblast-derived iCMs gained a chromatin status similar to cardiomyocytes, at least in some cardiac specific genes. Noteworthy, cardiac fibroblast-derived iCMs exhibited spontaneous contraction, spontaneous cytosolic Ca^{2+} oscillations, and electrical activity form single-cell extracellular recording resembling those observed in neonatal cardiomyocytes (Ieda et al., 2010).

Cardiac fibroblasts transduced ex vivo with GATA4, Mef2c Tbx5, and DsRed to be readily identified by fluorescence, were also injected into the normal heart of immunosuppressed NOD-SCID mice. Despite being injected into the heart only 1 day after viral infection, transplanted cells expressed α-sarcomeric actinin and showed sarcomeric structures within 2 weeks (Ieda et al., 2010). These findings suggested that transduced cardiac fibroblasts can reprogram to cardiomyocytes upon transplantation in vivo.

Although these results were obtained following transplantation into a normal heart, the ability to reprogram endogenous cardiac fibroblasts into cardiomyocytes raises the potential to introduce the defined factors, or factors that mimic their effects, directly into infarcted hearts to reprogram the endogenous fibroblast population, which represents more than 50% of the cells, into new cardiomyocytes that can contribute to the overall contractility of the heart.

The generation of iPSCs and iCMs was received with huge interest both from researchers and the media, offering a potential alternative to costly and sometimes controversial ES cell research. Despite this enthusiasm, the fact that these cells were created via genetic engineering of the cell using viral vectors rendered them unsafe for any potential therapeutic use. However, research in the field has progressed at breakneck speed. Several methods were quickly developed to deliver transcription factor genes without viral vectors and the first iPSCs have already been generated with no genetic alteration, with a combination of epigenetic and non-genetic approaches, or by using recombinant proteins. Proteins can be delivered into cells in vitro and in vivo by conjugating them with a short peptide that mediates protein transduction, such as HIV tat and poly-arginine (Michiue et al., 2005). In addition, various solubilization and refolding techniques for processing inclusion body proteins expressed in E. coli to bioactive proteins have been developed to allow facile and large-scale production of therapeutic proteins. Whether these tools may be used to afford efficient reprogramming of cardiac fibroblasts in vivo within infarcted hearts, and whether such a goal may also be pursued by the aid of naturally occurring or synthetic molecules harboring signaling and transcriptional "transducing logics", remains to be elucidated. This will become a major area of inquiry in the near future, since succeeding in this purpose may drastically change the perspective to afford efficient cardiac regeneration in humans.

Evidence of Regenerated Myocardium: Conventional and Molecular Imaging

One of the most important accomplishments of modern medicine is the development of imaging techniques able to explore biochemical/molecular processes in the intact organism. Since the development of molecular biology and nanotechnology, imaging can be conducted not only to visualize gross anatomical structures, but also to monitor function and track substructures of cells or molecule dynamics. In our hands, we tested human ferritin heavy chain (hFTH) as an effective reporter gene for in vivo long-term tracking of stem cells by cardiac 1.5 T magnetic resonance imaging (MRI) in a rat model of myocardial infarction (Campan et al., 2011). Conventional and molecular MRI in vivo showed the effects of engrafted stem cells on regional contractile function and myocardial viability. Moreover, single-molecule fluorescence imaging approaches showed in vivo an increased dimerization of TGF-β type II receptors in hypertrophic cardiomyocytes during the remodeling process (He et al., 2011). Advances in cardiac combined imaging technologies also allowed the visualization of multidimensional and multifunctional data of remodeled and/or repaired heart in humans, and in animal models of failing heart (Lionetti et al., 2007). Several technologies can be used for non-invasive conventional and targeted imaging of regenerated myocardium in vivo, such as echocardiography, PET, single photon emission computed tomography (SPECT) and MRI. The myocardial repair/regeneration tends to replace dysfunctional and/or fibrotic tissue with functionally mature new cells, served by well-organized capillary networks, also in response to extracellular matrix (ECM) degradation products and paracrine release of soluble molecules into the myocardium (Lionetti et al., 2010a). PET modality is the gold standard approach for non-invasive evaluation of myocardial viability and blood flow in humans, as well as animal models of cardiac disease (Lionetti et al., 2007), respectively through the intravascular injection of ^{18}F-fluorodeoxyglucose (^{18}F-FDG) or C-11-acetate and ^{13}N-labeled ammonia (^{13}NH$_3$). Moreover, a recent study showed the utility of new PET radiotracers to monitor cell proliferation within viable tissue by using radiotracer such as 3′-deoxy-3′-[18F]-fluorothymidine (Grierson and Shields, 2000). MRI may also provide high-resolution anatomical images that allow accurate regional evaluation of myocardial structure and function, and detection of interstitial fibrosis following regenerative treatments in the heart. A significant advantage of MRI is that it provides detailed information about the regions surrounding injured myocardium (e.g. edema, lesion or inflammation), which may hinder the effective recovery of damaged tissues. However, some contrast techniques by MRI have low sensitivity. Combining PET with a high-resolution anatomic imaging modality, such as MRI, can solve the localization issue as long as the images from the two modalities are accurately coregistered. In our recent investigations, we employed a multi-modal imaging approach to investigate the regenerative regional effects of cellular (Simioniuc et al., 2011) and acellular (Lionetti et al., 2010b) treatment in infarcted heart. The acellular treatment of ischemic myocardium caused a replacement of capillary network and proper cellular compartment in the myocardial border zone, as respectively witnessed by ^{18}F-FDG and ^{13}NH$_3$ myocardial uptake, compared to untreated hearts. The replacement of myocardial structure maintained competent regional and global left ventricular function preventing the onset of heart failure.

Imaging technologies highlighting the effects of cardiac regenerative treatment(s) without stem cell transplantation should also have a significant clinical relevance. However, additional technological efforts are needed, since successful multimodal imaging of regenerated myocardium in vivo requires that an "intelligent" contrast agent exerts an "effect size" sufficient for regional detection by imaging hardware.

Conclusions

For many years the idea of regenerating the heart has been skeptically regarded. Although stem cells may hold promises for cardiovascular repair, we are still far away from a real myocardial regeneration that would imply a high-fidelity recapitulation of cardiogenesis within pluripotent elements in such a high-throughput fashion to overcome the low-yielding bias of the spontaneous process itself. So far, cardiac stem cell therapy is still hampered by remarkable obstacles, including poor cell viability, very low delivery efficiency, uncertain differentiating fate in vivo, the needs for ex vivo cell expansion and eventual preconditioning with differentiating agents with consequent delay in transplantation after the onset of a heart attack. Moreover, the clinical use of stem cells will be burdened in a near future with a number of interrelated challenges, including: (i) high-throughput bioprocess development and improved downstream processing problems; (ii) significant modification, improvement and re-testing of current strategies of stem cell culturing and cardiovascular commitment complying with all standards of Good Manufacturing Practice (GMP); (iii) analytical methodologies for control of GMP bioprocessing and differentiation efficiencies.

Recent acquirements within the field of cell signaling, epigenetics, and genome reprogramming may disclose new paradigms within the field of cardiovascular regenerative medicine. In the next few years, we will probably witness to the attempt of using chemistry, both naturally occurring peptides or synthetic molecules, to drive cardiac regeneration through a number of non-mutually exclusive approaches, including: (i) direct myocardial delivery of molecules (i.e. HBR) rescuing the infarcted myocardium, (ii) cell cycle reentry of cardiomyocytes within the myocardium, and (iii) in vivo direct cardiac reprogramming of myocardial fibroblasts without an intermediate iPSC step.

The field of regenerative medicine is moving extremely quickly, involving both clinical expectations and economical interests. In order to gain real perspectives for cardiac regeneration, we need to bring together cell biologists, clinicians, chemists, physics, and engineers to develop novel strategies providing affordable, clinically compliant manipulation of cell pluripotency within a damaged heart. Expanding our knowledge within this context may eventually pave the way to improve the health of millions of people suffering for heart failure.

References

Baudino TA, Carver W, Giles W, Borg TK (2006) Cardiac fibroblasts: friend or foe? Am J Physiol Heart Circ Physiol 291:H1015–H1026

Bersell K, Arab S, Haring B, Kuhn B (2009) Neuregulin1/ErbB4 signaling induces cardiomyocyte proliferation and repair of heart injury. Cell 138:257–270

Bonaros N, Rauf R, Schachner T, Laufer G, Kocher A (2008) Enhanced cell therapy for ischemic heart disease. Transplantation 86:1151–1160

Camenisch TD, Spicer AP, Brehm-Gibson T, Biesterfeldt J, Augustine ML, Calabro A Jr, Kubalak S, Klewer SE, McDonald JA (2000) Disruption of hyaluronan synthase-2 abrogates normal cardiac morphogenesis and hyaluronan-mediated transformation of epithelium to mesenchyme. J Clin Invest 106:349–360

Campan M, Lionetti V, Aquaro GD, Forini F, Matteucci M, Vannucci L, Chiuppesi F, Di Cristofano C, Faggioni M, Maioli M, Barile L, Messina E, Lombardi M, Pucci A, Pistello M, Recchia FA (2011) Ferritin as a reporter gene for in vivo tracking of stem cells by 1.5T cardiac MRI in a rat model of myocardial infarction. Am J Physiol Heart Circ Physiol. 300(6): H2238–50

Cleland JG, Freemantle N, Coletta AP, Clark AL (2006) Clinical trials update from the American Heart Association: REPAIR-AMI, ASTAMI, JELIS, MEGA, REVIVE-II, SURVIVE, and PROACTIVE. Eur J Heart Fail 8:105–110

Dilworth FJ, Fromental-Ramain C, Yamamoto K, Chambon P (2000) ATP-driven chromatin remodeling activity and histone acetyltransferases act sequentially during transactivation by RAR/RXR *in vitro*. Mol Cell 6:1049–1058

Engel FB, Hsieh PC, Lee RT, Keating MT (2006) FGF1/p38 MAP kinase inhibitor therapy induces cardiomyocyte mitosis, reduces scarring, and rescues function after myocardial infarction. Proc Natl Acad Sci USA 103:15546–15551

Grierson JR, Shields AF (2000) Radiosynthesis of 3′-deoxy-3′-fluoro-thymidine: 18F-FLT for imaging cellular proliferation in vivo. Nucl Med Biol 27:143–156

He KM, Fu YN, Zhang W, Yuan JH, Li ZJ, Lv ZZ, Zhang YY, Fang XH (2011) Single-molecule imaging revealed enhanced dimerization of transforming growth factor β type II receptors in hypertrophic cardiomyocytes. Biochem Biophys Res Commun. Epub ahead of print

Ieda M, Fu JD, Delgado-Olguin P, Vedantham V, Hayashi Y, Bruneau BG, Srivastava D (2010) Direct reprogramming of fibroblasts into functional cardiomyocytes by defined factors. Cell 142:375–386

Illi B, Scopece A, Nanni S, Farsetti A, Morgante L, Biglioli P, Capogrossi MC, Gaetano C (2005) Epigenetic histone modification and cardiovascular lineage programming in mouse embryonic stem cells exposed to laminar shear stress. Circ Res 96:501–508

Janssens S, Dubois C, Bogaert J, Theunissen K, Deroose C, Desmet W, Kalantzi M, Herbots L, Sinnaeve P, Dens J, Maertens J, Rademakers F, Dymarkowski S, Gheysens O, Van Cleemput J, Bormans G, Nuyts J, Belmans A, Mortelmans L, Boogaerts M, Van de Werf F (2006) Autologous bone marrow-derived stem-cell transfer in patients with ST-segment elevation myocardial infarction: double-blind, randomised controlled trial. Lancet 367: 113–121

Kuhn B, Del Monte F, Hajjar RJ, Chang YS, Lebeche D, Arab S, Keating MT (2007) Periostin induces proliferation of differentiated cardiomyocytes and promotes cardiac repair. Nat Med 13:962–969

Lai L, Bohnsack BL, Niederreither K, Hirschi KK (2003) Retinoic acid regulates endothelial cell proliferation during vasculogenesis. Development 130:6465–6474

Lionetti V, Guiducci L, Simioniuc A, Aquaro GD, Simi C, De Marchi D, Burchielli S, Pratali L, Piacenti M, Lombardi M, Salvadori P, Pingitore A, Neglia D, Recchia FA (2007) Mismatch between uniform increase in cardiac glucose uptake and regional contractile dysfunction in pacing-induced heart failure. Am J Physiol Heart Circ Physiol 293:H2747–H2756

Lionetti V, Bianchi G, Recchia FA, Ventura C (2010a) Control of autocrine and paracrine myocardial signals: an emerging therapeutic strategy in heart failure. Heart Fail Rev 15: 531–542

Lionetti V, Cantoni S, Cavallini C, Bianchi F, Valente S, Frascari I, Olivi E, Aquaro GD, Bonavita F, Scarlata I, Maioli M, Vaccari V, Tassinari R, Bartoli A, Recchia FA, Pasquinelli G, Ventura C (2010b) Hyaluronan mixed esters of butyric and retinoic acid affording myocardial survival and repair without stem cell transplantation. J Biol Chem 285:9949–9961

Lunde K, Solheim S, Aakhus S, Arnesen H, Abdelnoor M, Forfang K (2005) ASTAMI investigators. Autologous stem cell transplantation in acute myocardial infarction: the ASTAMI randomized controlled trial. Intracoronary transplantation of autologous mononuclear bone marrow cells, study design and safety aspects. Scand Cardiovasc J 39: 150–158

Meyer GP, Wollert KC, Lotz J, Steffens J, Lippolt P, Fichtner S, Hecker H, Schaefer A, Arseniev L, Hertenstein B, Ganser A, Drexler H (2006) Intracoronary bone marrow cell transfer after myocardial infarction: eighteen months' follow-up data from the randomized, controlled BOOST (BOne marrOw transfer to enhance ST-elevation infarct regeneration) trial. Circulation 113:1287–1294

Michiue H, Tomizawa K, Wei FY, Matsushita M, Lu YF, Ichikawa T, Tamiya T, Date I, Matsui H (2005) The NH2 terminus of influenza virus hemagglutinin-2 subunit peptides enhances the antitumor potency of polyarginine-mediated p53 protein transduction. J Biol Chem 280:8285–8289

Nakamura T, Mizuno S, Matsumoto K, Sawa Y, Matsuda H, Nakamura T (2000) Myocardial protection from ischemia/reperfusion injury by endogenous and exogenous HGF. J Clin Invest 106:1511–1519

Novoyatleva T, Diehl F, van Amerongen MJ, Patra C, Ferrazzi F, Bellazzi R, Engel FB (2010) TWEAK is a positive regulator of cardiomyocyte proliferation. Cardiovasc Res 85:681–690

Orlic D, Kajstura J, Chimenti S, Jakoniuk I, Anderson SM, Li B, Pickel J, McKay R, Nadal-Ginard B, Bodine DM, Anversa P (2001) Bone marrow cells regenerate infarcted myocardium. Nature 410:701–705

Savani RC, Cao G, Pooler PM, Zaman A, Zhou Z, DeLisser HM (2001) Differential involvement of the hyaluronan (HA) receptors CD44 and receptor for HA-mediated motility in endothelial cell function and angiogenesis. J Biol Chem 276:36770–36778

Simioniuc A, Campan M, Lionetti V, Marinelli M, Aquaro GD, Cavallini C, Valente S, Di Silvestre D, Cantoni S, Bernini F, Simi C, Pardini S, Mauri P, Neglia D, Ventura C, Pasquinelli G, Recchia FA (2011) Placental stem cells pre-treated with hyaluronan-butyric-retinoic ester to cure infarcted pig hearts: a multimodal study. Cardiovasc Res. Epub ahead of print

Takahashi K, Yamanaka S (2006) Induction of pluripotent stem cells from mouse embryonic and adult fibroblast cultures by defined factors. Cell 126:663–676

Ventura C, Branzi A (2006) Autocrine and intracrine signaling for cardiogenesis in embryonic stem cells: a clue for the development of novel differentiating agents. Handb Exp Pharmacol 174:123–146

Ventura C, Zinellu E, Maninchedda E, Maioli M (2003) Dynorphin B is an agonist of nuclear opioid receptors coupling nuclear protein kinase C activation to the transcription of cardiogenic genes in GTR1 embryonic stem cells. Circ Res 92:623–629

Ventura C, Maioli M, Asara Y, Santoni D, Scarlata I, Cantoni S, Perbellini A (2004) Butyric and retinoic mixed ester of hyaluronan. A novel differentiating glycoconjugate affording a high throughput of cardiogenesis in embryonic stem cells. J Biol Chem 279:23574–23579

Ventura C, Cantoni S, Bianchi F, Lionetti V, Cavallini C, Scarlata I, Foroni L, Maioli M, Bonsi L, Alviano F, Fossati V, Bagnara GP, Pasquinelli G, Recchia FA, Perbellini A (2007) Hyaluronan mixed esters of butyric and retinoic acid drive cardiac and endothelial fate in term placenta human mesenchymal stem cells and enhance cardiac repair in infarcted rat hearts. J Biol Chem 282:14243–14252

Wheatley SC, Isacke CM, Crossley PH (1993) Restricted expression of the hyaluronan receptor, CD44, during postimplantation mouse embryogenesis suggests key roles in tissue formation and patterning. Development 119:295–306

Wobus AM, Kaomei G, Shan J, Wellner MC, Rohwedel J, Ji G, Fleischmann B, Katus HA, Hescheler J, Franz WM (1997) Retinoic acid accelerates embryonic stem cell-derived cardiac differentiation and enhances development of ventricular cardiomyocytes. J Mol Cell Cardiol 29:1525–1539

Chapter 37

Allogeneic Transplantation of Fetal Membrane-Derived Mesenchymal Stem Cells: Therapy for Acute Myocarditis

Shin Ishikane, Hiroshi Hosoda, Kenichi Yamahara, Makoto Kodama, and Tomoaki Ikeda

Abstract Acute myocarditis is an acute inflammatory disease of the myocardium for which there is currently no specific treatment. Inflammatory cells also play a role in the onset of myocarditis. Mesenchymal stem cells (MSC) have immunomodulatory properties, which make them an attractive cell source for treatment of myocarditis, given the importance of the inflammatory component in this disorder. Autologous transplantation of bone marrow-derived MSC (BM-MSC) significantly reduced myocardial inflammation and cardiac dysfunction in a rat model of acute autoimmune myocarditis by reducing inflammation and stimulating angiogenesis. However, BM aspiration procedures are invasive and can yield low numbers of MSC after processing. Recently, the focus has been on allogeneic MSC transplantation, and fetal membranes (FMs) as an alternative source of MSC are expected to provide a large number of cells. We demonstrated that allogeneic FM-derived MSC (FM-MSC) transplantation also reduced myocardial inflammatory cell infiltration and cardiac dysfunction in a rat model of acute autoimmune myocarditis and that myosin-responsive T cell proliferation and activation were suppressed by FM-MSC. The transplantation of allogeneic FM-MSC did not elicit any lymphocyte proliferative response despite their allogeneic origin. Although further experiments are needed to apply the current results to human cell therapy, allogeneic FM-MSC transplantation may provide a new therapeutic strategy for the treatment of acute myocarditis. This review focuses on the immunomodulatory effects of MSC and discusses the potential of allogeneic FM-MSC transplantation therapy in acute myocarditis.

Keywords Myocarditis · Mesenchymal stem cells · FM-MSC · EAM · HGF · Immunomodulatory

Introduction

Acute myocarditis is a nonischemic heart disease characterized by myocardial inflammation and interstitial edema. The disease results in rapidly progressing heart failure, arrhythmia, and sudden death. The major long-term consequence is dilated cardiomyopathy with chronic heart failure. Common viral infections are the most frequent cause of myocarditis, but other pathogens, hypersensitivity reactions, and systemic and autoimmune diseases have also been implicated. Although the early evidence showing the efficacy of immunoglobulin and interferon therapies appeared promising, these results have yet to be confirmed in randomized controlled clinical trials. The current treatment options are restricted to supportive care for patients with heart failure and arrhythmia. The lack of a specific treatment and the potential severity of the illness emphasize the importance of developing new effective therapeutic strategies for myocarditis.

Mesenchymal stem cells (MSC) are multipotent stem cells present in the bone marrow (BM), adipose, and many other tissues, which can differentiate into a variety of cells including adipocytes, osteocytes, chondrocytes, endothelial cells, and myocytes (Pittenger et al., 1999). MSC are a promising cell source for

T. Ikeda (✉)
Department of Regenerative Medicine and Tissue Engineering, National Cardiovascular Center Research Institute, Suita, Osaka 565-8565, Japan
e-mail: tikeda@hsp.ncvc.go.jp

regenerative therapies. We reported that the autologous administration of BM- or adipose tissue-derived MSC improves cardiac function in rat models of dilated cardiomyopathy (Nagaya et al., 2005), myocardial infarction (Miyahara et al., 2006), and acute autoimmune myocarditis (Ohnishi et al., 2007). However, there are several limitations in using an autologous cell source, including the invasiveness of collection procedures, inadequate cell numbers, and donor-site morbidity, and the functionality of precursor cells has been questioned in patients with cardiovascular risk factors. An alternative source of MSC that could provide large quantities of cells would be advantageous. One way to circumvent these limitations could be to use allogeneic MSC. If allogeneic MSC could be isolated from healthy young donors and had a therapeutic effect comparable to autologous MSC, they would be considered a superior new cell source because it would be possible to overcome the problems noted above, and wider clinical applications of cell therapy would become available. Therefore, we focused on fetal membranes (FMs), which are generally discarded as medical waste after delivery, as an alternative source of autologous MSC. Several studies reported that human FMs contain multipotent cells similar to BM-MSC that are easy to expand (In't Anker et al., 2004; Portmann-Lanz et al., 2006). We reported that the allogeneic transplantation of FM-derived MSC (FM-MSC) induces therapeutic angiogenesis in a rat model of hind limb ischemia (Ishikane et al., 2008). MSC have been reported to induce immune tolerance, and we confirmed that the transplantation of FM-MSC did not elicit any lymphocyte proliferative response despite their allogeneic origin. Recently, we reported that allogeneic FM-MSC transplantation ameliorated cardiac dysfunction and induced immunomodulatory and anti-inflammatory effects in a rat model of acute autoimmune myocarditis (Ishikane et al., 2010). To date, only four studies of the therapeutic effects of MSC transplantation in myocarditis, including our reports, have been published (Table 37.1). In this review, we focus on the immunosuppressive properties of MSC, and discuss the potential of allogeneic FM-MSC transplantation therapy for acute myocarditis.

Table 37.1 Reported studies of mesenchymal stem cell therapy in animal models of myocarditis

Animal model	Transplanted cells	Number of transplanted cells	Method of transplantation	Efficacy of MSC	References
Myosin-induced myocarditis in rats	Allogeneic FM-MSC	5×10^5 cells	Intravenous injection	Improvement of cardiac function Immunomodulation Antifibrosis Anti-inflammation	Ishikane et al. (2010)
Myosin-induced myocarditis in rats	Autologous BM-MSC	3×10^6 cells	Intravenous injection	Improvement of cardiac function Neovascularization Antiapoptosis Anti-inflammation VEGF and HGF secretion	Ohnishi et al. (2007)
Myosin-induced myocarditis in rats	Autologous BM-MSC	5×10^6 cells	Intramyocardial injection	Improvement of cardiac function Neovascularization Inflammatory cytokine suppression HGF secretion	Okada et al. (2007)
Coxsackievirus B3-induced myocarditis in mice	Xenogeneic BM-MSC	1×10^6 cells	Intravenous injection	Improvement of cardiac function Immunomodulation Antifibrosis Anti-inflammation Antiapoptosis Antivirus	Van Linthout et al. (2010)

Abbreviations: BM-MSC, bone marrow-derived mesenchymal stem cells; FM-MSC, fetal membrane-derived mesenchymal stem cells; MSC, mesenchymal stem cells

Experimental Model of Autoimmune Myocarditis

Patients with myocarditis present a variety of clinical manifestations, such as heart failure, arrhythmia, or circulatory collapse. Although myocarditis often follows viral infection, its pathogenesis is not fully understood. There is substantial evidence suggesting that autoimmune responses to heart antigens, particularly cardiac myosin, following viral infection may contribute to the disease process (Lauer et al., 1994).

An experimental autoimmune myocarditis (EAM) model in Lewis rats, produced by immunization with cardiac myosin, is characterized by extremely severe myocardial lesions and multinucleated giant cells, and it has been reported that the pathogenesis of both human giant-cell myocarditis and viral myocarditis resembles that of EAM (Kodama et al., 1990). This EAM is triphasic and comprises an antigen-priming phase on days 0–13, an autoimmune response phase on days 14–21, and a reparative phase thereafter that is associated with a chronically dilated cardiomyopathy phenotype. Although the pathogenesis of EAM has not been fully clarified, severe inflammatory cell infiltration is a characteristic of the disease.

In the rat model of EAM, T cells are activated and expanded in response to treatment with a fragment of cardiac myosin, and activated T cells and macrophages are then recruited to target the affected cardiomyocytes. The migration of activated T cells into the myocardium is considered the initial process of EAM. Fuse et al. (2003) reported that induction of acute autoimmune myocarditis is associated with systemic helper T cell 1 (Th1) dominance, while recovery is related to systemic helper T cell 2 (Th2) dominance. The Th1/Th2 balance accurately reflects the course of the disease and adjustment of the Th1/Th2 balance may lead to better treatments for acute myocarditis.

Autologous BM-MSC Transplantation for Acute Autoimmune Myocarditis

We reported the therapeutic effects of autologous BM-MSC transplantation in EAM (Ohnishi et al., 2007). The intravenous transplantation of Lewis rat-derived BM-MSC (3×10^6 cells/animal, 1 week after myosin administration) attenuated the increase in CD68-positive inflammatory cells and monocyte chemoattractant protein-1 (MCP-1) expression in myocardium that is seen in the Lewis EAM model. Pathology results showed that cardiac necrosis, granulation, edema, and fibrosis were decreased at 2 weeks after transplantation. Autologous BM-MSC transplantation improved heart failure, as demonstrated by improvement of hemodynamic and echocardiographic results, and increased the capillary density in the EAM myocardium. However, when PKH26 dye-labeled BM-MSC were transplanted intravenously in EAM rats, only a small fraction of endothelial cells and cardiomyocytes were positive for PKH26 at 2 weeks after transplantation. These results suggest that BM-MSC transplantation-induced neovascularization may have contributed to the improvement of cardiac function in the EAM, but the role of differentiation of transplanted BM-MSC to endothelial cells or cardiomyocytes appears to be largely insignificant in this improvement.

Our in vitro experiments demonstrated that MCP-1 stimulation of cardiomyocytes resulted in an increase in cell injury and apoptosis, whereas BM-MSC-derived conditioned medium attenuated these effects. BM-MSC secreted large amounts of angiogenic and antiapoptotic factors such as vascular endothelial growth factor, hepatocyte growth factor (HGF), insulin-like growth factor-1, and adrenomedullin. These results showed that MSC had cardioprotective effects by acting in a paracrine manner. Okada et al. (2007) reported that intramyocardial transplantation of autologous BM-MSC improved cardiac systolic function in EAM rats. The cardiac inflammatory lesions were decreased, and capillary density was increased by autologous BM-MSC transplantation. Autologous BM-MSC transplantation enhanced expression of HGF and inhibited expression of interleukin (IL)-2, IL-6, and IL-10 mRNAs in the EAM myocardium. These therapeutic effects were associated with enhancement of HGF secretion by transplanted BM-MSC. HGF is known to function in angiogenesis and myocyte regeneration and to possess antifibrotic activities. These results indicate that autologous BM-MSC transplantation causes therapeutic effects in a paracrine manner, and may be a useful tool in therapy of acute myocarditis. However, a waiting period is required to allow preparation of an adequate number of cells for transplantation of autologous BM-MSC. Because acute myocarditis is often associated with rapidly progressive heart failure, this delay in transplantation of autologous BM-MSC may not be appropriate. Therefore, an alternative cell source is needed that can be adaptable to use in the acute phase of myocarditis.

Fetal Membrane-Derived MSC

Human FMs, which are generally discarded as medical waste after delivery, have been shown recently to be rich sources of MSC. Because fetal tissues are routinely discarded postpartum, FMs (including amnion and chorion membranes) have proved to be inexpensive and easily obtained with virtually limitless availability, removing any need for mass tissue banking. Human amnion membrane-derived MSC (hAM-MSC) were isolated for the first time from AM of the second and third trimester of gestation by In't Anker et al. (2004) who demonstrated their potential for differentiation to osteogenic and adipogenic cells. Later, Portmann-Lanz et al. (2006) demonstrated their capacity for differentiation to chondrogenic, myogenic, and neurogenic lines. In 2007, Alviano et al. (2007) confirmed this finding and gave the first evidence of the angiogenic potential of hAM-MSC. A large number of MSC can be obtained from human FM and a prompt supply becomes possible by banking these cells. If FM-MSC can be used in allogeneic transplantation, FM-MSC may be a useful source for cell transplantation and regenerative medicine.

MSC are positive for major histocompatibility complex (MHC) class I but negative for MHC class II and for costimulatory factors such as CD40, CD80, and CD86, so are considered to be nonimmunogenic (Chamberlain et al., 2007). Allogeneic MSC transplantation has been used in several preclinical and clinical studies where allogeneic MSC were not rejected in the absence of immunosuppression. In our study, FM-MSC had a similar immunophenotype to BM-MSC and did not provoke alloreactive lymphocyte proliferation in vitro (Ishikane et al., 2008). In allogeneic FM-MSC transplantation to the hind limb

Table 37.2 Comparison of the characteristics of FM-MSC and BM-MSC observed in our studies

FM-MSC	Characteristic	BM-MSC
Noninvasive	MSC harvest procedure	Invasive
Placenta	Donor tissue	Adult bone marrow
High	Number of obtained cells	Low
CD11−, CD29+, CD31−, CD34−, CD45−, CD73+, CD90+, MHC class I+, MHC class II−	Immunophenotype	CD11−, CD29+, CD31−, CD34−, CD45−, CD73+, CD90+, MHC class I+, MHC class II−
Adipogenic Osteogenic Chondrogenic	In vitro multipotency	Adipogenic Osteogenic Chondrogenic
VEGF, HGF	Growth factor secretion	VEGF, HGF, IGF-1, adrenomedullin
In acute myocarditis: not induced In hind limb ischemia: induced	Angiogenesis	In acute myocarditis: induced In hind limb ischemia: induced
Low	Engraftment of transplanted cells	Low
Vascular endothelial cells: none Myocardium: none	In vivo differentiation	Vascular endothelial cells: very low or none Smooth muscle cells: very low Myocardium: very low
Evade	Alloreactive T cell activation (rejection)	Evade
Suppress	CD4+ T cell activation (immunomodulatory effect)	Suppress
Suppress	Fibrosis	Suppress
Suppress	Inflammatory cell infiltration	Suppress

Abbreviations: BM-MSC, bone marrow-derived mesenchymal stem cells; FM-MSC, fetal membrane-derived mesenchymal stem cells; HGF, hepatocyte growth factor; IGF-1, insulin-like growth factor-1; MSC, mesenchymal stem cells; MHC, major histocompatibility complex; VEGF, vascular endothelial growth factor muscles, a slight T cell infiltration was observed at the site of allogeneic FM-MSC injection, but the degree of infiltration was less marked than that following allogeneic splenic lymphocyte transplantation and was equivalent to that induced by autologous BM-MSC. These results suggest that FM-MSC can evade T cell alloreactivity and may be successfully transplanted across MHC barriers (Table 37.2).

Allogeneic FM-MSC Transplantation for Acute Autoimmune Myocarditis

To evaluate the therapeutic effects of allogeneic FM-MSC transplantation in acute myocarditis, FM-MSC obtained from MHC-mismatched ACI rats (5×10^5 cells/animal, 1 week after myosin administration) were transplanted intravenously into Lewis EAM rats. At 2 weeks after transplantation, this intravenous allogeneic transplantation of FM-MSC reduced fibrosis, edema, necrosis, granulation and eosinophil infiltration in the hearts exhibiting EAM (Fig. 37.1) (Ishikane et al., 2010) and significantly attenuated infiltration of inflammatory cells (CD68-positive monocytes/macrophages) and MCP-1 expression in the myocardium. The hemodynamic and echocardiographic results showed significant improvement of cardiac function as a result of allogeneic FM-MSC transplantation. The extent of the improvement was in the range of 30–60% in the indices of the level of dysfunction, which is equivalent to that observed in our previous study of autologous BM-MSC transplantation. However, we could not detect an increase in capillary density in the EAM myocardium. Transplanted green fluorescent protein (GFP)-positive cells were detected in the heart tissue 1 day and 1 week after intravenous transplantation of GFP-expressing FM-MSC, although only a few engrafted cells were found. At 4 weeks after transplantation, we could not find GFP-positive cells among the differentiated vascular endothelial cells and cardiomyocytes in the EAM myocardium of rats transplanted with allogeneic FM-MSC. These low levels of engraftment and differentiation of intravenously transplanted cells are in agreement with another report (Barbash et al., 2003). These results suggest that the main therapeutic effects of the transplanted allogeneic FM-MSC in the heart in EAM are not the result of their angiogenic effect or differentiation.

Immunomodulatory Effects of MSC

In addition to the immune phenotype of MSC, their immunomodulatory properties have received considerable attention in recent years. MSC have been demonstrated to have broad anti-inflammatory effects on both the innate and the adaptive immune systems, and are potent inhibitors of T cell activation and proliferation (Di Nicola et al., 2002), dendritic cell maturation (Jiang et al., 2005), and proliferation and cytotoxic activity of natural killer cells (Spaggiari et al., 2006). Recent clinical studies found that intravenous injection of BM-MSC ameliorates acute graft-versus-host disease (Le Blanc et al., 2008). Interestingly, the suppression of T cell proliferation by MSC shows no immunological restriction, insofar as similar suppressive effects were observed with cells that were either autologous or allogeneic to the responder cells. The immunoregulatory potency of hAM-MSC has also been reported (Wolbank et al., 2007).

In our study, allogeneic transplantation of FM-MSC significantly reduced the infiltration of T cells (CD3-positive cells) into EAM hearts. Some of the intravenously transplanted FM-MSC were found in the heart, lung, spleen, and liver. It is interesting that the number of transplanted cells in the spleen, the hub of T cell immunoreactivity, was greater at 1 week after transplantation than at 1 day after transplantation. In the T-lymphocyte proliferation assay, splenic T lymphocytes derived from allogeneic FM-MSC-transplanted EAM even 2 weeks after the transplantation of FM-MSC had a reduced proliferative response to myosin compared with the response of splenic T lymphocytes from untransplanted EAM. In addition, proliferation of activated T-lymphocytes was suppressed by coculture with allogeneic FM-MSC in vitro. Okada et al. (2007) reported that Th2-type cytokine expression in EAM was increased by HGF, whereas Th1-type cytokine expression was suppressed by intramyocardial transplantation of autologous BM-MSC. Increased expression of HGF may reduce the severity of EAM by suppressing the Th1 response. Van Linthout et al. (2010) reported that MSC could improve murine acute coxsackievirus B3-induced myocarditis via their immunomodulatory properties in a nitric oxide-dependent manner. Several other independent reports have suggested prostaglandin E2 (PGE2), indoleamine 2,3-dioxygenase, IL-6, IL-10,

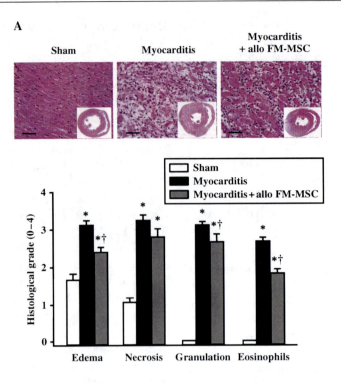

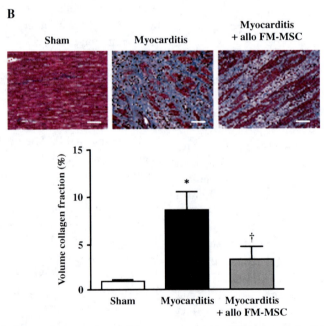

Fig. 37.1 Histopathological changes in acute myocarditis at 2 weeks after transplantation induced by transplantation of allogeneic FM-MSC. (**a**) Myocardial sections showed markedly less inflammation in the allogeneic FM-MSC transplanted group than in the untransplanted myocarditis group. *Insets* are transverse sections of the myocardium. The semiquantitative histological grade of edema and eosinophil infiltration were markedly decreased in the allogeneic FM-MSC transplanted group. (**b**) Myocardial fibrosis, (**c**) CD68-positive macrophage/monocyte infiltration, and (**d**) CD3-positive T cell infiltration were markedly reduced by allogeneic FM-MSC transplantation. Scale bars = 50 μm. Data are expressed as mean ± SEM. *$P < 0.05$ vs. the sham group; †$P < 0.05$ vs. the untreated myocarditis group

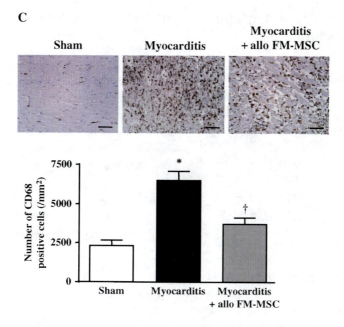

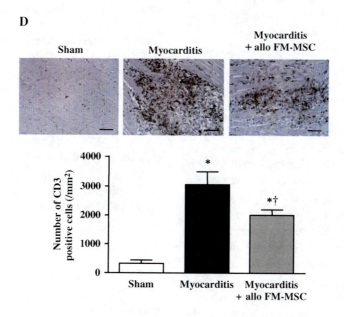

Fig. 37.1 (continued)

heme oxygenase-1, and galectin are among the molecules involved in the inhibition of T cell proliferation by MSC (Aggarwal and Pittenger 2005; Chabannes et al., 2007; Meisel et al., 2004; Sioud et al., 2011). In addition, MSC-affected accessory cells such as T-regulatory cells may be involved in the immunosuppression (Djouad et al., 2003). The induction of T-regulatory cells by MSC involves not only direct contact between MSC and CD4 cells, but also the secretion of soluble factors such as PGE2 (English et al., 2009). These results suggest that the immunomodulatory effects of allogeneic FM-MSC transplantation are mediated by both direct cell–cell contact and by secretion of soluble factors.

Potency of MSC Sheet Transplantation Therapy for Heart Failure

As discussed above, MSC transplantation has attractive possibilities as a tool for myocarditis therapy. However, further experiments are needed to apply the current results with MSC to human cardiomyoplasty, because their ameliorating effect on cardiac function is not necessarily enough for clinical use. To date, intravenous and intramuscular injections have been used in cell transplantation therapy, but the engraftment rate of transplanted MSC by these routes was very low (Ishikane et al., 2008, 2010). Although in EAM some of the intravenous transplanted MSC were found in the lung, heart, spleen, and liver at 1 week after transplantation, these engrafted cells could not be detected 4 weeks after transplantation. Most homing and engraftment studies have demonstrated little, if any, long-term (>1 week) engraftment of MSC after systemic administration (Parekkadan and Milwid, 2010). Studies have shown that the majority of administered MSC (>80%) immediately accumulate in the lung and are cleared with a half-life of 24 h. Thus, although intravenous cell transplantation is very convenient, it is not suitable for transplantation of large numbers of cells. We administered a low number of FM-MSC to avoid pulmonary embolism. Thus, a more effective transplantation route is needed to enhance the cardiac functional improvement.

Recently, cell sheet engineering has received attention as a method for heart tissue repair. Okano et al., have developed engineered cell sheets with scaffoldless tissue engineering by using temperature-responsive culture dishes (Yamada et al., 1990). These cell sheets allow for cell-to-cell connections and maintain the presence of adhesion proteins. The cell sheets preserve the extracellular matrix proteins deposited on the basal surface of the cultured cells. These adhesive proteins play an important role in enhancing the attachment between stacked cell sheets and also between cell sheets and the myocardial surface, thereby allowing for stable fixation of the cell sheet constructs to the target tissues. The cell sheets can readily be transferred and grafted to the scarred myocardium without additives or suturing. Memon et al. (2005) demonstrated that layered skeletal myoblast sheets transplanted to infarcted rat hearts were able to enhance left ventricular contraction, reduce fibrosis, and prevent left ventricular dilation. Kondoh et al. (2006) showed that in hamsters with dilated cardiomyopathy, myoblast sheet graft implantation improved cardiac performance and prolonged life expectancy, in association with a reduction in myocardial fibrosis. In our study in rats, adipose tissue-derived MSC sheets improved cardiac function in damaged hearts, with reversal of cardiac wall thinning and prolonged survival after myocardial infarction (Miyahara et al., 2006). These cell sheets allow transplantation of many more cells than intramyocardium or intravenous needle injection. Transplantation of MSC sheets or combined therapy with these sheets and systemic intravenous injection may result in more effective treatment of myocarditis.

Conclusions

This review shows the potential of allogeneic transplantation of FM-MSC for the treatment of acute myocarditis. Myocarditis is the end result of both myocardial infection and autoimmunity that causes active inflammatory destruction of myocytes. It is expected that allogeneic FM-MSC transplantation will be an effective therapy for acute myocarditis with rapidly progressive heart failure. The beneficial effects of allogeneic FM-MSC transplantation may be mainly attributable to the suppression of T-lymphocyte activation and anti-inflammatory effects. Although further experiments are needed to apply the current results to human cardiomyoplasty, we predict the development of allogeneic FM-MSC transplantation therapy for the treatment of severe acute myocarditis.

References

Aggarwal S, Pittenger MF (2005) Human mesenchymal stem cells modulate allogeneic immune cell responses. Blood 105:1815–1822

Alviano F, Fossati V, Marchionni C, Arpinati M, Bonsi L, Franchina M, Lanzoni G, Cantoni S, Cavallini C, Bianchi F, Tazzari PL, Pasquinelli G, Foroni L, Ventura C, Grossi A, Bagnara GP (2007) Term amniotic membrane is a high throughput source for multipotent mesenchymal stem cells with the ability to differentiate into endothelial cells in vitro. BMC Dev Biol 7:11

Barbash IM, Chouraqui P, Baron J, Feinberg MS, Etzion S, Tessone A, Miller L, Guetta E, Zipori D, Kedes LH, Kloner RA, Leor J (2003) Systemic delivery of bone marrow-derived mesenchymal stem cells to the infarcted myocardium: feasibility, cell migration, and body distribution. Circulation 108:863–868

Chabannes D, Hill M, Merieau E, Rossignol J, Brion R, Soulillou JP, Anegon I, Cuturi MC (2007) A role for heme oxygenase-1 in the immunosuppressive effect of adult rat and human mesenchymal stem cells. Blood 110: 3691–3694

Chamberlain G, Fox J, Ashton B, Middleton J (2007) Concise review: mesenchymal stem cells: their phenotype, differentiation capacity, immunological features, and potential for homing. Stem Cells 25:2739–2749

Di Nicola M, Carlo-Stella C, Magni M, Milanesi M, Longoni PD, Matteucci P, Grisanti S, Gianni AM (2002) Human bone marrow stromal cells suppress T-lymphocyte proliferation induced by cellular or nonspecific mitogenic stimuli. Blood 99:3838–3843

Djouad F, Plence P, Bony C, Tropel P, Apparailly F, Sany J, Noel D, Jorgensen C (2003) Immunosuppressive effect of mesenchymal stem cells favors tumor growth in allogeneic animals. Blood 102:3837–3844

English K, Ryan JM, Tobin L, Murphy MJ, Barry FP, Mahon BP (2009) Cell contact, prostaglandin E(2) and transforming growth factor beta 1 play non-redundant roles in human mesenchymal stem cell induction of CD4+CD25(High) forkhead box P3+ regulatory T cells. Clin Exp Immunol 156: 149–160

Fuse K, Kodama M, Ito M, Okura Y, Kato K, Hanawa H, Aoki S, Aizawa Y (2003) Polarity of helper T cell subsets represents disease nature and clinical course of experimental autoimmune myocarditis in rats. Clin Exp Immunol 134: 403–408

In't Anker PS, Scherjon SA, Kleijburg-van der Keur C, de Groot-Swings GM, Claas FH, Fibbe WE, Kanhai HH (2004) Isolation of mesenchymal stem cells of fetal or maternal origin from human placenta. Stem Cells 22:1338–1345

Ishikane S, Ohnishi S, Yamahara K, Sada M, Harada K, Mishima K, Iwasaki K, Fujiwara M, Kitamura S, Nagaya N, Ikeda T (2008) Allogeneic injection of fetal membrane-derived mesenchymal stem cells induces therapeutic angiogenesis in a rat model of hind limb ischemia. Stem Cells 26:2625–2633

Ishikane S, Yamahara K, Sada M, Harada K, Kodama M, Ishibashi-Ueda H, Hayakawa K, Mishima K, Iwasaki K, Fujiwara M, Kangawa K, Ikeda T (2010) Allogeneic administration of fetal membrane-derived mesenchymal stem cells attenuates acute myocarditis in rats. J Mol Cell Cardiol 49:753–761

Jiang XX, Zhang Y, Liu B, Zhang SX, Wu Y, Yu XD, Mao N (2005) Human mesenchymal stem cells inhibit differentiation and function of monocyte-derived dendritic cells. Blood 105:4120–4126

Kodama M, Matsumoto Y, Fujiwara M, Masani F, Izumi T, Shibata A (1990) A novel experimental model of giant cell myocarditis induced in rats by immunization with cardiac myosin fraction. Clin Immunol Immunopathol 57:250–262

Kondoh H, Sawa Y, Miyagawa S, Sakakida-Kitagawa S, Memon IA, Kawaguchi N, Matsuura N, Shimizu T, Okano T, Matsuda H (2006) Longer preservation of cardiac performance by sheet-shaped myoblast implantation in dilated cardiomyopathic hamsters. Cardiovasc Res 69:466–475

Lauer B, Padberg K, Schultheiss HP, Strauer BE (1994) Autoantibodies against human ventricular myosin in sera of patients with acute and chronic myocarditis. J Am Coll Cardiol 23:146–153

Le Blanc K, Frassoni F, Ball L, Locatelli F, Roelofs H, Lewis I, Lanino E, Sundberg B, Bernardo ME, Remberger M, Dini G, Egeler RM, Bacigalupo A, Fibbe W, Ringdén O (2008) Mesenchymal stem cells for treatment of steroid-resistant, severe, acute graft-versus-host disease: a phase II study. Lancet 371:1579–1586

Meisel R, Zibert A, Laryea M, Gobel U, Daubener W, Dilloo D (2004) Human bone marrow stromal cells inhibit allogeneic T-cell responses by indoleamine 2,3-dioxygenase-mediated tryptophan degradation. Blood 103:4619–4621

Memon IA, Sawa Y, Fukushima N, Matsumiya G, Miyagawa S, Taketani S, Sakakida SK, Kondoh H, Aleshin AN, Shimizu T, Okano T, Matsuda H (2005) Repair of impaired myocardium by means of implantation of engineered autologous myoblast sheets. J Thorac Cardiovasc Surg 130: 1333–1341

Miyahara Y, Nagaya N, Kataoka M, Yanagawa B, Tanaka K, Hao H, Ishino K, Ishida H, Shimizu T, Kangawa K, Sano S, Okano T, Kitamura S, Mori H (2006) Monolayered mesenchymal stem cells repair scarred myocardium after myocardial infarction. Nat Med 12:459–465

Nagaya N, Kangawa K, Itoh T, Iwase T, Murakami S, Miyahara Y, Fujii T, Uematsu M, Ohgushi H, Yamagishi M, Tokudome T, Mori H, Miyatake K, Kitamura S (2005) Transplantation of mesenchymal stem cells improves cardiac function in a rat model of dilated cardiomyopathy. Circulation 112: 1128–1135

Ohnishi S, Yanagawa B, Tanaka K, Miyahara Y, Obata H, Kataoka M, Kodama M, Ishibashi-Ueda H, Kangawa K, Kitamura S, Nagaya N (2007) Transplantation of mesenchymal stem cells attenuates myocardial injury and dysfunction in a rat model of acute myocarditis. J Mol Cell Cardiol 42:88–97

Okada H, Suzuki J, Futamatsu H, Maejima Y, Hirao K, Isobe M (2007) Attenuation of autoimmune myocarditis in rats by mesenchymal stem cell transplantation through enhanced expression of hepatocyte growth factor. Int Heart J 48: 649–661

Parekkadan B, Milwid JM (2010) Mesenchymal stem cells as therapeutics. Annu Rev Biomed Eng 12:87–117

Pittenger MF, Mackay AM, Beck SC, Jaiswal RK, Douglas R, Mosca JD, Moorman MA, Simonetti DW, Craig S, Marshak DR (1999) Multilineage potential of adult human mesenchymal stem cells. Science 284:143–147

Portmann-Lanz CB, Schoeberlein A, Huber A, Sager R, Malek A, Holzgreve W, Surbek DV (2006) Placental mesenchymal stem cells as potential autologous graft for pre- and perinatal neuroregeneration. Am J Obstet Gynecol 194: 664–673

Sioud M, Mobergslien A, Boudabous A, Floisand Y (2011) Mesenchymal stem cell-mediated T cell suppression occurs through secreted galectins. Int J Oncol 38:385–390

Spaggiari GM, Capobianco A, Becchetti S, Mingari MC, Moretta L (2006) Mesenchymal stem cell-natural killer cell interactions: evidence that activated NK cells are capable of killing MSCs, whereas MSCs can inhibit IL-2-induced NK-cell proliferation. Blood 107:1484–1490

Van Linthout S, Savvatis K, Miteva K, Peng J, Ringe J, Warstat K, Schmidt-Lucke C, Sittinger M, Schultheiss HP, Tschope C (2010) Mesenchymal stem cells improve murine acute coxsackievirus B3-induced myocarditis. Eur Heart J. doi:10.1093/eurheartj/ehq467

Wolbank S, Peterbauer A, Fahrner M, Hennerbichler S, van Griensven M, Stadler G, Redl H, Gabriel C (2007) Dose-dependent immunomodulatory effect of human stem cells from amniotic membrane: a comparison with human mesenchymal stem cells from adipose tissue. Tissue Eng 13:1173–1183

Yamada M, Koeda T, Kikuchi H, Nasu M, Isagozawa S, Mukaida H, Yosida H, Ahsan R, Otokida K, Kato M (1990) Evaluation of increasing digital blood flow during early period of air-cooled cold test (in Japanese). Kokyu To Junkan 38:571–576

Chapter 38

Patients with Cancer or Hematopoietic Stem Cell Transplant: Infection with 2009 H1N1 Influenza

Gil Redelman-Sidi

Abstract In 2009, emergence of a new influenza A strain of swine origin resulted in the first influenza pandemic since 1968. The virus, termed 2009 H1N1 influenza, was found to have unique virological and clinical characteristics. Among patients with cancer or hematopoietic stem cell transplant, 2009 H1N1 influenza is associated with a high frequency of lower respiratory tract involvement and hospitalization, and can result in severe outcomes. Neuraminidase inhibitors are the treatment of choice, although cases of oseltamivir resistance are increasingly being reported. Prevention is crucial, and can be achieved through a combination of infection control, vaccination and use of chemoprophylaxis.

Keywords H1N1 · Hematopoietic stem cell transplant · Lower respiratory tract (LRT) · Lymphocytopenia · RT-PCR · Oseltamivir · H275Y

Introduction

During the spring of 2009, a novel influenza A (H1N1) virus of swine origin emerged as a cause of human infection in Mexico. The virus was found to contain a unique combination of gene segments, with six genes deriving from triple-reassortant North-American swine virus lineages, and two from Eurasian swine virus lineages (Garten et al., 2009). After initially spreading to the United States and Canada, the virus disseminated worldwide, causing the first influenza pandemic since 1968.

Seasonal influenza among patients with malignancies or hematopoietic stem cell transplant (HSCT) has been associated with a high risk of lower respiratory tract (LRT) involvement and mortality. As the 2009 H1N1 influenza pandemic was evolving, it was unknown whether this was also true for the 2009 H1N1 influenza strain. This chapter reviews the available data on the characteristics of 2009 H1N1 influenza infection among patients with cancer or HSCT, and provides guidelines for treatment and prevention.

Pathophysiology

Viral Shedding

In uncomplicated infection with 2009 H1N1 influenza, nasopharyngeal viral RNA loads peak on the day of onset of symptoms, and decline gradually afterward. Most patients do not have detectable virus in the nasopharyngeal secretions for more than 1 week after the onset of symptoms. Several risk factors appear to be associated with prolonged shedding. Giannella et al. (2010) found that both immunosuppression and need for mechanical ventilation were independently associated with prolonged (≥ 7 days) viral shedding. Others have found younger age and severe pulmonary involvement to be predictive of prolonged nasopharyngeal shedding (To et al., 2010a, b).

G. Redelman-Sidi (✉)
Memorial Sloan-Kettering Cancer Center, New York, NY 10065, USA
e-mail: redelmansidi@hotmail.com

Shedding may also be prolonged among patients with cancer or HSCT recipients. In a study by Souza et al. (2010) viral shedding was prolonged among critically ill patients with cancer who required mechanical ventilation due to 2009 H1N1 infection; among 10 patients requiring mechanical ventilation, 5 had viral shedding for at least 11 days with a maximal shedding period of 63 days. In this study, samples from the patients with the longest duration of viral shedding, that were positive by real-time reverse-transcriptase polymerase chain reaction (RT-PCR), were also positive by culture, implying that the viruses were viable and infectious. Studies showing prolonged shedding among HSCT recipients suggest that, apart from immunosuppression, resistance to antivirals appears to be an important contributing factor; oseltamivir resistance was detected in a large proportion of viral isolates from HSCT recipients with prolonged shedding (Anton et al., 2010; Espinosa-Aguilar et al., 2011; Mohty et al., 2011).

Immune Response

The immune reaction to influenza infection comprises of innate and adaptive immune responses. The innate immune system is the first and oldest line of defense against invading pathogens. It recognizes pathogen-associated molecular patterns by different families of pattern recognition receptors, which create a fast and broadly reactive response that changes the infected tissue into an alerted state. In the case of influenza, innate responses are primarily triggered by recognition of viral nucleic acids by endosomal TLR3 and TLR7, by cytoplasmic RNA helicase RIG-I, and by nucleotide-binding domain and leucine-rich-repeat-containing proteins such as NOD2 (Wu et al., 2011).

The adaptive immune response to influenza infection can be divided to humoral and cellular responses. The humoral, or antibody-based, response is needed to prevent infection of the host. The cellular response is more important in late stages of infection, and is essential to eliminate virus-infected cells, which present virus-derived peptides through MHC class I molecules.

In immunocompetent persons, levels of serum neutralizing antibodies rise promptly after infection with 2009 H1N1 influenza. In contrast, patients with cancer or HSCT may exhibit an attenuated immune response to 2009 H1N1 influenza infection. Garland et al. found that only 6 of 11 patients with hematologic malignancies infected with 2009 H1N1 mounted an antibody response after infection, compared to 4 of 4 otherwise healthy adults. Cellular response in patients with hematologic malignancies appeared similarly attenuated; H1N1-specific T cells were detected in only 2 of 8 evaluable patients with hematologic malignancies compared with 4 of 4 controls (Garland et al., 2010).

Pathological Features

The main histopathological findings that have been described in fatal cases of 2009 H1N1 infection in the general population are diffuse alveolar damage with hyaline membrane formation, tracheitis, and necrotizing bronchiolitis. Alveolar hemorrhage, pulmonary vascular congestion, hemophagocytosis, pulmonary thromboemboli and myocarditis can also be seen (Harms et al., 2010).

The pathological features of fatal 2009 H1N1 infection among patients with cancer or HSCT appear largely similar to those in the general population. In one fatal case in a HSCT recipient, the pathological findings consisted of severe diffuse alveolar damage, extensive intraalveolar hemorrhage, formation of hyaline membranes, and viral cytopathic effects in alveolar epithelial cells, with no visible immune inflammatory response (Abdo et al., 2011). Hajjar et al. (2010) described the autopsies of five patients with cancer who died of 2009 H1N1 infection. The main feature was diffuse alveolar damage with variable degrees of hemorrhage. Alveolar and interstitial edema, hyaline membranes and reactive pneumocytes were commonly seen. Bacterial lung cultures were positive for *Streptococcus pneumoniae* in four of five cases. In addition to the pulmonary findings, all patients had acute tubular necrosis of the kidneys to some extent.

Epidemiology

2009 H1N1 influenza virus infection in the northern hemisphere peaked during the spring of 2009, with a second peak occurring during the fall of 2009 and the winter of 2010. It has remained prevalent during the influenza season of 2010–2011.

Like seasonal influenza, 2009 H1N1 is thought to be transmissible by 3 routes: contact exposure, droplet exposure, and airborne exposure. Evidence from experiments in animal models suggests that 2009 H1N1 influenza is more easily transmitted by droplet exposure than by airborne exposure compared to seasonal influenza (Maines et al., 2009). Children likely acquire and transmit infection more readily (Carcione et al., 2011). In a study of 2009 H1N1 influenza among HSCT recipients, household exposure to ill children was suggested to be a risk factor for acquiring infection (Mohty et al., 2011).

It is difficult to assess if patients with cancer or HSCT are at increased risk for acquiring 2009 H1N1 influenza compared to the general population. In a report describing all confirmed cases of 2009 H1N1 infection among patients with cancer or HSCT in a New-York cancer center during the spring of 2009, 11% of tested individuals were positive for 2009 H1N1 (Redelman-Sidi et al., 2010). This study showed significantly higher rates of 2009 H1N1 influenza diagnosis in patients with hematologic conditions compared to patients with solid tumors (17 and 7%, respectively), suggesting that patients with hematologic conditions are more susceptible to acquiring symptomatic influenza infection, or conversely, are more likely to be tested. In a report of 2009 H1N1 among HSCT recipients at a Swiss hospital, ~20% of tested patients were positive. In a nosocomial outbreak of 2009 H1N1 in a pediatric oncology unit an attack rate of 35% for confirmed cases and 50% for all cases (suspected and confirmed) was estimated (Chironna et al., 2010).

Clinical Manifestations

The incubation period for 2009 H1N1 influenza is estimated to be between 1 and 7 days. Viral shedding typically starts a day prior to the onset of symptoms. Similar to immunocompetent patients, most patients with 2009 H1N1 infection and cancer or HSCT present with upper respiratory tract symptoms, consisting of fever, cough, nasal congestion, sore throat, and myalgia. The frequency of 2009 H1N1 symptoms among patients with cancer or HSCT is shown in Table 38.1.

The frequency of LRT involvement (as determined by imaging) in patients with cancer or HSCT varies in different studies, ranging between 27 and 56% (Table 38.2). Radiologic findings include interstitial opacities, lobar infiltrates, or bilateral diffuse alveolar involvement. Corticosteroid use at baseline may predispose to LRT involvement; Espinosa-Aguilar et al. found that the use of ≥ 20 mg/day of prednisone equivalent at the time of diagnosis was associated with increased risk of LRT involvement by imaging (Espinosa-Aguilar et al., 2011).

Lymphocytopenia is a common, albeit nonspecific, finding among patients with cancer or HSCT presenting with 2009 H1N1 infection. In one study, lymphocytopenia (absolute lymphocyte count ≤ 200 cells/mL) on presentation was associated with increased risk of hospitalization (Redelman-Sidi et al., 2010). In the study by Espinosa-Aguilar et al. (2011) a trend towards an association of lymphocytopenia with LRT involvement was seen (71 vs 31%), although this did not achieve statistical significance.

Diagnosis

Any patient with cancer or HSCT who presents with new onset of upper or lower respiratory symptoms during a period of influenza activity in the community should be evaluated for influenza. Upper respiratory samples should be obtained from all patients by means of a nasal wash or a nasopharyngeal swab. In immunocompromised patients with evidence of LRT involvement, an endotracheal or bronchial aspirate should be obtained if possible. LRT specimens may have higher diagnostic yield for 2009 H1N1 than upper respiratory samples in this setting (Blyth et al., 2009), and additionally, could allow testing for concomitant pathogens.

Samples obtained can be tested by rapid antigen tests, direct or indirect immunofluorescence assays, viral culture or RT-PCR. In the general population, rapid antigen tests appear to have limited sensitivity for the detection of 2009 H1N1 influenza, and do not differentiate between subtypes of influenza A. Culture, while relatively sensitive, and able to identify additional respiratory viruses, takes several days to yield a result. Real-time RT-PCR is the most sensitive test for the diagnosis of 2009 H1N1. It has a rapid turnabout time, and can distinguish between

Table 38.1 Clinical symptoms of 2009 H1N1 infection among patients with cancer or hematopoietic stem cell transplant

	Redelman-Sidi et al. (2010)	Espinosa-Aguilar et al. (2011)	Girmenia et al. (2011)	Rihani et al. (2011)	Liu et al. (2010)	Total
Number of patients	45	27	21	39	27	159
Study setting	Single center Patients with cancer or hematologic conditions	Two centers Adult HSCT recipients	Single center Patients with hematologic conditions	Single center HSCT recipients	Single center Patients with hematologic malignancies and HSCT recipients	
Fever	41 (91%)	25 (93%)	21 (100%)	30 (77%)	19 (70%)	136 (86%)
Cough	42 (93%)	26 (96%)	16 (76%)	35 (90%)	23 (85%)	142 (89%)
Headache	2 (4%)	6 (22%)	NR	NR	NR	8 (10%)
Rhinorrhea	27 (60%)	12 (44%)	14 (67%)	18 (46%)	12 (44%)	83 (52%)
GI symptoms[a]	7 (16%)	7 (26%)	NR	5 (13%)	5 (19%)	24 (17%)
Sore throat	11 (24%)	10 (37%)	11 (52%)	20 (51%)	8 (30%)	42 (26%)
Dyspnea	8 (18%)	16 (59%)	NR	7 (18%)	11 (41%)	42 (30%)
Myalgia	5 (11%)	14 (52%)	NR	15 (38%)	4 (15%)	38 (27%)

NR, not reported; HSCT, Hematopoietic Stem Cell Transplant
[a]GI symptoms include nausea, vomiting or diarrhea

2009 H1N1 influenza and other subtypes of influenza A. Commercially available multiplex RT-PCR assays have the added advantage of being able to identify additional respiratory viruses.

The sensitivity of the different tests, among patients with cancer or HSCT, has been examined in several studies. As in the general population, the sensitivity of rapid antigen tests and immunofluorescence assays is limited. In one study, in which a case of 2009-H1N1 influenza was defined by a positive RT-PCR, the sensitivities of the rapid antigen test, direct immunofluorescence assay (DFA) and viral culture were 56, 68 and 86% respectively (Redelman-Sidi et al., 2010). In a study among HSCT recipients, the sensitivity of an indirect immunofluorescence assay was 61% compared to RT-PCR (George et al., 2011). In a third study among patients with hematologic malignancies, DFA was positive in 78% of patients with 2009 H1N1 influenza infection (Liu et al., 2010). Given the relatively poor sensitivities of rapid antigen tests and immunofluorescence assays for the diagnosis of 2009 H1N1 infection, empiric treatment should be considered for patients with high clinical suspicion, regardless of negative results. In such cases, confirmatory testing with viral culture, or, preferably, RT-PCR, could be done.

Treatment

Analysis of 2009 H1N1 influenza showed that it was inherently resistant to the adamantane group of antivirals due to an S31N mutation in the M2 gene, but susceptible to neuraminidase inhibitors (Garten et al., 2009). Apart from a few exceptions (see below), the virus has remained susceptible to oseltamivir. Accordingly, the treatment of choice for 2009 H1N1 influenza has been either oral oseltamivir or inhaled zanamivir.

The recommended doses of neuraminidase inhibitors for the treatment of 2009 H1N1 influenza infection in adults are two 5-mg inhalations (10 mg total) twice daily for inhaled zanamivir, and 75 mg twice daily for oral oseltamivir, for a total of 5 days. While no evidence exists to support this practice, some experts have suggested using higher doses (150 mg twice daily) for a longer duration (10 days) in immunocompromised patients, such as HSCT recipients or patients with profound lymphocytopenia (Casper et al., 2010).

As with seasonal influenza, treatment should be started as early as possible after symptom onset. Rodriguez et al. prospectively examined the impact of early (≤48 h) treatment with oseltamivir on critically

Table 38.2 Frequency of different outcomes of 2009 H1N1 infection among patients with cancer or hematopoietic stem cell transplant

	Redelman-Sidi et al. (2010)	Espinosa-Aguilar et al. (2011)	Paganini et al. (2011)	Rihani et al. (2011)	Mohty et al. (2011)	Amayiri and Madanat (2011)	Caselli et al. (2010)	Liu et al. (2010)
Number of patients	45	27	24	39	10	76	62	27
Setting	Single center Patients with cancer or hematologic conditions	Two centers Adult HSCT recipients	Single center Children with cancer	Single center HSCT recipients	Single center Adult HSCT recipients	Single center Children with cancer	Nine centers Children with cancer	Single center Patients with hematologic malignancies and HSCT recipients
LRT involvement	8 of 29 (27%) with radiographic assessment	14 of 25 (56%) with radiographic assessment	10 (42%)	8 of 28 (29%) with radiographic assessment	5 (50%)	11 of 30 (37%) with radiographic assessment	NR	10 (37%)
Hospitalization	17 (37%)	NR	NR	15 (38%)	5 (50%)	39 (51%)	39 (63%)	16 (59%)
Mechanical ventilation	0 (0%)	7 (26%)	6 (25%)	3 (8%)	3 (30%)	0 (0%)	1 (2%)	4 (15%)
ICU	1 (2%)	NR	6 (25%)	NR	NR	2 (3%)	1 (2%)	5 (19%)
Overall mortality	1 (2%)	9 (33%)	3 (12%)	2 (5%)	2 (20%)	0 (0%)	2 (3%)	3 (11%)
Influenza-related mortality	0 (0%)	6 (22%)	3 (12%)	2 (5%)	2 (20%)	0 (0%)	0 (0%)	2 (7%)

LRT, Lower respiratory tract; HSCT, Hematopoietic Stem Cell Transplant; NR, not reported ill patients with 2009 H1N1 influenza infection. Among their patients, 6% of whom had hematological conditions, early treatment was independently associated with reduced ICU mortality (OR = 0.44; 95% CI 0.22–0.90) compared to late treatment (Rodriguez et al., 2011). Early treatment has the additional benefit of shortening duration of shedding, potentially reducing the chance for transmission (Ling et al., 2010). While treatment benefit is almost certainly greatest when started within 48 h of symptom onset, it is likely that patients with severe illness benefit even when treatment is started later in the course of disease.

During the 2009 H1N1 pandemic, the FDA temporarily authorized the use of peramivir, an investigational intravenous (IV) neuraminidase inhibitor, for use in hospitalized patients not responding to either oral or inhaled antiviral therapy, or for those in whom oral or inhaled therapy was not expected to be effective. It should be noted that the H275Y neuraminidase mutation, which confers resistance to oseltamivir, also confers in-vitro resistance to peramivir; peramivir should therefore not be used for treatment of oseltamivir-resistant isolates.

The histidine to tyrosine mutation at residue 275 of the neuraminidase protein (H275Y) is the most commonly reported mutation conferring resistance to oseltamivir. Cases of oseltamivir resistance due to the H275Y mutation have been described in 2009 H1N1 influenza isolates from patients with cancer or HSCT. In some of these cases resistance emerged during the course of treatment with oseltamivir (Anton et al., 2010; Elbahlawan et al., 2011). Immunocompromised hosts, such as patients with cancer or HSCT, are at increased risk for emergence of an oseltamivir-resistant strain during treatment, due to a combination of prolonged viral shedding, extended duration of exposure to oseltamivir, and incomplete viral suppression. Oseltamivir-resistant strains can also be acquired by transmission from patients to patient; Moore et al. (2011) described transmission of oseltamivir-resistant 2009 H1N1 among eight patients in a hematology unit.

Zanamivir remains effective in oseltamivir-resistant cases. Patients with mild disease can be treated with inhaled zanamivir. For critically ill patients with oseltamivir-resistant 2009 H1N1 influenza, treatment options are limited. There have been several reports of successful treatment using an intravenous form of zanamivir in such cases (Kidd et al., 2009; Elbahlawan et al., 2011). Intravenous zanamivir is not currently licensed for use, but is available on a compassionate-use basis.

As mentioned above, bacterial co-infections are a common complication of 2009 H1N1 influenza infection. Patients with evidence of LRT involvement should be carefully evaluated for the presence of bacterial co-pathogens, and initiation of empiric treatment should be strongly considered in critically ill or severely immunocompromised patients.

Outcome

The outcomes of 2009 H1N1 influenza infection among patients with cancer or HSCT vary considerably in different studies (Table 38.2). While several studies reported low rates of ICU admission and mortality (Caselli et al., 2010; Redelman-Sidi et al., 2010; Amayiri and Madanat, 2011), others have reported severe disease, with high rates of mechanical ventilation and death in this population (Hajjar et al., 2010; Espinosa-Aguilar et al., 2011; Mohty et al., 2011; Paganini et al., 2011). These differences are likely explained by several factors. First, the populations described in different studies are highly heterogenous, and include children and elderly patients, patients with solid tumors and patients with hematologic malignancies, and patients receiving intensive chemotherapy versus patients on no active treatment; in studies describing HSCT recipients there is substantial diversity in time elapsed from transplant, presence of graft versus host disease (GVHD) and use of immunosuppressive agents. Second, there is heterogeneity in the timing of administration of treatment with a neuraminidase inhibitor from onset of symptoms. Third, it is possible that there is a selection bias, if in some studies the diagnosis of 2009 H1N1 influenza infection was more frequently entertained in sicker patients, whereas in other studies testing was administered liberally.

Choi et al. (2011) recently conducted a retrospective study comparing the severity of seasonal influenza A to cases of 2009 H1N1 influenza among HSCT recipients. Using a multivariate analysis, they found that 2009 H1N1 influenza was more likely to result in lower respiratory tract involvement and hypoxemia, although mortality rates did not differ. Similarly, the analysis by Paganini et al. (2011) in children with cancer revealed increased risk of hypoxemia, ICU admission and need for mechanical ventilation among patients with 2009 H1N1 influenza infection compared to seasonal influenza A infection; mortality was not significantly different between the two groups.

No parameters currently exist to predict which patients with cancer or HSCT would be more likely to incur severe disease with 2009 H1N1 infection. The only factor found to be associated with mortality among HSCT recipients infected with 2009 H1N1 influenza, in the study by Espinosa-Aguilar et al. (2011), was the use of ≥20 mg/day of prednisone equivalent at the time of diagnosis.

Prevention

Three main strategies exist to prevent 2009 H1N1 influenza infection among patients with cancer or HSCT: infection control measures, vaccination, and prophylactic use of antivirals.

Infection Control

Infection control measures consist of isolation of contagious patients, and prevention of disease transmission from patients' contacts. For seasonal influenza and other respiratory viruses, frequent hand washing was shown to be the most effective measure to prevent transmission, particularly when applied to children in the same household as the patient. In the inpatient setting, use of barriers, including masks, gloves, and gowns, is also effective. For hospitalized patients with 2009 H1N1 influenza infection, isolation precautions should be strictly maintained until symptoms resolve, and repeat virologic studies are negative; viral shedding in this population can be prolonged, even in the absence of symptoms.

Vaccination

Vaccination is aimed at patients, as well as their close contacts, including healthcare workers.

The main concern in vaccinating patients with cancer or HSCT is that they may be unable to mount an adequate immune response to the vaccine. Bate et al. (2010) evaluated response to two doses of an inactivated, adjuvant-containing 2009 H1N1 influenza vaccine among 54 children with cancer. Seroconversion was documented in 44% of the patients. In the univariate analysis, patients receiving chemotherapy were less likely to respond, as were children with hematologic malignancy compared to those with solid tumors. Engelhard et al. (2011) evaluated response to an inactivated, adjuvant-containing 2009 H1N1 influenza vaccine among HSCT recipients, and found a 41% seroconversion rate after two doses of the vaccine. Issa et al. (2011) found that among vaccinated HSCT recipients, the likelihood of a seroprotective titer increased the further the patients was from transplant, and was lower for patients who had received rituximab in the preceding year.

Although response rates may be low, inactivated influenza vaccine should be recommended for all patients with cancer or HSCT. Additionally, all family members and other close contacts should receive yearly vaccination unless contraindicated. If a family member or close contact receives a live vaccine, they should take care to avoid contact with the patient in the 7 days after vaccination. Healthcare workers with direct patient contact should also be vaccinated against the circulating influenza strains.

Antivirals

A third strategy for prevention of 2009 H1N1 influenza is prophylaxis with a neuraminidase inhibitor. Prophylaxis can be given following exposure to an individual with confirmed 2009 H1N1 influenza infection. The recommended oseltamivir dose for post-exposure prophylaxis in adults is 75 mg daily for at least 10 days. Some experts have advocated using a dose of 75 mg twice daily for post-exposure prophylaxis in this population, as incomplete suppression of viral replication could result in emergence of an oseltamivir-resistant strain (Casper et al., 2010).

Another approach is to give prophylaxis to all patients at risk during an outbreak. This tactic was used by George et al. (2011) during the 2009 H1N1 pandemic. After the occurrence of several cases of infection among HSCT recipients in their center, all 2009 H1N1-negative patients undergoing HSCT with reduced intensity conditioning received prophylaxis with oseltamivir 75 mg daily for 10 days. None of the 6 patients treated with this strategy developed 2009 H1N1 influenza infection in the 100 days after transplant.

References

Abdo A, Alfonso C, Diaz G, Wilford M, Rocha M, Verdecia N (2011) Fatal 2009 pandemic influenza A (H1N1) in a bone marrow transplant recipient. J Infect Developing Countries 5:132–137

Amayiri N, Madanat F (2011) Retrospective analysis of pediatric cancer patients diagnosed with the pandemic H1N1 influenza infection. Pediatr Blood Cancer 56:86–89

Anton A, Lopez-Iglesias AA, Tortola T, Ruiz-Camps I, Abrisqueta P, Llopart L, Marcos MA, Martinez MJ, Tudo G, Bosch F, Pahissa A, de Anta MT, Pumarola T (2010) Selection and viral load kinetics of an oseltamivir-resistant pandemic influenza A (H1N1) virus in an immunocompromised patient during treatment with neuraminidase inhibitors. Diagn Microbiol Infect Dis 68:214–219

Bate J, Yung CF, Hoschler K, Sheasby L, Morden J, Taj M, Heath PT, Miller E (2010) Immunogenicity of pandemic (H1N1) 2009 vaccine in children with cancer in the United Kingdom. Clin Infect Dis 51:e95–e104

Blyth CC, Iredell JR, Dwyer DE (2009) Rapid-test sensitivity for novel swine-origin influenza A (H1N1) virus in humans. N Engl J Med 361:2493

Carcione D, Giele CM, Goggin LS, Kwan KS, Smith DW, Dowse GK, Mak DB, Effler P (2011) Secondary attack rate of pandemic influenza A(H1N1) 2009 in Western Australian households, 29 May-7 August 2009. Euro Surveill 16:19765

Caselli D, Carraro F, Castagnola E, Ziino O, Frenos S, Milano GM, Livadiotti S, Cesaro S, Marra N, Zanazzo G, Meazza C, Cellini M, Arico M (2010) Morbidity of pandemic H1N1 influenza in children with cancer. Pediatr Blood Cancer 55:226–228

Casper C, Englund J, Boeckh M (2010) How I treat influenza in patients with hematologic malignancies. Blood 115:1331–1342

Chironna M, Tafuri S, Santoro N, Prato R, Quarto M, Germinario CA (2010) A nosocomial outbreak of 2009 pandemic influenza A(H1N1) in a paediatric oncology ward in Italy, October-November (2009) Euro Surveill 15:19454

Choi SM, Boudreault AA, Xie H, Englund JA, Corey L, Boeckh M (2011) Differences in clinical outcomes following 2009 influenza A/H1N1 and seasonal influenza among hematopoietic cell transplant recipients. Blood 117:5050–5056

Elbahlawan L, Gaur AH, Furman W, Jeha S, Woods T, Norris A, Morrison RR (2011) Severe H1N1-associated acute respiratory failure in immunocompromised children. Pediatr Blood Cancer. Published online February 4, 2011

Engelhard D, Zakay-Rones Z, Shapira MY, Resnick I, Averbuch D, Grisariu S, Dray L, Djian E, Strauss-Liviatan N, Grotto I, Wolf DG, Or R (2011) The humoral immune response of hematopoietic stem cell transplantation recipients to AS03-adjuvanted A/California/7/2009 (H1N1)v-like virus vaccine during the 2009 pandemic. Vaccine 29:1777–1782

Espinosa-Aguilar L, Green JS, Forrest GN, Ball ED, Maziarz RT, Strasfeld L, Taplitz RA (2011) Novel H1N1 influenza in hematopoietic stem cell transplantation recipients: two centers' experiences. Biol Blood Marrow Transplant 17:566–573

Garland P, de Lavallade H, Sekine T, Hoschler K, Sriskandan S, Patel P, Brett S, Stringaris K, Loucaides E, Howe K, Marin D, Kanfer E, Cooper N, Macdonald D, Rahemtulla A, Atkins M, Danga A, Milojkovic D, Gabriel I, Khoder A, Alsuliman A, Apperley J, Rezvani K (2010) Humoral and cellular immunity to primary H1N1 infection in patients with hematological malignancies and following stem cell transplantation. Biol Blood Marrow Transplant 17:632–639

Garten RJ, Davis CT, Russell CA, Shu B, Lindstrom S, Balish A, Sessions WM, Xu X, Skepner E, Deyde V, Okomo-Adhiambo M, Gubareva L, Barnes J, Smith CB, Emery SL, Hillman MJ, Rivailler P, Smagala J, de Graaf M, Burke DF, Fouchier RA, Pappas C, Alpuche-Aranda CM, Lopez-Gatell H, Olivera H, Lopez I, Myers CA, Faix D, Blair PJ, Yu C, Keene KM, Dotson PD Jr, Boxrud D, Sambol AR, Abid SH, St George K, Bannerman T, Moore AL, Stringer DJ, Blevins P, Demmler-Harrison GJ, Ginsberg M, Kriner P, Waterman S, Smole S, Guevara HF, Belongia EA, Clark PA, Beatrice ST, Donis R, Katz J, Finelli L, Bridges CB, Shaw M, Jernigan DB, Uyeki TM, Smith DJ, Klimov AI, Cox NJ (2009) Antigenic and genetic characteristics of swine-origin 2009 A(H1N1) influenza viruses circulating in humans. Science 325:197–201

George B, Ferguson P, Kerridge I, Gilroy N, Gottlieb D, Hertzberg M (2011) The clinical impact of infection with swine flu (H1N109) strain of influenza virus in hematopoietic stem cell transplant recipients. Biol Blood Marrow Transplant 17:147–153

Giannella M, Alonso M, Garcia de Viedma D, Roa PL, Catalan P, Padilla B, Munoz P, Bouza E (2010) Prolonged viral shedding in pandemic influenza A(H1N1): clinical significance and viral load analysis in hospitalized patients. Clin Microbiol Infect. Published online October 14, 2010

Girmenia C, Mercanti C, Federico V, Rea M, De Vellis A, Valle V, Micozzi A, Latagliata R, Breccia M, Morano SG, Brunetti GA, Sali M, Delogu G, Foa R, Alimena G, Gentile G (2011) Management of the 2009 A/H1N1 influenza pandemic in patients with hematologic diseases: a prospective experience at an Italian center. Acta Haematol 126:1–7

Hajjar LA, Mauad T, Galas FR, Kumar A, da Silva LF, Dolhnikoff M, Trielli T, Almeida JP, Borsato MR, Abdalla E, Pierrot L, Filho RK, Auler JO Jr, Saldiva PH, Hoff PM (2010) Severe novel influenza A (H1N1) infection in cancer patients. Ann Oncol 21:2333–2341

Harms PW, Schmidt LA, Smith LB, Newton DW, Pletneva MA, Walters LL, Tomlins SA, Fisher-Hubbard A, Napolitano LM, Park PK, Blaivas M, Fantone J, Myers JL, Jentzen JM (2010) Autopsy findings in eight patients with fatal H1N1 influenza. Am J Clin Pathol 134:27–35

Issa NC, Marty FM, Gagne LS, Koo S, Verrill KA, Alyea EP, Cutler CS, Koreth J, Armand P, Ho VT, Antin JH, Soiffer RJ, Baden LR (2011) Seroprotective titers against 2009 H1N1 influenza A virus after vaccination in allogeneic hematopoietic stem cell transplantation recipients. Biol Blood Marrow Transplant 17:434–438

Kidd IM, Down J, Nastouli E, Shulman R, Grant PR, Howell DC, Singer M (2009) H1N1 pneumonitis treated with intravenous zanamivir. Lancet 374:1036

Ling LM, Chow AL, Lye DC, Tan AS, Krishnan P, Cui L, Win NN, Chan M, Lim PL, Lee CC, Leo YS (2010) Effects of early oseltamivir therapy on viral shedding in 2009 pandemic influenza A (H1N1) virus infection. Clin Infect Dis 50:963–969

Liu C, Schwartz BS, Vallabhaneni S, Nixon M, Chin-Hong PV, Miller SA, Chiu C, Damon L, Drew WL (2010) Pandemic (H1N1) 2009 infection in patients with hematologic malignancy. Emerg Infect Dis 16:1910–1917

Maines TR, Jayaraman A, Belser JA, Wadford DA, Pappas C, Zeng H, Gustin KM, Pearce MB, Viswanathan K, Shriver ZH, Raman R, Cox NJ, Sasisekharan R, Katz JM, Tumpey TM (2009) Transmission and pathogenesis of swine-origin 2009 A(H1N1) influenza viruses in ferrets and mice. Science 325:484–487

Mohty B, Thomas Y, Vukicevic M, Nagy M, Levrat E, Bernimoulin M, Kaiser L, Roosnek E, Passweg J, Chalandon Y (2011) Clinical features and outcome of 2009-influenza A (H1N1) after allogeneic hematopoietic SCT. Bone Marrow Transplant. Published online March 21, 2011

Moore C, Galiano M, Lackenby A, Abdelrahman T, Barnes R, Evans MR, Fegan C, Froude S, Hastings M, Knapper S, Litt E, Price N, Salmon R, Temple M, Davies E (2011) Evidence of person-to-person transmission of oseltamivir-resistant pandemic influenza A (H1N1) 2009 virus in a hematology unit. J Infect Dis 203:18–24

Paganini H, Parra A, Ruvinsky S, Viale D, Baumeister E, Bologna R, Zubizarreta P (2011) Clinical features and outcome of 2009 influenza A (H1N1) virus infections in children with malignant diseases: a case-control study. J Pediatr Hematol Oncol 33:e5–e8

Redelman-Sidi G, Sepkowitz KA, Huang CK, Park S, Stiles J, Eagan J, Perlin DS, Pamer EG, Kamboj M (2010) 2009 H1N1 influenza infection in cancer patients and hematopoietic stem cell transplant recipients. J Infect 60:257–263

Rihani R, Hayajneh W, Sultan I, Ghatasheh L, Abdel-Rahman F, Hussein N, Hussein A, Al-Zaben A, Sarhan M, Saad M (2011) Infections with the 2009 H1N1 influenza virus among hematopoietic SCT recipients: a single center experience. Bone Marrow Transplant. Published online January 17, 2011

Rodriguez A, Diaz E, Martin-Loeches I, Sandiumenge A, Canadell L, Diaz JJ, Figueira JC, Marques A, Alvarez-Lerma F, Valles J, Baladin B, Garcia-Lopez F, Suberviola B, Zaragoza R, Trefler S, Bonastre J, Blanquer J, Rello J (2011) Impact of early oseltamivir treatment on outcome in critically ill patients with 2009 pandemic influenza A. J Antimicrob Chemother 66:1140–1149

Souza TM, Salluh JI, Bozza FA, Mesquita M, Soares M, Motta FC, Pitrowsky MT, de Lourdes Oliveira M, Mishin VP, Gubareva LV, Whitney A, Rocco SA, Goncalves VM, Marques VP, Velasco E, Siqueira MM (2010) H1N1pdm influenza infection in hospitalized cancer patients: clinical evolution and viral analysis. PLoS One 5:e14158

To KK, Chan KH, Li IW, Tsang TY, Tse H, Chan JF, Hung IF, Lai ST, Leung CW, Kwan YW, Lau YL, Ng TK, Cheng VC, Peiris JS, Yuen KY (2010a) Viral load in patients infected with pandemic H1N1 2009 influenza A virus. J Med Virol 82:1–7

To KK, Hung IF, Li IW, Lee KL, Koo CK, Yan WW, Liu R, Ho KY, Chu KH, Watt CL, Luk WK, Lai KY, Chow FL, Mok T, Buckley T, Chan JF, Wong SS, Zheng B, Chen H, Lau CC, Tse H, Cheng VC, Chan KH, Yuen KY (2010b) Delayed clearance of viral load and marked cytokine activation in severe cases of pandemic H1N1 2009 influenza virus infection. Clin Infect Dis 50:850–859

Wu S, Metcalf JP, Wu W (2011) Innate immune response to influenza virus. Curr Opin Infect Dis 24:235–240

Index

A
Abdo A, 352
Abematsu M, 214
Abnormal and normal HSCs, qualitative differences between, 37–38
Activins, 95–101
Actor B, 76
Acute autoimmune myocarditis, allogeneic FM-MSC transplantation for, 345
Acute myocardial infarction (AMI), 169
　pathogenesis, 172–173
Acute myocarditis therapy, 341–348
　autologous BM-MSC transplantation for, 344
Adachi Y, 39–40
Adams GB, 52
Adipogenesis, 317
Adipogenic unipotency, 269–274
Adipose-derived stem cells (ASCs), 269–274, 315–320
　ASCs/PRP combination therapy, 319–320
　availability of, 315–316
　differentiation capacity of, 317
　human cardiac muscle cells generation from, 269–274
　　co-culture with cardiomyocytes, 272–273
　　differentiation media, 271–272
　　epigenetic modification, 271
　　in vitro cardiac differentiation, 270–271
　　in vivo cardiac differentiation, 273–274
　isolation of, 316
　molecular characterization of, 317–318
　for regenerative medicine, 315–320
Adult brain, neurogenesis in, 211–212
Adult intestine, Hedgehog signaling in, 97–98
Adult neurogenesis in Alzheimer's disease, 261–262
　aneuploidy cells, 262–263
　and neural stem cells, 260–261
Adult stem cells
　evaluation, 174–175
　reprogramming, *see* Reprogramming adult stem cells
Advanced Cell Technology, Inc. (ACT), 242
ADVANCED-SET, filtering device 2, 7–10
　bone marrow fluid
　　injecting, 9
　　processing, 9
　materials, 7
　methods, 8–10
　　priming, 9
　　processing protocol for, 8
　　set-up, 8
　　syringes preparation, 8
Afanasyeva M, 40
Agata H, 308–309
Age-related macular degeneration (AMD), 299
Aggarwal R, 222
Aggarwal S, 347
Aging effect on murine HSCs frequency, 20
Ai J, 173
Akaike's information criterion (AIC), 16, 19
Akala OO, 18–19
Akita S, 279
Akopian V, 73
Alagumuthu M, 286
Aldehyde dehydrogenase (ALDH), 145–152
　ALDH1, 139
　effect on murine HSCs frequency, 22–23
Aldhous P, 69
Al-Hajj M, 138, 234
Alimoghaddam K, 29
Alkaline phosphatase (ALP) activity, 309
　staining for count ALP-positive iPS colonies, 92

Allison DD, 187
Allogeneic MSCs
　in graft-versus-host disease treatment, 249–257
　　clonal allogeneic MSCs, 252–255
　　immunogenicity of, 256
　　immunosuppressive drugs effects, 256
Allogeneic transplantation of FM-MSCs, 341–348
Allografts, 278
Alper J, 61
Alpha-fetoprotein (AFP), 43–48
Alvarez-Buylla A, 211, 260
Alviano F, 344
Alzheimer's disease (AD), adult neurogenesis in, 259–263
　aneuploidy cells, 262–263
　and neural stem cells, 260–261
Amato MA, 293
Amayiri N, 356
Amino N, 139
Amit M, 116
Amor S, 192
Amphiregulin (AREG), 234
Amyloid plaques, 283–289
Amyotrophic lateral sclerosis (ALS), 241–246
　cell-delivery into ALS lesions, difficulty in, 245
　clinical trials of cell transplantation for, 243–244
　regenerative therapy for, 242
　transplantation research for, 243
Ancestim, 54
Anderson DH, 260
Anderson DR, 15, 17
Aneuploid newly generated neuronal cells, 262–263
Aneuploidy cells, 262–263
Angiogenesis, 212–213, 220
Anon, 61
Antifibrotic patterning, 331–338
Anton A, 352, 356
Antonucci I, 193
Anversa P, 269
Aoki H, 291, 294
Appelbaum FR, 39
Arachnoid membrane, 283–289
Arai F, 222
Arai T, 242
Arendt T, 262
Arminan A, 188
Armstrong L, 151
Arnhold S, 294
Arvidsson A, 211–212

Asahara T, 220
Aspiration method (AM), 37–40
Asplund K, 191
Asselin-Labat ML, 234
Astrocytes, 211–216
Atochin DN, 192
Atrial natriuretic peptide (ANP), 175, 271
Aubin JE, 309
Auclair BA, 99
Autogenous bone grafts, 278
Autologous BM-MSC transplantation for acute autoimmune myocarditis, 344
Autologous stem cell transplantation (ASCT), 54
Autologous transplantation, 303
Awano T, 245
5-Azacytidine (5-aza), 150, 179–180, 271
Azuara V, 271

B

Bacigalupo A, 252
Bagley J, 224–225
Baglioni S, 288
Baharvand H, 115
Bajpai R, 114
Baker PS, 291, 293
Ball L, 252
Ballen KK, 52
Bandari PS, 31
Bao S, 128, 146
Baraniak PR, 193
Barbash IM, 345
Barker N, 97
Barker RA, 245
Baron R, 40
Barret's metaplasia, 176
Basic fibroblast growth factor (bFGF), 212
Basic helix-loop-helix (bHLH), 302
BASIC-SET, filtering device 1, 4–7
　materials, 4
　methods, 4–7
　　priming, 5
　　processing protocol for, 6
　　processing the bone marrow fluid, 5
　　set-up, 5
　　syringes preparation, 5
　　washing, 5
Bate J, 357
Baudino TA, 129, 336
Beauchamp JR, 324

Beaumont TL, 76
Behfar A, 177–178
Bendall SC, 158
Ben-Porath I, 132
Bensinger W, 52, 55
Ben-Yosef D, 61, 64
Bergmann O, 270
Bersell K, 335
Bertram L, 260
Bessa PC, 278
Beyer J, 55
Bharti K, 304
Bianco C, 155–162, 165
Bienz M, 96, 100
Biernat W, 76
Birkenhäger JC, 309
Bitgood MJ, 97
Black WC, 234
Bladder cancer, 164–165
Blank U, 222
Blanton MW, 320
Blau HM, 325
Bliss TM, 193
Blume KG, 39
Blyth CC, 353
Bmp/activin signaling pathways, 99–100
B-myosin heavy chain (b-MHC), 175
Bock C, 132, 245
Boeras DI, 263
Boerman RH, 76
Bomken S, 294
Bonaros N, 332
Bone defects, repair, 277–280
Bone marrow (BM), 27–35, 51–59
Bone marrow stromal cells (BMSCs), 3–12, 269–274, 308
    dexamethasone effect on, 308–310
    factors affecting, 312
    heterogeneous responses of, 307–313
    isolation from bone marrow, 3–12
        See also Filtering device/method
    osteogenic induction of, 308
    recombinant BMP-2 effect on, 310–312
Bone marrow transplantation (BMT), 37
    intravenously injected (IV-BMT), 39
    novel BMT (PM+IBM-BMT) *vs.* conventional BMT, 39–40
Bone mineral density (BMD), 38
Bonnefoix P, 25

Bonnefoix T, 13–15, 17, 19, 22, 25
Borlongan CV, 192–193, 195
Borstlap J, 62
Bovolenta P, 300
Boyer LA, 129
Bøyum A, 3
Braam SR, 114
Brain SD, 30
Brain, omental placement on, 286–287
Brain-derived neurotrophic factor (BDNF), 212
Branzi A, 332
Bratincsák A, 195
Breast cancer risk, 231–238
    cancer stem cells and tumor progression, 234–236
    See also Somatic breast stem cells
Breast cancer, 162
Bregni M, 39
Brennan C, 75, 128
Bromodeoxyuridine (BrdU)-labeling, 261
Broome CS, 30, 32
Brown AB, 261
Brown GC, 291
Brown JP, 208
Broxmeyer HE, 54
Brun A, 263
Brundin P, 261
Bryder D, 222
Brzezinski JAt, 302
Buckingham M, 170
Buckingham ME, 188
Buffo A, 212
Buhnemann C, 213
Bunce C, 291
Burdick JA, 187
Burke DZ, 176
Burkus JK, 311
Burnham KP, 15–16
Burns A, 258
Buske C, 18–19
Busser J, 262
Bustinza-Linares E, 151
Butt AM, 212

C
Calabrese C, 151
Calcitonin gene-related peptide (CGRP) role in cord blood (CB) stem cells, 31–32
    SP and CGRP on expansion, 32–33
    SP and CGRP together in, 32

Calcitonin gene-related peptide (CGRP) role (*cont.*)
    SP/CGRP on cell adhesion molecule expression, 33–34
Callanan M, 14–15, 17, 19, 22, 25
Calmont A, 177
Calvi LM, 52
Camenisch TD, 332
Cameron HA, 260
Campan M, 337
Cancedda R, 279
Cancer, Cripto-1 and, 159–160
Cancer stem cells (CSCs), 75–80, 137–142, 231–238, 294–295
    Cripto-1 and, 158–159
    Myc in, 132–134
    See also Somatic breast stem cells
Cannaday J, 283
Capanna R, 310
Capiod JC, 213
Caplan AI, 3, 83
Carcione D, 353
Cardiac cells characterization, 170–173
    cell markers involved in heart development, 171
    embryo-molecular features, 170
    intercalated discs, 171
    morphofunctional features, 170–172
    myocardiocyte cytoskeleton, 171–172
    protein filaments types, 171
        actin filaments, 171
        intermediate filaments, 171
        microtubules, 171
    sarcoplasmic reticulum, 171
Cardiac gene markers expressions, 188–189
Cardiac muscle-derived cells, 269–270
Cardiac regeneration, fundamentals of, 173–176
    adult cell, 174
Cardiac regenerative medicine without stem cell transplantation, 331–338
    direct cardiac reprogramming, 336–337
    rapid and sustained cardiovascular repair, 333–335
    regenerated myocardium, 337–338
    resuming cardiomyocyte proliferation, 335–336
Cardiac stem cells, 174
Cardiogenesis, 331–338
Cardiomyocytes, 169–182, 269–274, 323–328, 331–338
Cardiomyogenic differentiation
    CD44 role in, 187–188
    rMSCs CD44 surface markers in, 185–189

Cardiomyopathies, 331–338
Cardiomyoplasty, 323–328
Cardiopoiesis, 177
    guided, 177–178
Cardiovascular diseases (CVDs) treatment, 169
    First Heart Field (FHF), 170
    Second Heart Field (SHF), 170
Carlomagno F, 141
Carlsson T, 245
Carro MS, 77, 78
Cartwright P, 129
Carvajal-Vergara X, 65
Caselli D, 356
Casiraghi F, 256
Casper C, 354, 357
Caterson EJ, 3
Caulfield JB, 269
Caulfield T, 243
Caveolin-1 (Cav-1), 235
CD133 gene, 145–152
    location, 148
    structure, 147–148
        human CD133, 149
    transcript size of, 148
CD44 surface markers of mesenchymal stem cells, 186–189
    in cardiomyogenic differentiation, 187–188
Cell-based therapy for stroke, 193–194
Cell-conditioned medium (CM), 111–117
Cell lines, 61–73
Cell markers in heart development, 171
Cellular cardiomyoplasty, 323–328
    skeletal muscle-derived stem cells in, 323–328
Cellular extract methodology, 180–181
Cellular replacement therapy, 241–246
    cell resource, 245–246
    limitations, 241
    in neurodegenerative diseases using iPSCs, 241–246
Cellular reprogramming by Myc, 131–132
Central nervous system (CNS), 191–196, 211–216, 241–246, 291–297, 299
Cerberal cortex after stroke, 211–216
    See also under Neurogenesis
Cerebral ischemia, exogenous neural stem cell transplantation after, 213–214
Cerebrovascular diseases, 191–196
Cervello I, 194
Cervical cancer, 163

Index

Chabannes D, 347
Chacko DM, 302–303
Chamberlain G, 344
Chan JY, 107
Chan RW, 194
Chan WK, 256
Chang TC, 130
Charbord P, 185
Charles N, 151
Chemokine receptor 4 (CXCR4), 288
Chemokines, stem cell mobilization with, 57–58
Chen AE, 112
Chen FP, 236
Chen L, 256
Chen X, 310
Chetrite GS, 232
Chien KR, 174
Childs R, 39
Chironna M, 353
Cho NH, 195
Cho RH, 20
Choi SM, 356
Choi YS, 270–273
Chondrogenesis, 307–313, 317
Choo AB, 295
Christman JK, 179
Chua KN, 223, 225
Chung C, 187
Chung Y, 112
Chute JP, 22, 24
Clarke CL, 232
Clarke DL, 79
Clarke MF, 146
Clarke RB, 232, 235–236
Cleland JG, 333
Clevers H, 96, 100
Clinical applications of HSCs, 226–227
Clinical-grade MSCs, 250–252
    isolation, 250–252
        gradient centrifugation method, 251
        production methods for, 250–252
        subfractionation culturing method, 251
Clonal allogeneic MSCs, 252–255
Clonally-expanded MSCs derived from tooth germs
    cryopreservation, 86–87
    isolation and expansion, 86
    thawing of, 87
Clonally-expanded MSCs, iPS cells generation from, 89–92

Cocciadiferro L, 159
Coculture method, 178–179
Cohen PA, 34
Cole MF, 158
Coles BL, 303
Collecting the cell harvest solution, 9
Coller BS, 107
Collins CA, 325
Colon cancer, 163–164
Colony forming count, 27–35
Colony-forming unit (CFU) assay, 10
Comyn O, 291
Cone-rod homeobox (Crx), 302
Cones, 299–305
Conjugated equine oestrogens (CEE), 236
Connexion, 323–328
Connolly ES, Jr., 193
Connor S, 61
Corcoran KE, 34
Cord blood hematopoietic stem cells (CB-HSCs), 27–35
    calcitonin gene-related peptide (CGRP) role, 31–32
    cell adhesion molecule expression, modulation, 29–30
    disadvantage of, 28
    expansion, growth factor cocktail for, 28–29
        cytokines in, 28
    neuropeptides in, 30
    optimum growth factor cocktail, clinical importance of, 34–35
    SP and CGRP on expansion, 32–33
    SP and CGRP together in, 32
    SP/CGRP on cell adhesion molecule expression, 33–34
    substance P (SP) role, 31
Cotterman R, 129
Couillard-Despres S, 208
Cox HM, 30
Cramer EM, 318
Cripto-1, 155–165
    cancer and, 159–160
    cancer stem cells and, 158–159
    embryonic development and, 156–157
    embryonic stem cells and, 157–158
    EMT and, 159
    expression in human tumors, 162–165
        bladder cancer, 164–165
        breast cancer, 162

Cripto-1 (*cont.*)
    cervical cancer, 163
    colon cancer, 163–164
    digestive system tumors, 163–164
    endometrial cancer, 162–163
    gall bladder cancer, 164
    gastric cancer, 163
    leiomyosarcoma of uterus, 163
    nasopharyngeal cancer, 165
    ovarian cancer, 162
    pancreatic cancer, 164
    reproductive system, 162–163
    skin carcinomas, 165
    testicular cancer, 163
    uveal melanoma, 164
  human Cripto-1, 155–156
  oncogenic activities in vitro, 160
  oncogenic activities in vivo, 161–162
  signaling pathways activated by, 160–161
Crypts, 95
Cullen BR, 106
Current good manufacturing process (cGMP), 111
Curtis MA, 260
Cyclophosphamide (CY), 55–56
Cyclosporine A (CsA), 256
Cytokeratin 5 (CK5), 237
Cytokines
  in HSCs expansion, 222
  stem cell mobilization with, 55–58

D

Da Cruz L, 304
Dahlmann-Noor A, 291, 293
Dai WD, 278
Dalerba P, 138
Dalton S, 129–130, 132
D'Andrea D, 156
Dang CV, 128
Darsalia V, 211–213
Das H, 222–223, 225–226
Das T, 302
De Biase P, 310
De Castro NP, 155–165
DeCarvalho AC, 77, 79
Decitabine, 150
Del Bue M, 320
Demirer T, 57
Denning-Kendall P, 28–29
Density gradient method, 3

Dental pulp stem cells (DPSCs), 83–92
Desert hedgehog (Dhh), 97
Deshpande DM, 245
Desmosomes, 323–328
Dexamethasone effect on human BMSCs, 308–310
    glucocorticoids, 308–309
Dezawa M, 213
Diabetic retinopathy (DR) or glaucoma, 299
Di Bari MG, 159
Diefenderfer DL, 309, 311
Diethylaminobenzaldehyde (DEAB), 22–23
Digestive system tumors, 163–164
Dilworth FJ, 332
Di Nicola M, 345
Ding HL, 260
Ding S, 224
Ding YC, 256
Dinsdale J, 212
DiPersio JF, 58
D'Ippolito G, 3
Djouad F, 347
DNA methylation, 148–150
DNA methyltransferase (DNMT), 145–152, 179
Doetsch F, 207, 212
Doi A, 132
Dominici M, 252, 287, 308
Donor lymphocyte infusion (DLI) for malignant tumors treatment, 39
Donor MSCs recruitment, strategies for, 38
Donovan PJ, 292
Dore-Duffy P, 212
Doublecortin (DCX), 199–209
Double-immunofluorescence staining for nestin, 201–204, 207
Double-spin method, 319
Drago H, 195
Draper JS, 113
Dravid G, 29
Drowley L, 328
Duan X, 259
Dubois B, 259
Ductal carcinoma-in-situ (DCIS), 231–238
Dugan MJ, 56
Dulbecco's modified Eagle's medium (DMEM), 43–48, 120, 316–320
Dulbecco's modified Eagle's medium-low glucose (DMEM-lg), 272
Dumont JE, 138
Durukan A, 192

E

Early onset form of AD (EOAD), 259–263
Ebert AD, 61, 242
Eby BW, 318
Eden A, 148
Eden J, 232
Eden JA, 232–237
Efe JA, 182
Elbahlawan L, 356
ELDA software, 14
Ellerström C, 114
Embryoid body (EB) formation in vitro, 122–123
Embryo-molecular features, 170
Embryonic development, Cripto-1 and, 156–157
Embryonic germ cells (EGCs), 127–133
Embryonic stem cells (ESC), 43–48, 83–92, 127–133, 223, 241–242
    clinical trials using ESC-derived cells, 242
    Cripto-1 and, 157–158
    See also Human embryonic stem cells (hESCs)
Emsley HC, 192
Endogenous fibroblasts within infarcted tissue, direct cardiac reprogramming of, 336–337
Endometrial cancer, 162–163
Endometrial regenerative cells (ERC), 194–195
Endometrium, stem cells derived from, 194–195
Endosteal niche, 104
Endothelial cells (ECs), 220
    mesenchymal-derived, 277–280
        vascular ECs (VEC), 279
    stalk cells, 220
    tips cells, 220
Endothelial progenitor cells (EPCs), 179, 224, 279
Engel FB, 335
Engelhard D, 357
England T, 214
English K, 348
Enhanced green fluorescent protein (EGFP), 43–48, 106
Epiblast stem cells (EpiSCs), 127–133
Epithelial-mesenchymal interaction, 95–101
Epithelial to mesenchymal transition (EMT), 101, 140, 156
    Cripto-1 and, 159
Epithelium, 95–101
Erbas B, 234
Erickson GR, 317
Eriksson PS, 260–261
Espina V, 235
Espinosa-Aguilar L, 352–354, 356
Esteve P, 300
Esumi T, 38
Evans WH, 3
Ex vivo expansion of HSCs, 219–228
    biomaterials in, 223–224
    cytokines in, 222
    genetic factors in, 222
    growth factors in, 222
    nanofiber-mediated, 221
    See also under Ischemia, ex vivo expanded HSCs for
Exogenous endothelial progenitor cells (EPCs), 220
Exogenous neural stem cell transplantation after cerebral ischemia, 213–214
Experimental autoimmune myocarditis (EAM), 343–348
Extracellular matrix (ECM), 75–80, 277–280
Eye field transcription factors (EFTF), 300

F

^{18}F-fluorodeoxyglucose (^{18}F-FDG), 337
Fagin JA, 141
Familial adenomatous polyposis (FAP), 96
Fedde KN, 309
Fedorovich NE, 279
Feedback loop, 95–101
Feeder dependent culture of hESCs, 113
Feeder-free culture of hESCs, 113–114
Ferguson RL, 287
Fernandes G, 40
Fernandez PC, 128
Ferri CP, 260
Fetal bovine serum (FBS), 113, 119–124
Fetal membrane-derived MSCs (FM-MSCs), 341–348
    allogeneic FM-MSC transplantation, 345
    allogeneic transplantation of, 341–348
        autoimmune myocarditis, 343
        reported studies, 342
    autologous BM-MSC transplantation for acute autoimmune myocarditis, 344
    fetal membrane-derived MSC, 344–345
    MSC sheet transplantation therapy for heart failure, 348
Fetus, 231–238
Fibroblast growth factor (FGF)-4, 219
Fibroblast growth factor-inducible molecule 14 (FN14), 335
Fibronectin (FN), 223

Field LJ, 172
Filgrastim, 53
Filipcik P, 260
Filtering device/method, 3–12
    assessment, 10–12
        colony forming units, 11
        colony-forming unit (CFU) assay, 10
        FACS, double staining, 11
        FACS, single staining, 11
        fluorescence-activated cell sorting (FACS) analysis, 10
        processing time and isolated numbers, 11
    for BMSCs isolation from bone marrow, 3–12
        density gradient method, 3
        filtering device 1 (BASIC-SET), 4–7
        filtering device 2 (ADVANCED-SET), 7–10
        harvesting bone marrow, 4
        mononuclear cells (MNCs) separation from RBCs, 3
        processing protocol for ADVANCED-Set, 8
        processing protocol for BASIC-Set, 6
First Heart Field (FHF), 170
Flomenberg N, 58
Flow cytometric analyses, 48
Flt3-ligand (FL), 222
Fluorescence-activated cell sorting (FACS), 10, 146, 249–257
Folkman J, 219
Follicular carcinoma (FTC), 137–142
Forde SP, 34
Fouts K, 324
Francipane MG, 141
Francois M, 256
Franke K, 223, 225
Fraser JK, 270, 316
Frecha C, 105
Freije WA, 77
Friedenstein AJ, 10, 248, 278, 308
Fukuhara S, 272
Fukumitsu K, 43
Fukutani Y, 260
Functional hepatocyte-like cells, human ESCs differentiation into, 43–48
Fuse K, 343
Fusetti M, 259

G

Gage FH, 199, 211, 259–260
Galanis E, 76
Gall bladder cancer, 164
Gao J, 245
Gap-junctions formation, 326–327
García-Gómez I, 288
Garcia-Rostan G, 141
Garcia-Verdugo JM, 211
Garland P, 352
Garten RJ, 351–354
Gastric cancer, 163
Gastroepiploic arteries, 283–289
GATA4, 269–274
Gaudet F, 148
Gaustad KG, 181, 272
Gearhart J, 111, 292
Gearhart J, 292
Geiger H, 20
Genbacev O, 113
George B, 354, 357
Gerecht S, 186–187
Germ cell stem cells (GSCs), 128
Gertz M, 51, 55–56
Ghatpande S, 188
Ghods AJ, 79
Ghostine S, 324
Giannella M, 351
Gibelli B, 138
Ginestier C, 139, 147, 235
Girmenia C, 354
Glasgow's modified Eagle's medium (GMEM), 123
Glaucoma, 291–297, 299–305
Glial fibrillary acidic protein, 75–80
Glioblastoma (GBM), 75–80
    mesenchymal gene expression in, 76–78
Gliosarcoma (GS) stem cells, 75–80
    epithelial to mesenchymal transition (EMT), 78
    glial and mesenchymal differentiation, 75–80
        in experimental models, 78–79
    mesenchymal metaplasia, 76
Gluckman E, 28
Glucocorticoids, 308–309
Glycosylation, 185–189
GM-CSF, 283–289
Goker H, 252
Goldgaber D, 260
Goldsmith HS, 284, 286–287
Golebiewska A, 104
Goodell MA, 147
Gould E, 261
Gradient centrifugation method, 251

Graft-versus-host disease (GvHD), 28, 39, 356
    allogeneic MSCs in treatment of, 249–257
        clinical experiences in, 252–255
        clonal allogeneic MSCs, 252–255
        nonclonal MSCs in, 252–255
Graft-versus-leukemia reaction (GvLR), 39
Graft-versus-tumor (GvT), 39
Granulocyte colony-stimulating factor (G-CSF), 51–59
Granulocyte-macrophage colony stimulating factor (GM-CSF), 288
Granulopesis, 30
Greco SJ, 31
Green fluorescence protein transgenic (GFP-Tg) mouse, 325
Greiser CM, 236
Grierson JR, 337
Gronthos S, 10, 12, 84
Gross GC, 261
Growth factor cocktail for CB-HSCs expansion, 28–29
Gruss P, 291
Guan K, 128
Guhr A, 63–64, 66, 70
Guided cardiopoiesis, 177–178
Gunzer K, 54
Guo K, 38
Gupta R, 219
Gurney ME, 243
Gustafson L, 263
Guzman R, 194
Gyrus, 211–216

H

Haas R, 55
Hadad I, 320
Hagege AA, 326
Hajjar LA, 352
Håkelien AM, 180
Halbleib M, 317
Halvorsen YD, 317
Hamada S, 162, 164
Han SJ, 76
Hanna J, 128, 131
Haque MS, 260
Hara A, 292, 294–295, 297
Hara J, 286
Haraguchi N, 146
Haramis AP, 99

Harb N, 114
Hardwick JC, 99
Harms PW, 352
Harris MB, 312
Harrison JR, 309
Harrison P, 318
Harzenetter MD, 30, 32
Hatzopoulos AK, 324
He KM, 337
Heart disease treatment, *see* Cardiovascular diseases (CVDs) treatment
Hedgehog pathway, 95–101
    in adult intestine, 97–98
    desert hedgehog (Dhh), 97
    Indian hedgehog (Ihh), 97
    intestinal stem cells, 95–101
        during development, 97
    sonic hedgehog (Shh), 97
Hellstrom M, 185, 187
Hematopoietic niche, 52
    endothelial niche, 52
    endosteal niche, 52
Hematopoietic progenitor cells (HPCs), 51–59
Hematopoietic stem cell transplantation (HSCT), 249
Hematopoietic stem cells (HSCs), 13–25, 37–40, 220
    frequency estimation, 13–25
        See also Limiting dilution competitive repopulation assays (LDCRA)
    MHC restriction between HSCs and MSCs, 38
    See also Human HSCs
Hennig AK, 302
Heparan sulphate proteoglycan (HSPG), 160
Hepatocyte growth factor (HGF), 43–48, 219, 331–338, 341–348
Hepatocyte-like cells, 43–48
Herbert KE, 54
Herpes simplex virus-thymidine kinase (HSV-tk) gene, 295
Herrera MB, 185–186
Herrup K, 262
Hess DA, 22
Hess DC, 192
Heterogenicity of human cells for therapeutic use, 312–313
Hicok KC, 316–317
Hida N, 195
Himburg HA, 13, 222

2009 H1N1 influenza, 351–358
  clinical manifestations, 353
  diagnosis, 353–354
  epidemiology, 352–353
  outcome, 356–357
  pathological features, 352
  pathophysiology, 351–352
    immune response, 352
    viral shedding, 351–352
  prevention, 357–358
    antivirals, 357–358
    infection control, 357
    vaccination, 357
  treatment, 354–356
    H275Y, 356
    neuraminidase inhibitors for, 354
    Zanamivir, 356
Hirami Y, 304
Histidine to tyrosine mutation at residue 275 (H275Y), 356
Hochedlinger K, 291, 304
Hodgson JG, 79
Hoechst-stained endometrium cells, 194
Hollier BG, 159
Homeobox genes (HOXB4), 222
Homeostasis, 95–101
Homing processes, 29
Hoogduijn MJ, 256
Hoppo T, 43
Horackova M, 326
Hormone replacement therapy (HRT), 236
Horn P, 3
Horwitz EM, 250
Horwitz KB, 232, 237
Hough SR, 158
Houghton J, 40
Hovatta O, 113
Hu Q, 304
Hu Y, 14
Huang JI, 317
Human adipose stem cells (hASCs), 181
Human cardiac muscle cells generation, 269–274
  See also Adipose-derived stem cells (ASCs)
Human clonal MSC, 249–257
Human Cripto-1, 155–156
  structure of, 156
Human embryonic stem cells (hESCs), 43–48, 111–117

differentiation into endodermal cells (Step 1), 45–46
differentiation into functional hepatocyte-like cells, 43–48
  AFP-producing endodermal cells induction, 44
  culture protocol, 44
  maturation into functional hepatocytes, 44
existing hESCs lines, 62–65
expansion
  in suspension, 116
  rock inhibitor and, 115
feeder dependent culture of, 113
feeder-free culture of hESCs, 113–114
hESC lines derivation, 112–113
  from inner cell masses (ICMs), 112
  prospects for, 116–117
human ESC-derived endodermal cells maturation (Step 2), 46
MLSGT20 cells preparation, 46
murine CD45−CD49F±Thy1$^+$gp38$^+$mesenchymal cells, primary culture of, 46–48
passaging hESCs, 114
  xeno-free condition, 114
static culture of, 111–117
suspension culture of, 111–117
undifferentiated hESCs in adherence culture, maintenance, 115
use of hESCs cell lines in international research, 69–73
  National Stem Cell Bank (NSCB), 70
Xeno-free culture media, 112
Human ferritin heavy chain (hFTH), 337
Human hES transplantion into mouse retina, 291–297
  See also Retinal transplantation of hESc/iPS into mouse
Human HSCs, 18–24
  LDCRA of, 18–24
    vent-like homeobox gene *VENTX* effect on, 18–24
Human induced pluripotent stem cells (hiPSCs), 61–73
  existing hiPSC lines, 62–65
    by the end of 2009, 66
  hESCreg registry, 62
  NIH Guidelines for Human Stem Cell Research, 62
  pre-implantation genetic diagnosis (PGD), 64
  public documentation of hiPSC lines, lack of, 63

published research, cell lines and their use in, 61–73
  1998–2009, 66
  from 2003 to 2008, 69
  from 2005 to 2009, 71
  research on, status and impact of, 61–73
Human mesenchymal stem cells (hMSC), 243, 332
Human pluripotent stem cells
  extent of research on, 65–68
  international research impact on, 68–69
    journal impact factor, 68
Human third molars preparation for MSCs isolation/clonally-expansion, 86–87
Human thyroid cancer stem cells, 137–142
Human tumors, Cripto-1 expression in, 162–165
  See also under Cripto-1
Human umbilical vein ECs (HUVECs), 279
Humayun MS, 302
Humphrey RK, 129
Hung LY, 173
Hung SC, 250
Huntington's disease (HD), 241–246
Hurlbut JB, 61
Hurn PD, 192
Hutcheson KA, 324
Hutton JF, 29
Hyaluronan mixed ester of butyric and retinoic acids (HBR), 332
Hyaluronic acid (HA), 186–187
Hydrogel, 185–189
Hyperpolarization, 180
Hypoxia, 151–152
Hyun I, 245

I

Ichioka N, 38
Ieda M, 182, 336–337
Ikebukuro K, 38
Ikeda E, 83–84, 86
Ikeda H, 304
Ikehara S, 37–40
Ikushima H, 149
Ilangumaran S, 187
Illi B, 271, 332
Imai Y, 107
Immunocytochemical staining, 122–123
Immunofluorescence staining for nestin, 201–205
Immunomodulatory effects of MSCs, 345–348
Immunosuppressive drugs effect on MSCs, 256
Induced pluripotent stem cells (iPSCs), 128, 131–133, 336–337
  See also Human induced pluripotent stem cells (hiPSCs)
In vitro cardiac differentiation, 270–271
In vitro differentiation, iPS cells, 122–124
  embryoid body formation in vitro, 122–123
  neural differentiation of marmoset iPS cells, 123–124
In vivo cardiac differentiation, 273–274
In't Anker PS, 342, 344
Inaba M, 39
Indian hedgehog (Ihh), 97
Induced pluripotent stem (iPS) cells, 145–152, 241–246
  generation from alkaline phosphatase (ALP) staining, 92
  generation from clonally-expanded MSCs, 89–92
  generation from mesenchymal stromal cells, 83–92
    clonally-expanded MSCs, 86
    cryopreservation of clonally-expanded MSCs, 86–87
    equipment, 85–86
    human third molars preparation, 86–87
    materials, 84–86
    plat-A packaging cells, expansion, and cryopreservation of, 88–89
    procedure, 86
    reagents, 84
    reagents set up, 85
    SNL feeder cells, preparation, 87–88
    tissue preparation, 84
    vectors, 84
  See also Marmoset iPS generation
Inflammation in stroke, 192–193
Injecting the cell harvest solution, 9
Injury-induced neural stem/progenitor cells, support survival of, 212–213
Inner cell mass (ICM), 127–133
Inoue T, 301–303
Integrin role in HSCs function, 106–108
  inside-out signaling, 107
  outside-in signaling, 107
  reconstitution capacities of KSL HSCs, 107
Interleukin (IL)-3, 222
Intestinal stem cells, 95–101
  self-renewal and differentiation of, 95–101
    Bmp/activin signaling pathways, 99–100

Intestinal stem cells (*cont.*)
    See also Hedgehog pathway
  Wnt signaling and, 96–97
Intra-bone marrow (IBM)-BMT method, 37–38
Intravenously injected BMT (IV-BMT), 39
Iqbal K, 260
Iruela-Arispe ML, 220
Isasi RM, 62
Ischemia, ex vivo expanded HSCs for, 219–228
  angiogenesis mechanism, 220
  preclinical applications, 224–226
  sources of HSCs, 220–221
Ishida T, 38
Ishii T, 43–44, 46
Ishikane S, 342, 344, 348
Isidori A, 54
Islam MO, 147
Issa NC, 357
Ito K, 4
Ito M, 124
Itoh T, 199–200, 202, 206–208
Iwanami A, 124
Iwasaki K, 79

J

Jaenisch R, 292
Janssens S, 333
Jelski W, 139
Jiang XX, 37, 345
Jiang Y, 3
Jin K, 259, 261
Jin R, 192
Jin ZB, 291, 301, 304
Joggerst SJ, 324
Jordan CT, 132, 145–147
Joshi DD, 31
Joyner JC, 250
Judson RL, 130
Jung B, 100

K

Kadiyala S, 309
Kajstura J, 269, 270
Kakudo N, 316–317, 319
Kalaycio M, 56
Kalirai H, 235–236
Kamo N, 43
Kaneda H, 38
Kaneko Y, 261

Kang HJ, 58
Kang J, 260
Kannan RY, 279
Karamboulas C, 271
Karasawa JTH, 286
Karl MO, 305
Karussis D, 243
Karyotypic analysis, 122
Katoh K, 302
Kauser K, 175
Kawakami M, 30
Kawamura K, 277
Kawamura M, 37–38
Kawamura T, 271
Kawasaki H, 123
Kayali AG, 288
Kebriaei P, 255
Kedinger M, 98
Keller G, 323
Kelly DL, 129
Kempermann G, 260
Kenney NJ, 161
Kent DG, 25
Kibschull M, 113
Kidd IM, 356
Kiel MJ, 109
Kim D, 292
Kim H, 260, 277
Kim HS, 115
Kim J, 129, 131
Kim KJ, 312
Kim M, 270
Kim MS, 4
Kim S, 279
Kim SY, 193
Kingsbury MA, 262
Kitamura T, 84
Kleindorfer D, 191
Klimanskaya I, 112, 114
Klonisch T, 139, 141
Knockout mice, 231–238
Knockout serum replacement (KSR), 111–117
Knoppers BM, 62
Knudson W, 186–187
Koc ON, 250
Kodach LL, 100
Kodama M, 343
Koestenbauer S, 158
Kohn DB, 105

Koike Y, 39
Koketsu D, 211
Kolf CM, 77
Kolterud A, 98
Komitova M, 202, 207–208, 261
Kondo T, 212
Kondoh H, 348
Kondziolka D, 194, 214
Kopen GC, 249
Kordower JH, 246
Korinek V, 98
Kosinski C, 98–99
Koyanagi M, 179
Krawetz R, 112, 116
Krist LFG, 284
Kroll TG, 138
Kuan WL, 245
Kuhn B, 335
Kuo YR, 256
Kuroda Y, 3
Kushida T, 38–39
Kuznetsov SA, 312
Kwong FN, 312

L
LaBarge MA, 325
Labosky PA, 128
LaFerla FM, 259
Laflamme MA, 323
Lai L, 332
LaIuppa JA, 223, 225
Lakowski J, 301, 303
LaMarca HL, 232, 234
Lamba DA, 291, 293–294, 301, 304
Lan L, 138
Landry P, 106
Langer R, 278
Lapidot T, 52–53
Late onset form of AD (LOAD), 259–263
Lathia JD, 151
Lauer B, 343
Laughlin MJ, 23
Lawrence MG, 160
Lazarus HM, 250
L-Calc (StemCell Technologies) software, 14
Le Blanc K, 250, 255–256, 345
Leber's congenital amaurosis (LCA), 299
Lecanda F, 311
Lee CC, 160
Lee G, 242
Lee J, 78–79
Lee JA, 317
Lee JS, 151
Lee SH, 279
Lee SJ, 252
Lee ST, 193
Lee WC, 271
Lees CW, 98–99
Lefort N, 294
Leiomyosarcoma of uterus, 163
Leker RR, 212
Lemoli RM, 51, 53
Lemonnier M, 188
Lendahl U, 261
Lenograstim, 54
Lentiviral vectors (LVs), 103–109, 292
    as effective viral vector system for HSCs, 105–106
    selfinactivating (SIN) vector systems, 105
    in target gene expression inhibition, 106
    third-generation LVs production, 105
Leobon B, 324
Lepore AC, 243
Lerner UH, 30
Lévesque JP, 52
Levine AD, 66–67, 72
Levkovitch-Verbin H, 291, 293
Li J, 263, 310
Li L, 104–105
Li W, 261
Li X, 112, 115
Li XJ, 242
Li Y, 31, 223, 225
Liang Y, 20–21
Licznerska BE, 232
Lieberman KA, 76
Liebermann-Meffert D, 283–285
Liechty KW, 249
Lim JH, 250
Limiting dilution competitive repopulation assays (LDCRA), 13–25
    HSCs frequency estimation by, 13–25
    modeling, with multi-cell Poisson models (MCPM), 14–18
        concept and principles, 14–18
    multi-cell Poisson models (MCPM) of, 18
        human HSCs, 18–24
        murine HSCs, 18
Lin CH, 129–130

Lin Y, 220
Ling LM, 356
Lionetti V, 333–334, 338
Liscic RM, 245
Lister R, 61, 73
Litbarg N, 284, 288
Litingtung Y, 97
Liu B, 29
Liu C, 354–355
Liu D, 140
Liu H, 120
Liu JW, 280
Liu Y, 271
Locker M, 303, 305
Loeffler M, 95
Loeser RF, 186–187
Lois C, 260
Lorenzini S, 58
Löser P, 61–66, 68, 70, 72
Losordo DW, 220
Louis DN, 75–76
Louissaint A Jr, 213
Lovett M, 277
Lower respiratory tract (LRT), 351–358
Lu J, 29
Ludwig T, 114
Lui S, 236
Luijendijk RW, 288
Lumbosacral arachnoiditis, 283–289
Lunde K, 333
Luong MX, 62
Lutterbach J, 75–76
Lymphocytopenia, 353
Lysine-specific demethylase 1 (LSD1), 130

M

MacLaren RE, 294, 301–303
Macrophage colony stimulating factor (M-CSF), 288
Madanat F, 356
Madison BB, 98–99
Maines TR, 353
Maiorana A, 288
Major histocompatibility complex (MHC), 37–40
Makino S, 271
Maleic anhydride (MA) substrate, 223
Malignant tumors treatment, IBM-BMT and DLI for, 39
Malynn BA, 129

Mammary tumor virus promoter (MMTV-Cripto-1 mice), 161
Mani SA, 149
Maragakis NJ, 245
Marg S, 108
Markowitz S, 100
Marmont AM, 37
Marmoset iPS generation, 119–124
  established iPS cells, characterization, 122–123
    immunocytochemical staining, 122–123
    karyotypic analysis, 122
    reverse transcription-PCR, 122
  teratoma formation, 124
  using six transcription factors (method), 119–124
    picking colonies, 120–122
    virus infection of marmoset cells, 120
    virus production, 120
  in vitro differentiation, 122–124
Marquardt T, 291
Martelli ML, 141
Marx RE, 318–319
Masuda H, 194
Matsui W, 139
Mauney JR, 279
McCord AM, 151
McCormick J, 66–68
McCormick JB, 66–68, 70
McCredie KB, 51
McCulloch CAG, 309
McDermott SP, 24
McDevitt TC, 193
McKeever PE, 78–79
McMahon AP, 97, 99, 182
McMahon JM, 182
Mcniece IK, 35
Medroxyprogesterone acetate (MPA), 236
Medullary thyroid carcinoma (MTC), 137–142
Meinel L, 279
Meis JM, 75–77
Meisel R; 347
Melkoumian Z, 112, 114
Memon IA, 348
Menasche P, 326
Mendes SC, 308
Meng G, 112–113, 115
Meng X, 194–195
Menstrual blood stem-like cells, 191–196
  stroke therapy using, 191–196
    cell-based therapy, 193–194

inflammation in stroke, 192–193
practical issues, 195–196
stem cells derived from endometrium, 194–195
targets for stem cells in stroke, 193
Mercier I, 235
Mesenchymal differentiation, 75–80
Mesenchymal drift, 78
Mesenchymal gene expression in glioblastoma, 76–78
Mesenchymal stem cells (MSCs), 37, 176–177, 249–257, 278–280
  bone defects repair, 277–280
    autogenous bone grafts, 278
    tissue engineering strategies, 278
  donor MSCs recruitment, strategies for, 38
  HSCs and, MHC restriction between, 38
  immunology activity, 175–176
  immunomodulatory effects of, 345–348
  iPSs generation from, 83–92
  mesenchymal-derived endothelial cells, 277–280
  paracrine activity, 175–176
  See also Allogeneic MSCs; Clinical-grade MSCs
Meshorer E, 130
Metcalf JP, 352
Methotrexate (MTX), 295
Meyer GP, 333
Meyer JS, 291
Meyer N, 128
Miao D, 278
Micalizzi DS, 159
Michiue H, 337
Migliore L, 262–263
Mikkelsen, T, 77
Mikkelsen TS, 131–132
Mikos AG, 278
'Milky spots', 284–285
Miller CR, 76
Miller MW, 261
Mills CR, 255
Milwid JM, 175, 348
Min JY, 323
Misteli T, 130
Mistry AS, 278
Mitsios JV, 108
Miura K, 244, 246
Miura M, 83
Miyahara Y, 270, 342, 348
Miyan JA, 30, 32
Mizugishi K, 213
Mizuno D, 308, 311–312

Mobilization, stem cell, 51–59
  biology of, 52–53
    stress-induced signals, 52
  with chemokines, 57–58
  with cytokines alone, 57
  with cytokines plus chemotherapy, 55–57
  factors affecting, 55
  hematopoietic niche, 52
  mobilization agents available, 53–54
    ancestim, 54
    filgrastim, 53
    lenograstim, 54
    pegfilgrastim, 54
    plerixafor, 54
    sarmograstim, 53
  and regenerative medicine, 58–59
Model-averaged HSC frequency estimate, computation, 16
  statistical validity of, checking, 17
Mohr JC, 223
Mohty B, 352–353
Mommaas B, 221
Monocyte chemoattractant protein-1 (MCP-1), 344
Mononuclear cells (MNCs), 3, 280
Montini E, 105
Moore C, 356
Moore KL, 170
Morel AP, 151
Moretti A, 65
Morita E, 245
Morita S, 84
Morita Y, 13, 25
Morkel M, 162
Morrison SJ, 109
Moser M, 107
Moursi AM, 278
Mouse embryonic fibroblasts (MEFs), 113, 119–124
Moyamoya disease, 283–289
Mueck AO, 237
Müller FJ, 63, 73
Multi-cell Poisson models (MCPM), 13–14
  hypothesis, 15
  model-averaged HSC frequency estimate, computation, 16
Multiple myeloma (MM), 54
Multipotent MSCs, 307–313
Multipotent stromal/stem cells, 249–257
Muramoto GG, 22–23

Murine CD45−CD49F±Thy1+gp38+mesenchymal cells, primary culture of, 46–48
Murine embryonic development, 127–133
Murine HSCs, LDCRA of, 18
   aging effect on, 20
   aldehyde dehydrogenase effect on, 22–23
   direct injection into NOD/SCID mice bone marrow effect on, 24
   prostaglandin E2 (PGE2) effect on, 20
   Trp53/p16^{Ink4a}/p19^{Arf} gene deletion effect on, 18
Murphy JF, 185–187
Murphy MP, 195
Murry CE, 269, 323
Myc target genes, 127–133
   in cancer stem cells, 132–134
      therapy implications, 133
   cellular reprogramming by, 131–132
   function, general modes, 128–129
   as a multifaceted regulator of pluripotency and reprogramming, 127–133
      Myc family of proteins, 128
      pluripotent stem cells regulation by, 129–131
         Oct4, Sox2 and Nanog (OSN) regulators, 129
Mycophenolic acid (MPA), 256
Myocardial infarction, 331–338
   stem cells in, 175
Myocardial regeneration, 269–274
   in vivo, stem cells use in, 176
Myocardiocyte cytoskeleton, 171–172

N

Nadal-Ginard B, 269
Nagaya N, 342
Najm FJ, 128
Nakagami H, 270
Nakagawa M, 83, 244
Nakagomi N, 213–214
Nakamura T, 38, 207, 212, 334
Nakanishi C, 176
Nakatomi H, 212
Nakatsuji N, 48, 246
Nakauchi H, 104
Nakayama D, 212–213
Narayanasami U, 56
Nasopharyngeal cancer, 165
Nauta AJ, 256
Negative regulator of Wnt signaling, 98–99
Neumann M, 242
Neural differentiation
   of marmoset iPS cells in vitro, 123–124
   retinal transplantation inducing, 291–297
Neural stem cells (NSCs), 199–209, 259–263
Neurodegenerative diseases, 241–246
Neurogenesis, 211–216
   in adult brain, 211–212
   in cerberal cortex after stroke, 211–216
      angiogenesis, 212–213
      clinical trials to enhance, 214–216
      exogenous neural stem cell transplantation, 213–214
      injury-induced neural stem/progenitor cells, support survival of, 212–213
Neurogenin1, 331–338
Neurokinin-A (NK-A), 31
Neuropeptides in hematopoesis, 30
Neutrophils, 52, 191–196
Newman M, 260
Niches, 52
   endosteal niche, 52
   endothelial niche, 52
Nieswandt B, 108
Nikiforova M, 137–138
Nikiforov YE, 137–138
Nilsson M, 206
Nishimura M, 37, 260
Nishisho I, 96
^{13}N-labeled ammonia (^{13}NH$_3$), 337
N-methyl-Daspartate (NMDA), 294
NOD/SCID mice bone marrow, direct injection, effect on murine HSCs frequency, 24
Nonclonal MSCs, 252–255
Non-Hodgkin Lymphoma (NHL), 54
Normal and abnormal HSCs, qualitative differences between, 37–38
Normal myocardium, cell replacement in, 172–173
Normal stem cells transplantation, rationale for, 37–40
North TE, 13, 20, 22
Notch pathway, 235–236
Novoyatleva T, 335
Nowakowski RS, 261
Nowell PC, 236
Nüsslein-Volhard C, 97
Nygren JM, 224

O

O'Brien CA, 147
OCT-4, 295
Oct4, Sox2 and Nanog (OSN) regulators, 129

Oda Y, 83, 87, 92
Odorico JS, 323
Oestrogen receptor knockout mice (ERKO), 234
Offerhaus GI, 96
Ogaeri T, 106
Oh SK, 116
Ohgushi H, 83, 278
Ohmori T, 103–109
Ohnishi S, 342, 344
Okada H, 344
Okita K, 83
Okuda T, 261
Oligodendrocyte progenitor cells (OPCs), 242
Olivetti G, 269
Omentum, 283–289
    anatomy, 284–285
    arterial vascularization of, 285
    embryology, 284–285
    in injured tissue repair, 283–289
    in reparative medicine, 285–287
        omental placement on brain, 286–287
        omental placement on spinal cord, 287
    omental stem cells, 287–289
    structure, 284–285
        adipose-rich areas, 284
        thin translucent membranes, 284
Oncogenic transformation, signaling activated by cripto-1 during, 160–161
Ontogenetic stage of donor cells for retinal repair, 302–303
Organ transplantation, IBM-BMT for, 38
Orlic D, 272, 324, 331
Orthodenticle homeobox 2 (Otx2), 302
Osakada F, 291, 304
Osawa M, 23
Oseltamivir, 351–358
O'Shaughnessy L, 283
Osteoblasts, 185–189
Osteoclasts, 52
Osteogenesis, 317
Osteogenic reagents, 307–313
Ostergaard K, 186
Oswald J, 280
Osyczka AM, 309, 311–312
Ouyang HW, 278
Ovarian cancer, 162
Owen-Smith J, 66–68
Oyaizu N, 37
Oyama T, 271

P

p160-Rho-associated coiled kinase (ROCK), 115
    and hESC expansion, 115
Padykula HA, 194
Pagani FD, 324
Paganini H, 356
Palmer TD, 260
Pan Y, 302, 306
Pancreatic cancer, 164
Papadeas ST, 245
Papillary carcinoma (PTC), 137–142
Parathyroid hormone, 51–59
Parekkadan B, 175, 348
Parent JM, 199
Park DH, 192
Park JW, 141
Parkinson's disease, 241–246
Parrilla-Reverter G, 291
Pasek M, 171–172
Pasqualini JR, 232
Passaging hESCs, 114
Patah PA, 35
Patani N, 234
Patel AN, 193–195
Patrick CW Jr, 317
Pearce DJ, 139
Pegfilgrastim, 54
Peichev M, 220
Pekny M, 206
Pelus LM, 51, 57
Peng X, 108, 109
Penn LZ, 128
Perán M, 181
Pérez Romero C, 169
Perfusion method, 37–40
Periostin, 335
Peripheral blood mononuclear cell (PBMC), 256
Peripheral blood, 27–35
Perron M, 301–302
Perry JR, 76
Persaud TVN, 170
Petersen BE, 249
Peterson EA, 3
Petit A, 260
Petrich BG, 108
Petrini M, 40
Phillips BW, 116
Phillips HS, 75, 77
Phinney DG, 249, 308–309

Phosphate buffered saline (PBS), 121, 316
Picard-Riera N, 206–207
Pinho MdFB, 288
Pittenger MF, 4, 249, 341, 347
Planat-Benard V, 270, 272, 317
Plasminogen activator, 191–196
Plat-A packaging cells
   cryopreservation of, 88–89
   expansion of, 88–89
   passaging of, 88
   thawing of, 88
Platelet-rich plasma (PRP), 315–320
   ASCs/PRP combination therapy, 319–320
   characteristics, 318
   collection technique of, 319
   processing technique of, 319
      double-spin method, 319
      single-spin method, 318
   for regenerative medicine, 315–320
Plerixafor, 54, 56
Plotnikov EY, 179
Pluchino S, 261
Pluripotent stem cells, 61–73, 127–128
Pochampally R, 10
Ponti D, 235
Portmann-Lanz CB, 342, 344
Potten CS, 95
Pouzet B, 324
Prasher VP, 260
Pre-implantation genetic diagnosis, 61–73
Prentice RL, 233
Preprotachykinin-I gene (PPT-I), 31
Presenilin 1 (PSEN1), 260
Prianishnikov VA, 194
Pries R, 186
Prokhorova TA, 292
Prostaglandin E2 (PGE2), 20–22
Purton LE, 13–14

Q
Qiu Q, 279
Qualtrough D, 100
QuantiTect Reverse Transcription kit (Qiagen), 122
Querfurth HW, 259

R
Rafii S, 58
Rajala K, 112, 114
Ramalho-Santos M, 97

Rameshwar P, 27, 30–32
Randomised controlled trial (RCT), 236
Rangappa S, 179, 272
Rao AS, 141
Rao SG, 29
Rat mesenchymal cell (rMSCs) CD44 surface markers, 185–189
   in cardiomyogenic differentiation, 185–189
      cardiac gene markers expressions, 188–189
Ratajczak MZ, 40
Rawat VPS, 18, 20
Rawls AS, 106
Recombinant BMP-2 effect on human BMSCs, 310–312
Reddi AH, 310
Redelman-Sidi G, 353–354
Regenerated myocardium, 337–338
   conventional imaging, 337–338
   molecular imaging, 337–338
Regeneration therapy
   for ALS, 242
   IBM-BMT for, 38–39
   stem cell mobilization and, 58–59
Regional wall motion score (RWMS), 325–326
Reh TA, 305
Reilly GC, 311
Reinecke H, 323–324
Reis RL, 279
Reis RM, 76
Rengo G, 173
Reparative medicine, omentum in, 285–287
   omental placement on brain, 286–287
   omental placement on spinal cord, 287
   surgical applications, 285–287
Repopulation of HSCs after transplantation, 103–109
   HSCs fate after transplantation, 104–105
   integrin in, 106–108
   vinculin role in, 103–109
   See also Lentiviral vectors (LVs)
Reproductive system tumors, 162–163
Reprogramming adult stem cells, 169–182
   transdifferentiation methodology for, 169–182
      cellular extract methodology, 180–181
      coculture method, 178–179
      fibroblasts to cardiomyocytes, 182
      hyperpolarization, 180
      molecular mechanisms in, 177
      viral vectors, 181–182

Retinal repair, stem cells for, 299–305
    adult retina for autologous transplantation, 303
    from basic to applied biology, 299–305
    generating cell diversity in retina, 300–302
    iPS era, 303–304
    ontogenetic stage of donor cells for, 302–303
Retinal transplantation of hESc/iPS into mouse, 291–297
    cell types for, 292–293
    neural differentiation induced by, 291–297
    retinal regeneration by hES/iPS Cells, 293–294
    teratoma suppression, strategies for, 295–297
    teratomas derived from hES/iPS cells, 294
Retinitis pigmentosa (RP), 299
Retroviral vectors, 292
Reubinoff BE, 122
Reverse transcription-PCR, 122
Reyes M, 250
Reynolds BA, 260
Ricci-Vitiani L, 79
Rice AC, 199
Richards M, 113
Rickard DJ, 250
Rihani R, 354
Rizzino A, 129
Roberts DJ, 99
Robinson S, 27–29
Rodriguez A, 356
Rodríguez JJ, 261
Rods, 299–305
Roeder I, 13, 20
Roh JD, 278
Romieu-Mourez R, 256
Rose N, 40
Rosen JM, 232, 234
Rosenzweig A, 250
Roukis TS, 318
Rouwkema J, 279
RTK/RAS/ERK signaling pathway, 151
Rubart M, 172
Rubinson DA, 106
Russo J, 233
Rutka JT, 79

S

Sacchetti B, 308
Safford KM, 317
Saha K, 61
Saino O, 212
Salem HK, 83, 308
Salman H, 208
Salvati M, 76
Sandmaier B, 39
Santos MI, 279
Saporta S, 213
Sarcomere, 169–182
Sarcoplasmic reticulum, 171
Sarmograstim, 53
Sasaki E, 119–121
Savani RC, 187, 332
Savitz SI, 214
Sbano P, 256
Scadden DT, 13, 52
Schabitz WR, 212
Schachinger V, 227
Scharfman HE, 212
Schlingensiepen KH, 150
Schmidek HH, 79
Schmitz N, 55
Schwarz EJ, 249
Schwarz F, 311
Scott CT, 62, 70, 72
Seale P, 324
Second Heart Field (SHF), 170
Selective-oestrogen receptor modulators (SERMs), 236
Selfinactivating (SIN) vector systems, 105
Selleri C, 53
Seong JM, 278
Sermon KD, 64–65
Sex-determining region Y-Box 2 (SOX2), 201–202
Shachaf CM, 133
Shahrokhi S, 29, 32–34
Shankle WR, 286
Sharp J, 242
Shattil SJ, 107
Shatz CJ, 291
Sheehan JP, 311
Shepherd RM, 59
Shi S, 156, 250
Shi YJ, 130
Shields AF, 337
Shim WS, 272
Shimotsuma M, 285
Shin HY, 213
Shizuru JA, 13, 24
Shmelkov SV, 148
Short hairpin RNA, 103–109

Shyu WC, 214
Siddappa R, 309
Side population, 145–152
Sikavitsas VI, 279
Silk fibroin (SF), 185
Silva F, 193, 195
Silva GV, 224
Simioniuc A, 338
Singh A, 284, 288–289
Singh AM, 130
Singh H, 116
Singhatanadgit W, 318
Single photon emission computed tomography (SPECT), 337
Single-spin method, 318
Sioud M, 347
Siwko SK, 233
Six transcription factors/method, 119–124
   See also under Marmoset iPS generation
Skeletal muscle interstitium derived multipotent stem cells (SKMI-DMSCs), 323–328
   in cellular cardiomyoplasty, 323–328
      cardiac differentiation, 327–328
      gap-junctions formation, 326–327
      spontaneous synchronous contraction in vitro, 326–327
   complete differentiation into cardiomyocytes in vivo, 325–326
   differentiation potential of, 325
   isolation of, 324–325
   localization of, 324–325
Skin carcinomas, 165
Slack JM, 176
Smith K, 129–130, 132
Smith KN, 130
Smith SE, 318
Smits AM, 180
Smyth GK, 14
SNL feeder cells
   cryopreservation of, 88
   mitomycin C treatment, 88
   passaging, 88
   preparation of, 87–88
   thawing of, 87–88
Solchaga LA, 278
Somatic breast stem cells, 231–238
   and clinical medicine, 236–238
   normal, 232–233
   pregnancy and, 232–233

Song L, 176, 284
Song SU, 250
Sonic hedgehog (Shh), 97
Sorlie T, 234
Sotthibundhu A, 261
Sources of HSCs, 220–221
Souza TM, 352
Spaggiari GM, 345
Spinal cord, omental placement on, 287
Spontaneous cerebral stroke in rats, 199–209
   new neurons differentiation from neural stem cells, 199–209
      dividing and proliferating cells, labeling, 200
      double-immunofluorescence staining for nestin, 201–202
      experimental and control groups, 200
      immunohistochemistry, 200–201
      methods, 200–205
      quantification of DCX-positive cells, 203
      quantitation of positive cells, 202–203
      SVZ observation in SHRSP after stroke, 203–205
      triple-immunofluorescence staining for nestin, 202
Srour EF, 104
St George-Hyslop PH, 260
Stadtfeld M, 292, 304
Stage-specific embryonic antigen 1 (SSEA-1), 122, 288
Stagg J, 256
Stalk cells, 220
Stamm C, 226
Stassi G, 140
Statistical single-hit Poisson model (SHPM), 13–14
   ELDA software, 14
   L-Calc (StemCell Technologies) software, 14
   and multi-cell Poisson model, comparison, 16
Stefanick ML, 236
Steiner D, 112, 116
Stem cell bank, 61–73
Stem cell disorders (SCDs) concept, 37–40
   IBM-BMT
      for organ transplantation, 38
      for regeneration therapy, 38–39
   IBM-BMT + donor lymphocyte infusion (DLI) for malignant tumors treatment, 39
   MHC restriction between HSCs and MSCs, 38

normal and abnormal HSCs, qualitative differences between, 37–38
novel BMT (PM+IBM-BMT), 39–40
Stem cell factor (SCF), 222
Stem cell mobilization, *see* Mobilization, stem cell
Stem cell niches, 232
Stem Cell Registry of the European Union (hESCreg), 62
Stem cells from human exfoliated deciduous teeth (SHED), 83–92
Stem cells in stroke, targets for, 193
Stojkovic P, 113
Storms RW, 22
Strauss S, 242
Strem BM, 317–318
Strizzi L, 159–161, 163
Strohsnitter WC, 233
Stroke therapy, 191–196
See also under Menstrual blood stem-like cells
Stroke-prone spontaneously hypertensive rats (SHRSP), 200–202
Ström S, 112
Stromal cell-derived factor-1 (SDF-1), 52, 288
Subfractionation culturing method, 251
Substance P (SP) role in cord blood (CB) stem cells, 31
SP and CGRP on expansion, 32–33
SP and CGRP together in, 32
SP/CGRP on cell adhesion molecule expression, 33–34
Subventricular zone (SVZ), 211–216, 259–263
Suemori H, 45, 122
Sugarman J, 292
Sugawara A, 122
Suh S, 284
Sun HC, 279
Sun JS, 278
Sun Y, 161–162
Sundelacruz S, 180
Superoxide dismutase 1 (SOD1), 243
Suppressors cytokine signalling (SOCS), 140
Sutherland RL, 232
Suzuki Y, 39
Svendsen CN, 61
Swaroop A, 302
Swiontkowski MF, 311
Szilvassy SJ, 14

T
Tabu K, 148–151
Taguchi A, 211–213
Takada K, 38, 107
Takahashi K, 61, 67, 69, 83, 119–120, 128–129, 132, 242, 273, 304–305, 323, 336
Takahashi T, 272
Takahashi Y, 243
Takano T, 138–139
Takenaka Y, 4
Tallini G, 138
Tamaki T, 324–325, 327
Tamura Y, 309
Tan MY, 185
Tanzi RE, 260
Taswell C, 14
Tatlisumak T, 192
Taupin P, 260–263
Taylor DA, 324
Taylor HS, 195
Taymor K, 62
Tchkonia T, 287
Tenenbaum HC, 309
Teratoma, 323–328
derived from hES/iPS cells, 294
formation, 124
suppression, strategies for, 295–297
Terzic A, 177
Tesar PJ, 127
Tesio M, 53
Testicular cancer, 163
Than S, 37
Thiemermann C, 83
Thiery JP, 78, 159
Thomas D, 138
Thomas ED, 39
Thomas T, 138
Thomson JA, 61, 68, 70, 111, 114, 122, 241
Thonhoff JR, 243
Thored P, 207–208
Thrombocytes, 315–320
Thrombopoietin (TPO), 222
Thyroid cancer, 137–142
emerging concepts in, 139–140
fetal cell, 139
new therapeutic strategies for, 140–141
thyroid cancer multi-step hypothesis, 139
See also Human thyroid cancer stem cells
Thyroid stem cells (TSCs), 138–139

Ting AY, 238
Tips cells, 220
Tissue culture polystyrene (TCPS), 223
Tissue engineering, 307–313
TNF-related weak inducer of apoptosis (TWEAK), 335–336
To KK, 351
Tobita M, 319–320
Toda H, 213
Todaro M, 138–140
Toma C, 249
Tomioka I, 119, 121–123
Tomita S, 271
Toni N, 260
Tooth germ progenitor cells (TGPCs), 83–92
Torella D, 169, 173
Torres LB, 119
Tosh D, 176
Toyoda M, 288
Transdifferentiation methodology, 176–177
    for adult stem cells reprogramming, 169–182
        See also Reprogramming adult stem cells
    molecular mechanisms in, 177
Transforming growth factor (TGF)-β, 51–59, 315–320
Transplant patients, 351–358
    See also 2009 H1N1 influenza
Transplantation research for ALS, 243
Transplantation therapy, 243–245
    HSCs fate after, 104–105
        endosteal niche, 104
        lodging in bone marrow environment 'niche', 104
        vascular niche, 104
        See also Repopulation of HSCs after transplantation
    hurdles in, 243–245
        ethical issues, 243
        functional efficacy, 244–245
        robust supply, 243–244
        safety, 244
Trastuzumab, 235
Traumatic brain injury (TBI), 199
Treatment with plasminogen activator (tPA), 191
Tremmel M, 186–187
Trichopoulos D, 231, 233
Trichostatin A, 271
Trimethylated histone H3 of lysine 27 (H3K27me3), 336

Triple-immunofluorescence staining for nestin, 202, 206
'Triple negative' tumour, 234
Tropepe V, 303
Troponin, 169–182
Trumpp A, 104, 109
Tse HF, 226
Tse, WT, 250
Tso CL, 77–78
Tsumura A, 150
Tuan RS, 176
Tumor stem cell (TSC), 145–152
    concepts of, 146
    detection of, 146–147
    DNA methylation, 148–150
    hypoxia, 151–152
    multipotential stem cells, 146
    RTK/RAS/ERK signaling pathway, 151
    self-renewing stem cells, 146

U

Ucar D, 139
Uccelli A, 250
Ueda Y, 40
Ueno NT, 39
Undifferentiated anaplastic thyroid carcinoma (UTC), 137–142
Urist MR, 310
Uterus, leiomyosarcoma of, 163
Uveal melanoma, 164

V

Vacanti JP, 278
Valarmathi MT, 280
van den Boom M, 187
van den Brink GR, 96–98
van Dop WA, 97–99
van Harmelen V, 288
van Laake LW, 323
van Linthout S, 347
van Vliet P, 180
van Zant G, 20
Varnat F, 98, 101
Vascular endothelial growth factor (VEGF)-1, 219
Vascular niche, 104
Vasculogenesis, 220
Ventura C, 331–332
Verfaillie CM, 29, 250
Verhaak RG, 75, 77–79

Vescovi AL, 79
Vesicular glutamate transporter 1 (VGLUT1), 296
Viczian AS, 302
Villa-Diaz LG, 112, 114
Villi, 95–101
Vinculin role in HSCs repopulation, 103–109
    importance, 108
Viral shedding, 351–352
Viral vectors, 181–182
Visvader JE, 159
von Heimburg D, 317
von Recum H, 279
von Willebrand Factor (vWF), 334

W

Wagers AJ, 224
Wakitani S, 249
Waller EK, 250
Wang FS, 152
Wang H, 32
Wang JF, 260
Wang LC, 98
Wang NK, 291
Wang T, 272
Wang XP, 260
Wang ZX, 133
Washing, 9
Watanabe K, 112, 115, 155, 158–159, 165
Watt SM, 34, 107
Wechselberger C, 159, 161
Wei CL, 158
Weinstein RS, 309
Weiss S, 260
Weissman IL, 13, 24
Welch HG, 234
West EL, 302–303
Wheatley SC, 332
Whey acidic protein (WAP) promoter, 161
Wieschaus E, 97
Wilkosz S, 284
Williams DA, 35
Wilms' tumor antigen 1 (WT-1), 288
Wilson A, 13, 52, 104, 109
Winitsky SO, 328
Winkler IG, 53–54
Witkiewicz AK, 235
Wnt signaling
    and intestinal stemcell, 96–97
    negative regulator of, 98–99

Wobus AM, 61, 332
Wolbank S, 345
Wolff EF, 195
Woodbury D, 249
Wormald R, 291
Wright DE, 51
Wu S, 128, 352
Wu H, 32
Wu S, 352
Wu W, 352
Wu WL, 286
Wu Z, 160

X

Xiong Y, 199
Xu C, 113–114
Xue JH, 212
Xue JJ, 182
Xu H, 170
Xu J, 191
Xu Y, 115

Y

Yagyuu T, 83
Yahata T, 24
Yamada M, 348
Yamada Y, 182
Yamagiwa H, 278
Yamanaka S, 83, 119–120, 128, 132, 146, 246, 304, 336, 338
Yamazaki S, 52, 153
Yang MC, 185, 188
Yang Y, 262
Yao S, 114
Yasuchika K, 47
Yauch RL, 100–101
Yin T, 104–105
Ylöstalo J, 312
Yokota T, 108
Yokoyama A, 212
Yoo SW, 212
Yoon J, 188
Yoon YS, 250
Yoshimura K, 318
You H, 148
Young MJ, 293
Yu HY, 280
Yu J, 61, 67, 69, 292
Yu Y, 261

Z

Zabierowski SE, 147
Zacharias WJ, 98–99
Zanamivir, 356
Zannettino AC, 12
Zarzeczny A, 243
Zhai QL, 29
Zhang C, 261
Zhang FB, 271
Zhang P, 138–139
Zhang QX, 284
Zhang ZG, 213
Zheng Y, 29
Zhong Z, 196
Zhou B, 170
Zhou H, 128
Zhou J, 185–186, 280
Zhu D, 242
Zhu H, 186–187
Zhu W, 137, 141
Ziabreva I, 261
Ziegler Wh, 108
Zohar R, 250
Zon LI, 13, 18
Zuk PA, 270, 287, 315–317

Printed by Publishers' Graphics LLC
MO20120730